CESO-ZA

DEPARTMENT OF THE ARMY
U.S. Army Corps of Engineers
Washington, D.C. 20314-1000

EM 385-1-1

Manual
No. 385-1-1

15 September 2008

Safety

SAFETY AND HEALTH REQUIREMENTS

1. Purpose. This manual prescribes the safety and health requirements for all Corps of Engineers activities and operations.

2. Applicability. This manual applies to Headquarters, US Army Corps of Engineers (HQUSACE) elements, major subordinate commands, districts, centers, laboratories, and field operating activities (FOA), as well as USACE contracts and those administered on behalf of USACE. Applicability extends to occupational exposure for missions under the command of the Chief of Engineers, whether accomplished by military, civilian, or contractor personnel.

3. References.

   a. 29 Code of Federal Regulation (CFR) 1910

   b. 29 CFR 1926

   c. 29 CFR 1960

   d. Executive Order (EO) 12196

   e. Federal Acquisition Regulation (FAR) Clause 52.236-13

This manual supersedes EM 385-1-1, 3 November 2003

f. Department of Defense Instruction (DODI) 6055.1

g. Army Regulation (AR) 40-5

h. AR 385-10.

4. General.

a. The provisions of this manual implement and supplement the safety and health standards and requirements referenced above. Where more stringent safety and occupational health standards are set forth in these requirements and regulations, the more stringent standards shall apply.

b. Mission applicability introduced in paragraph 2 above shall include the following:

(1) Construction contract work under the provisions of FAR Clause 52.236-13. Contractors shall comply with the latest version of EM 385-1-1 (including interim changes) that is in effect on the date of solicitation. Prior to making an offer, bidders should check the HQUSACE Safety and Occupational Health web site (see paragraph c) for the latest changes. No separate payment will be made for compliance with this paragraph or for compliance with other safety and health requirements of this contract. Note: Existing contracts will continue to apply the provisions of the previous edition of this manual until contract completion.

(2) Service, supply, and research and development contracting actions. Compliance with this manual shall be a contract requirement for such activities unless technical representatives (in coordination with safety and health professionals) advise that special precautions are not appropriate due to extremely limited scope of services or similar. However, it is understood that this manual in its entirety may be too complex for the type of work being performed under these contracts. These contractors may reference Appendix A, paragraph 11 for limited scope Accident Prevention Plan (APP).

(3) Contracting actions for hazardous, toxic, and radioactive waste site investigation, design, or remediation activities. Compliance with this manual shall be a contract requirement.

c. Changes. All interim changes (changes made between publication of new editions) to this manual, and the effective date of change, will be posted on the Safety and Occupational Health Office website:http://www.usace.army.mil/CESO/Pages/Home.aspx and in USACE Electronic bid Sets. Hard copies of this manual are available from the local contracting official.

d. Interpretations. Within the Corps of Engineers, interpretations to the requirements contained within this manual shall be executed in accordance with the process contained in Appendix M. Interpretations will apply only to the specific situation in question and may not be used as a precedent to determine the meaning of a requirement as it may apply to another circumstance.

e. Variances and Waivers. Within the Corps of Engineers, variances and waivers to provisions of this manual require the approval of the Chief of Safety and Occupational Health, HQUSACE. Variances or waivers shall provide an equal or greater level of protection, shall be substantiated with a hazard analysis of the activity and shall be documented and forwarded through channels to Chief of Safety and Occupational Health, HQUSACE. The process for requesting variances or waivers is contained in Appendix N.

f. Activities performed OCONUS. Some of the technical requirements of this manual may not be applicable to overseas activities due to conflicting circumstances, practices, and laws or regulations of the locality or the unavailability of equipment. In such instances, means other than the ones specified in this manual may be used to achieve the required protection. In such instances, a hazard analysis must be developed to document that the required protection will be achieved by the alternate means.

g. Unless otherwise indicated, when publications are referenced in this manual, the most recent edition is to be used.

h. The use of underlining in this manual indicates new or changed text from the 2003 version.

i. Supplementation of this manual is not authorized except as published by the Safety and Occupational Health Office, HQUSACE.

(1) Local USACE organizations may develop Standard Operating Procedures (SOPs) to implement the provisions contained within this manual, but may not implement new requirements without the specific approval of HQUSACE.

(2) Locally developed Safety and Health Requirements will not be included in contract requirements without the approval of HQUSACE.

FOR THE COMMANDER:

STEPHEN L. HILL
Colonel, Corps of Engineers
Chief of Staff

EM 385-1-1
15 Sep 08

TABLE OF CONTENTS

Section   **Page**

1. Program Management 1
    A. General 1
    B. Indoctrination and Training... 13
    C. Physical Qualification of Employees 15
    D. Accident Reporting and Recordkeeping....................... 17
    E. Emergency Planning 19
    F. Emergency Operations... 20

2. Sanitation.. 21
    A. General Requirements 21
    B. Housekeeping 21
    C. Drinking Water 21
    D. Non-Potable Water... 23
    E. Toilets... 24
    F. Washing Facilities 28
    G. Showers... 28
    H. Change Rooms 29
    I. Clothes Drying Facilities 29
    J. Food Service... 29
    K. Waste Disposal 30
    L. Vermin Control.. 31

3. Medical and First-Aid Requirements 33
    A. General 33
    B. First-Aid Kits.. 36
    C. First-Aid Stations and Infirmaries 39
    D. Personnel Requirements and Qualifications 40

4. Temporary Facilities 43
    A. General 43
    B. Access/Haul Roads 46

5. Personal Protective and Safety Equipment........................ 49
    A. General 49

    B. Eye and Face Protection 51
    C. Hearing Protection and Noise Control 60
    D. Head Protection 63
    E. <u>Protective Footwear</u> 65
    F. <u>High-Visibility Apparel</u> 66
    <u>G.</u> Respiratory Protection 67
    H. <u>Full Body Harnesses, Lanyards and Lifelines</u> 72
    <u>I.</u>   Electrical Protective Equipment 73
    <u>J.</u>   Personal Flotation Devices 77
    K. Lifesaving and Safety Skiffs 80

6. Hazardous <u>or Toxic</u> Agents and Environments 83
    A. General 83
    B. Hazardous <u>or Toxic Agents</u> 85
    C. Hot Substances 93
    D. Harmful Plants, Animals, and Insects 96
    E. Ionizing Radiation 97
    F. Nonionizing Radiation and Magnetic and
       Electric Fields 108
    G. Ventilation and Exhaust Systems 111
    H. Abrasive Blasting 112
    <u>I.</u>   <u>Inclement Weather and Heat/Cold Stress
       Management</u> 119
    <u>J.</u>   Cumulative Trauma Prevention 125
    <u>K.</u> Indoor Air Quality (IAQ) Management 126
    <u>L.</u> <u>Control of Chromium (VI) Exposure</u> 129
    M. <u>Crystalline Silica</u> 130

7. Lighting 139
    A. General 139

8. Accident Prevention Signs, Tags, Labels, Signals,
   Piping System Identification, and Traffic Control 143
    A. Signs, Tags, Labels, and Piping Systems 143
    B. Signal Systems, Personnel, and Procedures 153
    C. Traffic Control 154

9. Fire Prevention and Protection 167
    A. General 167

B. Flammable and Combustible Liquids 172
C. Liquefied Petroleum Gas (LP-Gas) 179
D. Temporary Heating Devices 184
E. First Response Fire Protection 190
F. Fixed Fire Suppression Systems 195
G. Firefighting Equipment 196
H. Fire Detection and Employee Fire Alarm Systems 197
I. Fire Fighting Organizations - Training and Drilling 198
J. Fire Patrols 199
K. USACE Wild Land Fire Control 199

10. Welding and Cutting 203
A. General 203
B. Respiratory Protection 205
C. Fire Protection 207
D. Oxyfuel Gas Welding and Cutting 209
E. Arc Welding and Cutting 212
F. Gas Metal Arc Welding 214

11. Electrical 215
A. General 215
B. Arc Flash 219
C. Overcurrent Protection, Disconnects, and Switches .. 221
D. Grounding 222
E. Temporary Wiring and Lighting 227
F. Operations Adjacent to Overhead Lines 230
G. Batteries and Battery Charging 232
H. Hazardous (Classified) Locations 234
I. Power Transmission and Distribution 237
J. Underground Electrical Installations 254
K. Work in Energized Substations 255
L. Communication Facilities 256

12. Control of Hazardous Energy 257
A. General 257
B. Training 261
C. Periodic Inspections 262
D. Locks and Tags 262
E. Application and Removal of Locks and Tags 263

EM 385-1-1
15 Sep 08

13. Hand and Power Tools 267
    A. General 267
    B. Grinding and Abrasive Machinery 269
    C. Power Saws and Woodworking Machinery 271
    D. Pneumatic Tools 273
    E. Explosive-Actuated Tools 274
    F. Chain Saws 276
    G. Abrasive Blasting Machinery 276
    H. Power-Driven Nailers and Staplers 277

14. Material Handling, Storage, and Disposal 279
    A. Material Handling 279
    B. Material Storage 280
    C. Housekeeping 283
    D. Debris Nets 284
    E. Material Disposal 285

15. Rigging 287
    A. General 287
    B. Personnel Qualifications 288
    C. Multiple Lift Rigging (MLR) 289
    D. Wire Rope 291
    E. Chain 295
    F. Fiber Rope (Natural and Synthetic) 297
    G. Slings 299
    H. Rigging Hardware 301

16. Cranes and Hoisting Equipment 307
    A. General 307
    B. Personnel Qualifications 311
    C. Classification of Equipment and Training of Operators
       (USACE-Owned and Operated Cranes and
       Hoists Only 319
    D. Inspection Criteria 321
    E. Safety Devices and Operational Aids 335
    F. Testing 340
    G. Operation 343
    H. Critical Lifts 353

iv

	I. Environmental Considerations	356
	J. Lattice, Hydraulic, Crawler-, Truck-, Wheel-, and Ringer-Mounted Cranes	357
	K. Portal, Tower, and Pillar Cranes	359
	L. Floating Cranes, Floating Derricks, Crane Barges, and Auxiliary Shipboard Mounted Cranes	363
	M. Overhead and Gantry Cranes	371
	N. Monorails and Underhung Cranes	372
	O. Derricks	372
	P. Handling Loads Suspended from Rotorcraft	374
	Q. Material Hoists	376
	R. Pile Drivers	380
	S. Hydraulic Excavators, Wheel/Track/Backhoe Loaders Used to Transport/Hoist Loads with Rigging	383
	T. Crane-Supported Personnel (Work) Platforms	387

17. Conveyors 399
    A. General 399
    B. Operation 405

18. Motor Vehicles, Machinery and Mechanized Equipment, All Terrain Vehicles, Utility Vehicles and other Specialty Vehicles 409
    A. General 409
    B. Guarding and Safety Devices 411
    C. Operating Rules 417
    D. Transportation of Personnel 421
    E. Motor Vehicles (for Public Roadway Use) 422
    F. Trailers 424
    G. Machinery and Mechanized Equipment 424
    H. Drilling Equipment 433
    I. All Terrain Vehicles (ATVs) 437
    J. Utility Vehicles 439
    K. Specialty Vehicles 442

19. Floating Plant and Marine Activities 445
    A. General 445
    B. Access 458

- C. Marine Fall Protection Systems 461
- D. Main Deck Perimeter Protection 461
- E. Marine Railing Types... 464
- F. Launches, Motorboats, and Skiffs 468
- G. Dredging 471
- H. Scows and Barges 474
- I. Navigation Locks and Vessel Locking 475

20. Pressurized Equipment and Systems 477
    - A. General 477
    - B. Compressed Air and Gas Systems 481
    - C. Boilers and Systems 485
    - D. Compressed Gas Cylinders 486

21. Fall Protection.. 491
    - A. General 491
    - B. Training 493
    - C. Fall Protection Program 494
    - D. Controlled Access Zones 495
    - E. Fall Protection Systems.. 495
    - F. Covers 499
    - G. Safety Net Systems 500
    - H. Personal Fall Protection Systems 502
    - I. Ladder-Climbing Devices (LCDS)......................... 509
    - J. Scaffolds, Aerial Lift Equipment and Moveable Work Platforms... 509
    - K. Warning Line Systems (WLS) 510
    - L. Safety Monitoring Systems (SMS) 511
    - M. Rescue Plan and Procedures… 511
    - N. Working Over or Near Water 512

22. Work Platforms and Scaffolding....................................... 515
    - A. General 515
    - B. Scaffolds - General... 517
    - C. Metal Scaffolds and Towers 524
    - D. Wood Pole Scaffolds 528
    - E. Suspended Scaffolds 533
    - F. Hanging Scaffolds 544
    - G. Form and Carpenter's Bracket Scaffolds 549

EM 385-1-1
15 Sep 08

    H. Horse Scaffolds 552
    I. Pump Jack Scaffolds 552
    J. Adjustable Scaffolds 555
    K. Crane-Supported Work (Personnel) Platforms 555
    L. Elevating Work Platforms 555
    M. Vehicle-Mounted Elevating and Rotating Work
       Platforms (Aerial Devices/Lifts) 557
    N. Mast Climbing Work Platforms 560
    O. Roofing Brackets 562
    P. Stilts 562

23. Demolition 565
    A. General 565
    B. Debris Removal 568
    C. Wall Removal 570
    D. Floor Removal 571
    E. Steel Removal 572
    F. Mechanical Demolition 572

24. Safe Access, Ladders, Floor & Wall Openings, Stairs and
    Railing Systems 575
    A. Safe Access – General 575
    B. Ladders 578
    C. Handrails 582
    D. Floor, Wall and Roof Holes and Openings 583
    E. Stairways 585
    F. Ramps, Runways and Trestles 587
    G. Personnel Hoists and Elevators 588

25. Excavations and Trenching 589
    A. General 589
    B. Safe Access 595
    C. Sloping and Benching 597
    D. Support Systems 598
    E. Cofferdams 602

26. Underground Construction (Tunnels), Shafts, and
    Caissons 613

    A. General 613
    B. Hazardous Classifications 622
    C. Air Monitoring, Air Quality Standards, and
       Ventilation... 624
    D. Fire Prevention and Protection......................... 630
    E. Drilling 634
    F. Shafts 635
    G. Hoisting.. 636
    H. Caissons 637
    I. Compressed Air Work....................................... 638
    J. Underground Blasting 639

27. Concrete, Masonry, Steel Erection and Residential Construction 643
    A. General 643
    B. Concrete and Masonry Construction 644
    C. Formwork and Shoring..................................... 646
    D. PreCast Concrete Operations 650
    E. Lift-Slab Operations... 651
    F. Structural Steel Assembly 653
    G. Systems-Engineered Metal Buildings 672
    H. Masonry Construction Roofing......................... 676
    I. Roofing 677
    J. Residential Construction 678

28. Hazardous Waste Operations and Emergency Response (HAZWOPER)... 681
    A. General 681
    B. Site Safety and Health Plan (SSHP) 681
    C. Responsibilities 685
    D. Training 686
    E. Medical Surveillance 690
    F. RCRA TSD Facilities 691
    G. Facility or Construction Project Emergency
       Response... 691

EM 385-1-1
15 Sep 08

29. Blasting 695
    A. General 695
    B. Transportation of Explosive Materials 700
    C. Handling of Explosive Materials 703
    D. Electromagnetic Radiation 704
    E. Vibration and Damage Control 705
    F. Drilling and Loading 707
    G. Wiring 710
    H. Firing 712
    I. Post-Blast Procedures 714
    J. Underwater Blasting 715

30. Diving Operations 717
    A. General 717
    B. Diving Operations 729
    C. SCUBA Operations 733
    D. Surface Supplied Air (SSA) Operations 735
    E. Mixed-Gas Diving Operations 737
    F. Equipment Requirements 738
    G. Scientific Snorkeling 744

31. Tree Maintenance and Removal 747
    A. General 747
    B. Tree Climbing 750
    C. Felling 753
    D. Brush Removal and Chipping 755
    E. Other Operations and Equipment 757

32. Airfield and Aircraft Operations 763
    A. Airfields - General 763
    B. Aircraft 766

33. Munitions and Explosives of Concern (MEC) Encountered
    During USACE Activities 767
    A. General 767
    B. MEC Examples 768

ix

EM 385-1-1
15 Sep 08

<u>34. Confined Space Entry</u> 789
    <u>A. Confined Spaces – Non-Marine Facilities</u> 789
    <u>B. Work Performed in Confined and Enclosed Spaces on Ships and Vessels</u> 795

Appendices
A – Minimum Basic Outline for Accident Prevention Plans A-1
B – Emergency Operations B-1
C – BLANK C-1
D – Assured Equipment Grounding Conductor Program D-1
E – BLANK E-1
F – BLANK F-1
G – BLANK G-1
H – BLANK H-1
I – Crane Testing Requirements for Performance Tests I-1
J – BLANK J-1
<u>K</u> – BLANK K-1
<u>L</u> – BLANK L-1
M – USACE Process for Requesting Interpretations M-1
N – USACE Process for Requesting Waivers/Variances N-1
<u>O</u> – Manning Levels for Dive Teams O-1
<u>P</u> – <u>Safe Practices of Rope Access Work</u> P-1
<u>Q</u> – Definitions Q-1
<u>R</u> – Metric Conversion Table R-1
<u>S</u> – References and Resources S-1
T – BLANK T-1
<u>U</u> – Floating Plant/Marine Railing Types U-1

Acronyms Acronyms-1

<u>**Index**</u> Index-1

Figures
1-1 – Position Hazard Analysis 6
1-2 – Activity Hazard Analysis 10
5-1 – Personal Flotation Devices 79
8-1 – Sign and Tag Signal Word Headings 156
8-2 – Example Tag Layout 157
8-3 – Example Sign Layout 161

EM 385-1-1
15 Sep 08

8-4 – Radio Frequency Warning Symbol 163
8-5 – Laser Caution Sign 164
8-6 – Laser Warning Sign 164
8-7 – Radiological Warning Symbol 165
8-8 – Slow-Moving Vehicle Emblem 165
8-9 – Accident Prevention Tags 166
15-1 – Wire Rope Clip Spacing (Not to be used for slings) 292
15-2 – Wire Rope Clip Orientation (Not to be used for slings) 293
15-3 – Hooks 304
16-1 – Crane Hand Signals 349
16-2 – Helicopter Hand Signals 377
16-3 – Hydraulic Excavating Equipment used to Hoist 386
22-1 – Hanging Scaffold 548
25-1 – Sloping and Benching 605
25-2 – Trench Shields 611
25-3 – Trench Jacks 612
29-1 – Power Firing Systems for Series and Parallel Series
       Firing Systems 698
29-2 – Recommended Installation of Shooting Station and
       Accessory Arrangement for Using Arcontroller 698
33-1   Grenades 769
33-2   Projectiles 773
33-3   Mortars 775
33-4   Rockets 776
33-5   Guided Missiles 778
33-6   Bombs 779
33-7   Practice Bombs 780
33-8   Dispensers 781
33-9   Submunitions 782
33-10 Pyrotechnics 784
33-11 Items that Might Contain Chemical Warfare Materiel 758
U-1   Type A Railings U-1
U-1   Type B Railings U-2
U-1   Type C Railings U-3

Tables
2-1 – Minimum Toilet Facilities (Other than Construction Sites) ... 26
2-2 – Minimum Toilet Facilities (Construction Sites) 28
3-1 – Minimum Quantity Requirements for Basic Unit Packages .. 38

5-1 – Eye and Face Protector Selection Guide	53
5-2 – Required Shades for Filter Lenses and Glasses in Welding, Cutting, Brazing, and Soldering	59
5-3 – Permissible Non-DOD Noise Exposures	61
5-4 – Permissible DOD Noise Exposures	63
5-5 – Standards for Electrical Protective Equipment	74
6-1 – Occupational Dose Rates	100
6-2 – Laser Safety Goggle Optical Density Requirements	109
6-3 – Abrasive Blasting Media: Silica Substitutes	113
6-4 – Wind Chill Temperature Table	124
6-5 – Time to Occurrence of Frostbite in Minutes or Hours	124
6-6 – U.S. Guidelines and Limits for Occupational Exposure to Crystalline Silica	132
7-1 – Minimum Lighting Requirements	141
8-1 – Accident Prevention Sign Requirements	158
8-2 – Accident Prevention Color Coding	160
8-3 – Identification of Piping Systems	162
9-1 – Maximum Allowable Size of Containers and Tanks for Flammable and Combustible Liquids	175
9-2 – Outside Storage of LP-Gas Container and Cylinder Minimum Distances	182
9-3 – Temporary Heating Device Clearances	186
9-4 – Fire Extinguisher Distribution	191
11-1 – Minimum Clearance from Energized Overhead Electric Lines	231
11-2 – Hazardous (Classified) Locations	236
11-3 – AC Live Work Minimum Approach Distance	239
15-1 – Number of Clips and the Proper Torque Necessary to Assemble Wire Rope Eye Loop Connections with a Probable Efficiency Not More Than 80%	294
15-2 – Allowable Chain Wear	296
16-1 – Crane and Derrick Inspection Frequency	325
16-2 – Wire Rope Removal and Replacement Criteria	334
16-3 – Minimum Clearance from Energized Overhead Electric Lines	354
19-1 – Fire Extinguisher Requirements for Launches/Motorboats	470
21-1 – Safety Net Distances	500
22-1 – Selection Criteria for Planking and Platforms	519

EM 385-1-1
15 Sep 08

22-2 – Maximum Intended Load 519
22-3 – Wood Plank Selection.. 522
22-4 – Single Wood Pole Scaffolds 529
22-5 – Independent Wood Pole Scaffolds 531
22-6 – Ladder-Type Platforms 540
22-7 – Form Scaffolds 550
22-8 – Minimum Dimensions for Horse Scaffold Members 552
25-1 – Soil Classification 603
27-1 – Erection Bridging for Short Span Joists 667
27-2 – Erection Bridging for Long Span Joists........................... 669
29-1 – Energy Ratio and Peak Particle Velocity Formula 706
30-1 – Umbilical Markings.. 741
I-1 – Crane Performance Testing Requirements -
   No-Load Tests I-2
I-2 – Crane Performance Testing Requirements -
   At-Load Tests I-6
O-1 – Dive Team Composition, SCUBA, Untethered,
   0 to 100 ft (0 to 30.5 m)... O-1
O-2 – Dive Team Composition, SCUBA, Tethered with
   Communications, 0 to 100 ft (0 to 30.5 m) O-2
O-3 – Dive Team Composition, Surface Supplied Air,
   0 to 100 ft (0 to 30.5 m) O-2
O-4 – Dive Team Composition, Surface Supplied Air,
   101 to 190 ft (31.8 to 57.9 m).. O-3
O-5 – Dive Team Composition, Surface Supplied Mixed Gas
   Diving... O-4

BLANK

EM 385-1-1
15 Sep 08

SECTION 1

PROGRAM MANAGEMENT

01.A GENERAL

01.A.01 No person shall be required or instructed to work in surroundings or under conditions that are unsafe or dangerous to his or her health.

01.A.02 The employer is responsible for initiating and maintaining a safety and health program that complies with the US Army Corps of Engineers (USACE) safety and health requirements.

01.A.03 Each employee is responsible for complying with applicable safety and occupational health requirements, wearing prescribed safety and health equipment, reporting unsafe conditions/activities, preventing avoidable accidents, and working in a safe manner.

01.A.04 Safety and health programs, documents, signs, and tags shall be communicated to employees in a language that they understand.

01.A.05 Worksites with non-English speaking workers shall have a person(s), fluent in the language(s) spoken as well as English, on site when work is being performed, to interpret and translate as needed.

01.A.06 The Contractor shall erect and maintain a safety and health bulletin board in a commonly accessed area in clear view of the on-site workers. The bulletin board shall be continually maintained and updated and placed in a location that is protected against the elements and unauthorized removal. It shall contain, at minimum, the following safety and health information:

a. A map denoting the route to the nearest emergency care facility;

b. Emergency phone numbers;

c. A copy of the most up-to-date Accident Prevention Plan (APP) shall be mounted on or adjacent to the bulletin board, or a notice on the bulletin board shall state the location of the APP. The location of the APP shall be accessible on the site by all workers;

d. A copy of the current Activity Hazard Analysis/analyses (AHA) shall be mounted on or adjacent to the bulletin board, or a notice on the bulletin board should state the location of the AHAs. The location of the AHAs shall be accessible on the site by all workers;

e. The Occupational Safety and Health Administration (OSHA) Form 300A, <u>Summary of Work Related Injuries and Illnesses</u>, shall be posted, in accordance with OSHA requirements, <u>from February 1 to April 30 of the year following the issuance of this form. It shall be</u> mounted on or adjacent to the bulletin board, which shall be accessible on the site by all workers;

f. A copy of the Safety and Occupational Health deficiency tracking log shall be mounted on or be adjacent to the bulletin board or a notice on the bulletin board shall state the location where it may be accessed by all workers upon request; **> See 01.A.12.d.**

g. Safety and Health promotional posters;

h. Date of last lost workday injury;

i. OSHA Safety and Health Poster.

01.A.07 USACE Project Managers (PMs), in accordance with the Safety and Occupational Health Reference Document contained in the USACE Business Manual, shall ensure that a safety and

EM 385-1-1
15 Sep 08

occupational health plan is developed <u>for funded projects</u> and incorporated into each Project Management Plan (PMP)/Program Management Plan (PrgMP). <u>The PM shall collaborate with the customer on project safety goals and objectives and subsequently communicate these through the PMP/PrgMP safety and occupational health plan and Project Delivery Team (PDT) meetings.</u>

01.A.08 USACE PDT shall develop the safety and occupational health plan to be incorporated in the PMP and is responsible for assuring that safety and occupational health requirements are properly addressed and executed throughout the life cycle of each project.

> a. <u>The PDT shall ensure that identified hazards, control mechanisms, and risk acceptance are formally communicated to all project stakeholders.</u>
>
> b. <u>Unified Facilities Guide Specification (UFGS) for Safety and Health (currently 01 35 26)</u> shall be used in all USACE contract work and those contracts administered on behalf of the USACE under the provisions of FAR Clause 52.236-13.
>
> c. <u>Military Construction (MILCON) Transformation contracts will include the Federal Acquisition Regulation (FAR) Clause 52.236-13 as well as the Model Request for Proposal (RFP).</u>

01.A.09 For USACE activities where USACE employees are engaged in functions other than routine office or administrative duties, a project safety and health plan shall be developed, implemented, and updated as necessary.

> a. Such activities include operations and maintenance; recreational resource management; in-house conducted environmental restoration (investigation, design, and remediation); surveying, inspection, and testing; construction management; warehousing; transportation; research and development; and other activities when the Government Designated Authority (GDA) and the <u>command's local Safety</u>

EM 385-1-1
15 Sep 08

and Occupational Health Office (SOHO) agree on the benefit of such a program for accident prevention.

b. The project safety and health plan shall address applicable items listed in Appendix A in addition to the USACE Command's safety and occupational health program requirements.

c. For Hazardous Waste Operations and Emergency Response (HAZWOPER) sites, refer to Section 28 for Site Safety and Health Plan (SSHP) guidance.

01.A.10 A position hazard analysis (PHA) shall be prepared, updated as necessary, documented by the supervisor, and reviewed by the command's SOHO for each USACE position as warranted by the hazards associated with the position's tasks. A generic PHA may be used for groups of employees performing repetitive office/administrative tasks where the primary hazards result from ergonomic challenges, lighting conditions, light lifting and carrying tasks, and indoor air quality. *> See Figure 1-1 for an outline of a PHA. An electronic version of a PHA may be found on the HQUSACE Safety Office Website.*

a. The GDA, using the advice of the SOHO, shall determine the need for analysis of each position within his or her area of responsibility.

b. In developing the analysis for a particular position, supervisors should draw upon the knowledge and experience of employees in that position in addition to the SOHO.

c. A complete PHA document shall indicate that the hazards, control mechanisms, Personal Protective Equipment (PPE) and training required for the position were discussed with the employee, and the PHA shall be signed by the supervisor and employee. A PHA shall contain a copy of the employee's training certificate of completion for all required training.

EM 385-1-1
15 Sep 08

d. Supervisors shall review the contents of PHAs with employees upon initial assignment to a position, and at least annually or whenever there is a significant change in hazards.

01.A.11 Before initiation of work at the job site, an APP shall be reviewed and found acceptable by the GDA.

a. The APP shall contain appropriate appendices (for example, a SSHP for hazardous waste site cleanup operations, a Lead Compliance Plan when working with lead, or an Asbestos Hazard Abatement Plan when working with asbestos).

b. The APP shall be written in English by the Prime Contractor and shall articulate the specific work and hazards pertaining to the contract. The APP shall also implement in detail the pertinent requirements of this manual.

c. APPs shall be developed and submitted by the Contractor in the format provided in Appendix A of this manual. The Contractor shall address each of the elements/sub-elements in the outline contained in Appendix A in the order that they are provided in the manual. If an item is not applicable because of the nature of the work to be performed, the Contractor shall state this exception and provide a justification. **> See Appendix A.**

d. For limited scope supply, service and R&D contracts, the Contracting Officer and local SOHO may authorize an abbreviated APP. **> See Appendix A, paragraph 11 for details.**

e. The APP shall be developed by Qualified personnel and then signed in accordance with Appendix A, paragraph 1. The Contractor shall be responsible for documenting the Qualified person's credentials.

f. For contract operations, the Contractor's APP shall be job-specific and should include work to be performed by subcontractors. In addition, the APP should state measures to

EM 385-1-1
15 Sep 08

be taken by the Contractor to control hazards associated with materials, services, or equipment provided by suppliers.

g. Updates to the APP shall be reviewed and approved by the GDA.

FIGURE 1-1

POSITION HAZARD ANALYSIS (PHA)

POSITION HAZARD ANALYSIS (PHA) FOR USACE EMPLOYEE	
NAME: (Print - Last, First, MI): JOB SERIES: _____ JOB TITLE: _____ JOB NUMBER (SF52): _____	Prepared by: (Print Name – Last, First, MI): Reviewed by (SSHO): _____ Date (mo) _ _ (day) _ _ (year) _ _ _ _

COMMAND NAME & ORGANIZATION CODE: _____

PRIMARY DUTY LOCATION: _____

Clearances Required

EM OPS Team First Aid/CPR Respirator CDL Crane Operator Diver HTRW Other
☐ ☐ ☐ ☐ ☐ ☐ ☐ ☐

POSITION TASKS	SAFETY AND/OR OCCUPATIONAL HEALTH HAZARDS*	RECOMMENDED CONTROLS
1.	1.	1.
2.	2.	2.
3.	3.	3.
4.	4.	4.
5.	5.	5.
6.	6.	6.
7.	7.	7.

*Note - Examples of potential hazards are as follows:

Safety: trenching, electrical, slips, trips, fall hazards, etc.

Physical Agent: Exposure to heat/cold, noise, stress, vibration, radiation, etc.

Chemical: Exposure to solvents, cadmium, paints, welding fumes, pesticides, etc.

Biological: Exposure to bloodborne pathogens, poison ivy, insects, fungi, etc.

FIGURE 1-1 (Continued)

POSITION HAZARD ANALYSIS (PHA)

EQUIPMENT, MATERIALS, CHEMICALS TO BE USED	INSPECTION REQUIREMENTS	TRAINING REQUIREMENTS
List for each task [include Material Safety Data Sheets(MSDSs)]	List inspection requirements for each work task	List safety/health training requirements
1.	1.	1.
2.	2.	2.
3.	3.	3.
4.	4.	4.
5.	5.	5.
6.	6.	6.
7.	7.	7.
8.	8.	8.
9.	9.	9.
10.	10.	10.

This analysis serves as the hazard assessment required by Sections 01, 05, and 06 of EM 385-1-1, U.S. Army Corps of Engineers Safety and Health Requirements Manual. The employee covered by this analysis has been instructed in the tasks to be performed, the hazards to be encountered, the potential adverse effects of exposure to such hazards and the controls to be used. He/she has received adequate training specifically related to safe work practices, administrative and engineering controls and personal protective equipment (PPE) to be used in order to ensure assigned work tasks are conducted in a safe and healthful manner. He/she has demonstrated an understanding of the safety and health equipment and PPE to be used to include its limitations, useful shelf-life, how to properly don, doff, adjust, and wear required PPE, and how to properly care for, inspect, maintain, store, and dispose of such equipment. Attached is documentation of the training received, dates of such training, and the subject matter taught.

Supervisor Signature _____ Employee Signature _____

Date ___/___/_____   Date ___/___/_____

01.A.12 Inspections.

a. The APP or the USACE project safety and health plan shall provide for frequent safety inspections/<u>audits</u>, conducted by a Competent Person, of the work sites, material, and equipment to ensure compliance with the plan and this manual. <u>These inspections/audits shall be documented in writing and available upon request to the GDA. They shall include the name of the inspector, date, and all findings.</u>

b. In addition, Contractor Quality Control (QC) personnel - as part of their QC responsibilities - shall conduct and document daily safety and occupational health inspections in their daily QC logs.

c. Identified safety and health issues and deficiencies, and the actions, timetable, and responsibility for correcting the deficiencies, shall be recorded in inspection reports. Follow-up inspections to ensure correction of any identified deficiencies must also be conducted and documented in inspection reports.

d. The Contractor shall establish a safety and occupational health deficiency tracking system that lists and monitors the status of safety and health deficiencies in chronological order. The list shall be posted on the project safety bulletin board, be updated daily, and should provide the following information:

(1) Date deficiency identified;

(2) Description of deficiency;

(3) Name of person responsible for correcting deficiency;

(4) Projected resolution date;

(5) Date actually resolved.

EM 385-1-1
15 Sep 08

e. The Contractor shall immediately notify the GDA of any OSHA or other regulatory agency inspection and provide GDA an opportunity to accompany the Contractor on the inspection. (The inspection will not be delayed due to non-availability of the GDA.) The Contractor shall provide the GDA with a copy of any citations or reports issued by the inspector and any corrective action responses to the citation(s) or report(s).

01.A.13 <u>Contractor-Required AHA</u>. Before beginning each work activity involving a type of work presenting hazards not experienced in previous project operations or where a new work crew or sub-contractor is to perform the work, the Contractor(s) performing that work activity shall prepare an AHA. *> See Figure 1-2 for an outline of an AHA. <u>An electronic version AHA may be found on the HQUSACE Safety Office Website.</u>*

a. AHAs shall define the activities being performed and identify the work sequences, the specific anticipated hazards, site conditions, equipment, materials, and the control measures to be implemented to eliminate or reduce each hazard to an acceptable level of risk.

b. Work shall not begin until the AHA for the work activity has been accepted by the GDA and discussed with all engaged in the activity, including the Contractor, subcontractor(s), and Government on-site representatives at preparatory and initial control phase meetings.

c. The names of the Competent/Qualified Person(s) required for a particular activity (for example, excavations, scaffolding, fall protection, other activities as specified by OSHA and this manual) shall be identified and included in the AHA. Proof of their competency/qualification shall be submitted to the GDA for acceptance prior to the start of that work activity.

d. The AHA shall be reviewed and modified as necessary to address changing site conditions, operations, or change of competent/qualified person(s).

EM 385-1-1
15 Sep 08

(1) If more than one Competent/Qualified Person is used on the AHA activity, a list of names shall be submitted as an attachment to the AHA. Those listed must be Competent/Qualified for the type of work involved in the AHA and familiar with current site safety issues.

(2) If a new Competent/Qualified Person (not on the original list) is added, the list shall be updated (an administrative action not requiring an updated AHA). T he new person shall acknowledge in writing that he or she has reviewed the AHA and is familiar with current site safety issues.

FIGURE 1-2

ACTIVITY HAZARD ANALYSIS (AHA)

Date Prepared: _____

Project Location: _____

Prepared By: _____

Job/Task: _____

Reviewed By: _____

JOB STEPS	HAZARDS	CONTROLS	RAC
Identify the principal steps involved and the sequence of work activities.	Analyze each principal step for potential hazards.	Develop specific controls for potential hazards.	Assign Appropriate Risk Assessment Code (RAC) per AR 385-10.
EQUIPMENT	TRAINING	INSPECTIONS	
List equipment to be used in the work activity.	List training requirements.	List inspection requirements.	

EM 385-1-1
15 Sep 08

01.A.14 <u>USACE-Required AHAs</u>. An AHA shall be prepared and documented for each USACE activity as warranted by the hazards associated with the activity. Generally, an AHA should be prepared for all field operations.

    a. The <u>supervisor</u>, utilizing the recommendations of the SOHO, should determine the need for an AHA for each activity within his or her area of responsibility.

    b. In developing the AHA for a particular activity, USACE supervisors should draw upon the knowledge and experience of employees in that activity as well as the <u>SOHO</u>.

    c. The Government uses this process to assess and manage the risks associated with the project.

01.A.15 To ensure compliance with this manual, the Contractor may be required to prepare for review specific safety and occupational health submittal items. These submittal items may be specifically required by this manual or may be identified in the contract or by the Contracting Officer's Representative (COR). All safety and occupational health submittal items shall be written in English and provided by the Contractor to the GDA.

01.A.16 The COR or a designated representative shall immediately stop work when an employee is deemed to be in imminent danger of serious injury or loss of life. **> See Federal Acquisition Regulation (FAR) Clause 52.236-13(d).**

<u>01.A.17 Site Safety and Health Officer (SSHO). The Contractor shall employ a minimum of one Competent Person at each project site to function as the SSHO, depending on job complexity, size and any other pertinent factors.</u>

    <u>a. The SSHO shall be a full-time responsibility unless specified differently in the contract. The SSHO shall report to a senior project (or corporate) official.</u>

b. The SSHO(s), as a minimum, must have completed the 30-hour OSHA Construction safety class or as an equivalent, 30 hours of formal construction safety and health training covering the subjects of the OSHA 30-hour course (see Appendix A, paragraph 4.b) applicable to the work to be performed and given by qualified instructors. *> The SSHO is also required to have five (5) years of construction industry safety experience or three (3) years if he possesses a Certified Safety Professional (CSP) or safety and health degree.*

c. An SSHO (or a Designated Representative, as identified in the APP/AHA and as deemed appropriate/equivalent to SSHO by the GDA) shall be on-site at all times when work is being performed.

d. The SSHO shall be responsible for managing, implementing and enforcing the Contractor's Safety and Health Program in accordance with the accepted APP.

e. SSHOs shall maintain this competency through 24 hours of formal safety and health related coursework every four (4) years.

> For limited service contracts, for example, mowing (only), park attendants, rest room cleaning, the Contracting Officer and Safety Office may modify SSHO requirements and waive the more stringent elements of this section.
> See Appendix A, paragraphs 4 and 11.

> For complex or high hazard projects, the SSHO shall have a minimum of ten (10) years of safety-related work with at least five (5) years experience on similar type projects.

01.A.18 The Prime Contractor is responsible for ensuring subcontractor compliance with the safety and occupational health requirements contained in this manual.

EM 385-1-1
15 Sep 08

01.A.19 Collateral Duty Safety Personnel. USACE organizations may be augmented by Collateral Duty (Army civilian) safety personnel. Collateral duty safety personnel shall:

a. Be appointed through written orders;

b. Have met the requirements of 29 CFR 1960.58, training of collateral duty safety and health personnel and committee members, before reporting to duty;

c. Give their safety duties proper priority;

d. Report directly to their unit manager concerning safety–related matters;

e. Coordinate activities with their supporting SOHO.

01.B INDOCTRINATION AND TRAINING

01.B.01 A Qualified Person(s) shall conduct all training required by this manual. All training shall correspond to American National Standards Institute (ANSI) regulation Z490.1.

01.B.02 Employees shall be provided with safety and health indoctrination prior to the start of work as well as continuous safety and health training to enable them to perform their work in a safe manner. All training, meetings and indoctrinations shall be documented in writing by date, name, content and trainer.

01.B.03 Indoctrination and training should be based upon the existing safety and health program of the Contractor or Government agency, as applicable, and shall include but not be limited to:

a. Requirements and responsibilities for accident prevention and the maintenance of safe and healthful work environments;

b. General safety and health policies and procedures and pertinent provisions of this manual;

c. Employee and supervisor responsibilities for reporting all accidents;

d. Provisions for medical facilities and emergency response and procedures for obtaining medical treatment or emergency assistance;

e. Procedures for reporting and correcting unsafe conditions or practices;

f. Job hazards and the means to control/eliminate those hazards, including applicable PHAs and/or AHAs;

g. Specific training as required by this manual.

01.B.04 All visitors to USACE Government- or Contractor-controlled sites presenting hazardous conditions shall be briefed by a Qualified Person on the hazards to be expected on the site and the safety and health controls required (for example, hard hat, foot protection, etc.). The person in charge of the site shall ensure that all visitors entering the site are properly protected and are wearing or provided with the appropriate PPE. Site personnel should maintain a stock of common PPE, such as hard hats, eye protection, ear plugs, and reflective vests, for use by visitors. The site manager shall provide an escort for all visitors while on site. A visitor sign-in log shall be maintained on site.

01.B.05 Safety meetings shall be conducted to review past activities, plan for new or changed operations, review pertinent aspects of appropriate AHA (by trade), establish safe working procedures for anticipated hazards, and provide pertinent safety and health training and motivation.

a. Meetings shall be conducted at least once a month for all supervisors on the project location and at least once a week for all workers by supervisors or foremen.

b. Meetings shall be documented, including the date, persons in attendance, subjects discussed, and names of individual(s) who conducted the meeting. Documentation shall be maintained and copies furnished to the GDA on request.

c. The GDA shall be informed of all scheduled meetings in advance and be invited to attend.

01.B.06 Emergency situations.

a. The employer shall provide training in handling emergency situations that may arise from project activities or equipment operation.

b. All persons who may have occasion to use emergency and rescue or lifesaving equipment shall be familiarized with the equipment location, trained in its proper use, be instructed in its capabilities and limitations, and medically qualified for its use.

01.C PHYSICAL QUALIFICATIONS OF EMPLOYEES

01.C.01 All persons shall be physically, medically, and emotionally (ready, willing and able) qualified for performing the duties to which they are assigned. Some factors to be considered in making work assignments are strength, endurance, agility, coordination, and visual and hearing acuity.

a. At a minimum, employees shall meet the physical requirements for specific job tasks and hazards as required by OSHA guidelines, Department of Transportation (DOT) regulations, and U.S. Coast Guard (USCG) requirements.

b. Medical documentation shall be recorded using applicable medical screening and/or medical history and examination forms and shall be maintained in accordance with 5 CFR 293 and Privacy Act requirements.

01.C.02 While on duty, employees shall not use or be under the influence of alcohol, narcotics, intoxicants, or similar mind-altering substances.

EM 385-1-1
15 Sep 08

> a. Employees found to be under the influence of or consuming such substances will be immediately removed from the job site. Contractors shall enforce the drug-free workplace requirements.
>
> b. Any employee under a physician's treatment and taking prescribed narcotics or any medication that may prevent one being ready, willing and able to safely perform position duties shall provide a medical clearance statement to his supervisor.

01.C.03 Operators of any equipment or vehicle shall be able to read and understand the signs, signals, and operating instructions in use.

01.C.04 Operators are not be permitted to operate beyond the following limits:

> a. Operators of equipment, such as hoisting equipment and draglines, mobile construction equipment, electrical power systems, hydropower plants, industrial manufacturing systems, hydraulically operated equipment, powered vessels, and boats, shall not be permitted to exceed twelve (12) hours of duty time in any 24-hour period, including time worked at another occupation. A minimum of eight (8) consecutive hours shall be provided for rest in each 24-hour period.
>
> b. Operators of motor vehicles, while on duty, shall not operate vehicles for a continuous period of more than ten (10) hours in any 24-hour period; moreover, no employee, while on duty, may operate a motor vehicle after being in a duty status for more than twelve (12) hours during any 24-hour period. A minimum of eight (8) consecutive hours shall be provided for rest in each 24-hour period.

01.C.05 Compressed-air workers.

> a. No person is permitted to enter a compressed-air environment until examined by a licensed physician and found to be physically qualified to engage in such work.

EM 385-1-1
15 Sep 08

b. Any person working in a compressed-air environment who is absent from work for ten (10) or more days, or is absent due to sickness or injury, shall not resume work until reexamined by a licensed physician, and found to be physically qualified to work in a compressed-air environment.

c. After a person has been continuously employed in compressed-air for a period designated by a physician, but not to exceed one (1) year, that person shall be reexamined by a physician to determine if he/she remains physically qualified to engage in compressed-air work.

d. All other requirements for compressed-air work should be as specified in the contract technical provisions.

01.D ACCIDENT REPORTING AND RECORDKEEPING

01.D.01 All accidents occurring incidentally to an operation, project, or facility for which this manual is applicable shall be investigated, reported, and analyzed as prescribed by the GDA.

a. Employees are responsible for reporting all injuries or occupationally related illnesses as soon as possible to their employer or immediate supervisor.

b. Employers and immediate supervisors are responsible for reporting all injuries to the GDA <u>as soon as reasonably possible but no later than</u> 24 hours.

c. No supervisor may decline to accept a report of injury from a subordinate.

01.D.02 An accident that has, or appears to have, any of the consequences listed below shall be immediately reported to the GDA. The following accidents shall be investigated in depth to identify all causes and to recommend hazard control measures. The GDA shall immediately notify the SOHO of all serious accidents and subsequently follow-up with official accident reports as prescribed by regulation. **Contractors are responsible for**

notifying OSHA when one or more of their employees are seriously injured.

   a. Fatal injury/<u>illness</u>;

   b. Permanent totally disabling injury/<u>illness</u>;

   c. Permanent partial disabling injury/<u>illness</u>;

   d. Three or more persons <u>hospitalized as inpatients as a result of a single occurrence</u>;

   e. <u>$200,000 or greater accidental property</u> damage or damage in an amount specified by USACE in current accident reporting regulations

   f. Arc Flash Incident/Accident; or

   <u>g. USACE aircraft destroyed or missing.</u>

01.D.03 Except for rescue and emergency measures, the accident scene shall not be disturbed until it has been released by the investigating official. The Contractor is responsible for obtaining appropriate medical and emergency assistance and for notifying fire, law enforcement, and regulatory agencies. The Contractor shall assist and cooperate fully with the GDA conducting the Government investigation(s) of the accident.

01.D.04 Daily records of all first-aid treatments not otherwise reportable shall be maintained on prescribed forms and furnished to the GDA upon request.

01.D.05 In addition to any other applicable requirements within this section on contract operations, the Prime Contractor shall:

   a. Maintain records of all exposure and accident experience incidental to the work (this includes exposure and accident experience of the Prime Contractor and subcontractors and, at a minimum, these records shall include exposure work hours and

EM 385-1-1
15 Sep 08

a log of occupational injuries and illnesses - OSHA Form 300 or equivalent as prescribed by 29 CFR 1904); provide a current copy of OSHA Form 300 or equivalent to the GDA upon request;

b. Maintain health hazard assessment documentation and employee exposure monitoring to chemical, biological, and physical agents as required by Section 06. Provide this information to employees who are characterized by these assessments and exposure monitoring in accordance with OSHA requirements. Immediately notify the GDA of any exposure in excess of the limits specified in Section 06 and the hazard control measures that have been taken to reduce or eliminate such exposures.

c. Submit project work hours to the COR monthly <u>in the format</u> provided by the COR. Work hours include all hours on the project where an employee is in an on-duty pay status.

01.E EMERGENCY PLANNING

01.E.01 Emergency plans to ensure employee safety in case of fire or other emergency shall be prepared, in writing, and reviewed with all affected employees. Emergency plans shall be tested to ensure their effectiveness.

a. Plans shall include escape procedures and routes, critical plant operations, employee accounting following an emergency evacuation, rescue and medical duties, means of reporting emergencies, and persons to be contacted for information or clarification.

b. On-site emergency planning shall be integrated with off-site emergency support. (Documentation of specific on-site emergency services shall be made and may include written agreements, memoranda for record, telephone conversation logs, etc.) The emergency services provider should be offered an on-site orientation of the project and associated hazards.

EM 385-1-1
15 Sep 08

01.E.02 Planning for any operation shall include the total system response capabilities to minimize the consequences of accidents or natural disaster and shall consider communications, rescue, first aid, medical, emergency response, emergency equipment, and training requirements.

01.E.03 The number of persons permitted in any location shall correspond to rescue and escape capabilities and limitations.

01.E.04 Emergency alert systems shall be developed, tested, and used to alert all persons likely to be affected by existing or imminent disaster conditions and to alert and summon emergency responders.

01.E.05 Emergency telephone numbers and reporting instructions for ambulance, physician, hospital, fire, and police shall be conspicuously and clearly posted at the work site.

01.E.06 Employees working alone in a remote location or away from other workers shall be provided an effective means of emergency communications. This means of communication could include a cellular phone, two-way radios, hard-line telephones or other acceptable means. The selected communication shall be readily available (easily within the immediate reach) of the employee and shall be tested prior to the start of work to verify that it effectively operates in the area/environment. An employee check-in/check-out communication procedure shall be developed to ensure employee safety.

01.F EMERGENCY OPERATIONS.

01.F.01 In addition to the other pertinent parts of this manual, Civil Disaster Emergency Operations for floods, earthquakes, and hurricanes shall be conducted in accordance with Appendix B for both USACE and Contractor activities.

EM-385-1-1
15 Sep 08

SECTION 2

SANITATION

02.A GENERAL REQUIREMENTS. Employers shall establish and maintain <u>hygienic</u> sanitation provisions for all employees in all places of employment as specified in the following paragraphs.

<u>02.B HOUSEKEEPING</u>

<u>02.B.01 Places of employment shall be kept as clean as possible, taking into consideration the nature of the work. Regular cleaning shall be conducted in order to maintain safe and sanitary conditions in the workplace.</u>

<u>02.B.02 The floor of every workroom shall be kept as dry as possible. Drainage shall be maintained where wet processes are used, and false floors, platforms, mats, or other dry standing places shall be provided, when possible. Appropriate footwear shall also be provided.</u>

<u>02.B.03 To facilitate cleaning, every floor, working place, and passageway shall be kept free from protruding nails, splinters, loose boards, clutter, and unnecessary holes and openings.</u>

<u>02.C DRINKING WATER</u>

<u>02.C.01 An adequate supply of potable water shall be provided in all places of employment, for both drinking and personal cleansing.</u>

02.C.<u>02</u> Cool <u>drinking</u> water shall be provided during hot weather.

   a. Drinking water shall be provided at all Continental United States (CONUS) fixed facilities according to the

EM 385-1-1
15 Sep 08

requirements of the Safe Drinking Water Act, as amended, and all applicable Federal, state, and local regulations. Refer to 40 Code of Federal Regulations (CFR) 141 and 40 CFR 143, for updates to the national drinking water regulations. Refer to individual state and local regulations, as applicable, for updates in those regulations. CONUS facilities classified as suppliers of water:

(1) Shall comply with substantive and procedural requirements pursuant to 40 CFR 141;

(2) Shall meet any state and local regulations that are more stringent than the Federal regulations; and

(3) Shall ensure that the sanitary control and surveillance of water supplies and that the chlorination and fluoridation are conducted according to applicable guidelines.

b. Outside the Continental Unites States (OCONUS), drinking water at military fixed facilities shall be provided in compliance with country-specific Final Governing Standards (FGS) or, in the absence of FGS, the National Primary Drinking Water Regulations (NPDWR) as outlined in the Overseas Environmental Baseline Guidance Document (OEBGD), Department of Defense Instruction (DODI) 4715.5-G. In addition, the sanitary control and surveillance of water supplies and the chlorination and fluoridation shall be conducted according to applicable Department of Defense (DOD) Component guidelines, or if more stringent, the host nation requirements.

c. Drinking water for _temporary_ field activities shall be provided according to the procedures defined in Army Regulation (AR) 700-136, Field Manual (FM) 10-52, FM 21-10/Marine Corps Reference Publication (MCRP) 4-11.1D, and Technical Bulletin, Medical, (TB MED) 577.

EM-385-1-1
15 Sep 08

d. Drinking water on all Army floating vessels shall be provided according to 40 CFR 141 and chapter 6 of Navy Medical (NAVMED) P-5010-010-LP-207-1300.

02.C.03 Only approved potable water systems may be used for the distribution of drinking water. Construction trailers and other temporary or semi-permanent facilities shall be properly connected to the local municipal water supply unless the remoteness of the location makes this prohibitive. When unable to connect into the municipal supply, temporary potable water systems shall be utilized, with the services provided by a licensed potable water contractor. "Reclaimed water" (treated wastewater) use in potable systems is strictly prohibited.

02.C.04 Drinking water shall be dispensed by means that prevent contamination between the consumer and the source.

02.C.05 Portable drinking water dispensers shall be designed, constructed, and serviced to ensure sanitary conditions; shall be capable of being closed; and shall have a tap. Any container used to distribute drinking water shall be clearly marked "**DRINKING WATER**" and may not be used for other purposes.

02.C.06 Open containers such as barrels, pails, or tanks, or any container (whether with or without a fitted cover) from which the water is dipped or poured are prohibited for drinking water.

02.C.07 Fountain dispensers shall have a guarded orifice.

02.C.08 Use of a common cup (a cup shared by more than one worker) and other common utensils is prohibited. Employees shall use cups when drinking from portable water coolers/containers. Unused disposable cups shall be kept in sanitary containers and a waste receptacle shall be provided for used cups.

02.D NON-POTABLE WATER

EM 385-1-1
15 Sep 08

02.D.01 Outlets dispensing non-potable water shall be conspicuously posted **"CAUTION - WATER UNSAFE FOR DRINKING, WASHING, OR COOKING"**. Outlets dispensing non-potable water at Corps Dumping Stations within campgrounds may, in lieu of this requirement, be posted in accordance with USACE's Engineering Pamphlet (EP) 310-1-6A and EP 310-1-6B.

02.D.02 There shall not be any cross-connection, open or potential, between a system furnishing potable water and a system furnishing non-potable water.

02.D.03 Non-potable water may be used for cleaning work areas, except food processing and preparation areas and personal service rooms, provided this non-potable water does not contain concentrations of chemicals, fecal coli form, or other substances which could create unsanitary conditions or be harmful to employees.

02.E TOILETS

02.E.01 **General**. Toilets shall be present in all places of employment and shall contain the following: **Exception:** The requirements of this subdivision do not apply to mobile crews or to normally unattended work locations if employees working at these locations have transportation readily available to nearby toilet and/or washing facilities which meet the other requirements of this paragraph):

a. Separate toilet facilities, in toilet rooms, shall be provided for each sex and shall be provided in all places of employment according to Table 2-1;

b. Each lavatory shall be equipped with hot and cold running water, or tepid running water;

c. Hand soap or similar cleansing agents shall be provided;

d. Individual hand towels or sections thereof, of cloth or paper, warm air blowers or clean individual sections of continuous cloth toweling, convenient to the lavatories, shall be provided;

e. All lavatories shall be provided with an adequate supply of toilet paper and a holder for each seat;

f. Each toilet shall be contained within an individual compartment and equipped with a door and separated from other toilet fixtures by walls or partitions sufficiently high to ensure privacy;

g. Toilet facilities shall be constructed so that the interior is lighted;

h. Separate toilet rooms for each sex need not be provided if toilet rooms can only be occupied by one person at a time, can be locked from the inside, and contain at least one toilet seat;

i. Where such single-occupancy rooms have more than one commode, only one commode in each toilet room may be counted;

j. Washing and toilet facilities shall be cleaned regularly and maintained in good order;

k. Each commode shall be equipped with a toilet seat and toilet seat cover. Each toilet facility - except those specifically designed and designated for females - shall be equipped with a metal, plastic or porcelain urinal trough; and

l. Adequate ventilation shall be provided and all windows and vents shall be screened; seat boxes shall be vented to the outside (minimum vent size 4 in (10.1 cm)) with vent intake located 1 in (2.5 cm) below the seat.

TABLE 2-1

MINIMUM TOILET FACILITIES
(OTHER THAN CONSTRUCTION SITES)

Number of employees	Minimum number of Toilets[1]
1 to 15	One (1)
16 to 35	Two (2)
36 to 55	Three (3)
56 to 80	Four (4)
81 to 110	Five (5)
111 to 150	Six (6)
Over 150	Refer to Note [2]

NOTE: [1] Where toilet facilities will not be used by women, urinals may be provided instead of commodes, except that the number of commodes in such cases shall not be reduced to fewer than 2/3 of the minimum number specified.
[2] One additional toilet fixture for each additional 40 employees.

02.E.02 Construction Sites. Toilet facilities on construction sites shall be provided as follows (the requirements of this subsection do not apply to mobile crews or to normally unattended work locations if employees working at these locations have transportation immediately available to nearby toilet facilities):

a. Where sanitary sewers are not available, job sites shall be provided with chemical toilets, re-circulating toilets, or combustion toilets unless prohibited by state/local codes;

b. Each toilet facility shall be equipped with a toilet seat and toilet seat cover. Each toilet facility - except those specifically designed and designated for females - shall be equipped with a metal, plastic, or porcelain urinal trough. All shall be provided with an adequate supply of toilet paper and a holder for each seat;

c. Toilets shall be provided for each sex according to Table 2-2. Separate toilet rooms for each sex need not be provided if toilet rooms can only be occupied by one person at a time, can be locked from the inside, and contain at least one toilet seat;

d. Where it is not practical to provide running water, hand sanitizers may be used as a substitute for running water. (Many hand sanitizers contain flammable liquids and personnel shall be trained regarding their use, storage and safety precautions.);

e. Toilet facilities shall be constructed so that the occupants are protected against weather and falling objects; all cracks shall be sealed, and the door shall be tight-fitting, self-closing, and capable of being latched;

f. Adequate ventilation shall be provided and all windows and vents shall be screened; seat boxes shall be vented to the outside (minimum vent size 4 in (10.1 cm)) with vent intake located 1 in (2.5 cm) below the seat;

g. Toilet facilities shall be constructed so that the interior is lighted; and

h. Provisions for routinely servicing and cleaning all toilets and disposing of the sewage shall be established before placing toilet facilities into operation. The method of sewage disposal and the placement location selected shall be in accordance with Federal, state, and local health regulations.

EM 385-1-1
15 Sep 08

TABLE 2-2
MINIMUM TOILET FACILITIES
(CONSTRUCTION SITES)

Number of employees	Minimum number of Toilets[1]
20 or fewer	One (1)
20 or greater	One (1) toilet seat and One (1) urinal per 40 workers.
200 or greater	One (1) toilet seat and One (1) urinal per 50 workers.

NOTE: [1]Where toilet facilities will not be used by women, urinals may be provided instead of commodes, except that the number of commodes in such cases shall not be reduced to fewer than 2/3 of the minimum number specified.

02.E.03 Employees working in temporary field conditions, in mobile crews or in normally unattended work locations shall be provided at least one toilet facility unless transportation to nearby toilet facilities is readily available.

02.F WASHING FACILITIES

02.F.01 Washing facilities shall be provided at toilet facilities and as needed to maintain healthful and sanitary conditions.

02.F.02 Each washing facility shall be maintained in a sanitary condition and provided with water (either hot and cold running water or tepid running water), soap, and individual means of drying. If it is not practical to provide running water, hand sanitizers may be used as a substitute.

02.F.03 Washing facilities shall be in close proximity to the worksite.

02.G SHOWERS

02.G.01 Washing facilities for persons engaged in the application of paints, coatings, herbicides, insecticides, or

EM-385-1-1
15 Sep 08

other operations where contaminants may be harmful shall be at or near the work site and shall be equipped in order to enable employees to remove such substances.

02.G.02 Whenever showers are required by a particular standard, the showers shall be provided in accordance with the following:

    a. One shower shall be provided for every ten employees (or fraction thereof) of each sex, who are required to shower during the same shift;

    b. Body soap or other appropriate cleansing agents convenient to the showers shall be provided;

    c. Showers shall be equipped with hot and cold water feeding a common discharge line; and

    d. Employees who use showers shall be provided with individual clean towels.

02.H CHANGING ROOMS. Whenever employees are required by a particular standard to wear protective clothing, changing rooms shall be equipped with separate storage facilities for both street clothes and protective clothing.

02.I CLOTHES DRYING FACILITIES. If working clothes are provided by the employer and become <u>contaminated</u>, wet or are washed between shifts, provision shall be made to ensure that such clothing is <u>decontaminated, clean,</u> and dry before reuse.

02.J FOOD SERVICE

02.J.01 All cafeterias, restaurants, mess facilities, and related facilities on areas, projects, or installations shall be established, operated, and maintained in compliance with the health and sanitation recommendations of the United States

EM 385-1-1
15 Sep 08

Public Health Service and applicable state and local regulations.

02.J.02　All employee food service facilities and operations shall be conducted in accordance with sound hygienic principles.

02.J.03　In all places of employment where all or part of the food service is provided, the food dispensed shall be wholesome, free from spoilage, and shall be processed, prepared, handled, and stored in such a manner as to be protected against contamination.

02.J.04　No employee may be allowed to consume food or beverages in a toilet room or in any area exposed to a toxic material.

02.J.05　No food or beverages may be stored in toilet rooms or in an area exposed to a toxic material.

02.K　WASTE DISPOSAL

02.K.01　An adequate number of waste receptacles shall be provided in a food service area and used for the disposal of waste food. Receptacles shall be constructed of smooth, corrosion-resistant, easily cleanable, or disposable materials, provided with solid tight-fitting covers, emptied at least daily and maintained in a sanitary condition.

02.K.02　Receptacles used for putrescible solid or liquid waste or refuse shall be constructed in order to prevent leakage and to allow thorough cleaning and sanitary maintenance. Such receptacles shall be equipped with solid tight-fitting covers, unless they can be maintained in sanitary conditions without covers.

02.K.03　All sweepings, solid or liquid wastes, refuse, and garbage shall be removed in a manner which avoids creating a menace to health and should be discarded as often as

EM-385-1-1
15 Sep 08

necessary or appropriate to maintain sanitary conditions in the place of employment.

02.L VERMIN CONTROL

02.L.01 Every enclosed workplace shall be constructed, equipped, and maintained, as practicable as possible, in order to prevent the entrance or harborage of rodents, insects, or other vermin.

02.L.02 A continuing and effective extermination program shall be instituted when the presence of vermin is detected. The use of licensed exterminators/pest control personnel is required.

BLANK

EM 385-1-1
15 Sep 08

SECTION 3

MEDICAL AND FIRST-AID REQUIREMENTS

03.A GENERAL

03.A.01 Prior to the start of work, arrangements shall be made for medical facilities and personnel to provide prompt attention to injured employees and for consultation concerning occupational safety and health matters.

    a. An effective means of communication (hard-wired or cellular telephone, two-way radio, etc.) with #911 access or other emergency response source, and transportation to effectively care for injured workers shall be provided. Communication devices shall be tested in the area of use to assure functionality.

    b. The telephone numbers of physicians, hospitals, or ambulances shall be conspicuously posted, at a minimum, on the safety bulletin board and near the on-site project office telephones. <u>Medical facilities and personnel expected to treat injured employees shall be informed of the nature of the work to be performed and the injuries/illnesses prevalent on such jobsites.</u>

    c. A <u>highly visible</u> map delineating the best route to the nearest medical facility shall be prepared and posted on the safety bulletin board.

03.A.02 First-aid and cardiopulmonary resuscitation (CPR) availability.

    a. When a medical facility or physician is not accessible within five (5) minutes of an injury to a group of two (2) or more employees for the treatment of injuries, at least two (2) employees on each shift shall be qualified to administer first-aid and CPR. **> Minimum qualifications are listed in 03.D.**

EM 385-1-1
15 Sep 08

b. Individuals who are required to work alone in remote areas shall be trained in first-aid and shall be provided with an **effective** means of communication to call for assistance in the event of an emergency.

03.A.03 First-aid and medical facility requirements.

a. All projects, activities, installations, or contracts for which fewer than 100 persons are employed (greatest total number of employees on a shift) at the site of the work, and where neither a first-aid station nor an infirmary is available, shall be provided with a first-aid kit complying with the criteria contained in ANSI Z308.1. There shall be one first-aid kit for every 25 (or fewer) employees. In addition to the basic fill requirements of the first-aid kit, the employer, in consultation with a health care professional or competent first-aid person, shall evaluate the hazards found in the work environment to determine the necessity of optional fill contents.

b. All projects, activities, installations, or contracts for which more than 99 and fewer than 300 persons are employed (greatest total number of employees on a shift) at the site of the work, shall establish and equip, as directed by a Licensed Physician (LP), a first-aid station. In non-rural locations, medical clinics, hospitals, or doctors' offices, accessible within five (5) minutes of an injury may be approved for use provided the requirements of paragraph 03.A.03.a. are met.

c. Where tunnels are being excavated, a first-aid station and transportation facilities shall be provided so that treatment is available within five (5) minutes of the occurrence of an injury.

d. All projects, activities, installations, or contracts for which 300 or more persons are employed (greatest total number of employees on a shift) at the site of the work shall establish and equip, as directed by a licensed physician, an infirmary.

03.A.04 Should work activities present any potential exposure (of any part of the body) to toxic or corrosive materials, drenching

EM 385-1-1
15 Sep 08

and/or flushing facilities shall be provided in the work area for immediate emergency use. **> See Section 06.B.**

03.A.05 Before commencing use of epoxy resins, concrete, or other dermatitis-producing substances, employees shall be made aware of the manufacturers' skin protection recommendations. Barrier cream ointment or other skin protection measures recommended by the manufacturer for the specific exposure shall be available for use.

03.A.06 Employees designated as responsible for rendering first-aid or medical assistance shall be included in their employer's blood-borne pathogen program in accordance with 29 CFR 1910.1030 and shall:

> a. Be instructed in the sources, hazards, and avoidance of blood-borne pathogens and be provided the training specified in 29 CFR 1910.1030;
>
> b. Be provided with, and shall use and maintain, PPE (i.e., Breathing barrier, latex-free gloves, gowns, masks, eye protectors, and/or resuscitation equipment) when appropriate for rendering first-aid or other medical assistance to prevent contact with blood or other potentially infectious materials;
>
> c. Institute a site-specific blood-borne pathogen prevention program to include a site-specific Exposure Control Plan with provisions for engineering and administrative controls, Hepatitis B vaccination, PPE, training, recordkeeping, and a Post-Exposure Control Plan in the event of a blood-borne exposure. Post-exposure protocol shall include a plan to ensure **immediate** medical evaluation of exposed individual(s) per current recommendations of the Center for Disease Control (CDC) for human immuno-deficiency virus (HIV), Hepatitis B virus (HBV), Hepatitis C virus (HCV) and Hepatitis A virus (HAV).

03.A.07 Prior to the start of work outside the employee's normal geographical area, the employer shall inform employees of

EM 385-1-1
15 Sep 08

parasitic, viral and environmental diseases endemic to the geographical work location. Common diseases to consider are: Lyme Disease, West Nile Virus, Hantavirus, Histoplasmosis, Rocky-Mountain Spotted Fever, Dengue Fever, and Malaria.

    a. For guidance on the potential biological and environmental diseases in the work location, the employer shall consult the CDC Travel webpage, U.S. Army Center for Health Promotion and Preventive Medicine web site, and the health department in the local area.

    b. Information to be provided to the employee traveling in areas where such diseases are endemic shall include:

    (1) Modes of disease transmission;

    (2) Specific health risks associated with the disease;

    (3) Preventive measures such as available vaccines and PPE (gloves, eye and skin protection, respirator);

    (4) Appropriate work practices to prevent contact with infected agents (bird/rodent droppings, etc.), such as watering areas prior to dust-generating activities;

    (5) Vaccine information, to include information on the effectiveness, risk, and availability;

    (6) Safe removal of source where applicable;

    (7) Symptom recognition and medical referral.

03.B FIRST-AID KITS

03.B.01 <u>The performance requirements of the first aid containers shall be based on the storage area location of the first-aid kit and shall conform to ANSI Z308.1:</u>

a. Type I container is for permanently affixed indoor or atmosphere-controlled settings. Type 1 first-aid kits are required to meet the requirements of a ten (10)-unit container.

b. Type II and Type III first-aid kits shall, at a minimum, meet the requirements for a 16-unit container:

(1) Type II container is for portable indoor settings;

(2) Type III container is for portable outdoor settings.

c. The contents of the first-aid kit shall, at a minimum, contain the items detailed in Table 3-1.

d. First-aid kits shall be easily accessible to all workers and protected from the weather. The individual contents of the first-aid kits shall be kept sterile. First-aid kit locations shall be clearly marked and distributed throughout the site(s).

03.B.02 The contents of first-aid kits shall be checked by the employer prior to their use on site and at least every three (3) months when work is in progress to ensure that they are complete, in good condition, and have not expired.

EM 385-1-1
15 Sep 08

TABLE 3-1

REQUIREMENTS FOR BASIC UNIT PACKAGES

Unit first aid item	Minimum Size or Volume (metric)	Minimum Size or Volume (US)	Item quantity per unit package	Unit package size
*Absorbent Compress	206 cm^2	32 in^2	1	1
* Adhesive Bandage	2.5 x 7.5 cm	1 x 3 in	16	1
Antibiotic Treatment	0.9 g	1/32 oz	6	1
* Adhesive Tape	457.2 cm	5 yd (total)	1 or 2	1 or 2
* Antiseptic Swab	0.5 g	0.14 fl. oz.	10	1
Antiseptic Wipe	2.5 x 2.5 cm	1 x 1 in.	10	1
Antiseptic Towelette	157 cm^2	24 in^2	10	1
Aspirin, Individually Wrapped	325 mg		2	2
Bandage Compress (2 in.)	5 x 91 cm	2 x 36 in.	4	1
Bandage Compress (3 in.)	7.5 x 152 cm	3 x 60 in.	2	1
Bandage Compress (4 in.)	10 x 183 cm	4 x 72 in.	1	1
Burn Dressing	10 x 10 cm	4 x 4 in	1	1-2
* Burn Treatment	0.9	1/32 fl. oz.	6	1
CPR Barrier			1	1
Cold Pack	10 x 12.5 cm	4 x 5 in	1	1-2
Eye Covering, with means of attachment	19 cm^2	2.9 in^2	2	1
Eye Wash	30 ml	1 fl. oz total	1	2
Eye Wash & Covering, with means of attachment	30 ml total 19 cm^2	1 fl oz. Total 2.9 in^2	1 2	2
Gloves, latex free	XL	XL	1 pair	1
Gloves, latex free	L	L	1 pair	1
Roller Bandage (4 in.)	10 x 550 cm	4 in. x 6 yd.	1	1
Roller Bandage (2 in.)	5 x 550 cm	2 in. x 6 yd.	2	1
* Sterile pad	7.5 x 7.5 cm	3 x 3 in.	4	1
* Triangular Bandage	101 x 101 x 142 cm	40 x 40 x 56 in.	1	1

* Minimum mandatory contents for basic fill kit

EM 385-1-1
15 Sep 08

03.B.03 Automatic External Defibrillator (AED).

a. The placement of AEDs is optional (except for infirmaries, see 03.C.03.d) but highly recommended. The placement of AEDs on the worksite shall be preceded by an assessment of the time and distance to emergency medical services (EMS) and a justified need for such equipment.

b. An AED program shall include, at minimum:

(1) Training: First-aid attendants shall hold certification in first-aid and CPR from the American Red Cross (ARC), the American Heart Association (AHA), or from an organization whose training adheres to the standards of the International Liaison Committee on Resuscitation (as stated in writing), or from a LP. All classes shall contain a hands-on component. The certificate(s) shall state the date of issue and length of validity.

(2) Physician oversight and event assessment;

(3) Standard Operating Procedures (SOP) for EMS activation;

(4) Equipment Maintenance Program.

03.C FIRST-AID STATIONS AND INFIRMARIES

03.C.01 General.

a. For activities requiring a first-aid station or an infirmary, the type of facilities and equipment provided shall be determined after consideration is given to the proximity and quality of available medical services. The facilities and equipment shall also be in accordance with the recommendation of a licensed physician. Alternative facilities that provide the quantity and quality of services outlined in this section may be used if recommended by a LP.

EM 385-1-1
15 Sep 08

    b. Identification and directional markers shall be used to readily denote the location of all first-aid stations and infirmaries.

    c. Emergency lighting shall be provided for all first-aid stations and infirmaries.

03.C.02 A first-aid attendant shall be on duty in first-aid stations at all hours when work is in progress (except when on emergency calls).

03.C.03 Infirmaries.

    a. Infirmaries shall provide privacy, adequate lighting, climate control, adequate toilet facilities, hot and cold water, drainage, and electrical outlets. Walls and ceilings shall be finished with the equivalent of two coats of white paint; windows and doors shall be screened; floors shall be constructed with impervious materials.

    b. A properly equipped emergency vehicle, helicopter, or mobile first-aid unit shall be provided during work hours at sites requiring an infirmary. The emergency vehicle shall not be used for any other purpose, except in the case of a helicopter, which may be used for shift crew changes.

    c. A Registered Nurse (RN), a Licensed Physician's Assistant (LPA), a certified Emergency Medical Technician (EMT), or a Licensed Practical Nurse (LPN), if approved by a LP, shall be assigned on a full-time basis to each installation requiring an infirmary.

    d. Infirmaries shall be equipped with an AED.

03.D PERSONNEL REQUIREMENTS AND QUALIFICATIONS

03.D.01 All projects, activities, installations, or contracts on which 1,000 persons or more are employed (greatest total aggregate number of employees on a shift) shall have the full-time services of a LP. <u>A Nationally Registered Emergency Medical Technician</u>

EM 385-1-1
15 Sep 08

(NREMT) -Intermediate, NREMT - Paramedic, RN, LPN, or an LPA having direct communication with a LP may be used when a full-time physician is not available.

03.D.02 First-aid attendants shall hold certification in first-aid and CPR training from the ARC, the AHA, or from an organization whose training adheres to the standards of the International Liaison Committee on Resuscitation (as stated in writing) or from a LP. All classes shall contain a hands-on component. The certificate(s) shall state the date of issue and length of validity.

03.D.03 First-aid attendants, RNs, LPNs, LPAs and NREMT-Intermediates shall be under the direction of a LP.

03.D.04 Military personnel with equivalent qualifications may be used in lieu of the above personnel.

BLANK

EM 385-1-1
15 Sep 08

SECTION 4

TEMPORARY FACILITIES

04.A GENERAL

04.A.01 Plans for the layout of temporary construction buildings, facilities, fencing, and access routes and anchoring systems for temporary structures shall be submitted to and approved by the GDA. **> See 09.A.19 for temporary building spacing requirements; Section 11 for temporary power distribution approval requirements; and Section 24 for temporary ramp, trestle, scaffold, and platform approval requirements.**

04.A.02 The design and construction of temporary structures shall consider the following loadings (Reference American Society of Civil Engineers (ASCE) 7-98):

    a. Dead and live loads;

    b. Soil and hydrostatic pressures;

    c. Wind loads;

    d. Rain and snow loads;

    e. <u>Flood and ice loads;</u> and

    f. Seismic forces.

04.A.03 Trailers and other temporary structures used as field offices, as personnel housing, or for storage shall be anchored with rods and cables or by steel straps to ground anchors. The anchor system shall be designed to withstand winds and must meet applicable state or local standards for anchoring mobile trailer homes.

EM 385-1-1
15 Sep 08

04.A.04 Fencing and warning signs.

a. Temporary project fencing (or a substitute acceptable to the GDA and delineated in the APP) shall be provided on all projects located in areas of active use by members of the public, including those areas in close proximity to family housing areas and/or school facilities.

b. Fencing shall extend from grade to a minimum of 48 in (1.2 m) above grade and shall have a maximum mesh size of 2 in (50 mm). Fencing shall remain rigid/taut with a minimum of 200 lbs (.9 kN) of force exerted on it from any direction with less than 4 in (100 mm) of deflection.

c. Signs warning of the presence of construction hazards and requiring unauthorized persons to keep out of the construction area shall be posted on the fencing. At minimum, signs shall be posted every 150 ft (45.7 m). Fenced sides of projects that are less than 150 ft (45.7 m) shall, at minimum, have at least one warning sign. > *See also Section 8.*

d. Depending upon the nature and location of the project site, the GDA may determine that fencing is not required. This will be based on a risk analysis of public exposure and other project specific considerations, and will be included in the applicable AHA. In those locations where the GDA has determined fencing is not required, signs, warning of construction hazards, shall be conspicuously posted.

04.A.05 Temporary Work Camps (Floating plants excluded).

a. All sites used for temporary work camps shall be adequately drained. They shall not be subject to periodic flooding nor located within 200 ft (61 m) of swamps, pools, sink holes, or other surface collections of water unless adequate mosquito control methods have been implemented. The sites shall be graded, ditched, and rendered free from depressions in which water may become a nuisance.

EM 385-1-1
15 Sep 08

b. Sites shall be sized to prevent overcrowding of necessary structures.

C. The grounds and open areas surrounding the shelters shall be maintained free of rubbish, debris, waste paper, garbage, or other refuse.

d. Shelters will provide protection from the elements, and each room used for sleeping purposes shall contain at least 50 ft^2 (4.6 m^2) of floor space for each occupant and at least 7 ft-6 in (2.3 m) ceilings.

e. Beds, cots, or bunks, and suitable storage facilities (such as wall lockers for clothing and personal articles) shall be provided in every room used for sleeping purposes. Beds shall be spaced not closer than 36 in (91.4 cm) both laterally and end-to-end and shall be elevated at least 12 in (30.4 cm) from the floor. Double-decked bunk beds shall be spaced not fewer than 48 in (121.9 cm) both laterally and end-to-end with a minimum space of not fewer than 27 in (68.5 cm) between the upper and lower bunk. Triple deck bunks are prohibited.

f. Floors shall be constructed of wood, asphalt, or concrete. Wooden floors shall be of smooth and tight construction. Floors shall be kept in good repair.

g. <u>All wooden floors shall be elevated not less than 1-   ft (0.45 m) above the ground level at all points to prevent dampness, permit free circulation of air beneath, and for easier and safer maintenance.</u>

h. Living quarters shall be provided with windows that may be opened for purposes of ventilation.

i. All exterior openings shall be effectively screened with 16-mesh material and screen doors shall be equipped with self-closing devices.

EM 385-1-1
15 Sep 08

   j. Temporary sleeping quarters shall be heated, <u>cooled</u>, ventilated, lighted, and maintained in a clean and safe condition.

   k. Sleeping quarters must comply with applicable provisions of the National Fire Protection Agency (NFPA) 101 - <u>Life Safety Code</u>.

04.A.06 Unless otherwise indicated, throughout this manual, lumber dimensions are given in nominal sizes.

04.B ACCESS/HAUL ROADS

<u>04.B</u>.01 Access/haul roads shall be designed in accordance with current engineering criteria. Prior to construction, the Contractor shall provide the GDA with a copy of the <u>Access/Haul Road </u>plan for review and acceptance. Work on the haul road shall not commence until the GDA has accepted the plan. The plan shall address the following items:

   a. Equipment usage, traffic density, and hours of operation;

   b. Road layout and widths, horizontal and vertical curve data, and sight distances;

   c. Sign and signalperson requirements, road markings, and traffic control devices;

   d. Drainage controls;

   e. Points of contact between vehicles and the public, and safety controls at these points of contact;

   f. Maintenance requirements, including roadway hardness and smoothness and dust control; and

   g. Hazards adjacent to the road, such as bodies of water, steep embankments, etc.

EM 385-1-1
15 Sep 08

04.B.02 No employer shall move, or cause to be moved, any equipment or vehicle upon an access or haul road unless the roadway is constructed and maintained to safely accommodate the movement of the equipment or vehicle involved.

04.B.03 When road levels are above working levels, berms, barricades, or curbs shall be constructed to prevent vehicles overrunning the edge or end of embankment. Berms/curbs shall be constructed to one-half the diameter of the tires of the largest piece of equipment using the roadway.

04.B.04 Roadways shall have a crown and ditches for drainage. Water shall be intercepted before reaching a switch back or large fill and be led off.

04.B.05 Haul roads shall be constructed to widths suitable for safe operation of the equipment at the travel speeds proposed by the Contractor and accepted by the GDA.

04.B.06 All roads, including haul roads, shall be posted with maximum speed limits.

04.B.07 An adequate number of turn-outs shall be provided on single lane roads with two-way traffic. When turn-outs are not practical, the Contractor shall provide a traffic control system to prevent accidents.

04.B.08 Whenever possible, use a right-hand traffic pattern on two-way haul roads.

04.B.09 Curves.

   a. All curves shall have open sight lines and as great a radius as practical.

   b. Vehicle speed shall be limited on curves so that vehicles can be stopped within one-half the visible distance of the roadway.

c. The design of horizontal curves shall consider vehicle speed, roadway width and surfacing, and super elevation.

04.B.10 Grades.

a. When necessary, based on grade and machine and load weight, machines shall be equipped with retarders to assist in controlling downgrade descent.

b. Truck haul roads should be kept to less than a 10% grade. There should be no more than 400 ft (121.9 m) of grade exceeding 10%.

c. The maximum allowable grade shall not exceed 12%.

04.B.11 Lighting shall be provided as necessary.

04.B.12 Traffic control lights, barricades, road markings, signs, and signalpersons for the safe movement of traffic shall be provided in accordance with the DOT Federal Highway Administration's "*Manual on Uniform Traffic Control Devices*" and this Section.

04.B.13 Roadway hardness, smoothness, and dust control shall be used to maintain the safety of the roadway.

04.B.14 All roads shall be maintained in a safe condition and eliminate or control dust, ice, and similar hazards.

04.B.15 The deposition of mud and or other debris on public roads shall be minimized to the extent possible and in accordance with local requirements.

EM 385-1-1
15 Sep 08

SECTION 5

PERSONAL PROTECTIVE AND SAFETY EQUIPMENT

05.A GENERAL

05.A.01 Responsibilities.

a. The use of PPE is a control measure that is to be used only after a hazard evaluation identifies hazards associated with a particular job or activity, and it is determined that the hazards cannot be eliminated and/or controlled to an acceptable level through engineering design or administrative actions. Utilize process and engineering controls before PPE to protect employees.

b. Based on hazard evaluations conducted by supervisors, employers shall identity and select, and each affected employee shall use, PPE and safety equipment that will provide appropriate protection. *> See 29 CFR 1910.132*.

c. Employers shall communicate PPE and safety equipment decisions to each affected employee. Employees shall use all PPE and safety equipment that may be required to maintain their exposure within acceptable limits.

d. The employer will make all reasonable efforts to accommodate employees with religious beliefs that may conflict with determined PPE requirements. However, when reasonable efforts to accommodate employee's religious beliefs do not provide the necessary safe working environment (without PPE), then the employee must use the appropriate PPE or the employee will not be allowed to work in the area where the hazard requiring protection exists.

05.A.02 Employees shall be appropriately trained in the use and care of all required PPE and safety equipment.

EM 385-1-1
15 Sep 08

    a. Employees must be trained in and shall demonstrate an understanding of the following aspects of PPE prior to use: selection (for specific hazard); donning, doffing and adjusting; limitations and useful life; inspection and testing; and proper care including maintenance, storage and disposal.

    b. When the employer has reason to believe that any affected employee who has been trained does not have the understanding and skill required for the use of the PPE, the employer shall make certain that the employee receives the necessary re-training to acquire the appropriate skills.

    c. The employer shall verify through written certification that each affected employee has received and understood the required training. The written certification shall identify the name of each employee trained, the date(s) of the training, and the subjects taught.

05.A.03 A copy of the manufacturer's use, inspection, testing, and maintenance instructions shall be maintained with the PPE and safety equipment.

05.A.04 Personal protective and safety equipment shall be tested, inspected, and maintained in a serviceable and sanitary condition as recommended by the manufacturer.

    a. Defective or damaged equipment shall not be used. It shall be tagged as out of service and/or immediately removed from the work site to prevent use.

    b. Previously used PPE must be cleaned, disinfected, inspected, and repaired as necessary before issuing to another employee.

05.A.05 When employees provide their own safety equipment or PPE, the employer is responsible for assuring its adequacy in protecting against the hazard and its state of repair.

05.A.06 Minimum requirements.

EM 385-1-1
15 Sep 08

a. Employees shall wear clothing suitable for the weather and work conditions. For fieldwork (for example, construction sites, industrial operations and maintenance activities, emergency operations, regulatory inspections, etc.), at a minimum, this shall be:

(1) Short sleeve shirt;

(2) Long pants (excessively long or baggy pants are prohibited); and

(3) Leather or other protective work shoes or boots.

b. Protective equipment shall be of heat, fire, chemical, and/or electrical-resistive material when conditions require protection against such hazards.

05.A.07 Miners' lights and flashlights used around explosives, and in atmospheres likely to contain explosive vapors, dusts, or gases shall be approved by the Mine Safety and Health Administration (MSHA) or National Institute for Occupational Safety and Health (NIOSH) for use in such locations.

05.A.08 Persons involved in activities that subject the hands to injury (for example, cuts, abrasions, punctures, burns, chemical irritants, toxins, vibration, and forces that can restrict blood flow) shall select and use hand protection appropriate for the hazard in accordance with ANSI/International Safety Equipment Association (ISEA) 105.

05.A09 Protective leg chaps shall be worn by workers who operate chain saws. Protective leg chaps must meet the specifications in American Society for Testing and Materials (ASTM) Standard F1897.

05.B EYE AND FACE PROTECTION

05.B.01 Persons shall be provided with eye and face protection equipment, as outlined in Table 5-1, when machines or operations

EM 385-1-1
15 Sep 08

present potential eye or face injury from physical, chemical, or radiation agents.

a. Eye and face protection equipment shall meet the requirements of ANSI/ American Society of Safety Engineers (ASSE) Z87.1, and bear a legible and permanent "Z87" logo to indicate compliance with the standard.

b. Eye and face protection equipment shall be distinctly marked to facilitate identification of the manufacturer.

c. Employees shall use eye protection providing side protection.

05.B.02 When required by this regulation to wear eye protection, persons whose vision requires the use of corrective lenses in eyeglasses shall be protected by one of the following:

a. Prescription safety glasses providing optical correction and equivalent protection;

b. <u>Protective glasses with sideshields designed to fit over corrective lenses without disturbing the adjustment of the glasses;</u>

<u>c.</u> Goggles that can be worn over corrective lenses without disturbing the adjustment of the <u>glasses</u>, or

<u>d.</u> Goggles that incorporate corrective lenses mounted behind the protective lenses.

EM 385-1-1
15 Sep 08

TABLE 5-1

EYE AND FACE PROTECTOR SELECTION GUIDE

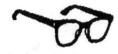

A. Spectacle, No sideshield

E. Spectacle, Non-Removable Lens

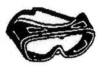

I. Cover Goggle, Direct Ventilation

B. Spectacle, Half Sideshield

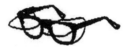

F. Spectacle, Lift Front

J. Cup Goggle, Direct Ventilation

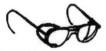

C. Spectacle, Full Sideshield

G. Cover Goggle, No Ventilation

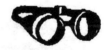

K. Cup Goggle, Indirect Ventilation

D. Spectacle, Detachable Sideshield

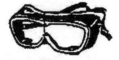

H. Cover Goggle, Indirect Ventilation

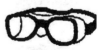

L. Spectacle, Headband Temple

EM 385-1-1
15 Sep 08

Table 5-1 (CONTINUED)

EYE AND FACE PROTECTOR SELECTION GUIDE

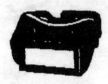

M. Cover Welding Goggle, Indirect Ventilation

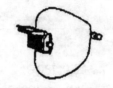

Q. Welding Helmet, Lift Front

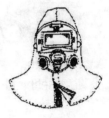

S. Respirator

N. Faceshield

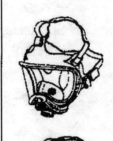

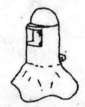

T1. Respirator

O. Welding Helmet, hand Hold

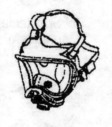

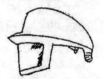

T2. Respirator

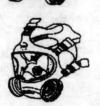

P. Welding Helmet, Stationary Window

R. Respirator

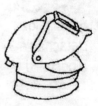

U. Respirator

EM 385-1-1
15 Sep 08

Table 5-1 (CONTINUED)

EYE AND FACE PROTECTOR SELECTION GUIDE

IMPACT: Chipping, grinding, machining, masonry work, riveting and sanding					
Assessment See Note (1)	**Protector Type**	**Protectors**	**Limitations**	**Not Recommended**
Flying fragments, objects, large chips, particles, sand, dirt, etc.	B, C, D, E, F, G, H, I, J, K, L, N	Spectacles, goggles, faceshields SEE NOTES (1)(3)(5)(6)(10) For severe exposures add N	Protective devices do not provided unlimited protection. SEE NOTE (7)	Protectors that do not provide protection from side exposure SEE NOTE (10) Filter or tinted lenses that restrict light transmittance, unless it is determined that a glare hazard exists. Refer to OPTICAL RADIATION.
HEAT: Furnace operations, pouring, casting, hot dipping, gas cutting, and welding				
Assessment See Note (1)	**Protector Type**	**Protectors**	**Limitations**	**Not Recommended**
Hot sparks	B, C, D, E, F, G, H, I, J, K, L, N	Faceshields, goggles, spectacles For severe exposure add N SEE NOTE (2)(3)	Spectacles, cup and cover type goggles do not provide unlimited facial protection SEE NOTE (2)	Protectors that do not provide protection from side exposure
Splash from molten metals	N	Faceshields worn over goggles H, K SEE NOTE (2)(3)		
High temperature exposure	N	Screen faceshields, reflective faceshields	SEE NOTE (3)	

Table 5-1 (CONTINUED)

EYE AND FACE PROTECTOR SELECTION GUIDE

CHEMICAL: Acid and chemical handling, degreasing, plating				
Assessment See Note (1)	**Protector Type**	**Protectors**	**Limitations**	**Not Recommended**
Splash	G, H, K N	For severe exposure add N	Ventilation should be adequate but protected from splash entry	Spectacles, welding helmets, hand shields
Irritating mists	G	Special purpose goggles	SEE NOTE (3)	

DUST: Woodworking, buffing, general industry conditions				
Assessment See Note (1)	**Protector Type**	**Protectors**	**Limitations**	**Not Recommended**
Nuisance dust	G, H, K	Goggles, eyecup and cover types	Atmospheric conditions and the restricted ventilation of the protector can cause the lenses to fog. Frequent cleaning may be required.	

OPTICAL RADIATION: Welding: electric arc				
Assessment See Note (1)	**Protector Type**	**Protectors**	**Limitations**	**Not Recommended**
O, P, Q	Typical filter lens shade		Protection from optical radiation is directly related to filter lens density. SEE NOTE (4). Select the darkest shade that allows adequate task performance.	Protectors that do not provide protection from optical radiation.

EM 385-1-1
15 Sep 08

NOTES:
(1) Care should be take to recognize the possibility of multiple and simultaneous exposure to a variety of hazards. Adequate protection against the highest level of each of the hazards must be provided.
(2) Operations involving heat may also involve optical radiation. Protection from both hazards shall be provided.
(3) Faceshields shall only be worn over primary eye protection.
(4) Filter lenses shall meet the requirements for shade designations in Table 5-2.
(5) Persons whose vision requires the use of prescription (Rx) lenses shall wear either protective devices fitted with prescription (Rx) lenses <u>with sideshields</u> or protective devices designed to be worn over regular prescription (Rx) eyewear.
(6) Wearers of contact lenses shall also be required to wear appropriate covering eye and face protection devices in a hazardous environment. It should be recognized that dusty and/or chemical environments may represent an additional hazard to contact lens wearers.
(7) Caution should be exercised in the use of metal frame protective devices in electrical hazard areas.
(8) Refer to ANSI/ASSE Z87-1, Section 6.5, Special Purpose Lenses.
(9) Welding helmets or hand shields shall be used only over primary eye protection.
(10) Non-sideshield spectacles are available for frontal protection only.

EM 385-1-1
15 Sep 08

05.B.03 Personnel who are considered blind in one eye and are working in other than administrative functions shall wear safety glasses with sideshields at all times.

05.B.04 Operations that require the use of, or exposure to, hot or molten substances (for example, babbitting, soldering, pouring or casting of hot metals, handling of hot tar, oils, liquids, and molten substances) shall require eye protection, such as goggles with safety lenses and screens for side protection, or face masks, shields, and helmets giving equal protection. Lens mountings shall be able to retain in position all parts of a cracked lens.

05.B.05 Operations that require handling of harmful materials (for example, acids, caustics, hot liquids, or creosoted materials) and operations where protection from gases, fumes, and liquids is necessary shall require the wearing of goggles with cups of soft pliable rubber and suitable faceshields, masks, or hoods that cover the head and neck, and other protective clothing appropriate to the hazards involved.

05.B.06 Operations where protection from radiant energy with moderate reduction of visible light is necessary, including welding, cutting, brazing, and soldering, shall require eye and face protection suitable to the type of work, providing protection from all angles of direct exposure, and with lenses of the appropriate shade. **> See Table 5-2.**

05.B.07 Glare-resistant glasses that comply with ANSI Z80.3 with an ultraviolet A-region (UVA) and ultraviolet B-region (UVB) 99% filtration shall be worn when conditions require protection against glare. <u>When conditions so warrant, polarized lenses shall also be considered.</u>

05.B.08 Tinted or automatically darkening lenses should not be worn when work tasks require the employee to pass often from brightly to dimly lighted areas.

EM 385-1-1
15 Sep 08

TABLE 5-2

REQUIRED SHADES FOR FILTER LENSES AND GLASSES IN WELDING, CUTTING, BRAZING, AND SOLDERING

OPERATION	SHADE NUMBER
Soldering	2
Torch Brazing	3 or 4
Cutting (light) up to 1 in (2.5 cm)	3 or 4
Cutting (medium) 1 to 6 in (2.5 to 15.2 cm)	4 or 5
Cutting (heavy) 6 in (15.2 cm) or more	5 or 6
Gas welding (light) up to 1/8 in (0.3 cm)	4 or 5
Gas welding (medium) 1/8 to 1/2 in (0.3 to 1.2 cm)	5 or 6
Gas welding (heavy) 1/2 in (1.2 cm) or more	6 or 8
Atomic hydrogen welding	10 – 14
Inert-gas metal-arc welding (nonferrous) - 1/16 to 5/32 in (0.1 to 0.4 cm) electrodes	11
Inert-gas metal-arc welding (ferrous) - 1/16 to 5/32 in (0.1 to 0.4 cm) electrodes	12
Shielded metal-arc welding - 1/16 to 5/32 in (0.1 to 0.4 cm) electrodes	10
Shielded metal-arc welding - 3/16 to 1/4 in (0.4 to 0.6 cm) electrodes	12
Shielded metal-arc welding - 5/16 to 3/8 in (0.7 to 0.9 cm) electrodes	14
Carbon arc welding	14

EM 385-1-1
15 Sep 08

05.C HEARING PROTECTION AND NOISE CONTROL

05.C.01 Sound-pressure level limits.

<u>a.</u> Non-DOD personnel shall be provided, as a minimum, protection against the effects of hazardous noise exposure whenever the sound-pressure level exceeds the limits and/or exposure times specified in Table 5-3.

<u>b.</u> DOD personnel shall be provided protection against the effects of hazardous noise exposure whenever sound-pressure levels exceed 85 decibels A-weighed [dB(A)] steady-state expressed as a time-weighted average (TWA) as specified in Table 5-4 or 140 dB(A) impulse.

05.C.02 Practical engineering or administrative controls shall be considered and used when personnel are subjected to sound-pressure levels exceeding the limits specified in Tables 5-3 <u>and 5-4.</u> When such controls fail to reduce sound-pressure levels to within the specified limit, PPE shall be selected, evaluated, provided, and used in accordance with the hearing conservation program.

05.C.<u>03</u> Hearing protection provided must be capable of reducing worker noise exposure below an 8-hour TWA of 85 dB(A). When hearing protection devices do not provide sufficient attenuation to reduce the worker noise exposure level below 85 dB(A), administrative control of exposure will be necessary.

TABLE 5-3

PERMISSIBLE NON-DoD NOISE EXPOSURES

(Contractor)

Duration/day (hours)	Sound-pressure level dB(A) slow response
8	90
6	92
4	95
3	97
2	100
1-1/2	102
1	105
	110
	115

When the daily noise exposure is composed of two or more periods of noise exposure of different levels, the combined effects should be considered rather than the individual effect of each. Exposure to different levels for various periods of time shall be computed according to the following formula:

$$C_n = T_1/L_1 + T_2/L_2 + ... + T_3/L_3$$

Where:

C = combined noise exposure factor,
T = the total time of exposure at a specified sound-pressure level (in hours), and
L = the total time of exposure permitted at that level (in hours), from Table 5-3.
If $C_n >= 1$, hearing protection is required.

EM 385-1-1
15 Sep 08

05.C.04 Whenever sound-pressure levels equal or exceed 85 dB(A) (measured as an 8-hour TWA), a continuing, effective hearing conservation program shall be administered in accordance with 29 CFR 1910.95. For DOD personnel the hearing conservation program shall conform to DODI 6055.12 and Department of the Army Pamphlet (DA Pam) 40-501.

05.C.05 When sound-pressure levels exceed 115 dB(A) steady-state, personal ear protection equivalent to the combination of earplugs and earmuffs shall be required.

05.C.06 Sound-pressure level measurements shall be made by qualified personnel using calibrated instruments.

05.C.07 Ear insert devices, to include disposable, preformed, or custom molded earplugs, shall be fitted to the exposed individual by an individual trained in such fitting and able to recognize the difference between a good and a poor fit. Plain cotton is not an acceptable protective device.

05.C.08 Noise hazard areas (areas in which sound-pressure levels exceed the limits specified in 05.C.01) shall be marked with caution signs indicating both the presence of hazardous noise levels and the requirement for hearing protection.

EM 385-1-1
15 Sep 08

Table 5-4
Permissible DoD Noise Exposures

(Government)

Duration/day (hours)	Sound-pressure level dB(A) slow response
No limit	80
9	84
8	85
4	88
3	90
1	95
	100
	105

05.D HEAD PROTECTION

05.D.01 All persons working in or visiting hard hat areas shall be provided with and required to wear Type I or Type II, Class G (General - low voltage electrical protection) or Class E (Electrical – high voltage electrical protection) headgear. For emergency response operations and other activities with greater need for side impact protection, Type II head protection is recommended. **> See Appendix B.**

 a. Hard hat areas <u>or activities</u> are those areas with potential hazard of head injury; in general, all construction areas are considered hard hat areas. <u>However, areas may be considered non-hard hat areas, or activities may be considered non-hard hat activities, if identified and properly documented in the associated AHA.</u> The identification and analysis of head hazards will be documented in an AHA, APP, or project safety and health plan, as appropriate.

EM 385-1-1
15 Sep 08

   b. Points of entry to a hard hat area shall have a sign warning of the requirement to wear hard hats.

05.D.02 All protective headgear shall meet the requirements of ANSI Z89.1.

   a. No modification to the shell or suspension is allowed except when such changes are approved by the manufacturer.

   b. Hard hats shall be worn with the bill facing forward <u>unless the GDA has determined exceptions for certain trades in order to accommodate appropriate mission accomplishments. Headgear must be designed to accommodate these needs.</u>

   c. Protective headgear worn near electric lines and equipment shall be Class E.

   d. No ball caps, knit caps, or other headdress shall be worn under the hard hat that could interfere with the fit or stability of the hard hat.

05.D.03 Protective headgear and components shall be visually inspected on a daily basis for signs of damage (dents, cracks, etc.) that might reduce the degree of safety integrity originally provided. Headgear will be periodically inspected for ultraviolet degradation as evidenced by cracking or flaking of the helmet.

05.D.04 Drilling holes or in any way changing the integrity of the hard hat is prohibited. <u>Alterations that will reduce the dielectric or impact strength will not be made.</u>

05.D.05 Protective headgear worn by USACE employees shall (in addition to complying with the preceding specifications) be:

   a. White in color and marked with a 1 in. (2.5 cm) band of red reflective material placed along the base of the crown with a 5 in. (12.7 cm) break in front. A red Corps of Engineers castle insignia will be centered at the front of the hat with the base of the insignia approximately   in (1.9 cm) above the base of the

EM 385-1-1
15 Sep 08

crown. Personnel may place their name above the insignia and their organization title below the insignia: the rank of military personnel should precede their name. An American Flag insignia may be worn on the back of the hard hat.

b. Requests for variations in color and marking to accommodate occupational specialties shall be submitted for consideration to HQUSACE Safety and Health Office.

c. Chin straps will be worn when wearers are subject to high wind conditions and/or working on elevated structures.

05.E PROTECTIVE FOOTWEAR.

05.E.01 Protective footwear that addresses the hazard(s) identified in the PHA/AHA shall be provided and worn.

05.E.02 All protective footwear shall meet ASTM F2412 and F2413 standards.

05.E.03 Add-on type devices, such as strap-on foot, toe or metatarsal guards, shall not be used as a substitute for protective footwear and must be demonstrated by the employer to be equally effective via independent testing data for these devices).

05.E.04 For activities in which USACE or contractor personnel or official visitors are potentially exposed to foot hazards, the applicable PHA/AHA, APP, or project safety and health plan shall include an analysis of, and prescribe specific protective measures to be taken for, reducing foot hazards.

05.E.05 Personnel shall, as a minimum, wear safety-toed boots meeting ASTM Standards F2412 and F2413 while working on construction sites unless it can be demonstrated by a PHA/AHA to the GDAs satisfaction that a different type of foot protection is required.

05.E.06 Footwear providing protection against impact and compressive forces, conduction hazards, electrical hazards,

EM 385-1-1
15 Sep 08

and sole puncture shall comply with the applicable requirements of ASTM F 2412-05 and F 2413-05. Footwear providing protection against impact and compression hazards shall be rated as I/75 and C/75.

a. Unexploded ordnance (UXO) personnel whose job tasks required protective footwear but require no metal parts in or on their footwear shall wear Conductive footwear (Cd) with protective toe cap/composite toe footwear.

b. Personnel participating in wild land fire management activities shall wear leather lace-up boots with slip-resistant soles, such as a hard rubber lug-type or tractor tread, a top height of 8 in (20.3 cm) or more with composite toes. Soles shall not be made of composition rubber or plastic, which have low melting points.

05.F HIGH-VISIBILITY APPAREL

05.F.01 High-visibility apparel meeting, at minimum, ANSI/ISEA 07-2004 Performance Class 2 requirements, shall be worn by workers (such as, but not limited to, signal persons, spotters, survey crews and inspectors) whenever:

a. Workers are exposed to vehicular or equipment traffic at speeds up to 45 mph (72.4 kph);

b. There is limited visibility of workers exposed to mobile/heavy equipment operations, vehicles, load handling, or other hazardous activities;

c. Reduced visibility conditions exist due to weather conditions, illumination, or visually complex backgrounds where ambient visibility is at least 50 ft (15.2 m); OR

d. Workers are involved in activities in close proximity to vehicular traffic with no protective barriers.

EM 385-1-1
15 Sep 08

05.F.02 If any or all of the following conditions exist, a determination shall be made by the SSHO, based on a risk assessment, as to whether Performance Class 3 high-visibility apparel is needed for higher visibility of workers. If so, they shall be worn by workers.

   a. Workers are exposed to vehicular or equipment traffic in excess of 45 mph (72.4 kph);

   b. Reduced visibility conditions exist due to weather conditions, illumination, or visually complex backgrounds where ambient visibility is less than 50 ft (15.2 m); OR

   c. Workers are performing tasks which divert attention from approaching vehicular traffic, traveling in excess of 45 mph (72.4 kph), as posted.

05.F.03 The apparel background material color shall be either fluorescent yellow-green, fluorescent orange-red, or fluorescent red (see ANSI/ISEA 107-2004). When choosing color, optimization of color conspicuity between the wearer and work environment shall be considered.

05.G RESPIRATORY PROTECTION

05.G.01 General. The use of respirators is required when occupational exposure levels exceed OSHA Permissible Exposure Limits (PELs) or American Conference of Governmental Industrial Hygienists (ACGIH) Threshold Limit Values (TLVs), and engineering or administrative exposure controls are not feasible to implement.

05.G.02 The voluntary use of dust masks (filtering face piece respirators) is permissible in atmospheres that are not hazardous. Prior to use of the voluntary respirators (including filtering face pieces), they must be evaluated and approved by the respiratory program administrator to ensure that the respirator use will in itself not create a hazard. If filtering face piece respirators are used, the

EM 385-1-1
15 Sep 08

employer shall provide the respirator users with the information contained in Appendix D of OSHA Standard 29 CFR 1910.134.

05.G.03 Written respiratory protection program. A written respiratory protection program shall be developed and implemented when respirators are used.

    a. All employees using respirators, with the exception of employees voluntarily using only filtering face pieces (NIOSH-approved dust masks), shall be included in the respiratory protection program.

    b. A respiratory protection program administrator with the technical qualifications (training and experience) and administrative authority to develop, implement and update (as necessary) the respiratory protection program shall be identified and so designated in the program.

    (1) The program administrator shall ensure that all respirator users (voluntary users included) comply with the requirements of the program.

    (2) Program Administrator Qualifications. The program administrator shall have the documented knowledge and experience to understand OSHA's respiratory protection standard (29 CFR 1910.134), evaluate respiratory hazards at the facility/project, select appropriate respirators based on facility/project hazards or potential hazard, and train employees on the use of selected respirators.

    c. Respiratory protection programs shall address each of the following topics:

    (1) Methods used to identify and evaluate workplace respiratory hazards;

    (2) Procedures for selecting respirators for use in the workplace;

EM 385-1-1
15 Sep 08

(3) Medical evaluations of employees required to use respirators;

(4) Fit testing procedures for tight-fitting respirators;

(5) Procedures for proper use of respirators in routine and reasonably foreseeable emergency situations;

(6) Procedures and schedules for cleaning, disinfecting, storing, inspecting, repairing, discarding, and otherwise maintaining respirators;

(7) Procedures to ensure adequate air quality, quantity, and flow of breathing air for atmosphere-supplying respirators;

(8) Training of employees in the respiratory hazards to which they are potentially exposed during routine and emergency situations;

(9) Training of employees in the proper use of respirators, including putting on and removing them, any limitations on their use, and their maintenance; and

(10) Procedures for regularly evaluating the effectiveness of the program.

(11) Project/facility specific voluntary use guidelines and a requirement for voluntary users to learn and understand the contents of 29 CFR 1910.134 Appendix D, Information for Employees Using Respirators When Not Required Under the Standard.

05.G.04 Medical evaluation. All employees, with the exception of employees voluntarily using filtering face pieces, shall be medically evaluated to ensure they are fit enough to wear the selected respirators. Evaluation options for respirator use are as follows:

a. Physical Examination. A physical examination for the purpose of clearing an employee to wear a selected respirator, supervised by a Board-Certified Occupational Medicine Physician. Medical clearances to wear respirators shall include the following:

(1) Telephone, e-mail, and physical address of the medical facility/provider;

(2) Printed name of the licensed, certified health care provider along with his/her signature;

(3) The statement of clearances or respiratory limitations only (no personal medical information shall be included. Employee identification shall not include the full social security number);

(4) Date of examination and date that clearance expires.

b. Respirator Medical Evaluation Service. An on-line, mail-in or in-person evaluation service for the purpose of clearing an employee to wear selected respirators may be used provided it is supervised by a Board-Certified Occupational Medicine Physician and based upon Appendix C to 29 CFR 1910.134, OSHA Respirator Medical Evaluation Questionnaire. Medical clearances to wear respirators shall include the information in (1) – (4) above.

c. Additional Medical Evaluations shall be provided when:

(1) An employee reports medical signs or symptoms that are related to the ability to use a respirator;

(2) A supervisor or the respirator program administrator informs the employer that an employee needs to be reevaluated;

(3) Information from the respiratory protection program, including observations made during fit testing and program evaluation, indicates a need for employee reevaluation;

(4) A change occurs in workplace conditions (e.g., physical work effort, protective clothing, temperature) that may result in a

EM 385-1-1
15 Sep 08

substantial increase in the physiological burden placed on an employee, OR

(5) It has been two years since the last medical evaluation.

05.G.05 Fit testing. Employees wearing respirators with tight-fitting face pieces [Supplied Air Respirators (SARs) and Self-Contained Breathing Apparatus (SCBAs) included] shall be fit tested to ensure that selected respirators achieve a proper face to face piece seal. Fit testing shall be performed before initial use of the selected respirator, whenever respirator size, make or model is changed, and at least annually thereafter. Fit testing requirements shall comply with respiratory protection program requirements.

05.G.06 Training and information. The program administrator or his designee shall provide respirator user training annually (or when requirements change significantly due to process changes or changes in site specific operations) to personnel using respirators at the facility or project. Annual training shall ensure that each employee using a respirator can demonstrate knowledge of the following topics:

a. Why the respirator is necessary and how improper fit, usage, or maintenance can compromise the protective effect of the respirator;

b. Limitations and capabilities of the respirator;

c. How to use the respirator effectively in emergency situations, including situations in which the respirator malfunctions;

d. How to Inspect, put on and remove, use, and check the seals of the respirator;

e. Procedures for maintenance and storage of the respirator;

f. How to recognize medical signs and symptoms that may limit or prevent the effective use of respirators; and

EM 385-1-1
15 Sep 08

g. The general requirements of the OSHA respirator standard at 29 CFR 1910.134.

05.G.07 Recordkeeping. Establish and retain written information regarding medical evaluations, fit testing, and the respirator program. The following shall be made available upon request:

a. Records of medical evaluations must be retained and made available, as needed;

b. Fit test records must be maintained for respirator users until the next fit test is administered. Establish a record of the Qualitative Fit Test (QLFT) and Quantitative Fit Test (QNFT) administered to an employee including:

(1) The name or identification of the employee tested;

(2) Type of fit test performed and name of the test administrator;

(3) Specific make, model, style, and size of respirator tested;

(4) Date of test; and

(5) The pass/fail results for QLFTs or the fit factor and strip chart recording or other recording of the test results for QNFTs.

c. Retain a written copy of the current respirator program.

05.H FULL BODY HARNESSES, LANYARDS, AND LIFELINES.

05.H.01 Full body harnesses, lanyards and lifelines are considered components of personal fall protection systems. Requirements for these components can be found in Section 21.H.05.

05.H.02 Lineman's equipment (electrically rated harnesses). The full body harness used around high voltage equipment or structures shall be an industry designed "Linemen's FP Harness" that will resist arc flashing. See 21.H.05.d.(2).

EM 385-1-1
15 Sep 08

05.I ELECTRICAL PROTECTIVE EQUIPMENT

05.I.01 Persons working on electrical distribution systems shall be provided with the appropriate electrical protective equipment. This equipment shall be inspected, tested, and maintained in safe conditions in accordance with Table 5-5.

05.I.02 Employees shall use rubber gloves, sleeves, blankets, covers, and line hoses as required by special conditions for work on energized facilities. Rubber goods provided to protect employees who work on energized facilities must meet ASTM F18 standards. Electrical workers' rubber insulating protective equipment shall be visually inspected for damage and defects prior to each use.

05.I 03 Rubber protective equipment must be subjected to periodic electrical tests. Rubber insulating gloves shall be inspected before first issue and every 6 months thereafter; rubber insulating blankets and sleeves shall be inspected before their first issue and every 12 months thereafter. Rubber insulating covers shall be inspected upon indication that insulating value is suspect (per 1910.137).

TABLE 5-5

STANDARDS FOR ELECTRICAL PROTECTIVE EQUIPMENT

SUBJECT	NUMBER AND TITLE
Head Protection	ISEA/ANSI Z89.1, *Requirements for Protective Headwear for Industrial Workers*
Eye and face protection	ANSI Z87.1, *Practice for Occupational and Educational Eye and Face Protection*
Gloves	ASTM D120-02a, *Standard Specification for Rubber Insulating Gloves*
Sleeves	ASTM D1051, *Standard Specification for Rubber Insulating Sleeves*
Gloves and sleeves	ASTM F496, *Standard Specification for In-Service Care of Insulating Gloves and Sleeves*
Leather protectors	ASTM F696, *Standard Specification for Leather Protectors for Rubber Insulating Gloves and Mittens*
Footwear	ASTM F1117, *Standard Specification for Dielectric Overshoe Footwear*
	ASTM 2412, *Standard Test Methods for Foot Protection* ASTM 2413, *Standard Specification for Performance Requirements for Foot Protection*
Visual inspection	ASTM F1236, *Standard Guide for Visual Inspection of Electrical Protective Rubber Products*
Apparel	ASTM F1506, *Standard Performance Specification for Flame Resistant Textile Materials for Wearing Apparel for Use by Electrical Workers When Exposed to Momentary Electric Arc and Related Thermal Hazards*

EM 385-1-1
15 Sep 08

05.I.04 Electric <u>arc</u> flash protection shall be provided for any person who enters the flash protection zone. **> See 11.B**. They must wear flame-resistant clothing and PPE, based on the incident exposure associated with the specific task. Refer to NFPA 70E for specific Hazard Risk Classifications and clothing/equipment requirements. **> Synthetic clothing such as acetate, nylon, polyester, rayon, either alone or in blends with cotton, may not be worn while in the flash protection zone.**

    a. Employees must wear protective eye equipment whenever there is a danger from electric arcs, flashes, flying objects, or electrical explosion.

    b. Employees must wear flame-resistant clothing whenever they may be exposed to an <u>arc</u> flash.

    <u>(1)</u> If used, flash suits and their closure design must permit easy and rapid removal.

    <u>(2)</u> The entire flash suit, including the window, must have energy-absorbing characteristics suitable for arc flash exposure.

    (3) Use clothing and equipment to maximize worker protection.

    <u>(4)</u> Clothing and equipment required by the degree of electrical hazard exposure can be worn alone or be integrated with normal apparel.

    <u>(5)</u> Protective clothing and equipment must cover associated parts of the body and all normal apparel that is not flame-resistant, while allowing movement and visibility.
> Synthetic materials that can melt next to skin shall not be worn.

    c. Employees must wear rubber-insulating gloves where there is a danger of hand or arm injury from electric shock or arc flash burns due to contact with energized parts. Gloves made from layers of flame-resistant material provide the highest level of

EM 385-1-1
15 Sep 08

protection. Leather glove protectors should be worn over voltage-rated rubber gloves.

d. Dielectric overshoes are required where electrically insulated footwear is used for protection against step and touch potential.

05.I.05 An air test shall be performed on electrical workers' rubber insulating gloves before each use.

05.I.06 Protective equipment of material other than rubber shall provide equal or better electrical and mechanical protection.

05.I.07 Live-Line (Hot-Line) Tools must be manufactured to meet ASTM F18 series as appropriate to the device and material. The insulating tool portion shall be made of fiberglass-reinforced plastic (FRP).

05.I.08 Only live-line tool poles having a manufacturer's certification to withstand at least the following test shall be used: 100 (kilo Volts) kV ac per ft (305 mm) of length for 5 minutes or 75 kV ac per ft (305 mm) for FRP tools. Records shall be maintained for all live-line tools to demonstrate satisfactory accomplishment of laboratory and shop test.

05.I.09 Wooden tools are not authorized for use. **> All wooden tools shall be replaced with FRP tools within 2 years of date of this manual.**

05.I.10 When using live-line tools, workers shall use voltage rated gloves and not place their hands closer than necessary to energized conductors or to the metal parts of the tool.

05.I.11 Only tools and equipment intended for live-line bare hand work should be used on transmission lines. The tools shall be kept dry and clean and shall be visually inspected before use each day.

05.I.12 See Section 05.H for requirements on lineman's personal fall protection equipment.

05.J PERSONAL FLOTATION DEVICES

05.J.01 Inherently buoyant Type III, Type V work vests, or better USCG-approved personal flotation devices (PFDs) shall be provided and properly worn (zipped, tied, latched, etc., in closed fashion) by all persons in the following circumstances: *> See 05.J.02; See Figure 5-1.*

   a. On floating pipelines, pontoons, rafts, or stages;

   b. On structures or equipment extending over or next to water except where guardrails, personal fall protection system, or safety nets are provided for employees;

   c. Working alone at night where there are drowning hazards, regardless of other safeguards provided;

   d. In skiffs, small boats, or launches, unless in an enclosed cabin or cockpit; or

   e. Whenever there is a drowning hazard.

05.J.02 Automatic-Inflatable PFDs Type V or better, USCG-approved for Commercial Use, may be worn by workers in lieu of inherently buoyant PFDs (See conditions 05.J.01.a-e above), provided the following criteria are met:

   a. PFDs are worn only by workers over 16 years of age and those who weigh 90 lb (40.8 kg) or more;

   b. An AHA must be performed for this activity;

   c. PFDs must be inspected, maintained, stowed and used only in accordance with the manufacturer's instructions (currently not intended to be used in areas of heavy construction or maintenance or where hot work (welding, brazing, cutting, soldering, etc.) is to be performed;

EM 385-1-1
15 Sep 08

    d. PFDs shall provide a 30-pound minimum buoyancy post-deployment;

    e. USACE employees shall comply with USACE's Auto-Inflatable Personal Flotation Device, Standards of Use Procedures, dated 1 July 2007.

    f. The USCG-approval for auto-inflatable PFD's is contingent upon the PFD being worn, not stowed. All auto-inflatable PFDs must be worn at all times drowning hazard exists.

05.J.03 All wearable PFDs shall be of a highly visible orange/reddish color. Each PFD shall have at least 31 in^2 (200 cm^2) of retroreflective material attached to its front side and at least 31 in^2 (200 cm^2) on its back side, per USCG requirements (46 CFR Part 25.25-15).

05.J.04 Each PFD shall be equipped with a USCG-approved automatically activated light. Lights are not required for PFDs on projects performed exclusively during daylight hours.

05.J.05 Before and after each use, the PFD shall be inspected for defects that would alter its strength or buoyancy.

05.J.06 Throwable devices (Type IV PFD).

    a. On USCG-inspected vessels, ring buoys are required to have automatic floating electric water lights (46 CFR 160).

    b. On all other floating plant and shore installations, lights on life rings are required only in locations where adequate general lighting (e.g., floodlights, light stanchions) is not provided. For these plants and installations, at least one life ring, and every third one thereafter, shall have an automatic floating electric water light attached.

    c. All PFDs shall be equipped with retroreflective tape in accordance with USCG requirements.

EM 385-1-1
15 Sep 08

FIGURE 5-1

PERSONAL FLOTATION DEVICES

Off-Shore Life Jacket (Type I PFD)
Best for open, rough or remote water, where rescue may be slow coming.

Near-Shore Buoyant Vest (Type II PFD)
Good for calm, inland water, or where there is a good chance of fast rescue

Flotation Aid (Type III PFD)
Good for calm, inland water, or where there is a good chance of fast rescue
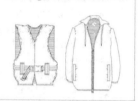

Throwable Device (Type IV PFD)
For calm, inland water with heavy boat traffic, where help is always nearby
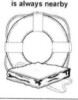

Special Use Devices (Type V PFD)
Only for special use or conditions
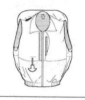

Inflatable Device (Type V Hybrid)
Only for special use or conditions
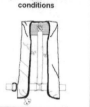

d. Life rings (rope attachment not required) and ring buoys (rope attachment required) shall be USCG-approved; shall have at least 70 ft (21.3 m) of 3/8 in (0.9 cm) of attached solid braid polypropylene, or equivalent. Throw bags may be used in addition to life rings or ring buoys. Life rings or ring buoys shall be readily available and shall be provided at the following places:

(1) At least one <u>not less than 20 in (51 cm) on each safety skiff up to 26 ft (7.9 m) in length (46 CFR 117.70).</u>;

EM 385-1-1
15 Sep 08

<u>(2)</u> At least one (1) 24 in (61 cm) in diameter on all motor boats longer than 26 ft (7.9 m) in length up to 65 ft (19.8 m) in length and for motor boats 65 ft (19.8 m) in length or longer, a minimum 3 life buoys of not less than 24 in (61 cm) and one additional for each increase in length of 100 ft (30.4 m) or fraction thereof; and

(3) At least one (1) at intervals of not more than 200 ft (60.9 m) on pipelines, walkways, wharves, piers, bulkheads, lock walls, scaffolds, platforms, and similar structures extending over or immediately next to water, unless the fall distance to the water is more than 45 ft (13.7 m), in which case a life ring shall be used. (The length of line for life rings at these locations shall be evaluated, but the length may not be less than 70 ft (21.3 m).)

05.J.07 At navigation locks, an analysis of the benefits versus the hazards of using floating safety blocks (blocks that may be quickly pushed into the water to protect individuals who have fallen in the water from being crushed by vessels) shall be made.

a. This analysis shall be documented as an AHA.

b. If the use of blocks is found acceptable, consideration shall be given to the size and placement of the blocks, the appropriate means of securing and signing the blocks, etc. When the use of blocks is found unacceptable, alternative safety measures shall be developed.

05.K LIFESAVING AND SAFETY SKIFFS

05.K.01 At least one skiff shall be immediately available at locations where employees work over or immediately next to water. Skiffs shall be kept afloat or ready for instant launching.

05.K.02 Personnel trained in launching and operating the skiff shall be readily available during working hours. Lifesaving personnel shall perform a lifesaving drill, including the launching and recovery of the skiff, before the initiation of work at the site and periodically

EM 385-1-1
15 Sep 08

thereafter as specified by the GDA (but at least monthly or whenever new personnel are involved).

05.K.03 Skiffs shall be kept afloat or ready for instant launching.

05.K.04 Required equipment must be onboard and meet or exceed USCG requirements and the requirements of Section 19 of this manual. Skiffs shall be equipped as follows:

    a. Four (4) oars (two (2) if the skiff is motor powered);

    b. Oarlocks attached to gunwales or the oars;

    c. One (1) ball-pointed boat hook;

    d. One (1) ring buoy with 70 ft (21.3 m) of 3/8 in (0.9 cm) solid braid polypropylene, or equivalent, line attached; and

    e. PFDs in number equaling the skiff rating for the maximum number of personnel allowed on board.

    f. **Fire Extinguisher.**

05.K.05 In locations where waters are rough or swift, or where manually operated boats are not practical, a power boat suitable for the waters shall be provided and equipped for lifesaving.

05.K.06 Skiffs and power boats shall have buoyant material capable of floating the boat, its equipment, and the crew.

05.K.07 On vessels (such as skiffs) without permanently mounted navigation lights, portable battery-operated navigation lights will be available and used for night operations.

BLANK

EM 385-1-1
15 Sep 08

SECTION 6

HAZARDOUS OR TOXIC AGENTS AND ENVIRONMENTS

06.A GENERAL

06.A.01 Exposure standards.

a. Exposure, through inhalation, ingestion, skin absorption, or physical contact, to any chemical, biological, or physical agent in excess of the acceptable limits specified in the most recently published ACGIH guideline, "*Threshold Limit Values and Biological Exposure Indices,*" or by OSHA, whichever is more stringent, shall be prohibited. For the purpose of this document, the term used for the most stringent standard is the Occupational Exposure Limit (OEL).

b. In case of conflicts between ACGIH and other standards or regulations referenced in this manual, the more stringent shall prevail.

c. The employer shall comply with all applicable standards and regulations to reduce contaminant concentration levels As Low As is Reasonably Achievable (ALARA).

d. Activities where occupational exposure to a chemical or biological agent is possible shall comply with current Department of Army (DA) safety and occupational health requirements for chemical and biological agents.

06.A.02 Hazard evaluation.

a. All operations, materials, and equipment shall be evaluated to determine the presence of hazardous environments or if hazardous or toxic agents could be released into the work environment.

EM 385-1-1
15 Sep 08

b. AHA and/or PHA shall be used for the evaluation. The analyses shall identify all substances, agents, and environments that present a hazard and recommend hazard control measures. Engineering and administrative controls shall be used to control hazards; in cases where engineering or administrative controls are not feasible, PPE may be used.

c. The analyses shall identify: that it serves as certification of hazard assessment; the workplace and activity evaluated; the name of the person certifying that the evaluation has been performed; and the date of the evaluation.

d. Operations, materials, and equipment involving potential exposure to hazardous or toxic agents or environments shall be evaluated by a qualified industrial hygienist, or other competent person, to formulate a hazard control program. This program must be accepted by the GDA before the start of operations.
> This evaluation shall be performed at least annually for USACE operations.

06.A.03 Testing and monitoring.

a. Approved and calibrated testing devices shall be provided to measure hazardous or toxic agents, and environments. Devices shall be labeled with calibration information (name of individual performing the calibration and date of current calibration). Calibration results shall be logged.

b. Individuals performing testing and monitoring shall be trained in hazards and testing and monitoring procedures. Testing devices shall be used, inspected, and maintained in accordance with the manufacturer's instructions, a copy of which shall be maintained with the devices.

c. NIOSH or OSHA sampling and analytical methods or other approved sampling and analytical methods shall be used. Laboratories used for analysis shall be accredited by nationally recognized bodies, such as the American Industrial Hygiene Association (AIHA), for the type of analysis performed.

EM 385-1-1
15 Sep 08

d. Determinations of the concentrations of, and hazards from, hazardous or toxic agents and environments shall be made by a qualified industrial hygienist or other competent person during initial startup and as frequently as necessary to ensure the safety and health of the work environment.

e. Records of testing/monitoring shall be maintained on site and shall be available to the GDA upon request.

06.A.04 The following methods shall be utilized for the control of exposure to hazardous or toxic agents and environments:

a. Substitution, if the substitute process or product is determined to provide the same outcome and to be less of a hazard;

b. Engineering controls (such as local/general ventilation), to limit exposure to hazardous or toxic agents and environments within acceptable limits;

c. Work practice controls, when engineering controls are not feasible or are not sufficient to limit exposure to hazardous or toxic agents and environments within acceptable limits, ;

d. Appropriate PPE (i.e., respirators, gloves, etc.) and associated programs shall be instituted when engineering, work practice controls or material substitution are not feasible or are not sufficient to limit exposure to hazardous or toxic agents.

06.B HAZARDOUS OR TOXIC AGENTS

06.B.01 Chemical Hazard Communication. A written hazard communication program shall be developed when the use of hazardous or toxic agents (any chemical which is a physical/health hazard) are procured, stored or used at a project site (per 29 CFR 1910.1200). The written hazard communication (hazcom) program shall address the following in project- specific detail:

a. Hazardous or Toxic Agent Inventory. A list of the hazardous or toxic agents with the following information:

(1) Explanation of how the agents are to be used at the project.

(2) For emergency response purposes, approximate quantities (e.g., liters, kilograms, gallons, pounds) that will be on site at any given time shall be provided for each material.

(3) A site map will be attached to the inventory showing where inventoried substances are stored.

(4) The inventory and site map will be updated as frequently as necessary to ensure accuracy.

b. Hazardous or Toxic Agent Labeling. Procedures for assuring that containers used to store and transport hazardous or toxic agents around the project site are appropriately labeled to communicate the physical and health hazards associated with the agents in the containers.

c. Material Safety Data Sheet (MSDS) Management. Procedures to ensure MSDSs are maintained at project site for each agent.

(1) Employees shall review MSDSs for specific safety and health protection procedures.

(2) Applicable information contained in the MSDS shall be incorporated in the AHA/PHAs or MSDS can be attached to the AHA/PHA for activities in which material will be used.

(3) The information will be followed in the use, storage, and disposal of material and selection of hazard control and emergency response measures.

d. Employee Information and Training. Procedures to ensure employees are trained initially and periodically when use of hazardous or toxic agents is altered or modified to accommodate changing on-site work procedures. Training shall cover the following topics:

EM 385-1-1
15 Sep 08

(1) Requirements and use of the hazcom program on the project;

(2) The location of all hazardous or toxic agents at the project;

(3) Identification and recognition of hazardous or toxic agents on the project;

(4) Physical and health hazards of the hazardous or toxic agents pertinent to project activities;

(5) Protective measures employees can implement when working with project-specific hazardous or toxic agents.

06.B.02 When engineering and work practice controls or substitution are either infeasible or insufficient, appropriate PPE and chemical hygiene facilities shall be provided and used for the transportation, use, and storage of hazardous or toxic agents.

a. When irritants or hazardous substances may contact skin or clothing, chemical hygiene facilities and PPE shall be provided. PPE may include suitable gloves, face/eye protection and chemical protective suits.

(1) The qualified industrial hygienist or other competent personnel shall determine the scope and type of protective equipment.

(2) Special attention shall be given to selecting proper chemical protection when working with materials designated with a "skin" notation by OEL. Such materials may produce systemic toxic effects through absorption through unbroken skin. **> See Section 5.**

b. When eyes or body of any person may be exposed to hazardous or toxic agents, suitable facilities for quick drenching or flushing of the eyes and body shall be provided in the work area for immediate emergency use and shall be no more than ten (10) seconds from the hazardous material. **> See ANSI Z358.1.**

(1) Emergency eyewash equipment must be provided where there is the potential for an employee's eyes to be exposed to corrosives, strong irritants, or toxic chemicals.

(2) The emergency eyewash equipment must irrigate and flush both eyes simultaneously while the operator holds the eyes open.

(3) The emergency eyewash equipment must deliver at least 0.4 gal (1.5 L) of water per minute for fifteen (15) minutes or more (minimum 6 gallons (22.7 L) water).

(4) Personal eyewash equipment may be used to supplement emergency washing facilities. They must not be used as a substitute. Personal eyewash fluids shall be visually inspected monthly to ensure they remain sanitary with no visible sediments.

(5) All plumbed emergency eyewash facilities and hand-held drench hoses shall be activated weekly and inspected annually to ensure that they function correctly and that the quality and quantity of water is satisfactory for emergency washing purposes.

06.B.03 Storage prior to transportation of hazardous chemicals, materials, substances and wastes shall be under the supervision of a qualified person.

a. Transportation, use, and storage of hazardous or toxic agents shall be planned and controlled to prevent contamination of people, animals, food, water, equipment, materials, and environment.

b. All storage of hazardous or toxic agents shall be in accordance with the recommendations of the manufacturer,

EM 385-1-1
15 Sep 08

OSHA and NFPA requirements and accessible only to authorized personnel.

c. Disposal of surplus or excess hazardous or toxic agents shall occur in a manner that will not contaminate or pollute any water supply, ground water, or streams; and will comply with Federal, State, and local regulations and guidelines.

d. Containers used to hold hazardous or toxic agents should not be used to hold other materials unless they have been managed or cleaned under hazardous waste and Department of Transportation (DOT) regulatory requirements.

e. Every hazardous or toxic agent being transported for disposal shall be transported with a copy of the substance's MSDS whenever applicable.

f. Persons who prepare shipments of hazardous chemicals, materials, substances and/or wastes that are defined as hazardous material under DOT regulations are required to be DOT trained, certified and issued an appointment letter in accordance with Defense Transportation Regulation 4500.9-R, Chapter 204.

06.B.04 A Process safety management program of highly hazardous chemicals shall be employed in accordance with 29 CFR 1910.119 or 29 CFR 1926.64 whenever a work activity involves:

a. A process that involves a chemical at or above the threshold quantities listed in Appendix A of the above-cited CFRs; or

b. A process that involves a flammable liquid or gas on site in one location in a quantity of 10,000 lb (4,535.9 kg) or more as defined in 29 CFR 1926.59(c), except:

(1) Hydrocarbon fuels used solely for workplace consumption as a fuel if such fuels are not part of a process containing another highly hazardous chemical covered by the standards

EM 385-1-1
15 Sep 08

cited above; or

(2) Flammable liquids stored in atmospheric tanks or transferred that are kept below their normal boiling point without benefit of chilling or refrigeration.

06.B.05 Lead and Asbestos Hazard Control Activities.

a. General. All projects will be evaluated for the potential to contact asbestos-containing material (ACM) and lead-based paint (LBP).

(1) If the evaluation shows the potential for activities to generate unacceptable occupational exposure to LBP, a written lead compliance plan shall be written. The lead compliance plan shall be in accordance with 29 CFR 1910.1025 and 29 CRF 1926.62.

(2) If the evaluation shows the potential for activities to disturb ACM, an asbestos abatement plan shall be developed. The asbestos abatement plan shall be in accordance with 29 CFR 1910.1001; 29 CFR 1926.1101; and 40 CFR 61, Subpart M.

(3) These plan(s) shall be developed as an appendix to the contract APP or, for USACE operations, the Project Safety Plan. The written plan(s) shall be submitted for acceptance by the GDA before beginning work.

b. Lead Compliance Plan. A lead compliance plan shall describe the procedures to be followed to protect employees from lead hazards while performing lead hazard control activities. The Plan shall address the following:

(1) A description of each work activity in which lead is emitted, to include equipment and materials used, controls in place, crew size, job responsibilities, operating procedures, and maintenance practices, work activity locations and lead-containing components keyed to the project drawings;

(2) Description of means to be used to achieve exposure compliance, including any engineering controls;

(3) Employee exposure assessment procedures to monitor and document employee lead exposure. Exposure monitoring shall include two types:

(a) Initial determination (may be omitted if there is sufficient objective/historical data showing action level compliance according to the requirements); and

(b) Continued exposure monitoring required as a result of initial exposure determinations.

(4) Protective clothing, housekeeping procedures to prevent spread of lead contamination both in and beyond the lead hazard control area, and hygiene facilities and practices to prevent employees from inadvertent ingestion of lead;

(5) Administrative controls to limit employee exposure to lead, including employee rotation schedule to be employed, if engineering controls or PPE fail to eliminate exposures exceeding the PEL;

(6) Medical surveillance procedures to monitor employee exposures and ensure fitness for wearing respiratory protection;

(7) Competent person and employee training required;

(8) Detailed sketches identifying lead hazard control areas, including decontamination areas and facilities, critical barriers, and physical and air distribution boundaries;

(9) Perimeter or other area air monitoring outside or adjacent to the regulated area;

(10) Security required for each lead hazard control area; and

(11) Waste generation, characterization, transportation, and disposal (including recordkeeping).

c. Asbestos Hazard Abatement Plan. An asbestos abatement plan shall describe procedures to be followed to protect employees from asbestos hazards while performing work that will disturb ACM. It shall address the following:

(1) A description of each activity where asbestos will be disturbed, to include the OSHA class of work, equipment required, controls to be used, crew size, job responsibilities, maintenance practices, and locations keyed to the project drawings;

(2) Method of notification of other employers at the worksite;

(3) Description of regulated areas, types of containment, decontamination unit plan, and engineering controls;

(4) Air monitoring: personal, environmental, and clearance. Employee exposure assessment procedures shall address monitoring and documenting employee exposures.

(a) An initial determination (may be omitted if there is sufficient objective/historical data showing compliance with the requirements);

(b) Continued exposure monitoring may be required as a result of initial exposure determinations;

(c) Environmental monitoring shall demonstrate the absence of asbestos fiber migration outside the regulated area; and

(d) Clearance monitoring to document that the area has met specified clearance criteria.

(5) PPE, including respirators and clothing;

(6) Housekeeping procedures addressing prevention of spread

EM 385-1-1
15 Sep 08

of contamination both in and beyond the regulated area;

(7) Hygiene facilities and practices;

(8) Competent person and employee training required;

(9) Medical surveillance, as required, to assess exposure and to monitor employee fitness to perform work tasks while wearing PPE to include respiratory protection devices;

(10) Waste generation, containerization, transportation, and disposal (including recordkeeping); and

(11) Security, fire, and medical emergency response procedures.

06.C HOT SUBSTANCES

06.C.01 Heating devices and melting kettles.

a. Heating devices and melting kettles shall be placed on firm, level, non-combustible foundations and shall be protected against traffic, accidental tipping, or similar hazards and, whenever possible, shall be placed downwind from employees or occupied buildings.

b. A method to contain uncontrolled spills of the heated material, which might be on fire, shall be developed. The placement of a fire retardant tarp under the kettle (or other effective means) shall be used.

c. A minimum of two (2) fire extinguishers, rated not less than 2A:20B:C, shall be available within 25 ft (7.6 m) of the working kettles. **> *Hot work permits shall be required on Government installations unless otherwise indicated by the GDA.***

d. The kettle operator must be trained in the proper operation of the kettle and have knowledge of the material being heated so

EM 385-1-1
15 Sep 08

as to not allow the material to be heated beyond the allowable temperature. A working thermometer shall be provided and used.

e. Heating devices and melting kettles shall not be left unattended when in use. When the kettle is heating material to the working temperature, the operator must be located on the same level as the kettle, be within eyesight and be within 25 ft (7.6 m) of the kettle. **> See 09.J.03.**

f. Bituminous-material melting kettles shall be provided with an effective tight fitting lid or hood, and a calibrated thermometer in operating condition.

(1) The temperature shall be maintained 25° below the flash point of the bituminous material.

(2) All melting kettles shall be sized for the job.

(3) The size and weight of the kettle must not exceed the structural capacity of the roof deck.

g. Bituminous-material melting kettles shall not be used or operated inside or within 25 ft (7.6 m) of combustible materials, including propane tanks stored or in use. The lid for the kettle should open away from the building.

h. The liquid propane container(s) used as the heat source shall be kept at least 10 ft (3 m) away from the kettle and shall be placed in an upright and secured position to insure it doesn't tip over.

i. Kettles shall be located so that means of egress is not restricted and shall be no closer than 10 ft (3 m) of egress path.

06.C.02 Enclosed areas in which hot substances are heated or applied shall be ventilated.

EM 385-1-1
15 Sep 08

06.C.03 Ladles, equipment, and material shall be moisture-free before being used or placed in heated material.

06.C.04 Flammable liquids with a flash point below 100° F (37.8° C) shall not be used to thin the mixture or to clean equipment.

06.C.05 Transporting and handling hot substances.

    a. Runways or passageways, clear of obstructions, shall be provided for all persons carrying hot substances.

    b. Hot substances shall not be carried up or down ladders.

    c. When hoists are used to raise or lower hot substances, attention shall be given to assuring that the hoisting mechanism is adequate for the loads imposed and is securely braced and anchored.

    d. All persons handling hot substances shall be provided protection against contact with, or exposure to radiant heat, glare, fumes, and vapors of the substances. At a minimum, roofers handling roofing materials shall be fully clothed including long sleeved shirts, shoes secured and at least 6 in (15 cm) in height, and gloves up to the wrist. > *See Section 5.*

    e. Containers for handling and transporting hot substances shall be of substantial construction (minimum 24-gauge sheet steel), free from any soldered joints or attachments, and shall not be filled higher than 4 in (10.1 cm) from the top.

    f. Piping used to transport hot substances shall have a entry and exit shut off valve and be made of flexible metallic hoses fitted with insulated handles. In cold climates, piping shall be insulated to prevent material from solidifying on the inside of the pipe.

06.C.06 An effective fire prevention program shall be described in the APP, AHA and maintained at the jobsite. All workers shall be trained in the specifics of the plan.

EM 385-1-1
15 Sep 08

06.D HARMFUL PLANTS, ANIMALS, AND INSECTS

06.D.01 Protection against hazards from insects <u>and/or animals harboring fleas or disease-carrying insects shall</u> include, as applicable, the following:

   a. PPE such as <u>netted</u> hoods, <u>leather work</u> gloves, and <u>high-top work</u> boots <u>worn in conjunction with trousers and long-sleeved shirts;</u>

   b. <u> Clothing treated at the factory with DEET or Permethrin are recommended in areas of high insect population;</u>

   c. Drainage or spraying of breeding areas;

   d. <u>Destroying or flagging (marking as hazard) of nests</u>;

   e. Smudge pots and aerosols for protecting workers <u>and</u> small areas;

   f. Elimination of <u>actions or</u> conditions that propagate insects or vermin;

   g. Extermination measures <u>by a certified pesticide applicator or, for over the counter items, following the instructions on the label</u>;

   h. Approved first-aid procedures for employees;

   i. Inoculation <u>against diseases known to be a local hazard</u>; and

   j. Instruction in recognition of the animals and insects and their common nesting habits, <u>aggressiveness, etc.</u>

06.D.02 <u>In areas where there is exposure to poisonous snakes or lizards, employees shall be required to:</u>

EM 385-1-1
15 Sep 08

a. Wear snake chaps or knee-high snake boots worn in conjunction with trousers and long-sleeved shirts;

b. Be trained in recognition of the snakes and their common nesting habits, aggressiveness, etc.; and

c. Be trained in the proper first aid procedures for bites.

06.D.03 In areas where employees are exposed to poisonous plants (e.g., poison ivy, oak, or sumac), the following protective measures, as applicable, shall be provided:

a. Removal or destruction of plants, where practical;

b. Appropriate protective clothing such as gloves;

c. Protective ointments;

d. Soap and water for washing exposed parts; and

e. Instruction in recognition and identification of the plants.

06.D.04 When burning poisonous plants, controls shall be instituted to prevent contact with or inhalation of toxic elements contained in the smoke.

06.E IONIZING RADIATION

06.E.01 Anyone who procures, uses, possesses, transports, transfers, or disposes of radioactive materials or radiation generating devices shall:

a. Notify, in writing, the GDA of the nature of the material or device, a description of intended use, the location of use and storage, and all transportation and disposal requirements;

b. Secure appropriate authorization or permit if a licensed or DOD regulated radiological device or radioactive material is to

EM 385-1-1
15 Sep 08

be used on a DOD installation (a lead time of at least 45 days should be allowed for obtaining a DOD authorization or permit);

c. Provide to the GDA a copy of all US Nuclear Regulatory Commission (NRC) or Agreement State licenses, the Army Radiation Authorization (ARA), Army Radiation Permit, and reciprocity forms (to include NRC Form 241), as applicable.

06.E.02 Qualified Personnel.

a. Operations involving radiation hazards or use of radioactive material or radiation generating devices shall be performed under the direct supervision of a Radiation Safety Officer (RSO), who is qualified and responsible for radiological safety.

b. The RSO will be technically qualified and will meet the experience, training, and education requirements listed below:

(1) Formally trained in radiation protection topics including the following: physics of radiation; radiation's interaction with matter; mathematics necessary for the subject matter; biological effects of radiation; type and use of instruments for detection, monitoring and surveying radiation; radiation safety techniques and procedures; and use of time, distance, shielding, engineering controls, and PPE to reduce radiation exposure;

(2) Hands-on training in the uses of equipment, instrumentation, procedures, and theory used in their unit;

(3) Knowledge of applicable regulations including those of the Nuclear Regulatory Commission before (NRC), U.S. Environmental Protection Agency (USEPA), U.S. Department of Energy (DOE), DOT and DOD, to include all applicable DOD Components, pertaining to radioactive materials, radiation generating devices, and radioactive and mixed waste; and

(4) Knowledge of the USACE Radiation Safety Program, and recordkeeping requirements for work with radioactive materials and radiation generating devices.

EM 385-1-1
15 Sep 08

06.E.03 Radiation Safety Program.

a. Operations involving radiation hazards, and users of radioactive material or radiation generating devices, shall develop and implement a Radiation Safety Program.

(1) The program shall be managed by the RSO and based on sound radiation safety principles that shall keep occupational doses and doses to the public ALARA.

(2) <u>The RSO is responsible for performing or ensuring the performance of an annual review of the program. Documentation of the review shall be retained for two (2) years</u>.

(3) A Radiation Safety Committee (RSC) shall be established in accordance with 10 CFR 20 and <u>DA PAM 385-24</u> as part of the Radiation <u>Safety</u> Program.

b. All personnel entering an area where radioactive material or radiation generating devices are used, and where there is a potential for an individual to receive a Total Effective Dose Equivalent (TEDE) of 100 millirem (mrem) or more in one (1) year, shall receive instruction in:

(1) The presence of the material or device;

(2) Health and safety problems associated with exposure to radiation, including the potential effects of radiation on a pregnant female, the fetus, or embryo;

(3) Precautions and controls used to control exposure;

(4) Proper use of instrumentation and dosimetry in the area;

(5) The Radiation Safety Program required in 06.E.03.a; and

(6) Their rights and responsibilities.

EM 385-1-1
15 Sep 08

c. The Radiation Safety Program will include plans and procedures for handling credible emergencies involving radiation and radioactive materials. This will include coordination with civilian and/or military emergency response organizations as necessary.

06.E.04 Dose Limits.

a. Occupational dose limits shall be based on the TEDE.
> See Table 6-1.

(1) An annual (i.e., per calendar year) limit that is the more limiting of: 5 rem [0.05 sieverts (Sv)] TEDE, or the sum of the deep dose equivalent and the committed dose equivalent to any individual organ or tissue of 50 rem (0.5 Sv), or 15 rem (0.15 Sv) to the lens of the eye, or 50 rem (0.05 Sv) shallow dose equivalent to the skin or any extremity.

TABLE 6-1

OCCUPATIONAL DOSE RATES

Body part	Annual limits with RSSO approval	Annual limits without RSSO approval	Suggested ALARA limits
Whole body	5 rem (0.05 Sv)	0.5 rem (0.005 Sv)	0.1 rem (0.001 Sv)
Individual organ	50 rem (0.5 Sv)	5 rem (0.05 Sv)	0.5 rem (0.005 Sv)
Lens of eye	15 rem (0.15 Sv)	1.5 rem (0.015 Sv)	0.15 rem (0.15 Sv)
Skin or extremity	50 rem (0.5 Sv)	5 rem (0.05 Sv)	0.5 rem (0.005 Sv)

(2) Without the written approval of the USACE Radiation Safety Staff Officer (RSSO), the annual occupational dose shall not exceed the more limiting of: 0.5 rem (0.005 Sv) TEDE, or the sum of the deep dose equivalent and the committed dose

EM 385-1-1
15 Sep 08

equivalent to any individual organ or tissue of 5 rem (0.05 Sv), or 1.5 rem(0.015 Sv) to the lens of the eye, or 5 rem (0.05 Sv) shallow dose equivalent to the skin, or any extremity.

(3) To keep doses ALARA, the user shall set administrative action levels below the annual dose limits. These action levels shall be realistic and attainable. Suggested action levels are the more limiting of: 0.1 rem (0.001 Sv) TEDE, or the sum of the deep dose equivalent and the committed dose equivalent to any individual organ or tissue of 0.5 rem(0.005 Sv), or 0.15 rem (0.0015 Sv) to the lens of the eye, or 0.5 rem (0.005 Sv) shallow dose equivalent to the skin or any extremity.

<u>(4) Any exposure in excess of an ALARA limit requires investigation by the RSO.</u>

b. <u>In accordance with DA PAM 385-24,</u> planned special exposures shall not be performed.

c. No employee under 18 years of age shall receive occupational exposure to ionizing radiation.

d. The dose to a declared pregnant employee shall not exceed 0.5 rem (0.005 Sv) during the entire gestation period and efforts shall be made to avoid variations in a uniform monthly exposure rate. If the dose to the embryo/fetus exceeds or is within 0.05 rem of 0.5 rem at the time of declaration, then dose to the embryo/fetus is limited to 0.05 rem for the remainder of gestation.

06.E.05 Radiation Monitoring, Surveys, and Dosimetry.

a. Users of radioactive material or radiation generating devices shall conduct surveys and monitoring to ensure occupational dose limits are not exceeded.

b. Instruments used for radiation monitoring and surveying shall be:

EM 385-1-1
15 Sep 08

(1) Available and used whenever radioactive material or radiation generating devices are used;

(2) Properly calibrated <u>at least annually</u> to a National Institute of Standards and Technology (NIST) traceable source;

(3) Appropriate for the type and intensity of the radiation surveyed;

(4) Operationally checked against a dedicated check source before each use; and

<u>(5) The RSO must maintain at least two survey instruments to accommodate maintenance and calibration downtime.</u>

c. Users of radioactive material or radiation generating devices and visitors or personnel performing work tasks in the area shall coordinate with the RSO for appropriate dosimetry use whenever any of the following situations exist:

(1) An individual enters a Radiation Area (> 5 mrem [50 microsieverts (μSv)] in any one (1) hour <u>at 1 ft (30 cm) from the radiation source</u>), or a High Radiation Area (> 100 mrem [1 mSv] in any one (1) hour <u>at 1 ft (30 cm) from the radiation source</u>), or a Very High Radiation Area (>500 rad [5 Gray (Gy)] in 1 hour <u>at 3.3 ft (1 m) from the radiation source</u>);

(2) An individual has the potential to receive greater than <u>the ALARA limits established pursuant to 06.E.04.a.(3)</u> in 1 year.

d. All external dosimetry shall be processed by a National Voluntary Laboratory Accreditation Program (NVLAP) certified laboratory. USACE personnel shall use <u>dosimetry provided by the Army Dosimetry Center</u>.

e. Users of unsealed radioactive material sources shall institute an internal dosimetry program:

EM 385-1-1
15 Sep 08

(1) When there is a potential for a employee to receive an internal dose of greater than 0.5 rem (5 mSv) per year;

(2) That is reviewed and approved by a qualified health physicist; and

(3) That contains provisions for a pre-exposure bioassay, a bioassay method capable of detecting internal radioactive materials, at a level below 10% of the annual limits of intake (ALI) listed in Appendix B of 10 CFR 20 for each radionuclide used, appropriate action levels for requiring additional bioassay, actions for individuals found to have internally deposited radioactive materials, and provisions for post-exposure bioassay.

06.E.06 Access, Storage, and Control.

a. All radiological devices and radioactive materials shall be designed, constructed, installed, used, stored, transported, and disposed of in such a manner to ensure personnel exposures are kept ALARA.

b. Users of radioactive materials or radiation generating devices shall post signs and control access to radiation areas in accordance with 06.E.08.

c. Where radiation levels exceed 2 mrem (20 µSv) in any 1 hour, users shall use engineering controls, shielding, access time limitation, and/or physical separation to keep doses to the public ALARA.

d. Users shall secure radioactive material and radiation generating devices against theft or unauthorized use.

e. Storage shall be in accordance with any license or permit requirements.

EM 385-1-1
15 Sep 08

f. Radioactive material and radiation generating devices, not in storage, shall be under constant control and surveillance.

g. Operations involving regulated radiation hazards or users of regulated radioactive material or radiation generating devices shall conduct surveys to ensure that the public dose limit of 0.01 rem (0.0001 Sv) is not exceeded.

06.E.07 Respiratory Protection and other Controls.

a. Users of radioactive material shall, to the extent practicable, institute process or engineering controls to limit concentrations of radioactive materials in air.

b. Where process or engineering controls are unable to control airborne radioactive material concentrations, users shall increase monitoring and limit intakes of radioactive materials through control of access, limitation of exposure times, use of respiratory protection equipment, or other controls.

c. The use of respiratory protection equipment shall be in compliance with 05.G of this manual, and shall be limited by the protection factors listed in Appendix A of 10 CFR 20.

06.E.08 Signs, Labels, and Posting Requirements.

a. The RSO shall post in a conspicuous location a sign or signs bearing the standard radiation symbol shown in Figure 8-7 and the following words:

(1) **"Caution, Radiation Area"** - areas where radiation field is equal to or greater than 5 mrem (0.05 mSv) in any 1 hour and less than 100 mrem (1 mSv) in any 1 hour at 30 cm from the radiation source;

(2) **"Caution, High Radiation Area"** - areas where radiation field is equal to or greater than 100 mrem (1 mSv) in any 1 hour at 12 in (30 cm) from the radiation source and less than 500

EM 385-1-1
15 Sep 08

rads (5 Gy) in any 1 hour <u>at 3.3 ft (1 m) from the radiation source</u>;

(3) **"Grave Danger, Very High Radiation Area"** - areas where the radiation field is equal to or greater than 500 rads (5 Gy) in any 1 hour;

(4) **"Caution, Airborne Radioactivity Area"** – <u>rooms, enclosures, or</u> areas where airborne radioactive material concentrations are greater than the derived air concentration (DAC) limits listed in 10 CFR 20, Appendix B <u>or where concentrations exist to such a degree that an individual present in the area without respiratory protective equipment could exceed, during the hours an individual is present in a week, an intake of 0.6% of the annual limit on intake (ALI) or 12 DAC-hours</u>; or

(5) **"Caution, Radioactive Material"** – <u>areas or</u> rooms where quantities of radioactive materials in excess of ten times the 10 CFR 20, Appendix C quantities are used or stored.

b. Users who receive or expect to receive a package containing radioactive material shall follow the package receipt procedures listed in 10 CFR 20.1906.

c. When a site has an NRC license, the RSO shall post an NRC Form 3 in a location visible to all employees who work with or around radioactive materials.

06.E.09 Radioactive Waste Disposal.

a. Radioactive sealed sources (and gauges) when no longer needed may be returned (transferred) to the manufacturer. The local USACE Command RSO <u>and the USACE RSSO</u> must be notified and any applicable licenses or permits amended or terminated.

EM 385-1-1
15 Sep 08

b. Radioactive waste disposal shall be coordinated with the GDA. For disposal actions specific to USACE operations and activities the GDA shall coordinate with the USACE Command RSO and the USACE Environmental and Munitions Center of Expertise.

c. Tritium (H-3) and Carbon-14 used in liquid scintillation counting, at concentrations below 0.05 microcuries per gram (μCi/g), may be disposed without regard to its radioactivity. (Note: Many liquid scintillation fluids are hazardous wastes and must be disposed of as such.)

06.E.10 Records.

a. All users of radioactive material or radiation generating devices shall prepare and maintain records of the Radiation Safety Program for three (3) years after termination of the license or permit.

b. For any individual <u>for whom monitoring was required by 06.E.05</u>, the RSO shall prepare and maintain documentation of that person's <u>occupational dose during the current year. The RSO shall also attempt to obtain records of cumulative occupational radiation dose.</u>

c. All users of radioactive material or radiation generating devices shall prepare and maintain records of all calculated or monitored radiation dose to individual members of the public so as to document compliance with 06.E.05.

06.E.11 Reports.

a. Any loss, theft, damage, or overexposure shall immediately upon discovery be reported to the RSO who will then file a report <u>(if required)</u> with NRC in accordance with the requirements of 10 CFR 20.

b. Incidents or accidents involving radioactive material or radiation generating devices shall be reported immediately to the RSO and the USACE RSSO.

c. Annual reports shall be issued by the RSO for each individual USACE radiation employee with the recorded or calculated dose assigned to the USACE individual for the year or specific work project. These shall be maintained in such a manner that accumulated exposure can be determined at a future date.

06.E.12 Transportation.

a. Users of radioactive material shall comply with the requirements of the DOT for inter- and intra-state transport contained in 49 CFR.

b. Persons who prepare shipments of radioactive materials that are defined as hazardous material under DOT regulations are required to be trained (49 CFR 173.1(b)), certified, and issued an appointment letter in accordance with DOD 4500.9-R, Chapter 204.

06.E.13 Medical surveillance. **> See Section 28 for requirements specific to work conducted under the provisions of 29 CFR 1910.120 and 29 CFR 1926.65.**

a. Medical examinations are not routinely required before occupational exposure to ionizing radiation. For USACE personnel, a medical examination shall be conducted in accordance with DA Pam 40-501, when deemed necessary, by a physician, the RSO, or other regulations. The RSO will coordinate with supporting medical personnel to help ensure that personnel receive appropriate occupational health surveillance.

b. All cases of overexposure and suspected ingestion or inhalation of radioactive materials shall be referred to a physician for examination.

EM 385-1-1
15 Sep 08

06.E.14 Radon.

a. Any structure, building or tunnel, wherein employees may be reasonably expected to be exposed to radon concentrations exceeding 7.5 picocuries per liter (pCi/L), shall be tested for radon. Where the radon concentration exceeds 7.5 pCi/L, requirements for exposure, SOPs, posting, training, medical records, record keeping and reporting shall apply, per 29 CFR 1910.1096. 29 CFR 1910.1096(c)(1) refers to Table 1 of Appendix B to 10 CFR 20. The Table 1 value for radon is 30 pCi/L.

b. USACE employees and USACE facilities will comply with testing, exposure, and mitigation guidance provided in AR 200-1.

06.F NONIONIZING RADIATION AND MAGNETIC AND ELECTRIC FIELDS

06.F.01 Lasers.

a. Only qualified and trained employees may be assigned to install, adjust, and operate laser equipment. Proof of qualification of the laser equipment operator shall be in the operator's possession during operation. <u>A qualified employee shall design or review for adequacy all radiation safety Standard Operating Procedure (SOP).</u>

b. Laser equipment shall bear a label to indicate make, maximum output, and beam spread.

c. Areas in which lasers are used shall be posted with standard laser warning signs. > *See Figures 8-5 and 8-6*

d. Employees whose work requires exposure to laser beams shall be provided with appropriate laser safety goggles that will protect for the specific wavelength of the laser and be of optical density adequate for the energy involved, as specified in Table 6-2. Protective goggles shall bear a label identifying the following data: the laser wavelengths for which use is intended, the optical density of those wavelengths, and the visible light transmission.

TABLE 6-2

LASER SAFETY GOGGLE OPTICAL DENSITY REQUIREMENTS

Intensity, continuous wave maximum power density (watts/cm^2)	Attenuation	
	Optical density	Attenuation factor
0.01	5	10,000
0.1	6	100,000
1.0	7	1,000,000
10.0	8	10,000,000

e. Beam shutters or caps shall be used, or the laser turned off, when laser transmission is not required. When the laser is left unattended for a period of time (e.g., during lunch hour, overnight, or at change of shifts) the laser shall be turned off.

f. Only mechanical or electronic means shall be used as a detector for guiding the internal alignment of the laser.

g. The laser beam shall not be directed at employees: whenever possible, laser units in operation shall be set above the heads of employees.

h. When it is raining or snowing or when there is dust or fog in the air, the operation of laser systems shall be prohibited (as practical); during such weather conditions employees shall be kept out of range of the areas of source and target.

i. Employee exposure to laser power densities shall be within the threshold limit values (TLVs) as specified by the ACGIH in "Threshold Limit Values and Biological Exposure Indices."

EM 385-1-1
15 Sep 08

j. Only Class 1, 2, or 3a lasers may be used as hand-held pointing devices. Lasers used as pointing devices (e.g., during briefings) shall not be directed toward employees and shall be handled and stored in accordance with the manufacturer's recommendations.

k. Suspected LASER eye injuries: Immediately evacuate personnel suspected of experiencing potentially damaging eye exposure from LASER radiation to the nearest medical facility for an eye examination. LASER eye injuries require immediate specialized ophthalmologic care to minimize long-term visual acuity loss

06.F.02 Radio frequency and electromagnetic radiation.

a. Ensure that no employee is exposed to electric or magnetic fields, radio frequency (RF) including infrared, ultraviolet, and microwave radiation levels exceeding the values listed in the ACGIH Threshold Limit Values and Biological Exposure Indices.

b. Routine use of RF protective clothing to protect personnel is prohibited.

(1) Protective equipment, such as electrically insulated gloves and shoes for protection against RF shock and burn, or for insulation from the ground plane, is permissible when engineering controls or procedures cannot eliminate exposure hazards.

(2) Users will identify, attenuate, or control potentially hazardous RF electromagnetic fields and other radiation hazards associated with electronic equipment by engineering design, administrative actions, or protective equipment, (in that order), or a combination thereof. Use process and engineering controls before personal protective equipment (PPE) to protect employees.

c. All personnel routinely working with RF emitting equipment where exposures may exceed TLVs will receive training in RF

EM 385-1-1
15 Sep 08

hazards, procedures for minimizing these hazards, and their responsibility to limit potential overexposures. Operator's manuals, Training Orders, Equipment SOPs, etc. will be available for all RF generating equipment and safety guidance will be followed.

d. Whenever personnel are potentially exposed to RF fields exceeding PELs, the fields will be measured and evaluated using Institute of Electrical and Electronics Engineers (IEEE) guidance. District and/or project safety personnel will use this information and document RF environments. Where multiple RF electromagnetic radiation emitters are located in fixed arrangements, RF evaluation data will include a determination of weighted contributions from expected simultaneously operated emitters.

0.6.G VENTILATION AND EXHAUST SYSTEMS

06.G.01 Portable and Temporary Ventilation Systems

a. All portable or temporary ventilation systems shall remove dusts, fumes, mists, vapors and gases away from the worker and the work environment or provide air to prevent an oxygen deficient atmosphere.

b. Portable or temporary ventilation systems shall be used as designed by the manufacturer. All hoses shall be only as long as the maximum allowed by the manufacturer to provide the required air flow at the supply or exhaust point. If adding or changing hoses, only hoses and/or connectors shall be used that are comparable and compatible with the hoses and connectors provided by the manufacturer.

c. Make-up air for air supply ventilation systems shall draw air free of contaminants and away from any potential contaminant source.

d. Any portable or temporary ventilation system and the locations the systems are to be used shall be approved by the

EM 385-1-1
15 Sep 08

GDA before use. Manufacturer information or design criteria shall be provided with the request for approval.

e. Airborne contaminants created by portable or temporary ventilation systems (such as drills, saws, and grinding machines) in concentrations exceeding acceptable safe limits shall be effectively controlled at the source. **< See 06.A.03.**

06.G.02 Ventilation systems shall be operated and maintained in such a manner to ensure the maintenance of a volume and velocity of exhaust air sufficient to gather contaminants and safely transport them to suitable points for removal.

06.G.03 Duration of operation.

a. Ventilation systems shall be operated continuously during operations when persons are exposed to airborne contaminants or explosive gases at or above acceptable safe limits as defined in 06.A.01 or as otherwise specified by this manual, referenced standards, or regulations.

b. Ventilation systems shall remain in operation for a time after the work process or equipment has ceased to ensure the removal of any contaminants in suspension or vaporizing into the air.

06.G.04 Local exhaust ventilation systems shall be periodically evaluated to ensure that proper contaminant capture, movement through the system and filtration or exhaust to the outside.

06.G.05 Dusts and refuse materials removed by exhaust systems or other methods shall be disposed of in a manner that will not create a hazard to employees or the public and in accordance with Federal, State, and local requirements.

06.H ABRASIVE BLASTING

06.H.01 Introduction. Silica sand shall NOT be used as an abrasive blasting media. Alternative abrasive blasting materials

EM 385-1-1
15 Sep 08

are available and listed in Table 6-3. Depending on the application, one of these alternative materials is suggested for use as an abrasive blasting media.

TABLE 6-3

ABRASIVE BLASTING MEDIA: SILICA SUBSTITUTES

APPLICATIONS	Media	ADVANTAGES
Cleaning Hard Metals (e.g. Titanium) Removing Metal Etch Glass Carve Granite	**ALUMINUM OXIDE**	Recyclable
General Paint Removal Stripping Aircraft Skins Cleaning Surfaces in Food Processing Plants Removing Paint from Glass	**BAKING SODA** (Sodium Bicarbonate)	Less Material Used/Less Cleanup Low Nozzle Pressures (35-90 PSI) Non-Sparking Water Soluble
General Paint, Rust & Scale Removal from Steel Paint Removal from Wood Exposure of Aggregates	**COAL SLAG**	Less Than 1% Free Silica Inert Fast Cutting Creates Anchor Profile
General Paint, Rust & Scale Removal from Steel Paint Removal from Wood	**COPPER SLAG**	Rapid Cutting
Deburring Paint & Rust Removal from Wood & Metal	**CORN COB GRANULES**	Low Consumption Low Dust Levels Biodegradable
Cleaning Aircraft Parts Cleaning Exotic Metals	**DRY ICE** (Carbon Dioxide)	No Residue Remains Minimal Cleanup
General Paint, Rust & Scale Removal from Steel	**GARNET**	Lower Nozzle Pressures (60-70 PSI) Low Dust Levels Fast Cleaning Rates Can be Recycled 6-7 Times Low Free Silica

EM 385-1-1
15 Sep 08

TABLE 6-3 (CONTINUED)

ABRASIVE BLASTING MEDIA: SILICA SUBSTITUTES

APPLICATIONS	Media	ADVANTAGES
Cleaning & Polishing Deburring	**GLASS BEADS**	Uniform Size and Shape Recyclable Provide High Luster Polished Surface
General Paint, Rust & Scale Removal from Steel	**NICKEL SLAG**	Rapid Cutting
Cleaning Soft Materials (e.g. Aluminum, Plastic, Wood) Cleaning Surfaces in the Petroleum Industry	**NUT SHELLS**	High Removal Speed Non-Sparking Low Consumption
Clean Light Mill Scale & Rust from Steel 2.5 MIL Profile & Finer	**OLIVINE**	Low Chloride Ion Level Low Conductivity

a. Abrasive blasting operations shall be evaluated to determine composition and toxicity of the abrasive and the dust or fume generated by the blasted material, including surface coatings. This determination shall be documented on the AHA (Activity Hazard Analysis) developed for the abrasive blasting activity.

b. Written operating procedures shall be developed and implemented for abrasive blasting operations, including pressurized pot procedures (filling, pressurizing, depressurizing, and maintenance and inspection). The procedures should be added as an appendix to the APP.

c. The concentration of respirable dust and fume in the breathing zone or persons exposed to the blasting operation shall be maintained in accordance with 06.A.01.

d. No employee will be allowed to work in abrasive blasting operations unless he has met the medical surveillance and training and experience, and has been provided the appropriate PPE.

e. All production and control systems used in a stationary abrasive-blasting process shall be designed or maintained to prevent escape of airborne dust or aerosols in the work environment and to ensure control of the abrasive agents.

f. Pressurized systems and components shall be inspected, tested, certified and maintained in accordance with the requirements of Section 20.

g. Engineering controls for noise and dust shall be considered even if they cannot reduce the exposures to the lowest Occupational Exposure Limit (OEL) but will significantly reduce noise and dust exposure to the employees.

06.H.02 Blast Cleaning Enclosures and Rooms:

a. Blast cleaning enclosures shall be exhaust ventilated in such a way that a continuous inward flow of air will be maintained at all openings in the enclosure during the blasting operation.

b. All air inlets and access openings shall be well baffled to prevent the escape of abrasive and the recommended continuous inward air velocity at the air inlets is a minimum of 250 fpm (4.6 kph).

c. Negative pressure should be maintained inside during blasting.

d. The rate of exhaust shall be sufficient to provide prompt clearance of the dust-laden air within the enclosure after cessation of the blasting.

e. Minimum recommended protective equipment of an abrasive blaster working inside a blasting room, in the open, in enclosed

EM 385-1-1
15 Sep 08

space, or outdoors is: safety boots or toe guards; durable coveralls, closeable at wrists, ankles, and other openings to prevent entry of abrasive dust and rubbing of such; respiratory, eye, and hearing protection; and gauntlet gloves.

f. If abrasive blasting is automated, the blast shall be turned off before the enclosure is opened. The exhaust system shall be run for a sufficient period of time to remove the dusty air within the enclosure to minimize the escape of dust into the workroom and prevent any health hazard.

g. In the room, a cleanup method other than broom sweeping or compressed air blowing should be used to collect the abrasive agent after blasting (e.g., vacuum cleaning). If the blasting agent is removed manually, appropriate personal protective equipment, including respiratory protection shall be worn and not removed until outside the blasting room.

06.H.03 Blasting without Enclosures.

a. If occasional but regular abrasive blasting must be performed inside a building without enclosures, respiratory protection shall be provided for all employees in the area. Portable engineering control devices shall be used at the location to collect the entire used abrasive agent as it is applied.

b. When airborne abrasive-blasting dust becomes sufficiently heavy in an area to cause a temporary safety hazard by reduced visibility, or discomfort to the unprotected employees not engaged in abrasive blasting, such operations in the affected area shall be discontinued until the airborne dust is removed by exhaust ventilation and the settled dust has been removed from the horizontal surfaces in the area. If such operations have to continue, appropriate respiratory protection shall be provided to those employees remaining in the area, provided visibility is adequate.

c. Abrasive materials shall not be allowed to accumulate on aisles and walkways to create a slipping hazard.

EM 385-1-1
15 Sep 08

d. If wet abrasive blasting is employed to reduce dust exposures, the aerosols produced and the dried residues that become airborne might be potential hazards and shall be considered.

06.H.04 Confined space. Abrasive blasting work conducted in a confined space shall be performed in accordance with Section 34 and 29 CFR 1910.146. If the space is mechanically ventilated, means shall be provided to collect dust before release to the open atmosphere.

06.H.05 Blasting Outdoors.

a. Blasters shall be protected in a manner equivalent to Section 05 and/or 29 CFR 1910.94(a)(5), whichever is more stringent.

b. Prudent care shall be taken to prevent the dust cloud from spreading to other work areas. Check with Local and State requirements which may add restrictions to outdoor abrasive blasting.

c. Hearing protection and respiratory protection shall be available to all other employees in the area if their presence is required.

06.H.06 Personal Protective Equipment (PPE).

a. Selection and use of PPE shall be in accordance with Section 05.

b. Air-supplied helmets, blast helmets/hoods, dust respirators, ear muffs, safety boots or toe guards, durable coveralls, closeable at wrists, ankles, and other openings, and safety glasses should be an individual issue item, identified with and used by only one employee. Such equipment may be reissued to another employee only after complete cleaning, repair, and decontamination.

c. Means shall be provided to clean and store air-supplied respiratory equipment after each shift of use. Storage shall be in a clean enclosure such as locker, footlocker, plastic container or zip-lock type bag. Employees shall be trained to maintain issued equipment in clean and good working condition.

d. Replacement of prescription or plano safety glasses shall be made if multiple pitting or etching is visible in the center of the lenses.

e. Replacement of faceplates in air-supplied helmets and blast helmets/hoods shall take place when a side-on light source produces obscuring visible reflections and glare from the etched spots and pit holes in the faceplate. Mylar coating, or similar transparent plastic material, is recommended to protect the glass or plastic faceplate.

f. Length of air hose may not be altered from the manufacturer's specifications.

g. Daily checks shall be performed by the wearer of PPE to maintain it in good working condition. Rips, tears, and openings of PPE that expose skin to abrasive agents shall be mended or replaced. Functional tests for leaks, proper respiration, and good connections shall be performed on the complete air-supply system.

h. Air supply - portable.

(1) The breathable air supplied to the blast helmet or hood shall be drawn from an oil and carbon monoxide free air compressor. The compressor used for blasting cannot be used for breathing air. Breathable air-supply system should be equipped, if possible, with audible alarm at the helmet or hood to warn the user of low air pressure.

(2) Hearing protection. Suitable hearing protection, capable of attenuating employee noise exposure below an 8-hour TWA of

EM 385-1-1
15 Sep 08

85 dB(A), shall be worn inside the blast helmet or hood unless hearing protection is an integral part of such helmet or hood.

(3) Heat stress. Cooling of breathable air, supplied to the blast helmets/hoods, should be considered depending on season and employee exposure to heat sources.

06.I INCLEMENT WEATHER AND HEAT/COLD STRESS MANAGEMENT

06.I.01 When there are warnings or indications of impending severe weather (heavy rains, thunderstorms, damaging winds, tornados, hurricanes, floods, lightning, etc.), weather conditions shall be monitored using a weather station that is part of the National Oceanic and Atmospheric Administration (NOAA) weather radio all hazards network or similar notification system. Appropriate precautions shall be taken to protect personnel and property from the effects of the severe weather. In areas with frequent inclement weather, the employer's APP or project safety plan shall include a discussion of:

    a. Severe weather triggers to alert the SHO to monitor weather conditions;

    b. Training on severe weather precautions, and actions;

    c. Identified area of retreat, preferably a substantial building.

06.I.02 Employers shall develop a comprehensive written activity/site-specific heat/cold stress monitoring plan, in accordance with this Section and using the exposure thresholds in ACGIH "Threshold Limit Values and Biological Exposure Indices" as guidance, and other references the employer determines applicable to protect employees exposed to temperature extremes. The plan shall be incorporated in the employer's APP or project safety and health plan and shall follow the guidelines of 06.I.04 of this manual.

EM 385-1-1
15 Sep 08

06.I.03 In hot environments, <u>the following guidelines will be followed to prevent heat related injury.</u>

   a. <u>D</u>rinking water shall be made available to employees and employees encouraged to frequently drink small amounts, e.g., one cup every 15-20 minutes; the water shall be kept reasonably cool. **> See Section 02.C.**

   b. <u>Tool box training in hot environments shall include training on the symptoms of heat related problems, contributing factors to heat related injuries, and prevention techniques.</u>

   c. <u>When possible, work should be scheduled for cooler periods during the day.</u>

   d. <u>Individuals shall be encouraged to take breaks in a cooler location, and use cooling devices as necessary, such as cooling vests, to prevent heat related injury. A buddy system shall be established to encourage fluid intake and watch for symptoms of heat related injury.</u>

   e. <u>SSHO shall monitor those individuals who have had a previous heat-related injury, are known to be on medication, or exhibits signs of possibly having consumed large amounts of alcohol in the previous 24 hours for signs, or indicating symptoms of heat related injuries.</u>

   f. <u>Individuals who are not acclimatized shall be allowed additional breaks. The period and number should be determined by the SSHO and provided to the supervisor and employee for implementation.</u>

06.I.04 In situations where heat stress may impact employee safety and health, employee acclimatization and workloads shall be assessed and work/rest regimens shall be established.

   a. For employees in permeable work clothing, Wet Bulb Globe Temperature (WBGT) Index or physiological monitoring shall be conducted and work/rest regimens established. <u>The SSHO</u>

EM 385-1-1
15 Sep 08

should assess the condition of the employees, specific weather conditions, work tasks, and other environmental factors and conditions to determine when to begin monitoring.

b. For employees in impermeable work clothing, only physiological monitoring shall be conducted, and work/rest regimens and fluid replacement schedules shall be established.

06.I.05 Where employees are exposed to solar radiation for short periods and there is the potential for sunburn or exposure for prolonged periods where long-term exposure could lead to health effects such as skin cancer, they shall be provided sun screen with a sun protection factor (SPF) appropriate for their skin type and exposure. Sunscreens shall be used only in accordance with the manufacturer's recommendations.

06.I.06 Employees working in air temperatures of -15 °F (-26 °C) or less shall use the work-/warm-up regimen specified in the ACGIH "Threshold Limit Values and Biological Exposure Indices."

06.I.07 At air temperatures of 36 °F (2 °C) or less, employees who become immersed in water or whose clothing becomes wet shall immediately change into dry clothing/ blankets and be treated for hypothermia. Blankets shall be included as part of the first aid equipment on such activities, and employees shall insure they have a change of clothing.

06.I.08 When manual dexterity is not required of a employee, he shall wear thermally protective gloves when exposed to the following temperatures.

    a. For light work, 40 °F (4 °C) and below; and

    b. For moderate and heavy work, 20 °F (-6.6°C) and below.

06.I.09 When fine work is required to be performed with bare hands for more than 10-20 minutes in an environment below 50 °F

(10 °C), procedures shall be established for keeping employees' hands warm.

06.I.10 Metal handles and control bars shall be covered by thermal insulating material at temperatures below 30 °F (–1 °C).

06.I.11 Cold weather sheltering and clothing requirements.

   a. If wind chill is a factor at a work location, the cooling effect of the wind shall be reduced by shielding the work area or requiring employees to wear an outer windbreak layer garment. An AHA and/or PHA shall be prepared as an attachment to the site-specific, cold-stress monitoring plan and shall identify specific controls to minimize employee exposure to extreme cold.

   b. Extremities, ears, toes, and nose shall be protected from extreme cold by proper clothing such as hats, gloves, masks, etc .

   c. Employees whose clothing may become wet shall wear an outer layer of clothing that is impermeable to water.

   d. Outer garments must provide for ventilation to prevent wetting of inner clothing by sweat.

   e. If clothing is wet, the employee shall change into dry clothes before entering a cold environment.

   f. Employees shall change socks and removable felt insoles at regular daily intervals or shall use vapor barrier boots.

   g. Due to the added danger of cold injury due to evaporative cooling, employees handling evaporative liquid (such as gasoline, alcohol, or cleaning fluids) at air temperatures below 40 °F (4 °C) shall take precautions to avoid soaking of clothing or contact with skin.

EM 385-1-1
15 Sep 08

h. Eyewear providing protection against ultraviolet light, glare, and blowing ice crystals shall be provided employees in snow- and/or ice-covered terrain.

06.I.12 Environmental monitoring shall be conducted as follows:

a. At air temperatures below 45 °F (7 °C) the temperature shall be monitored <u>a minimum of every eight (8) hours or as warranted</u>.

b. <u>At temperatures below 45°F (7 °C) and above 30 °F (-1 °C) the temperature and wind speed shall be monitored every four (4) hours or as warranted.</u>

c. At air temperatures below 30 °F (-1 °C) the temperature <u>and wind speed</u> shall be measured and recorded at least every four (4) hours <u>or more frequently if it begins to lower</u>.

d. The equivalent chill temperature and frost-bite precautions shall be determined by using Tables 6-4 and 6-5.

EM 385-1-1
15 Sep 08

TABLES 6-4 and 6-5

Wind Chill Temperature Table

Wind Speed (mph) ↓	Air Temperature (°F)																	
	40	35	30	25	20	15	10	5	0	-5	-10	-15	-20	-25	-30	-35	-40	-45
0	40	35	30	25	20	15	10	5	0	-5	-10	-15	-20	-25	-30	-35	-40	-45
5	36	31	25	19	13	7	1	-5	-11	-16	-22	-28	-34	-40	-46	-52	-57	-63
10	34	27	21	15	9	3	-4	-10	-16	-22	-28	-35	-41	-47	-53	-59	-66	-72
15	32	25	19	13	6	0	-7	-13	-19	-26	-32	-39	-45	-51	-58	-64	-71	-77
20	30	24	17	11	4	-2	-9	-15	-22	-29	-35	-42	-48	-55	-61	-68	-74	-81
25	29	23	16	9	3	-4	-11	-17	-24	-31	-37	-44	-51	-58	-64	-71	-78	-84
30	28	22	15	8	1	-5	-12	-19	-26	-33	-39	-46	-53	-60	-67	-73	-80	-87
35	28	21	14	7	0	-7	-14	-21	-27	-34	-41	-48	-55	-62	-69	-76	-82	-89
40	27	20	13	6	-1	-8	-15	-22	-29	-36	-43	-50	-57	-64	-71	-78	-84	-91
45	26	19	12	5	-2	-9	-16	-23	-30	-37	-44	-51	-58	-65	-72	-79	-86	-93
50	26	19	12	4	-3	-10	-17	-24	-31	-38	-45	-52	-60	-67	-74	-81	-88	-95

RISK OF FROSTBITE (see times on chart below)

GREEN   LITTLE DANGER (frostbite occurs in >2 hours in dry, exposed skin)
YELLOW   INCREASED DANGER (frostbite could occur in 45 minutes or less in dry, exposed skin)
RED   GREAT DANGER (frostbite could occur in 5 minutes or less in dry, exposed skin)

Time to occurrence of frostbite in minutes or hours
(In the most susceptible 5% of personnel.)

Wind Speed (mph) ↓	Air Temperature (°F)										
	10	5	0	-5	-10	-15	-20	-25	-30	-35	-40	-45
0	>2h	>2h	>2h	>2h	>2h	>2h	40	22	20	13	11	9
5	>2h	>2h	>2h	>2h	31	22	17	14	12	11	9	8
10	>2h	>2h	>2h	28	19	15	12	10	9	7	7	6
15	>2h	>2h	33	20	15	12	9	8	7	6	5	4
20	>2h	>2h	23	16	12	9	8	8	6	5	4	4
25	>2h	42	19	13	10	8	7	6	5	4	4	3
30	>2h	28	16	12	9	7	6	5	4	4	3	3
35	>2h	23	14	10	8	6	5	4	4	3	3	2
40	>2h	20	13	9	7	6	5	4	3	3	2	2
45	>2h	18	12	8	7	5	4	4	3	3	2	2
50	>2h	16	11	8	6	5	4	3	3	2	2	2

WET SKIN COULD SIGNIFICANTLY DECREASE THE TIME FOR FROSTBITE TO OCCUR.

*Source: USARIEM Technical Note "SUSTAINING HEALTH & PERFORMANCE IN COLD WEATHER OPERATIONS," October 2001

EM 385-1-1
15 Sep 08

06.I.13 If employees express a concern about their ability to work in a cold environment, they shall provide medical documentation on their ability to work in cold weather (30 °F (-1 °C) or below). If medical documentation is provided that shows they are suffering from diseases or taking medication that interferes with normal body temperature regulation or reduces tolerance to work in cold environments, they should be excluded from the cold weather tasks.

06.J CUMULATIVE TRAUMA PREVENTION

06.J.01 Work activities that require employees to conduct lifting, handling, or carrying; rapid and frequent application of high grasping forces; repetitive hand/arm manipulations; tasks that include continuous, intermittent, impulsive, or impact hand-arm vibration or whole body vibration; and other physical activities that stress the body's capabilities shall be evaluated by a competent person to ensure the activities are designed to match the capabilities of the employees.

06.J.02 When work activities that stress the body's capabilities are identified, the employer shall incorporate it in the AHA and identify it as a hazard in the SSHP/APP. The plan shall incorporate processes that recognize cumulative trauma hazards, isolate causative factors, inform and train employees, and implement controls.

06.J.03 Control measures to minimize hand-arm vibration shall include: the use of anti-vibration tools and/or gloves; implementation of work practices that keep the employee's hands and body warm and minimize the vibration coupling between the employee and the vibration tool; application of specialized medical surveillance to identify personnel susceptible to vibration and adherence to the TLV guidelines as specified in the ACGIH in "Threshold Limit Values and Biological Exposure Indices";.

EM 385-1-1
15 Sep 08

06.K INDOOR AIR QUALITY (IAQ) MANAGEMENT

06.K.01 Investigations. Supervisors will report employee concerns or complaints of IAQ problems to the facility manager/owner or other designated representative. That individual will be responsible for investigating and resolving the IAQ complaint in a timely manner and reporting back to the supervisor. For leased facilities, procedures for resolving IAQ issues should ultimately be investigated and resolved by the lessor. An industrial hygienist or other qualified and competent person will initiate an IAQ investigation using appropriate guidelines published by ACGIH; AIHA; ANSI; American Society of Heating, Refrigeration, and Air Conditioning Engineers (ASHRAE); USEPA; OSHA; NIOSH; or other Federal, DOD, State, local, and host nation requirements.

   a. Ensure building activities, such as painting, roof repairs, carpet installation and repair and other activities likely to involve usage of chemicals or solvents, are conducted after normal working hours where possible or in a manner that will prevent exposure to occupants.

   b. <u>Evaluate the condition of the air-handling system for proper operation, make-up air supply, blocked dampers or diffusers, cleanliness of ducts and filters, and standing water or wet areas.</u>

   c. Educate employees and supervisors concerning measures they can take to help maintain acceptable IAQ in their work areas. Employees shall be instructed not to make unauthorized modifications to the heating, ventilation, and air conditioning (HVAC) systems (i.e., blocking off vents, removing ceiling tiles).

06.K.02 Environmental tobacco smoke (ETS). Employees shall be protected from involuntary exposure to ETS in working and public living environments.

   a. Smoking shall be prohibited inside all DOD vehicles, aircraft, vessels, and work buildings.

EM 385-1-1
15 Sep 08

b. Designated smoking areas only in outdoor locations that are not commonly used or accessed by nonsmokers shall be provided. Receptacles will be provided in designated smoking areas for the containment of cigarette butts and other smoking by-products.

c. Designated smoking areas shall be located away from supplied-air intakes and building entryways/egresses to prevent ETS from entering occupied buildings and structures.

06.K.03 Mold Evaluation. Because mold can contribute to health problems ranging from minor irritation to serious debilitation if found in high quantities or improper locations, a mold assessment shall be performed when need is indicated.

a. Assessments/remediation shall be overseen by a person experienced in understanding both the properties of mold behaviors and building design or construction. This person may be an industrial hygienist, microbiologist, or a qualified mold inspector who has been certified by an independent IAQ certifying agency and/or who can demonstrate training and experience in the IAQ investigative field. Some states, local authorities and host nations also require this person to be licensed.

b. Assessment of potential mold hazards shall first be visual and based on criteria in the USACHPPM, TG 278, Industrial Hygiene Preventive Medicine Mold Assessment Guide, the EPA Indoor Air Quality Checklists, and guidance from AIHA. Bulk and/or air samples are generally not necessary to evaluate mold hazardous environments. In climates with high humidity, it may be necessary to perform both qualitative and quantitative air samples of indoor and outdoor locations in order to determine the extent of the impact on the building and to set a pre-remediation baseline.

c. Causes of mold (i.e., water leakages, seepages, drainage, HVAC/ insulation repaired, etc.) shall be addressed before completing mold remediation.

EM 385-1-1
15 Sep 08

06.K.04 Mold Remediation. If the assessment reveals mold remediation is required, then USACHPPM TG 277, Army Facilities Management Information Document on Mold Remediation Issues and any local, state, or host nation guidelines or regulations shall be used.

a. A remediation plan shall be written by a qualified mold expert and shall include: location and extent of the mold, description of conditions found (i.e. wet or dry), type of materials or 'substrate' that the mold is growing on, whether the substrate can be cleaned or must be removed, source or problem which created the mold, repair of building structure or component that is the source, and whether the mold contaminated area can be isolated from the remainder of the building and or its occupants. The plan shall also include, at a minimum, an AHA describing the steps involved in remediation, identified hazards, recommended controls, equipment and materials (i.e., fungicide or bleach used for removal), inspection requirements and training requirements.

b. Mold remediation should not be performed by the same entity that performed the evaluation.

c. Employees in the immediate area of the mold remediation shall be informed of the remediation, results of any testing, and symptoms of the hazard.

d. Post remediation air sampling shall be done in the immediate area and in any areas in the mold spore or vegetative air-pathway. Mold in areas above drop ceilings with combined air plenums shall have air samples taken within the plenum as well as in air-serviced areas. Air samples should be taken in the immediate area of remediation and analyzed by a laboratory in the AIHA Environmental Microbiology Laboratory Accreditation Program.

EM 385-1-1
15 Sep 08

06.L Control of Chromium (VI) Exposure

06.L.01 General. All activities which could generate chromium (VI) fumes, mists, or dusts shall be evaluated by an IH or SP to determine potential personnel exposure over the OSHA chromium (VI) standards. Typical operations where chromium exposures are high include: Portland cement greater than 20 parts per million (ppm) chromium, cutting or breaking up of cement surfaces, painting or paint removal operations, heating or welding on stainless steel, cutting or breaking up wood treated with preservatives, and handling or applying anti-corrosive substances or coatings.

   a. The evaluation may be objective or air sampling as described in CFR 1910.1026.

   b. The evaluation shall be added as an appendix to the APP and AHA.

06.L.02 To prevent exposure to Chromium (VI), the use of paints with chromium pigments, Portland cement with greater than 20 ppm chromium, or chromium/arsenic treated lumber shall be avoided when possible. Should chromium (VI) containing products be required, a justification and similar non-chromium (VI) product evaluation shall be conducted and submitted for review by the GDA.

06.L.03 If chromium containing compounds are used and the objective determination is inconclusive, before air sampling confirms the level of exposure, the employer shall comply with the requirements of 1910.1026, 1915.1026, or 1926.1126, whichever is applicable. At a minimum, employers shall provide appropriate PPE, respirators, washing facilities, and a lunch room/area clean from chromium dust and/or fume.

06.L.04 If air sampling confirms chromium (VI) exposure over the OEL, and there is no adequate substitute or work practice change (i.e., use of argon instead of carbon dioxide when arc welding), then the employer shall provide appropriate engineering controls,

EM 385-1-1
15 Sep 08

i.e., local HEPA filtered ventilation systems, medical surveillance, and air sampling as required by the applicable chromium (VI) standard. If adequate engineering controls are not feasible or appropriate due to the length of the task, then PPE shall be provided.

06.M CRYSTALLINE SILICA

06.M.01 Occupational Standards

a. Employee airborne exposure to crystalline silica shall not exceed the 8-hour TWA limit as specified by the ACGIH in their "Threshold Limit Values and Biological Exposure Indices" or by OSHA, whichever is more stringent. Table 6-3 provides U.S. guidelines and limits for occupational exposure to crystalline silica established by NIOSH, OSHA, MSHA, and ACGIH as of the date of this manual.

b. Mandatory requirements.

(1) Employee exposure shall be eliminated through the implementation of feasible engineering controls.

(2) After all such controls are implemented and they do not control to the OEL, each employer must rotate its employees to the extent possible in order to reduce exposure.

(3) When all engineering or administrative controls have been implemented, and the level of respirable silica still exceeds OEL, an employer rely on a respirator program pursuant to the mandatory requirements of Section 5 E. and 29 CFR 1910.134.

06.M.02 Monitoring.

a. Each employer who has a place of employment in which silica is occupationally produced, reacted, released, transported, stored, handled, or used shall inspect each workplace and work operation to determine if any employee may be exposed to silica at or above the OEL. This evaluation

EM 385-1-1
15 Sep 08

shall be documented in the AHA for the job/task to be completed.

b. Air monitoring and analysis. Sampling and analytical methods shall be in accordance with those specified in Section 6A.

TABLE 6-6

U.S. GUIDELINES AND LIMITS FOR OCCUPATIONAL EXPOSURE TO CRYSTALLINE SILICA

Reference	Substance	Guideline or limit (mg/m^3)
NIOSH	Crystalline silica: quartz, cristobalite, and tridymite as respirable dust	REL = 0.05 (for up to 10-hr workday during a 40-hr workweek
OSHA [29 CFR 1910.1000, Table Z-3]	Respirable crystalline silica, quartz	PEL = 10 / %quartz+2 (8-hr TWA)
	Respirable crystalline silica, cristobalite	PEL = half the value calculated from the formula for quartz
MSHA [30 CFR 56, 57, 70, 71]	Respirable quartz in underground and surface metal and nonmetal mines	PEL = 10 / %quartz+2 (8-hr TWA)
	Respirable crystalline silica present in concentrations greater than 5% in surface and underground coal mines	RDS = 10 / %quartz (8-hr TWA)
ACGIH [20062]	Respirable crystalline silica, quartz	TLV = 0.025 (8-hr TWA)
	Respirable crystalline silica, cristobalite	TLV = 0.025 (8-hr TWA)

REL = Recommended Exposure Limit - NIOSH
PEL = Permissible Exposure Limit - OSHA
RDS = Respirable Dust Standard - MSHA
TLV = Threshold Limit Value - ACGIH

EM 385-1-1
15 Sep 08

06.M.03 Medical Surveillance. Each employer shall institute a medical surveillance program for all employees who are exposed to airborne concentrations of silica above the OEL. The employer shall provide each employee a medical examination performed by or under the supervision of a licensed physician and shall provide the examination during the employee's normal working hours without cost to the employee. The content of the medical exam shall be determined by the physician based on the exposure records of the employee and guidance provided by NIOSH Standard DHS pub. No 92-102 Aug 1992 or OSHA Instruction CPL 2-2.7 Oct 30, 1972.

a. Medical examinations shall also be made available:

(1) At least annually for each employee exposed to airborne concentrations of silica above the OEL at any time during the preceding 6 months; and

(2) Upon notification by the employee that the employee has developed signs or symptoms commonly associated with chronic exposure to silica.

b. Where medical examinations are performed, the employer shall provide the examining physician with the following information:

(1) The reason for the medical examination requested;

(2) A description of the affected employee's duties as they relate to the employee's exposure;

(3) A description of any PPE used or to be used;

(4) The results of the employee's exposure measurements, if available; and

EM 385-1-1
15 Sep 08

(5) Upon request of the physician, information concerning previous medical examination of the affected employee.

c. Physician's written opinion. The employer shall obtain and furnish the employee with a written opinion from the examining physician containing the following:

(1) The signs or symptoms of silica exposure manifested by the employee, if any;

(2) A report on the findings of any medical tests completed.

(3) The physician's opinion as to whether the employee has any detected medical condition that would place the employee at increased risk of material impairment to the employee's health from exposure to silica or would directly or indirectly aggravate any detected medical condition;

(4) Any recommended limitation upon the employee's exposure to silica or the use of PPE; and

(5) A statement that the employee has been informed by the physician of any medical condition that requires further examination or treatment.

06.M.04 Training. Each employee who may be potentially exposed to silica shall be instructed at the beginning of his/her employment or assignment of potential silica exposure in the following:

a. Relevant symptoms; appropriate emergency procedures; and proper conditions and precautions for safe use or exposure;

b. To advise the employer of the development of the signs and symptoms of prolonged exposure to silica;

c. Specific nature of operations that could result in exposure to silica above the OEL, as well as safe work practices for the

EM 385-1-1
15 Sep 08

release of the silica and the types and function of engineering controls;

d. Proper housekeeping practices;

e. The purpose, proper use, and limitations of respirators;

f. A description of, and explain the purposes for, the medical surveillance program; and

g. The increased risk of impaired health due to the combination of smoking and silica dust exposure.

06.M.05 Respiratory Protection.

a. When the exposure limits to silica cannot be met by limiting the concentrations of silica in the work environment by engineering and administrative controls, an employer must use a respiratory protection program meeting the requirements of 29 CFR 1910.134 and Section 5.G. A respirator specified for use in higher concentrations of airborne silica may be used in atmospheres of lower concentrations.

b. Properly fitted particulate-filter respirators may be used for short, intermittent, or occasional dust exposures such as cleanup, dumping of dust collectors, or unloading shipments of sand at a receiving point when it is not feasible to control the dust by enclosure, exhaust ventilation, wetting, or other means.

06.M.06 Protective Clothing. Where exposure to airborne silica or other substances is above the OEL, work clothing shall be HEPA vacuumed before removal unless it is wet. Clothes shall not be cleaned by blowing or shaking.

06.M.07 Housekeeping.

a. To prevent the dispersal of silica dust, all exposed surfaces shall be maintained free of accumulation of silica dust.

b. Dry sweeping and the use of compressed air for the cleaning of floors and other surfaces shall be prohibited. If vacuuming is used the exhaust air shall be HEPA filtered to prevent generation of airborne respirable silica concentrations. Gentle washdown of surfaces is preferred.

c. Emphasis shall be placed upon preventive maintenance and repair of equipment, proper storage of dust producing materials, and collection of dusts containing silica. Sanitation shall meet the requirements of 29 CFR 1910.141.

06.M.08 Personal Hygiene Facilities and Practices..

a. All food, beverages, tobacco products, nonfood chewing products, and unapplied cosmetics shall be discouraged in work areas.

b. Employers shall provide adequate washing facilities to include water and soap.

06.M.09 Engineering Controls.

a. Dust suppression. Moisture, mists, fogs, etc., shall be added where such addition can substantially reduce the exposure to airborne respirable silica dust.

b. Ventilation. Where a local exhaust ventilation and collection system is used in a building, it shall be designed and maintained to prevent the accumulation or recirculation of airborne silica dust into the workplace. The system shall be inspected periodically. Adequate measures shall be taken to ensure that any discharge will not produce health hazards to the outside environment.

c. Additional control measures. When mobile equipment is operated in areas of potential silica exposure, engineering controls shall be provided to protect the operator from such exposure.

06.M.10 Itinerant Work. When employees are exposed to airborne silica at temporary work sites away from the primary worksite, emphasis shall be placed on respiratory protection, protective clothing, portable engineering controls, and provisions for personal hygiene and sanitation. Training of employees shall be provided to protect them as well as others from airborne silica dust exposure.

BLANK

SECTION 7

LIGHTING

07.A GENERAL

07.A.01 While work is in progress, offices, facilities, accessways, working areas, construction roads, etc., shall be lighted by at least the minimum light intensities specified in Table 7-1. <u>If lighting provided is questionable as to intensity, light monitoring shall be performed to insure proper light intensities are provided.</u>

07.A.02 Office lighting shall be in accordance with ANSI/ Illuminating Engineering Society of North America (IESNA) RP-1.

07.A.03 Roadway lighting shall be in accordance with ANSI/IESNA RP-8.

07.A.04 Marine lighting shall be in accordance with ANSI/IESNA RP-12.

07.A.05 Means of egress.

> a. Means of egress shall be illuminated, with emergency and non-emergency lighting, to provide a minimum of 1 footcandle (fc), [1 lumen per square foot (lm/ft^2)], (11 lux (lx), measured at the floor. **> *Reference NFPA 101.***

> b. The illumination shall be arranged so that the failure of any single lighting unit, including the burning out of an electric bulb, will not leave any area in total darkness, <u>impeding the means of egress.</u>

07.A.06 Lamps and fixtures will be guarded and secured to preclude injury to personnel. Open fluorescent fixtures will be provided with wire guards, lenses, tube guards and locks, or safety sockets that require force in the horizontal axis to remove the lamp.

EM 385-1-1
15 Sep 08

07.A.07 Lamps for general illumination shall be protected from accidental contact or breakage. Protection shall be provided by elevation of at least 7 ft (2.1 m) from normal working surface, suitable fixture or lamp holder with a guard. <u>Additionally, fixtures may be no closer than 18 in (0.5 m) to overhead sprinkler systems, if the building is so equipped, per NFPA Standards.</u>

<u>07.A.08 If work is to be performed at night, a night operations lighting plan shall be developed to ensure that all activities, areas and operations are adequately illuminated to perform work safely.</u>

<u>07.A.09 For temporary lighting, see Section 11.E.06.</u>

TABLE 7-1

MINIMUM LIGHTING REQUIREMENTS

Facility or function	Illuminance – lx (lm/ft^2)
Accessways - general indoor - general outdoor - exitways, walkways, ladders, stairs	 55 (5) 33 (3) 110 (10)
Administrative areas (offices, drafting and meeting rooms, etc.)	540 (50)
Chemical laboratories	540 (50)
Construction areas - general indoor - general outdoor - tunnels and general underground work areas (minimum 110 lx required at tunnel and shaft heading during drilling, mucking, and scaling)	 55 (5) 33 (3) 55 (5)
Conveyor routes	110 (10)
Docks and loading platforms	33 (3)
Elevators, freight and passenger	215 (20)
First-aid stations and infirmaries	325 (30)
Maintenance/operating areas/shops - vehicle maintenance shop - carpentry shop - outdoors field maintenance area - refueling area, outdoors - shops, fine detail work - shops, medium detail work - welding shop	 325 (30) 110 (10) 55 (5) 55 (5) 540 (50) 325 (30) 325 (30)
Mechanical/electrical equipment rooms	110 (10)
Parking areas	33 (3)
Toilets, wash, and dressing rooms	110 (10)
Visitor areas	215 (20)
Warehouses and storage rooms/areas - indoor stockroom, active/bulk storage - indoor stockroom, inactive - indoor rack storage - outdoor storage	 110 (10) 55 (5) 270 (25) 33 (3)
Work areas – general (not listed above)	325 (30)

BLANK

EM 385-1-1
15 Sep 08

SECTION 8

ACCIDENT PREVENTION SIGNS, TAGS, LABELS, SIGNALS, PIPING SYSTEM IDENTIFICATION AND TRAFFIC CONTROL

08.A. SIGNS, TAGS, LABELS AND PIPING SYSTEMS

08.A.01 Signs, tags, and labels shall be provided to give adequate warning and caution of hazards. They are provided to instruct and direct workers and the public.

08.A.02 All warning systems such as signs, tags, and labels shall be visible at all times when the hazard or problem exists, and shall be removed or covered when the hazard or problem no longer exists.

08.A.03 All employees shall be informed as to the meaning of the various signs, tags, and labels used throughout the workplace and any special precautions that may be required.

08.A.04 The safety and occupational health related signs in the USACE sign manual (EP 310-1-6a) have been determined to meet or exceed ANSI and/or OSHA requirements. USACE facilities shall use signs based upon the specifications in the USACE Sign Manual at permanent USACE-owned and USACE-operated sites. USACE employees and contractors may opt to use signs meeting either the OSHA or ANSI standards for temporary use during the life of a project.

08.A.05 Signs, Tags, Placards, Labels, and Piping Systems shall meet or exceed the following standards:

   a. USACE *Sign Standards Manual*, EP 310 1-6;

   b. 29 CFR 1910.145;

   c. ANSI/IEEE C95.2;

EM 385-1-1
15 Sep 08

    d. ANSI Z136.1;

    e. ANSI Z535.1;

    f. ANSI Z535.2;

    g. ANSI Z535.5;

    h. ANSI/ASME A13.1; and

    i. DOT Federal Highway Administration, *Manual on Uniform Traffic Control Devices for Streets and Highways* (MUTCD).

08.A 06 The type of sign or tag used in a particular situation shall be appropriate for the degree of hazard or intent of message. The Workplace Safety signs with Danger and Caution headings have standard legends that must be used exactly as shown in the USACE Sign Standards Manual. If a sign with a unique legend not appearing on pages 11-4 to 11-7 or in the UNICOR catalog is needed, the procedures detailed on page 1-13 should be followed. The sign legend shall be concise, easy to read and should contain enough information to be easily understood. *> See Figure 8-1 for Sign and Tag Signal Word Headings; Figure 8-2 for Example Tag Layout; Figure 8-3 for Example Sign Layout; Table 8-1 for Accident Prevention Sign Requirements.*

    a. DANGER SIGNS: Danger signs must conform to the following requirements:

    (1) Danger signs will be used only when the circumstances indicate an imminently hazardous situation that, if not avoided, **will** result in death or serious injury.

    (2) Signal word.

    (a) USACE Standard: The signal word "Danger" is white on a red background at the top of the sign.

(b) ANSI Alternate Standard: Danger signs must have the signal word "**DANGER**" in white letters placed at the top of a rectangular safety red background placed at the top of the sign. The safety alert symbol shall precede the signal word. The base of symbol shall be on the same horizontal level as the base of the letters of the signal word - the height equaling or exceeding the signal word height. *> See Figure 8-1.*

(c) OSHA Alternate Standard: As an alternative, Danger Signs may have "**DANGER**" in white letters on a safety red oval background with a white border on a black rectangular field. This distinctive panel shall appear in the uppermost portion of the sign. No other signal word or symbol shall be used within this distinctive shape and color arrangement.

(3) The message panel.

(a) USACE Standard: For workplace safety signs the lettering describing the specific danger is black letters on a white background. On other approved Danger Signs, the message is white lettering on a red background.

(b) OSHA or ANSI Alternate Standard: The lettering shall be black letters on a white background or white letters on a black background and the symbol/pictorial panel, if used, shall be square with a black safety red, or black and safety red symbol on a white background.

b. WARNING SIGNS: Warning signs must conform to the following requirements:

(1) Warning signs may be used only when the circumstances indicate a potentially hazardous situation that, if not avoided, **could** result in death or serious injury. The hazards may be the same as those associated with Danger signs but are of significantly less magnitude.

EM 385-1-1
15 Sep 08

(2) Signal Word.

(a) USACE Standard: On approved Warning Safety signs the signal word "Warning" appears in black lettering on a yellow-green background under a black top border. There are no Warning workplace safety signs in the Corps system.

(b) ANSI Standard: Warning signs must have the signal word "**WARNING**" in black letters on a rectangular range background placed at the top of the sign. The safety alert symbol shall precede the signal word. The base of symbol shall be on the same horizontal level as the base of the letters of the signal word – the height equaling or exceeding the signal word height. > *See Figure 8-1.*

(c) OSHA Standard Alternative: As an alternative, Warning Signs may have the signal word "**WARNING**" in black lettering within a safety orange truncated diamond on a black rectangular background. The distinctive panel shall be located at the uppermost portion of the sign. No other word or symbol shall be used within this distinctive shape or color arrangement.

(3) The message panel.

(a) USACE Standard: On approved Warning signs the message panel shall be in black lettering on a yellow-green background.

(b) OSHA or ANSI Alternate Standard: The message panel shall be in black lettering on a white background or white lettering on a black background. The message may, as an alternative, be in black letters on a safety orange background. The symbol/pictorial panel, if used, shall be square with a black symbol on a white background. The symbol panel used as an alternative may be square with a black symbol on an orange background.

c. CAUTION SIGNS: Caution signs must conform to the following requirements:

EM 385-1-1
15 Sep 08

(1) Caution signs may be used only when circumstances indicate a potentially hazardous situation that, if not avoided, **may** result in a minor or moderate injury. It may also be used to alert against unsafe practices that may result in property damage. The hazards may be the same as those associated with Danger signs but are of significantly less magnitude.

(2) Signal Word.

(a) USACE Standard: On Workplace Safety Signs the word "Caution" appears in yellow lettering on black bar at the top of the yellow message panel. On other approved Caution Safety Signs the signal word "Caution" appears in black lettering on a yellow-green background under a black top border.

(b) Alternate ANSI Standard: Caution signs must have the signal word "**CAUTION**" in black lettering on a rectangular yellow background placed at the top of the sign. The safety alert symbol shall precede the signal word if the hazard is a potential personal injury hazard. (The alert symbol is not used when the situation is used to indicate property damage hazards.) The base of the symbol shall be on the same horizontal level as the base of the letters of the signal word – the height shall equal or exceed the signal word height. **> See Figure 8-1.**

(c) Alternate OSHA Standard: As an alternative, caution signs may have the signal word "**CAUTION**" in safety yellow letters within a black rectangular background, and this distinctive panel shall be located in the uppermost portion of the sign. No other signal word or symbol shall be used with this distinctive color or signal shape arrangement.

(3) Message Panel.

(a) USACE Standard: The descriptive legend appears in black lettering on a yellow panel.

EM 385-1-1
15 Sep 08

(b) OSHA or ANSI Alternate Standard: The message panel shall be in black lettering on a white background or white lettering on a black background. The message may, as an alternative, be in black lettering on a safety yellow background. The symbol/pictorial panel, if used, shall be square with a black symbol on a white background. As an alternative, it may be square with a black symbol on a safety yellow background.

d. NOTICE SIGNS: Notice signs should conform to the following requirements:

(1) Notice signs may be used to indicate a statement of company policy directly or indirectly related to the safety of personnel or protection of property. The signal word SHOULD NOT be associated directly with a hazard or hazardous situation, and shall not be used in place of "Danger", "Warning", or "Caution." These signs are used to control or define access and circulation. They are used primarily for information and are not placed to identify a hazard.

(2) Notice signs shall have the signal word "Notice" in white lettering on a safety blue background on a rectangular field, and this distinctive panel shall be located in the uppermost portion of the visual alerting device. No other signal word or symbol shall be used within this distinctive shape and color arrangement.

(3) Message panel:

(a) General Standards for Workplace: The message shall be in safety blue or black letters on a white background. The symbol/pictorial panel, if used, shall be square with a safety blue or black symbol on a white background.

(b) USACE Alternative for Outdoor Use: Notice signs posted on USACE managed property for public viewing in areas accessible to the public, including recreation areas, may have white letters on blue background. Text for these custom signs shall be approved by the District Sign Manager. Other signs

EM 385-1-1
15 Sep 08

used to define access and use may include prohibition symbol signs or Restricted Area signs.

e. GENERAL SAFETY SIGNS: General safety signs should conform to the following requirements:

(1) General safety signs may be used to indicate general instructions relative to safe work practices, remind of proper safety procedures or indicate the location of safety equipment. These signs identify rules and facilities relating to health, first aid, medical equipment, sanitation, housekeeping practice and general safety information.

(2) Legend Panel: White signal word "Safety" on safety green header with black text on white panel.

f. FIRE SAFETY SIGNS: Fire safety signs shall conform to the following requirements:

(1) Fire safety signs may be used to indicate the location of emergency firefighting equipment. Fire extinguisher signs shall be placed where fire extinguishers cannot be directly seen from designated exit pathways. (NFPA 10 D2.2.2)

(2) These signs do NOT have a signal word.

(3) The message panel shall be in safety red letters on a white background in either a square or rectangular field. The symbol/pictorial panel, if used, shall be safety red on white or white on safety red.

g. DIRECTIONAL ARROW SIGNS: Directional arrow flow signs should conform to the following requirements:

(1) Directional arrow signs may be used to indicate the direction to emergency equipment, safety equipment, and other locations important to safety.

EM 385-1-1
15 Sep 08

(2) Directional signs that relate to accident prevention use a format similar to all other Workplace Safety signs. The header shall have white lettering on a black rectangular background. The arrow symbol shall be in black lettering on a white background.

h. COLORS: Color coding shall be in accordance with Table 8-2 of this manual. Color specifications for Corps safety signs are found in the USACE Sign Standards Manual.

i. Piping systems shall be identified. The identification of piping systems (including pipes, fittings, valves, and pipe coverings) shall be in accordance with Table 8-3 of this manual.

j. The RF radiation hazard-warning symbol specified in Figure 8-4 of this manual shall be used in the identification of RF radiation hazards.

k. Laser caution and warning signs shall be in accordance with ANSI Z136.1. *> See Figures 8-5 and 8-6 for examples.*

l. Ionizing radiation warning signs, labels, and signals shall contain the symbol show in Figure 8-7 of this manual.

m. Vehicles or equipment that, by design, move at 25 miles per hour (mph) (1.1 meters per second (m/s)) or less on public roads shall display the slow-moving vehicle emblem. *> See Figure 8-8.*

08.A.07 Safety sign finishes shall be of durable materials with colors in accordance with the <u>USACE Signs Standards Manual</u>, or ANSI Z535.1.

08.A.08 Safety signs shall be so placed to alert and inform the viewer in sufficient time to take appropriate evasive actions to avoid the potential harm from the hazard. They shall be legible, non-distracting, and not hazardous in themselves. They shall be <u>fabricated</u> with <u>retro</u>-reflective sheeting as appropriate for adequate visibility under normal and emergency operating conditions.

EM 385-1-1
15 Sep 08

08.A.09 Each container of hazardous material shall be labeled, tagged or marked with the identity of the material(s), appropriate hazard warnings, potential health effects and the name and address of the manufacturer, importer or other responsible party. **> See 06.B.01**

    a. Signs, placards, process sheets, batch tickets, operating procedures, or other written means may be used in lieu of affixing labels to stationary process containers if the alternative method identifies the containers to which it is applicable and conveys the information required above. The written information shall be readily available to employees in their work area throughout each work shift.

    b. Portable containers into which hazardous material(s) are transferred from labeled containers and which are intended only for the immediate use by the employee who performs the transfer are not required to be labeled. However, there shall be a means of indicating that the hazardous material has been used in the container.

08.A.10 Signs, tags and labels shall be located as close as safely possible to their respective hazards. Tags will be affixed by a positive means (such as wire, string, or adhesive) that prevents their loss or unintentional removal.

08.A.11 Signs, tags, and labels shall be legible and in English.

    a. <u>In areas where a significant percentage of the workforce or the visiting population speaks primarily in a foreign language, the use of symbol signs is strongly encouraged.</u> **> See USACE Sign Standards Manual, Section 8.**

    b. <u>When no symbols exist or where words are essential, two signs - one in English and one in the foreign language - should be placed side by side.</u>

EM 385-1-1
15 Sep 08

c. These signs will follow the same format: same overall size, letter size and style, color, and mounting.

d. Because of variations in dialect, the legends on non-English signs shall be developed at the local level.

e. Two languages should never appear on the same sign.
> See 01.A.04.

08.A.12 Signs shall be furnished with rounded or blunt corners and shall be free from sharp edges, burrs, splinters, or other sharp projections. The ends or heads of bolts or other fastening devices shall be located so that they are not a hazard.

08.A.13 Construction areas shall be posted with legible traffic signs at points of hazard in accordance with the MUTCD.

08.A.14 Signs required to be seen at night shall be reflectorized.

08.A.15 Accident prevention tags shall be used only as a temporary means of warning employees of an existing hazard, such as defective tools, equipment, and lockout. *> See Figure 8-9; See Section 12 for lockout/tagout requirements.*

08.A.16 Tags shall contain a signal word (either **"DANGER"** or **"CAUTION"**) and a major message (presented in either pictographs, written text, or both) to indicate the specific hazardous condition or the instruction to be communicated to the employee. The signal word shall be readable at a minimum distance of 5 ft (1.5 m) or such greater distance as warranted by the hazard. The signal word and major message shall be understandable to all employees who may be exposed to the hazard. *> See 08.A.05 for basic design criteria.*

08.A.17 Accident prevention tags shall be rectangular in shape and shall be no smaller than 3 in x 5 in (8 cm x 13 cm). The corners may be square cut, chamfered, or rounded.

EM 385-1-1
15 Sep 08

08.A.18 Kerosene lamps and open flame pots shall not be used for, or with, warning signs or devices.

08.A.19 Warning signs shall be placed on unattended Government-owned floating plant and land-based heavy equipment accessible to the public and shall read "**No Trespassing – U.S. Government Property**."

08.B SIGNAL SYSTEMS, PERSONNEL AND PROCEDURES

08.B.01 A standard signal system shall be used on all operations.

    a. Hand signals for crane operations shall conform to ANSI/ASME B30 series. > *See Figures 16-1.*

    b. Traffic flagging procedures shall be in accordance with the DOT Federal Highway Administration's MUTCD.

    c. For Marine signals, see Section 19 of this manual.

    d. For helicopter hand signals, see Figure 16-2 of this manual.

08.B.02 Standard hand signals shall be posted at the operator's position, signal control points and other points as necessary to inform those concerned.

08.B.03 Manual (hand) signals may be used when the distance between the operator and signal person is not more than 100 ft (30.4 m). Radio, telephone, or a visual and audible electrically-operated system shall be used when the distance between operator and signal person is more than 100 ft or when they cannot see each other.

08.B.04 A signal person shall be provided when the point of operation (includes area of load travel and area immediately surrounding the load placement) is not in full view of the vehicle, machine, or equipment operator; when vehicles are backed more than 100 ft (30.4 m); when terrain is hazardous; or when two or more vehicles are backing in the same area.

EM 385-1-1
15 Sep 08

08.B.05 A flag person or other controls shall be provided when operations or equipment on or next to a highway create a traffic hazard. An exception shall be made only when an adequate mechanical signaling or control device is provided for safe direction of the operation.

08.B.06 Where manual (hand) signals are used, only one person shall be designated to give signals to the operator. This signal person shall be located to see the load and be clearly visible to the operator at all times.

08.B.07 Flag signaling shall be accomplished by use of red flags at least 18 in (45.7 cm) square or sign paddles. In periods of darkness, red lights shall be used.

08.B.08 High visibility apparel shall be worn by flag and signal persons. > *See Section 05.F.*

08.B.09 Signal systems shall be protected against unauthorized use, breakage, weather, or interference; any malfunction shall be cause to stop all work.

08.B.10 Only persons who are competent and qualified by experience and/or training with the operations being directed shall be used as signal persons.

08.B.11 Signal persons shall back one vehicle at a time. While under control of a signal person, the driver shall not back or maneuver until directed and the driver shall stop when visual contact with the signal person is lost.

08.B.12 The signal person shall have a warning device of clear range and penetrating sound to warn persons when the load is coming in so they have time to get in the clear.

08.C TRAFFIC CONTROL

08.C.01 Traffic control shall be accomplished in accordance with DOT Federal Highway Administration's MUTCD.

EM 385-1-1
15 Sep 08

08.C.02 The Contractor shall conduct his operations in such a manner as to offer the least possible obstruction to the safe and satisfactory movement of traffic over the existing roads during the life of the contract.

08.C.03 The Contractor shall be responsible for providing, erecting, maintaining, and removing all traffic signs, barricades, and other traffic control devices necessary for maintenance of traffic.

08.C.04 All barricades, warning signs, lights, temporary signals, other devices, flagmen, and signaling devices shall meet or exceed the minimum requirements of the local DOT requirements.

08.C.05 Prior to the commencement of contract operations, the Contractor shall submit for acceptance the complete details of the proposed traffic control plan for the maintenance of traffic and access through the contract work area.

08.C.06 The Contractor shall coordinate with the GDA and obtain approval from local authorities prior to closing or restricting any roads.

08.C.07 Barricades, danger, warning and detour signs, as required, shall be erected before any roads are closed.

    a. When roads are temporarily closed to public access, barricades or gates shall be used that are highly visible in day or night conditions. At a minimum, barriers shall be coated with reflective paint or be applied with highly reflective tape on both sides, and be signed with R11-2, 'ROAD CLOSED'.

    b. Affected roads shall also be posted with appropriate warning signs a minimum of 100 ft (30.5 m) before the barrier by W20-3, DNG-11, WRN-24, or other appropriate signs from the MUTCD or EP 310-6-1a. Size and placement of signs depends on viewing distance and speed limit of roadway.

EM 385-1-1
15 Sep 08

FIGURE 8-1

SIGN AND TAG SIGNAL WORD HEADINGS

USACE	ANSI	OSHA
WARNING Warning	⚠ **WARNING** Warning	**WARNING** Warning
DANGER Danger	⚠ **DANGER** Danger	**DANGER** Danger
CAUTION Caution - Workplace Safety	⚠ **CAUTION** Caution	**CAUTION** Caution
CAUTION Caution - Undesignated Safety		
SAFETY Safety		
NOTICE Notice		

FIGURE 8-2

EXAMPLE TAG LAYOUT

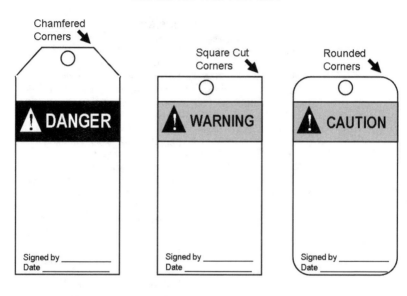

EM 385-1-1
15 Sep 08

TABLE 8-1

ACCIDENT PREVENTION SIGN REQUIREMENTS

TYPE	PURPOSE	DESIGN
DANGER	Indicates a specific immediate and grave danger, a hazard capable of producing irreversible damage or injury, and prohibition against harmful activity.	Layout as shown in Fig 8-1. Shall have "DANGER" in white letters at top of rectangular safety red background placed at top of sign. Safety alert symbol shall precede signal word. Base of symbol shall be on same horizontal level as base of letters of signal word-height equaling or exceeding signal word height. Alternate OSHA or ANSI requirement calls for lettering to be black letters on white background or white letters on black background and symbol/pictorial panel, if used, shall be square with black safety red, or black and safety red symbol on a white background. The USACE standard requires that the specific danger be described in black letters on a white background. On other approved Danger signs, the message is white lettering on a red background.
CAUTION	Call attention to a specific potential hazard capable of resulting in severe, but not irreversible, injury or damage.	Layout as shown in Fig 8-1. Shall have "CAUTION" in yellow on black background and lower panel for additional sign wording in black on a yellow background.

EM 385-1-1
15 Sep 08

TABLE 8-1 (Continued)

ACCIDENT PREVENTION SIGN REQUIREMENTS

TYPE	PURPOSE	DESIGN
GENERAL SAFETY	Includes notices of general practice and rules relating to health, first aid, medical equipment, sanitation, housekeeping, and general safety.	Layout as shown in Fig 8-1 or consisting of single panel. Shall have appropriate keyword as signal word in white on a green background in the upper panel and a lower panel for additional sign wording or symbols in black or green on a white background. Alternatively, the entire sign may be white letters on a green background.
FIRE AND EMERGENCY	Used only to label or points the way to fire extinguishing equipment, fires escapes and exits, gas shutoff valves, sprinkler drains, and emergency procedures.	Layout as shown in Fig 8-1 or consisting of a single red panel. Shall have the appropriate keyword as the signal word in white on a red background in the upper panel and a lower panel for additional sign wording or symbols in red on a white background. Alternatively, the entire sign may be white letters on a red background.
INFORMATION	Provide information of a general nature, such as designation of facilities or services, in order to avoid confusion or misunderstanding.	Layout as shown in Fig 8-1 or consisting of a single panel. Should have signal word "NOTICE" in white on blue background in upper panel and lower panel for additional wording or symbols in blue or black on a white background OR entire sign may be white letters on blue background.
EXIT	Used to indicate exits.	Lettered in legible letters, not less than 6 in (15.2 cm) high, on white field. The principal stroke of letters shall be at least 3/4 in (5.1 cm) in width.

EM 385-1-1
15 Sep 08

TABLE 8-2

ACCIDENT PREVENTION COLOR CODING

COLOR	PURPOSE
Red	Red shall be the color used for identifying dangerous conditions, emergency controls, fire detection equipment and fire suppression systems, and containers of flammable liquids.
Orange	Orange shall be the color used for designating dangerous parts of machines and energized equipment. Orange shall also be used for temporary traffic control signs in construction zones.
Yellow	Yellow shall be the color for designating conditions requiring caution, marking dangerous chemicals, marking physical hazards, and markings for ionizing radiation.
Green	Green shall be the color for designating safety equipment and operator devices and the location of first-aid and safety equipment (other than firefighting equipment).
Blue	Blue shall be the color used for designating information of a non-safety nature.
Purple	Purple shall be the color used to designate ionizing radiation hazards.

EM 385-1-1
15 Sep 08

FIGURE 8-3

EXAMPLE SIGN LAYOUT

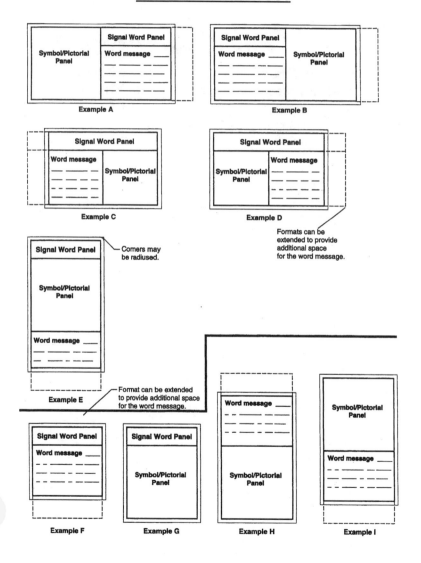

TABLE 8-3

IDENTIFICATION OF PIPING SYSTEMS

Outside diameter of pipe or covering	Length of color field "A"	Size of letters "B"
3/4 to 1 1/4 inches	8 inches	1/2 inch
1 1/2 to 2 inches	8 inches	3/4 inch
2 1/2 to 6 inches	12 inches	1 1/4 inch
8 to 10 inches	24 inches	2 1/2 inch
over 10 inches	32 inches	2 1/2 inch

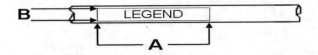

EM 385-1-1
15 Sep 08

FIGURE 8-4

RADIO FREQUENCY WARNING SYMBOL

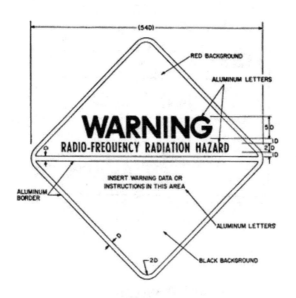

D = scaling unit

Lettering: ratio of letter height to thickness of letter lines
        Upper triangle: 5 to 1 = large
                                      6 to 1 = medium
        Lower triangle: 4 to 1 = small
                                      6 to 1 = medium
Symbol is square, triangles are right-angle isosceles

EM 385-1-1
15 Sep 08

FIGURE 8-5

LASER CAUTION SIGN

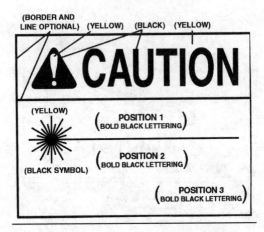

FIGURE 8-6

LASER WARNING SIGN

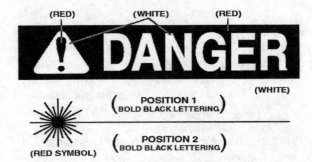

EM 385-1-1
15 Sep 08

FIGURE 8-7

RADIOLOGICAL WARNING SYMBOL

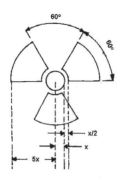

1. Cross-hatched area is to be magenta or purple.
2. Background is to be yellow.

FIGURE 8-8

SLOW-MOVING VEHICLE EMBLEM

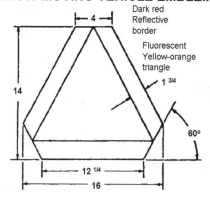

NOTE: All dimensions are in inches

EM 385-1-1
15 Sep 08

FIGURE 8-9

ACCIDENT PREVENTION TAGS

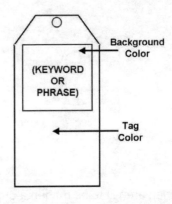

Keyword/Phrase	Keyword/Phrase Print Color	Background Color	Tag Color
"DANGER"	White in red oval	Black	White
"CAUTION"	Yellow	Black	Yellow
"DO NOT OPERATE	White	Red	White
"OUT OF ORDER"	White	Black	White
"DO NOT USE"			
Informational message or inspection	Black or green	N/A	Green & white OR White & black

EM 385-1-1
15 Sep 08

SECTION 9

FIRE PREVENTION AND PROTECTION

09.A GENERAL

09.A.01 A fire prevention plan shall be written for facilities and project sites. > *For Construction operations see NFPA 241; for Marine operations see 19.A.04.*

> a. It shall include, as a minimum: A list of the major workplace fire hazards; potential ignition sources; the types of fire suppression equipment or systems appropriate to the control of fire; assignments of responsibilities for maintaining the equipment and systems; personnel responsible for controlling the fuel source hazards; and housekeeping procedures, including the removal of waste materials.
>
> b. It shall be used to brief employees and emergency first responders on the fire hazards, the materials and processes to which they are exposed, and the emergency evacuation procedures.

09.A.02 An annual survey of the suitability and effectiveness of fire prevention and protection measures and facilities at each project or installation shall be made by a qualified person. Records of the survey findings and recommendations shall be retained on file at the project or installation.

09.A.03 When unusual fire hazards exist or fire emergencies develop, additional protection shall be provided as required by the GDA.

09.A.04 The GDA shall survey all activities and determine which require a hot work permit. > *See Sections 6.C and 10.C.*

09.A.05 Fires and open flame devices shall not be left unattended.

09.A.06 All sources of ignition shall be prohibited within 50 ft (15.2 m) of operations with a potential fire hazard. The area shall be conspicuously and legibly posted "**NO SMOKING, MATCHES, OR OPEN FLAME.**"

09.A.07 Smoking shall be prohibited in all areas where flammable, combustible, or oxidizing materials are stored. "**NO SMOKING, MATCHES, OR OPEN FLAME**" signs will be posted in all prohibited areas.

09.A.08 Areas where there is danger of underground fire shall not be used for the storage of flammable or combustible materials.

09.A.09 A barrier having a fire resistance rating equivalent to a listing of at least 1 hour shall segregate DOT-identified noncompatible materials that may create a fire hazard. For compressed gas cylinders see Section 20.D.

09.A.10 A good housekeeping program that provides for the prompt removal and disposal of accumulations of combustible scrap and debris shall be implemented on the site. Self-closing containers shall be used to collect waste saturated with flammable or combustible liquids. Only non-combustible or UL labeled nonmetallic containers may be used to dispose of waste and rubbish.

09.A.11 Measures must be taken to control the growth of tall grass, brush, and weeds adjacent to facilities. A break of at least 3 ft (0.9 m) shall be maintained around all facilities.

09.A.12 Paint-soiled clothing and drop cloths, when not in use, shall be stored in well-ventilated steel cabinets or containers.

09.A.13 Insulating material with a combustible vapor barrier shall be stored at least 25 ft (7.6 m) from buildings or structures. Only the quantity required for one day's use shall be permitted in buildings under construction.

EM 385-1-1
15 Sep 08

09.A.14 Disposal of combustible waste materials shall be in compliance with applicable fire and environmental laws and regulations.

09.A.15 Burning operations.

> a. Burning areas shall be established in coordination with the GDA and with the agency responsible for monitoring fire potential at the location of the proposed burning area.
>
> b. Burning operations shall be in compliance with Federal, State, and local regulations and guidelines.
>
> c. A sufficient force to control and patrol the burning operations shall be maintained until the last embers have been extinguished.
>
> d. Bump blocks shall be provided where trucks back to a fire or burning pit.
>
> e. Prescribed burning activities for natural resource management shall be conducted in accordance with guidelines set forth in Section 09.K.

09.A.16 Low-density fiberboard, combustible insulation, or vapor barriers with a flame spread rating greater than 25 shall not be installed in permanent buildings.

09.A.17 Temporary enclosures shall be covered with flame-resistant tarpaulins or material of equivalent fire-resistant characteristics.

09.A.18 When outside help is relied upon for fire protection, a written agreement shall be made, or a memorandum of record, stating the terms of the arrangement and the details for fire protection services, and shall be provided to the GDA.

EM 385-1-1
15 Sep 08

09.A.19 Temporary building spacing shall be <u>in accordance with the International Building Code (IBC)</u>.

09.A.20 Fire lanes providing access to all areas shall be established and maintained free of obstruction.

09.A.21 Vehicles, equipment, materials, and supplies shall not be placed so that access to fire hydrants and other firefighting equipment is obstructed.

09.A.22 Hazardous locations.

    a. Electrical lighting shall be the only means of artificial illumination in areas where flammable liquids, vapors, fumes, dust, or gases are present.

    b. All electrical equipment and installations in hazardous locations shall be in accordance with the National Electrical Code (NEC) for hazardous locations.

    c. Globes or lamps shall not be removed or replaced nor shall repairs be made on the electrical circuit until it has been de-energized.

09.A.23 <u>Sufficient</u> clearance shall be maintained around lights and heating units to prevent ignition of combustible materials.

09.A.24 All combustibles shall be shielded from the flames of torches used to cut or sweat pipe.

09.A.25 Precautions shall be taken to protect formwork and scaffolding from exposure to, and spread of, fire.

09.A.26 Fire protection in the construction process.

    a. Fire cut-offs shall be retained in buildings undergoing alterations or demolition until operations require their removal.

b. Where a water distribution system is required for the protection of buildings or other structures, water mains and hydrants shall be installed before or concurrent with the construction of facilities. Until the permanent system is in operation, an equivalent temporary system shall be provided.

c. Permanent (fixed) extinguishing equipment and water supply for fire protection shall be installed and in operable condition as soon as possible. The scheduling of sprinkler installation shall closely follow the building construction and, following completion of each story, shall be placed in service as soon as possible.

d. During demolition or alterations, existing automatic sprinkler systems shall be retained in service as long as reasonable. Modification of sprinkler systems to permit alterations or additional demolition should be expedited so that the system may be returned to service as quickly as possible. Sprinkler control valves shall be checked daily at close of work to ascertain that the protection is in service. The operation of sprinkler control valves is permitted only when approved by the GDA.

e. During the construction process, the construction of fire walls and exit stairways required for completed buildings shall have priority; fire doors, with automatic closing devices, shall be hung on openings as soon as practical.

09.A.27 Water supply and distribution facilities for fire fighting shall be provided and maintained in accordance with NFPA recommendations.

09.A.28 Recommendations of the NFPA shall be complied with in situations not covered in this section. Where local building codes are established, the more stringent requirements shall apply.

EM 385-1-1
15 Sep 08

09.B FLAMMABLE AND COMBUSTIBLE LIQUIDS

09.B.01 All storage, handling, and use of flammable and combustible liquids shall be in accordance with NFPA 30, NFPA 30A, or other applicable standards under the supervision of a qualified person.

09.B.02 All sources of ignition shall be prohibited in areas where flammable and combustible liquids are stored, handled, and processed. Suitable **NO SMOKING, MATCHES, OR OPEN FLAME** signs shall be posted in all such areas.

09.B.03 Fire protection requirements.

> a. At least one portable fire extinguisher rated 20-B:C shall be provided on all tank trucks or other vehicles used for transporting and/or dispensing flammable or combustible liquids.
>
> b. Each service or refueling area shall be provided with at least one fire extinguisher rated not less than 40-B:C and located so that an extinguisher shall be within 100 ft (30.4 m) of each pump, dispenser, underground fill pipe opening, and lubrication or service area.

09.B.04 Flammable liquids shall be kept in closed containers or tanks when not in use.

09.B.05 Workers shall guard carefully against any part of their clothing becoming contaminated with flammable or combustible fluids. They shall not be allowed to continue work if their clothing becomes contaminated, and they must remove or wet down the clothing as soon as possible.

09.B.06 No flammable liquid with a flash point (closed cup test) below 100 °F (37.7 °C) shall be used for cleaning purposes or to start or rekindle fires.

EM 385-1-1
15 Sep 08

09.B.07 Ventilation adequate to prevent the accumulation of flammable vapors to hazardous levels shall be provided in all areas where flammable and combustible liquids are handled or used.

09.B.08 Only labeled/listed (by a nationally-recognized testing laboratory) containers and portable tanks shall be used for the storage of flammable and combustible liquids.

    a. Metal containers and portable tanks (less than 660 gal (2.4 m^3) individual capacity) meeting the requirements of, and containing products authorized by, Chapter I, 49 CFR (U.S. DOT Hazardous Materials Regulations), Chapter 9 of the United Nations' *"Recommendations on the Transport of Dangerous Goods,"* or NFPA 386 shall be acceptable.

    b. Plastic containers meeting the requirements of, and used for petroleum products within the scope of, one or more of the following specifications shall be acceptable: ASTM F852, ASTM F 76, and ANSI/UL 1313.

    c. Plastic drums meeting the requirements of and containing products authorized by 49 CFR or by Chapter 9 of the United Nations' *"Recommendations on the Transport of Dangerous Goods"* shall be acceptable.

    d. Fiber drums that meet the requirements of Item 296 of the National Motor Freight Classification (NMFC) or Rule 51 of the Uniform Freight Classification (UFC) for Types 2A, 3A, 3B-H, 3B-L, or 4A and meet the requirements of and contain liquid products authorized either by Chapter I, 49 CFR (U.S. DOT Hazardous Materials Regulations) or by DOT exemption shall be acceptable.

09.B.09 Portable tanks (less than 660 gal (2.4 m^3) individual capacity) shall be provided with one or more devices installed in the top with sufficient emergency venting capacity to limit internal pressure under fire exposure conditions to 10 pounds per square inch (psi) (68.9 kilopascal (kPa)) gauge or 30% of the bursting pressure of the portable tank, whichever is greater.

EM 385-1-1
15 Sep 08

a. At least one pressure-actuated vent having a minimum capacity of 6000 ft^3 (170 m^3) of free air per hour shall be used. It shall be set to open at not more than 5 psi (35 kPa) gauge.

b. If fusible vents are used, they shall be actuated by elements that operate at a temperature not exceeding 300 °F (148.8 °C).

c. Where plugging of a pressure-actuated vent can occur, fusible plugs or venting devices that soften to failure at a maximum of 300 °F (148.8 °C) under fire exposure shall be permitted to be used for the entire emergency venting requirement.

09.B.10 The design, construction, and use of storage tanks containing flammable or combustible liquid shall be as specified in NFPA 30.

09.B.11 The maximum allowable size for a container or metal portable tank (less than 660 gal (2.5 m^3) individual capacity) shall not exceed the those shown in Table 9-1:

09.B.12 The design, construction, and use of storage cabinets, indoor storage areas, outdoor storage areas, hazardous materials storage lockers, and other occupancies shall be in accordance with NFPA 30 or, for marine applications, 46 CFR 147 covers use of cabinets and 46 CFR 92.05-10 specifies design and construction.

09.B.13 Flammable and combustible liquids in quantities greater than that required for 1 day's use shall not be stored in buildings under construction and not more than a 2 day supply shall be stored on paint barges.

TABLE 9-1

MAXIMUM ALLOWABLE SIZE OF CONTAINERS AND TANKS FOR FLAMMABLE AND COMBUSTIBLE LIQUIDS

Container type	Flammable Liquids Class			Combustible Liquids Class	
	IA	IB	IC	II	III
Glass	16 oz (473 mL)	32 oz (946 mL)	1 gal (3.8 L)	1 gal (3.8 L)	1 gal (3.8 L)
Metal (other than DOT drums) or approved plastic)	1 gal (3.8 L)	5 gal (19 L)	5 gal (19 L)	5 gal (19 L)	5 gal (19 L)
Safety cans	2 gal (7.6 L)	5 gal (19 L)	5 gal (19 L)	5 gal (19 L)	5 gal (19 L)
Metal drum (DOT) specification	8.1 ft^3 (0.23 m^3)	8.1 ft^3 (0.23 m^3)	8.1 ft^3 (0.23 m^3)	8.1 ft^3 (0.23 m^3)	8.1 ft^3 (0.23 m^3)
Approved metal portable tank	88.3 ft^3 (2.5 m^3)	88.3 ft^3 (2.5 m^3)	88.3 ft^3 (2.5 m^3)	88.3 ft^3 (2.5 m^3)	88.3 ft^3 (2.5 m^3)
Polyethylene DOT Spec 34, UN 1H1, or as authorized by DOT Exemption	1 gal (3.8 L)	5 gal (19 L)	5 gal (19 L)	8.1 ft^3 (0.23 m^3)	8.1 ft^3 (0.23 m^3)
Fiber drum NMFC or UFC Type 2A, Types 3A, 3B-H, or 3B-L, or Type 4A				8.1 ft^3 (0.23 m^3)	8.1 ft^3 (0.23 m^3)

EM 385-1-1
15 Sep 08

09.B.14 Flammable and combustible liquids shall not be stored in areas used for exits, stairways, or safe passage of people.

09.B.15 Safety cans and other portable containers for flammable liquids having a flash point at or below 73 °F (23 °C) shall be labeled/listed and painted red with a yellow band around the can and the name of the contents legibly indicated on the container.

09.B.16 Unopened containers of flammable and combustible liquids, such as paints, varnishes, lacquers, thinners, and solvents, shall be kept in a well ventilated location, free of excessive heat, smoke, sparks, flame, or direct rays of the sun.

09.B.17 In areas where flammable and combustible liquids are handled or stored, a self-closing metal refuse can, listed by a nationally recognized testing laboratory, shall be provided and maintained in good condition.

<u>09.B.18 Storage areas/tanks shall be surrounded by a curb, earthen dike or other equivalent means of containment of at least 6 in (.15 m) in height, or to a height that will contain the contents in the event of a leak. When dikes or curbs are used, provisions shall be made for draining off accumulations of ground or rain water or spills of flammable liquids. Drains shall terminate at a safe location and shall be accessible to operation under fire conditions. If fuel and oil storage areas are subject to the provisions of 40 CFR 112 (Spill Prevention Control and Countermeasures), those provisions shall apply as well.</u>

09.B.19 Where liquids are used or handled, provisions shall be made to promptly and safely dispose of leakage or spills.

09.B.20 Flashlights and electric lanterns used while handling flammable and combustible liquids shall be listed by a nationally recognized testing laboratory for the intended use.

09.B.21 Dispensing flammable and combustible liquids - general.

a. All pumping equipment used for the transfer of flammable and combustible liquids shall be listed by a nationally recognized testing laboratory or approved by, and labeled or tagged in accordance with, the Federal agency having jurisdiction, such as the DOT.

b. Flammable and combustible liquid dispensing systems shall be electrically bonded and grounded. All fuel tanks, hoses, and containers of 5 gal (18.9 L) or less shall be kept in metallic contact while flammable <u>and combustible</u> liquids are being transferred; transfer of flammable <u>and combustible</u> liquids in containers in excess of 5 gal shall be done only when the containers are electrically bonded.

c. Flammable or combustible liquids shall be drawn from, or transferred into, vessels, containers, or tanks within a building or outside only through a closed piping system, from safety cans, by means of a device drawing through the top, or from a container, or portable tanks, by gravity or pump, through an approved self-closing valve. Transferring by means of air pressure on the container or portable tanks is prohibited.

d. Areas in which flammable or combustible liquids are transferred in quantities greater than 5 gal (18.9 L) from one tank or container to another shall be separated from other operations by at least 25 ft (7.6 m) or a barrier having a fire resistance of at least 1 hour. Drainage or other means shall be provided to control spills. Natural or mechanical ventilation shall be provided to maintain the concentration of flammable vapor at or below 10% of the lower flammable limit.

e. Dispensing units shall be protected against collision damage by suitable means and permanent dispensing units shall be securely bolted in place.

f. Dispensing nozzles and devices for Class I liquids shall be listed.

g. Lamps, lanterns, heating devices, small engines, and similar equipment shall not be filled while hot: these devices shall be filled only in well ventilated rooms free of open flames or in open air and shall not be filled in storage buildings.

h. Dispensing devices shall be in all cases at least 20 ft (6 m) from any activity involving fixed sources of ignition.

09.B.22 Service and refueling areas.

a. Dispensing hoses shall be listed; dispensing nozzles shall be an approved automatic-closing type without a latch-open device.

b. Equipment using Class I liquid fuel shall be shut down during refueling, servicing, or maintenance: this requirement may be waived for diesel-fueled equipment serviced by a closed system with attachments designed to prevent spillage.

c. Dispensing of flammable fluids from tanks of 55 gal (0.20 m^3) capacity or more shall be by listed pumping arrangement. Transferring by air pressure on the container or portable tank is prohibited.

d. Clearly identified and easily accessible switch(es) shall be provided at a location remote from dispensing devices to shut off the power to all dispensing devices in an emergency.

e. A listed emergency breakaway device designed to retain liquid on both sides of the breakaway point shall be installed on each hose dispensing Class I liquids.

09.B.23 Tank cars/trucks.

a. Tank cars/trucks shall be spotted and not loaded or unloaded until brakes have been set and wheels chocked.

EM 385-1-1
15 Sep 08

b. Tank cars/trucks shall be attended for the entire time they are being loaded or unloaded. Precautions shall be taken against fire or other hazards.

c. Tank cars/trucks shall be properly bonded and grounded while being loaded or unloaded. Bonding and grounding connections shall be made before dome covers are removed on tank cars/trucks and shall not be disconnected until such covers have been replaced. Internal vapor pressure shall be relieved before dome covers are opened.

09.C LIQUEFIED PETROLEUM GAS (LP-GAS)

09.C.01 Storage, handling, installation, and use of LP-Gases and systems shall be in accordance with NFPA Standard 58 and USCG regulations, as applicable.

09.C.02 LP-Gas containers, valves, connectors, manifold valve assemblies, regulators, and appliances shall be of an approved type.

09.C.03 Any appliance that was originally manufactured for operation with a gaseous fuel other than LP-Gas and is in good condition may be used with LP-Gas only after it is properly converted, adapted, and tested for performance with LP-Gas.

09.C.04 Polyvinyl chloride and aluminum tubing shall not be used in LP-Gas systems.

09.C.05 Safety devices.

a. Every container and vaporizer shall be provided with one or more safety relief valves or devices. These valves and devices shall be arranged to afford free vent to the outside air and discharge at a point not less than 5 ft (1.5 m) horizontally from any building opening that is below the discharge point.

b. Container safety relief devices and regulator relief vents shall be located not less than 5 ft (1.5 m) in any direction from air

EM 385-1-1
15 Sep 08

openings into sealed combustion system appliances or mechanical ventilation air intakes.

c. Shut-off valves shall not be installed between the safety relief device and the container, or the equipment or piping to which the safety relief device is connected, except that a shut-off valve may be used where the arrangement of the valve is such that full required capacity-flow through the safety relief device is always afforded.

09.C.06 Container valves and accessories.

a. Valves, fittings, and accessories connected directly to the container, including primary shut off valves, shall have a rated working pressure of at least 250 psi (1723.6 kPa) gauge and shall be of material and design suitable for LP-Gas service.

b. Connections to containers (except safety relief connections, liquid level gauging devices, and plugged openings) shall have shutoff valves located as close to the container as practical.

09.C.07 Multiple container systems.

a. Valves in the assembly of multiple container systems shall be arranged so that replacement of containers can be made without shutting off the flow of gas in the system (this is not to be construed as requiring an automatic changeover device).

b. Regulators and low-pressure relief devices shall be rigidly attached to the cylinder valves, cylinders, supporting standards, building walls, or otherwise rigidly secured and shall be installed or protected from the elements.

09.C.08 LP-Gas containers and equipment shall not be used in unventilated spaces below grade in pits, below-decks, or other spaces where dangerous accumulations of heavier-than-air gas may accumulate due to leaks or equipment failure.

09.C.09 Welding is prohibited on LP-Gas containers.

EM 385-1-1
15 Sep 08

09.C.10 Dispensing.

a. Equipment using LP-Gas shall be shut down during refueling operations.

b. Filling of fuel containers for motor vehicles from bulk storage containers shall be performed not less than 10 ft (3 m) from the nearest masonry-walled building, not less than 25 ft (7.6 m) from the nearest building of other construction, and, in any event, not less than 25 ft from any building opening.

c. Filling, from storage containers, of portable containers or containers mounted on skids shall be performed no less than 50 ft (15.2 m) from the nearest building.

09.C.11 Installation, use, and storage outside buildings.

a. Containers shall be upright upon firm foundations or otherwise firmly positioned. Flexible connections (or other special fixtures) shall be provided to protect against the possibility of the effect of settlement on the outlet piping.

b. Containers shall be in a suitable ventilated enclosure or otherwise protected against tampering.

c. Storage outside buildings, of containers awaiting use, shall be located from the nearest building or group of buildings in accordance with Table 9-2.

TABLE 9-2

OUTSIDE STORAGE of LP-GAS CONTAINERS AND CYLINDERS

MINIMUM DISTANCES

Quantity of LP-Gas stored	Distance
Less than 500 lb (227 kg)	0 ft
500 lb (227 kg) 6,000 lb (2730 kg)	10 ft (3 m)
6,000 lb (2730 kg) 10,000 lb (4545 kg)	20 ft (6 m)
More than 10,000 lb (4545 kg)	25 ft (7.6 m)

d. Storage areas shall be provided with at least one approved portable fire extinguisher rated no less than 20-B:C.

09.C.12 Installation, use, and storage inside of buildings.

a. Storage of LP gas containers (empty or full) in industrial buildings (not normally frequented by the public) shall not exceed 300 lbs (2,598 ft^3 in vapor form). Empty containers which have been in LP-Gas service when stored inside, shall be considered as full containers for the purpose of determining the maximum quantity of LP-Gas permitted. **Exemption: A total of 5 one-pound propane cylinders may be stored indoors as long as they are stored away from exits and stairways, or in areas normally used for the safe exit of people.**

b. Containers stored inside shall not be located near exits, stairways, or in areas normally used for the safe exit of people.

c. Container valves shall be protected while in storage as follows: by setting into recess of container to prevent the possibility of it being struck if the container is dropped upon a

EM 385-1-1
15 Sep 08

flat surface, or by ventilated cap or collar fastened to the container capable of withstanding blow from any direction equivalent to that of a 30 lb (13.6 kg) weight dropped 4 ft (1.2 m).

d. Outlet valves of containers in storage shall be closed.

e. Storage locations shall be provided with at least one approved portable fire extinguisher having a minimum rating of 8-B:C.

f. Containers, regulating equipment, manifolds, pipe, tubing, and hose shall be located to minimize exposure to high temperatures or physical damage.

g. The maximum water capacity of individual containers shall be 245 lb (111.1 kg), nominal 100 lb (45.3 kg), LP-Gas capacity.

h. Containers having a water capacity greater than 2.5 lb (1.1 kg) (nominal 1 lb (0.4 kg) LP-Gas capacity that are connected for use shall stand on a firm and substantially level surface and, when necessary, shall be secured in an upright position. Systems using containers having a water capacity greater than 2.5 lb (1.1 kg) shall be equipped with excess flow valves internal either with the container valves or in the connections to the container valve outlets.

i. Regulators shall be directly connected to either the container valves or to manifolds connected to the container valves. The regulator shall be suitable for use with LP-Gas. Manifolds and fittings connecting containers to pressure regulator inlets shall be designed for at least 250 psi (1723.6 kPa) gauge service pressure.

j. Valves on containers having water capacity greater than 50 lb (22.6 kg) (nominal 20 lb (9 kg) LP-Gas capacity) shall be protected from damage while in use or storage.

EM 385-1-1
15 Sep 08

k. Hose shall be designed for a working pressure of at least 250 psi (1723.6 kPa) gauge. Design, construction, and performance of hose and connections shall have been suitability determined by listing by a nationally recognized testing agency. Hose length shall be as short as possible but long enough to permit compliance with spacing requirements without kinking, straining, or causing the hose to be so close to a burner as to be damaged by heat.

09.D TEMPORARY HEATING DEVICES

09.D.01 Only temporary heating devices approved by the GDA shall be used. Each heater should have a safety data plate permanently affixed by the manufacturer. The plate shall provide requirements or recommendations for:

a. Clearances from combustible materials;

b. Ventilation (minimum air requirements for fuel combustion);

c. Fuel type and input pressure;

d. Lighting, extinguishing, and relighting;

e. Electrical power supply characteristics;

f. Location, moving, and handling; and

g. Name and address of the manufacturer.

> *If this information is not available on a data plate, it shall be in writing at the job site.*

09.D.02 A positive operating procedure shall be established to assure the following:

a. Proper placement and servicing;

b. Safe clearance from combustible material;

c. Close surveillance;

d. Safe fuel storage and refueling;

e. Proper maintenance; and

f. Ventilation and determination of gaseous contamination or oxygen deficiency.

09.D.03 Heater installation and maintenance shall be in accordance with the manufacturer's instructions.

09.D.04 Open-flame heating devices having exposed fuel below the flame are prohibited.

09.D.05 Heaters, when in use, shall be set horizontally level, unless otherwise permitted by the manufacturer's specifications.

09.D.06 Heaters unsuitable for use on wood floors shall be so marked. When such heaters are used, they shall rest on suitable heat insulating material, such as concrete of at least 1 in (2.5 cm) thickness or equivalent; the insulating material shall extend 2 ft (0.6 m) or more in all directions from the edges of the heater.

09.D.07 Heaters used near combustible tarpaulins, canvas, or similar coverings shall be located at least 10 ft (3 m) from such coverings; coverings shall be securely fastened to prevent them from igniting or upsetting the heater due to wind action.

09.D.08 Heaters shall be protected against damage.

09.D.09 Installation of temporary heating devices shall provide minimum clearances to combustible materials as specified in Table 9-3.

TABLE 9-3

TEMPORARY HEATING DEVICE CLEARANCES

Heater type	Sides	Rear	Chimney connector
Room heater – circulating	11.8 in (30 cm)	11.8 in (30 cm)	17.7 in (45 cm)
Room heater – radiant	35.4 in (90 cm)	35.4 in (90 cm)	17.7 in (45 cm)

09.D.10 Fuel combustion space heating devices used in any enclosed building, room, or structure shall be vented by a flue pipe to the exterior of the structure.

    a. Fresh air shall be supplied, by natural or mechanical means, in sufficient quantities to ensure the health and safety of workers. Particular attention shall be given to areas where heat and fumes may accumulate.

    b. When heaters are used in confined spaces, precautions shall be taken to ensure proper combustion, maintenance of a safe and healthful atmosphere for workers, and limitation of temperature rise in the area. These precautions shall be addressed in the confined space entry permit. **> See 06.I.**

    c. Vent pipes shall be located a safe distance from flammables and combustibles. Where vent pipes pass through combustible walls or roofs, they shall be properly insulated and securely fastened and supported to prevent accidental displacement or separation.

09.D.11 When a heater is placed in operation, initial and periodic checks shall be made to ensure it is functioning properly.

09.D.12 Fuel combustion heater CO hazards.

EM 385-1-1
15 Sep 08

a. When heaters are used in enclosed or partially enclosed structures, CO shall be continuously monitored; or tests for the presence of CO shall be made within 1 hour of the start of each shift and at least every 4 hours (every 2 hours for solid fuel heaters) thereafter.

b. CO concentrations greater than 25 ppm (TLV) of air volume at worker breathing levels shall require extinguishing of the heater unless additional ventilation is provided to reduce the CO content to acceptable limits.

09.D.13 Personnel involved in fueling heaters shall be trained in, and thoroughly familiar with, the manufacturer's recommended safe fueling procedures.

09.D.14 Heaters shall be equipped with an approved automatic device to shut off the flow of fuel if the flame is extinguished (on liquid fuel heaters, barometric or gravity oil feed shall not be considered a primary safety control).

09.D.15 Spark arresters shall be provided on all smoke stacks or burning devices having forced drafts or short stacks permitting live sparks or hot materials to escape.

09.D.16 Solid fuel heaters are prohibited in buildings and on scaffolds.

09.D.17 Gas heaters - general.

a. All piping, tubing, and hose shall be leak tested using soap suds or other noncombustible detection means (tests shall not be made with a flame) after assembly and proven free of leaks at normal operating pressure.

b. Hose and fittings shall be protected from damage and deterioration.

c. All hose and fittings shall be checked to ensure that the type, capacity, and pressure ratings are as specified by the heater

EM 385-1-1
15 Sep 08

    manufacturer: hose shall have a minimum working pressure or 250 psi (1723.6 kPa) gauge and a minimum bursting pressure of 1250 psi (8618.4 kPa) gauge.

    d. All hose connectors shall be capable of withstanding, without leakage, a test pressure of 125 psi (861.8 kPa) gauge and shall be capable of withstanding a pull test of 400 lb (181.4 kg).

    e. Hose connectors shall be securely connected to the heater by mechanical means. Neither "slip-end" connectors (connections that allow the hose end to be held only by the friction of the hose material against the metal fitting of the unit) nor ring keepers (tightened over the hose to provide an increased force holding the hose to the metal fitting) are permitted.

09.D.18 Natural gas heaters. When flexible gas supply lines are used, the length shall be as short as practical and shall not exceed 25 ft (7.6 m).

09.D.19 Portable LP-Gas heaters > *See also 09.C.*

    a. If LP-Gas is supplied to a heater by hose, the hose shall not be less than 10 ft (3 m), nor more than 25 ft (7.6 m), in length.

    b. Heaters shall be equipped with an approved regulator in the supply line between the fuel cylinder and the heater unit. Cylinder connectors shall be provided with an excess flow valve to minimize the flow of gas in the event the fuel line ruptures.

    c. LP-Gas heaters having inputs above 50,000 British thermal unit (Btu) per hour shall be equipped with either a pilot, which must be lighted and proved before the main burner can be turned on, or an electronic ignition. [These provisions do not apply to portable heaters under 7,500 Btu per hour when used with containers having a maximum water capacity of 2.5 lb (1.1 kg)].

EM 385-1-1
15 Sep 08

d. Container valves, connectors, regulators, manifolds, piping, and tubing shall not be used as structural support for LP-Gas heaters.

e. Heaters, other than integral heater-container units, shall be located at least 6 ft (1.8 m) from any LP-Gas container (this shall not prohibit the use of heaters designed specifically for attachment to the LP-Gas container or to a supporting standard, provided they are designed and installed to prevent direct or radiant heat application from the heater into the containers). Blower and radiant type heaters shall not be directed toward any LP-Gas container within 20 ft (6 m).

f. If two or more heater-container units (of either the integral or non-integral type) are located in an unpartitioned area of the same floor, the container or containers of each unit shall be separated from the container or containers of any other unit by at least 20 ft (6 m).

g. When heaters are connected to containers for use in an unpartitioned area on the same floor, the total water capacity of containers, manifolded together for connection to a heater(s), shall not be greater than 735 lb (333.3 kg) (nominal 300 lb (136 kg) LP-Gas capacity). Such manifolds shall be separated by at least 20 ft (6 m).

09.D.20 Installation of heating equipment in service or lubrication areas.

a. Heating equipment installed in lubrication or service areas where there is no dispensing or transferring of flammable liquids shall be installed such that the bottom of the heating unit is at least 18 in (.5 m) above the floor and is protected from damage.

b. Heating equipment installed in lubrication or service areas where flammable liquids are dispensed shall be of a type approved for garages and shall be installed at least 8 ft (2.4 m) above the floor.

EM 385-1-1
15 Sep 08

09.E FIRST RESPONSE FIRE PROTECTION

09.E.01 Portable fire extinguishers shall be provided where needed as specified in Table 9-4. Fire extinguishers shall be inspected monthly and maintained as specified in NFPA 10. Records shall be kept on a tag or label attached to the extinguisher, on an inspection check list maintained on file, or by an electronic method that provides a permanent record. The date the inspection was performed and the initials of the person performing the inspection shall be recorded.

09.E.02 Approved fire extinguishers.

    a. Fire extinguishers shall be approved by a nationally recognized testing laboratory and labeled to identify the listing and labeling organization and the fire test and performance standard that the fire extinguisher meets or exceeds.

EM 385-1-1
15 Sep 08

TABLE 9-4

FIRE EXTINGUISHER DISTRIBUTION

	Occupancy					
	Low Hazard		Medium Hazard		High Hazard	
	Class A	Class B	Class A	Class B	Class A	Class B
Minimum rating for single extinguisher	2-A	5-B or 10-B[1]	2-A	10-B or 20-B	4-A	40-B or 80-B[2]
Maximum coverage (floor area) per unit of A-rating	3,000 ft^2	n/a	1,500 ft^2	n/a	1,000 ft^2	n/a
Maximum floor area for extinguisher	11,250 ft^2	n/a	11,250 ft^2	n/a	11,250 ft^2	n/a
Maximum travel distance to extinguisher	75 ft	30 ft for 5-B 50 ft for 10-B	75 ft	30 ft for 10-B 50 ft for 20-B	75 ft	30 ft for 40-B 50 ft for 80-B

(1) up to 3 foam extinguishers of at least 2 1/2 gal (9.5 L) capacity may be used to fulfill low hazard requirements
(2) up to 3 aqueous film foaming foam (AFFF) extinguishers of at least 2 1/2 gal (9.5 L) capacity may be used to fulfill high hazard requirements

Derived from NFPA 10
In multiple-story facilities, at least 1 extinguisher shall be adjacent to stairways. On construction and demolition projects, a 1/2 in (1.2 cm) diameter garden hose, not to exceed 100 ft (30.4 m) in length and equipped with a nozzle, may be substituted for a 2-A rated fire extinguisher provided it its capable of discharging a minimum of 5 gal (18.9 L) per minute with minimum hose stream range of 30 ft (9.1 m) horizontally. The garden hose lines shall be mounted on conventional racks or reels. The number of location of hose racks or reels shall be such that at least 1 hose stream can be applied to all points in the area.

EM 385-1-1
15 Sep 08

> b. Fire extinguishers shall be marked with their letter (class of fire) and numeric (relative extinguishing effectiveness) classification.
>
> c. Fire extinguishers using carbon tetrachloride or chlorobromomethane extinguishing agents are prohibited.
>
> d. Soldered or riveted shell self-generating foam or gas cartridge water-type portable extinguishers that are operated by inverting the extinguisher to rupture or initiate an uncontrollable pressure generating chemical reaction to expel the agent are prohibited.

09.E.03 Fire extinguishers shall be in a fully charged and operable condition and shall be suitably placed, distinctly marked, and readily accessible.

09.E.04 When portable fire extinguishers are provided for employee use in the workplace, the employer shall provide training (upon initial employment and at least annually thereafter) in the following:

> a. General principles of fire extinguisher use and the hazards involved with incipient stage fire fighting to all employees; and
>
> b. Use of the appropriate firefighting equipment to those employees designated in an emergency action plan to use firefighting equipment.

09.E.05 Approved fire blankets shall be provided and kept in conspicuous and accessible locations as warranted by the operations involved.

09.E.06 No fire shall be fought where the fire is in imminent danger of contact with explosives. All persons shall be removed to a safe area and the fire area guarded against intruders.

EM 385-1-1
15 Sep 08

09.E.07 Standpipe and hose system equipment.

a. Standpipes shall be located or otherwise protected against damage. Damaged standpipes shall be repaired promptly.

b. Reels and cabinets used to contain fire hose shall be designed and maintained to ensure the prompt use of the hose valve, hose, and other equipment. Reels and cabinets shall be conspicuously identified and used only for fire equipment.

c. Hose outlets and connections shall be located high enough above the floor to avoid their obstruction and to be accessible to employees. To ensure hose connections are compatible with support fire equipment, screw threads shall be standardized or adapters shall be provided throughout the system.

d. Standpipe systems shall be equipped with vinyl type or lined hoses of such length that friction loss resulting from water flowing through the hose will not decrease the pressure at the nozzle below 30 psi (206.8 kPa) gauge. The dynamic pressure at the nozzle shall be within 30 psi (206.8 kPa) gauge and 125 psi (861.8 kPa) gauge.

e. Standpipe hoses shall be equipped with basic spray nozzles with a straight stream to wide stream spray pattern. Nozzles shall have a water discharge control capable of functions ranging from full discharge to complete shutoff.

09.E.08 The following tests shall be performed on standpipe and hose systems before placing them in service:

a. Piping (including yard piping) shall be hydrostatically tested for at least 2 hours at not less than 200 psi (1378.9 kPa) (or at least 50 psi (344.7 kPa) in excess of normal pressure when the normal pressure is greater than 150 psi (1034.2 kPa)); and

b. Hose shall be hydrostatically tested with couplings in place at a pressure of not less than 200 psi (1378.9 kPa). This pressure shall be maintained for at least 15 seconds, but not more than

1 minute, during which time the hose shall not leak nor shall the jacket thread break.

09.E.09 Standpipe and hose system inspection and maintenance.

a. Water supply tanks shall be kept filled to the proper level except during repairs. When pressure tanks are used, proper pressure shall be maintained at all times except during repairs.

b. Valves in the main piping connections to the automatic sources of water supply shall be kept fully open at all times, except during repairs.

c. Hose systems shall be inspected at least annually and after each use to assure that all equipment is in place, available for use, and in operable condition.

d. When the system or any portion of the system is found not to be serviceable, it shall be removed for repair and replaced with equivalent protection (such as fire watches and extinguisher) until the repairs are complete.

e. Hemp and linen hoses shall be unracked, physically inspected for deterioration, and reracked using a different fold pattern at least annually.

09.E.10 The minimum water supply for standpipe and hose systems provided for the use of employees shall be sufficient to provide 100 gal (0.37 m^3) per minute for at least 30 minutes.

09.E.11 For all structures in which standpipes are required, or where standpipes exist in structures being altered, the standpipes shall be brought up as soon as practical and maintained as construction progresses so that they are always ready for fire protection use. There shall be at least one standard hose outlet at each floor.

09.E.12 For employees that may encounter incipient stage wild land fires, local safety programs shall provide basic training (upon initial employment and at least annually thereafter) in techniques commonly used to extinguish incipient stage wild land fires and the hazards associated with such fire fighting activities.

09.F FIXED FIRE SUPPRESSION SYSTEMS

09.F.01 Fixed fire suppression systems shall be designed, installed, and acceptance-tested in accordance with requirements of the NFPA.

09.F.02 Fixed fire suppression systems shall be inspected and maintained in accordance with UFC 3-600-02, *O&M: Inspection, Testing, and Maintenance of Fire Protection Systems"*. Inspection and maintenance dates shall be recorded on the container, on a tag attached to the container, or in a central location.

09.F.03 Automatic sprinkler systems shall be protected from damage.

09.F.04 Vertical clearance of at least 18 in (45.7 cm) shall be maintained between the top of stored material and sprinkler deflectors.

09.F.05 If a fixed extinguishing system becomes inoperable, the employer shall notify the employees and take necessary precautions to assure their safety until the system is restored to operating order.

09.F.06 Effective safeguards shall be provided to warn employees against entry into fixed extinguishing system discharge areas where the atmosphere remains hazardous to employee safety and health. Manual operating devices shall be identified as to the hazard against which they will provide protection.

09.F.07 Warning or caution signs shall be posted at the entrance to, and inside, areas protected by fixed extinguishing systems that use agents in concentrations known to be hazardous to employee safety and health.

09.F.08 Dry chemical fixed extinguishing systems.

   a. Dry chemical extinguishing agents shall be compatible with any foams or wetting agents with which they are used.

   b. Dry chemical extinguishing agents of different compositions shall not be mixed together.

   c. Dry chemical extinguishing systems shall be refilled with the chemical stated on the approval nameplate or an equivalent compatible material.

09.F.09 Gaseous agent fixed extinguishing systems.

   a. Agents used for initial supply and replenishment shall be of a type approved for the system's application.

   b. Employees shall not be exposed to toxic levels of the gaseous agent or its decomposition products.

09.F.10 When water and spray foam fixed extinguishing systems are used, the drainage of water shall be away from work areas and routes of emergency egress.

09.G FIREFIGHTING EQUIPMENT

09.G.01 Firefighting equipment shall be provided and installed in accordance with applicable NFPA <u>and</u> OSHA regulations.

09.G.02 No fire protection equipment or device shall be made inoperative or used for other purposes, unless specifically approved by the GDA.

09.G.03 If fire hose connections are not compatible with local firefighting equipment, adapters shall be made available.

EM 385-1-1
15 Sep 08

09.H FIRE DETECTION AND EMPLOYEE FIRE ALARM SYSTEMS

09.H.01 Fire detection and employee fire alarm systems shall be designed and installed in accordance with requirements of NFPA and OSHA.

09.H.02 Fire detection systems and components shall be restored to normal operating condition as soon as possible after each test/alarm. Spare devices and components shall be maintained in sufficient quantities for the prompt restoration of the system.

09.H.03 Fire detection systems shall be maintained in operable condition except during maintenance or repairs.

> a. Fire detectors and detector systems shall be tested and adjusted as often as necessary to maintain operability and reliability; factory calibrated detectors need not be adjusted after installation.
>
> b. Pneumatic and hydraulic operated detection systems installed after January 1, 1981, shall be equipped with supervised systems.
>
> c. The servicing, testing, and maintenance of fire detection systems shall be performed by a trained person knowledgeable in the operations and functions of the system.
>
> d. Fire detectors that need to be cleaned of dirt, dust, or other particulate matter to be fully functional shall be cleaned at regular intervals.

09.H.04 Fire detection systems and devices shall be protected from weather, corrosion, and mechanical and physical damage.

09.H.05 Fire detectors shall be supported independently of their control wiring or tubing.

09.H.06 An alarm system shall be established by the employer so that employees on the site and the local fire department can be alerted of an emergency.

09.H.07 Manually operated alarm actuation devices shall be conspicuous and accessible and inspected and maintained in operable condition.

09.H.08 The alarm shall be distinctive and recognizable as a signal to evacuate the work area or to perform actions designated in the emergency action plan.

> a. The alarm shall be capable of being perceived above ambient noise and light levels by all employees in the affected area.
>
> b. Tactile devices may be used to alert those employees who would not otherwise be able to recognize the audible or visual alarm.

09.H.09 Employees shall be instructed in the preferred means of reporting emergencies, such as manual pull box alarms, public address systems, or telephones.

> a. The alarm code and reporting instructions shall be conspicuously posted at phones and at employee entrances.
>
> b. Reporting and evacuating instructions shall be conspicuously posted.
>
> c. For work at installations that are equipped with radio wave fire alarm systems, a compatible fire alarm transmitter should be used at the construction site.

09.I FIREFIGHTING ORGANIZATIONS - TRAINING AND DRILLING

09.I.01 Firefighting organizations shall be provided to assure adequate protection to life and property. NFPA recommendations

EM 385-1-1
15 Sep 08

shall be used for determining type, size, and training of fire fighting organizations.

09.I.02 Fire brigade drills shall be held to assure a well-trained and efficient operating force. Records of such drills shall be maintained at the installation.

09.I.03 Demonstration and training in first-aid firefighting shall be conducted at intervals to ensure that project personnel are familiar with, and capable of operating, firefighting equipment.

09.J FIRE PATROLS

09.J.01 When watch personnel or guards are provided, they shall make frequent rounds through buildings and storage areas when work is suspended.

09.J.02 Smoke detectors shall be installed and maintained where personnel are quartered.

09.J.03 In any instance where combustible materials have been exposed to fire hazards (such as welding operations, hot metals, or open flame), a fire watch shall be assigned to remain at the location for at least one (1) hour after the exposure has ended.

09.K USACE WILD LAND FIRE CONTROL

09.K.01 At all USACE facilities and areas with potential exposure to wild land fire, whether prescribed or planned, a wild land fire management plan shall be developed. The plan, which is further detailed in EP 1130-2-540, shall address prescribed fire and wild fire prevention and suppression, shall include the following items, and shall be updated annually:

a. An individual prescribed fire burn plan procedure, as outlined in EP 1130-2-540, that requires individual burn plans to include an AHA and an on-site safety meeting to include discussion of predicted weather patterns, escape route(s), and safety zone(s);

b. An analysis of wild land fire causes and special wild fire hazards and risks;

c. Proposed measures to reduce wild fire occurrence and decrease fire damage;

d. Procedures for public education and wild fire prevention sign posting (including procedures for keeping the public informed of the current fire danger rating);

e. Provisions for cooperative efforts with all other neighboring wild land fire management protection agencies;

f. The in-house wild land fire management or control team organization and personnel roster, training and equipment requirements, and notification procedures;

g. A listing of cooperating agencies and notification procedures, (including any mutual aid agreements with adjacent fire departments and agencies);

h. A listing of additional available resources for work force, equipment, supplies, and facilities, and contracting or procurement information;

i. An up-to-date map(s) of the managed and/or protected area(s) that shows boundaries, roads, and other means of access, heliports, airports, water sources, special hazards, and special fire risks;

j. A listing of weather information sources;

k. Procedures for public notification; and

l. A pre-attack fire suppression plan as outlined in EP 1130-2-540.

EM 385-1-1
15 Sep 08

09.K.02 Wild land fire management teams and operations should be organized and conducted in accordance with the requirements of NFPA 1143.

   a. Wild land fire management team personnel shall, as a minimum, receive training that will include fire line safety, basic wild land fire behavior, basic wild land fire suppression tactics, communications procedures, first aid and use, limitations and care of protective and firefighting equipment.

   b. Firefighting equipment shall be maintained in working and ready condition.

   c. PPE, fire-resistant clothing, safety hard hats, safety toe (non steel-toe) leather boots, goggles, and fire resistant gloves, as required by NFPA 1143, part A.6.2.4.1 and NFPA 1977, shall be provided and maintained in working and ready condition. **> See also Section 5.**

   d. Employees engaged in fire management activities shall be examined, as part of their medical surveillance, by a physician and certified to be physically able to perform assigned fire management duties.

   e. Communication equipment shall be provided to personnel as necessary for coordination, control, and emergency needs.

09.K.03 Recommendations of NFPA 1143 shall be complied with in wild land fire situations not covered in this Section.

09.K.04 Wild land fire management teams shall consist of two or more qualified individuals.

BLANK

EM 385-1-1
15 Sep 08

SECTION 10

WELDING AND CUTTING

10.A GENERAL

10.A.01 Welders, cutters, and their supervisor shall be trained in the safe operation of their equipment, safe welding/cutting practices, and welding/cutting respiratory and fire protection.
> *AIHA publication "Welding Health and Safety: A Field Guide for OEHS Professionals" is recommended.*

10.A.02 All welding equipment shall be inspected before each use to ensure that all required safety devices and ancillary equipment are in place and properly functioning. Defective equipment shall be removed from service, replaced or repaired, and reinspected before again being placed in service.

10.A.03 Electrical and pressurized system requirements.

a. Welding cylinders and their use and maintenance shall meet the applicable requirements of Section 20.

b. Arc welding and cutting systems and their use shall meet the applicable requirements of this section.

10.A.04 Arc welding and cutting operations shall be shielded by noncombustible or flameproof screens that will protect employees and other persons working in the vicinity from the direct rays of the arc, sparks, molten metal, spatter, and chipped slag.

10.A.05 Cable, hoses, and other equipment shall be kept clear of passageways, ladders, and stairways.

10.A.06 Welding and cutting of hazardous materials.

a. When welding, cutting, or heating on steel pipelines containing natural gas, 49 CFR 192 shall apply.

EM 385-1-1
15 Sep 08

    b. Before welding, cutting, or heating is commenced on any surface covered by a preservative coating whose flammability is not known, a test shall be made to determine its flammability. Preservative coatings shall be considered highly flammable when scrapings burn with extreme rapidity.

    c. Preservative coatings shall be removed a sufficient distance from the area to be heated to ensure any temperature increase of the unstripped metal will not be appreciable; artificial cooling of the metal surrounding the heating area may be used to limit the area to be stripped.

    d. When welding, cutting, or heating toxic surface coatings (paints, preservatives, surface stripping chemicals, etc.) in enclosed spaces, all surfaces covered with the coatings shall be stripped of such for a distance of at least 4 in (10.1 cm) from the area of heat application or the employees shall be protected by airline respirators.

10.A.07 All structural welding performed on critical items, such as scaffolding, shoring, forms, ladders, piling, etc., as well as other critical items as designated by the GDA, shall only be performed by welders certified in accordance with American Welding Society (AWS) standards using qualified and approved welding practices and procedures (AWS certification or approved equivalent organization which trains to AWS standards).

10.A.08 Before heat is applied to a drum, container, or hollow structure, a vent or opening shall be provided for the release of any built-up pressure generated during the application of heat.

10.A.09 Employees performing welding, cutting, and heating work shall be protected by PPE appropriate for the hazards that they may encounter and based upon the results of an AHA conducted specifically for the welding, cutting, or heating operation that they will be performing. All required respiratory, eye and face, noise, head, foot, and skin protection equipment shall be selected and used in accordance with Section 5.

EM 385-1-1
15 Sep 08

10.A.10 All welding and cutting equipment and operations shall be in accordance with standards and recommended practices of <u>American National Standards Institute (ANSI)</u>/American Welding Society (AWS) Z49.1.

10.B RESPIRATORY PROTECTION

10.B.01 All welding, cutting, and heating operations shall be ventilated (natural or mechanical) such that personnel exposures to hazardous concentrations of airborne contaminants are within acceptable limits. *> See Section 6.*

10.B.02 Welding, cutting, and heating not involving conditions or materials described in this Section may normally be done without mechanical ventilation or respiratory protective equipment.

10.B.03 Either general mechanical or local exhaust ventilation shall be provided whenever welding, cutting, or heating is performed in a confined space. *> See 10.A.06.d and 10.B.05.*

10.B.04 Materials of toxic significance. Welding, cutting, or heating operations that involve or generate any of the substances listed below shall be performed in accordance with the following subparagraphs: Antimony, Arsenic, Barium, Beryllium, Cadmium, Chromium, <u>Chromium (VI),</u> Cobalt, Copper, Lead, Manganese, Mercury, Nickel, Ozone, Selenium, Silver, or Vanadium. *> See also 10.A.06.d.*

    a. Whenever these materials are encountered in confined spaces, local mechanical exhaust ventilation and personal respirat<u>ive equipment</u> shall be used.<u> The use of local mechanical exhaust ventilation systems that permit the re-entry of exhaust air back into the work area, or local exhaust which incorporate a system for the filtration and recirculation of exhaust air back into the work area shall not be permitted</u>.

    b. Whenever these materials, except beryllium<u> and chromium (VI)</u>, are encountered in indoor operations, local mechanical exhaust ventilation <u>systems that are sufficient to reduce and</u>

EM 385-1-1
15 Sep 08

maintain personal exposures to within acceptable limits shall be used. The use of local mechanical exhaust systems that permit the re-entry of exhaust air back into the work area, or that include a system for the filtration and the recirculation of exhaust air back into the work area are not permitted. When either beryllium or chromium (VI) is encountered in indoor operations, approved local mechanical exhaust ventilation systems and personal respiratory protection shall be used.

c. Whenever these materials, except beryllium and chromium (VI), are encountered in outdoor operations, and local mechanical exhaust ventilation systems sufficient to reduce and maintain personal exposures to within acceptable limits are not provided, then appropriate respiratory protective equipment shall be used.

d. Whenever beryllium and chromium (VI), are encountered in outdoor operations, the need for and type of engineering and work practice controls to be implemented, as well as the need for and type of respiratory protection to be provided shall be based upon the results of an initial worker exposure assessment and exposure determination with regards to these substances.

e. Workers may be exposed to hazardous concentrations of chromium (VI) while welding, cutting or performing hot work on stainless steel, high chrome alloys or chrome-coated metal, or during the application and removal of chromate-containing paints and other surface coatings. **> See OSHA's Standard for Hexavalent Chromium (Chromium (VI), 29 CFR 1926.1126.**

10.B.05 Welding, cutting, or heating operations that involve or generate fluorine or zinc compounds shall be performed in accordance with the following:

a. In confined spaces, local mechanical exhaust ventilation and personal respiratory protection sufficient to maintain exposures to within acceptable limits shall be used.

EM 385-1-1
15 Sep 08

b. In open spaces, sampling shall be performed to determine concentrations of fluorides or zinc compounds and the need for local exhaust ventilation and personal respiratory protection sufficient to maintain exposures to within acceptable limits.

10.B.06 Arc and gas cutting. Oxygen cutting using either an iron powder or chemical flux, gas-shielded arc cutting, and plasma cutting shall employ local mechanical exhaust ventilation or other means adequate to remove the fumes generated.

10.B.07 Other persons exposed to the same atmosphere as welders or cutters shall be protected in the same manner as welders or cutters.

10.C FIRE PROTECTION

10.C.01 Suitable fire extinguishing equipment of sufficient capacity shall be provided in the immediate vicinity of welding or cutting operations and maintained in a state of constant readiness for immediate use. Hot work permits shall be required on Government installations when welding, cutting, or heating operations are performed unless otherwise indicated by the GDA.

10.C.02 Before conducting welding or cutting operations, the area shall be surveyed to ensure it is free of the following hazards:

a. Proximate combustible materials,

b. The presence or possible generation of potentially explosive atmospheres (flammable gases, vapors, liquids, or dusts); and

c. The presence or nature of an oxygen-enriched atmosphere.

10.C.03 Hierarchy of fire control. Objects to be welded, cut, or heated shall be:

a. Moved to a location free of dangerous combustibles;

EM 385-1-1
15 Sep 08

    b. If the work cannot be moved, all moveable fire hazards in the vicinity shall be taken to a safe place (moved at least 35 ft (10.6 m) horizontally from the welding or cutting area) or the combustible material and construction shall be protected from the heat, sparks, and slag of welding;

    c. When welding or cutting must be done in a location where combustible or flammable materials are located, inspection and authorization by the GDA shall be required before such operations are begun (the location shall be checked for latent fires <u>by qualified fire watch personnel</u> after the work is completed).

10.C.04 When a welding, cutting, or heating operation is such that normal fire prevention precautions are not sufficient, additional <u>qualified fire watch</u> personnel shall be assigned to guard against fire and shall be instructed in anticipated fire hazards and how fire fighting equipment is to be used. **> See 09.J.03,**

10.C.05 When welding or cutting is to be done over combustible flooring, the flooring shall be protected by fire-resistant shielding, covered with damp sand, or kept wet. Where flooring is wet or damp, personnel operating arc welding or cutting equipment shall be protected from <u>potential</u> shock <u>hazards</u>.

10.C.06 Noncombustible barriers shall be installed below welding or burning operations in a shaft or raise,

10.C.07 Openings or cracks in walls, floors, or ducts within 35 ft (10.6 m) of the site <u>of welding or cutting operations</u> shall be tightly covered to prevent the passage of sparks to adjacent areas.

10.C.08 Where welding or cutting is to be done near walls, partitions, ceilings, or roofs of combustible construction, fire resistant guards shall be provided to prevent ignition.

10.C.09 Where welding or cutting is to be done on a metal wall, partition, ceiling, or roof, precautions shall be taken to prevent

EM 385-1-1
15 Sep 08

ignition, due to heat conduction or radiation, of combustibles on the other side.

10.C.10 Welding or cutting shall not be done on a metal partition, wall, ceiling, or roof with a combustible covering nor on walls or partitions of combustible sandwich-type panel construction.

10.C.11 Before welding or cutting drums, tanks, or other containers and equipment that have contained hazardous materials, the containers shall be thoroughly cleaned in accordance with NFPA 326 and ANSI/AWS F4.1.

10.C.12 Hot tapping or other welding or cutting on a flammable gas or liquid transmission or distribution pipeline shall be performed only by personnel qualified to make hot taps and only with the permission of the GDA.

10.C.13 When welding or cutting is to be conducted near a sprinkler head, a wet cloth or equivalent protection shall be used to cover the sprinkler head and then removed at the completion of the welding or cutting operation.

10.C.14 When welding or cutting in areas protected by fire detection and suppression systems, precautions shall be taken to avoid accidental initiation of these systems.

10.D OXYFUEL GAS WELDING AND CUTTING

10.D.01 Oxyfuel gas welding and cutting equipment shall be listed by a nationally-recognized testing laboratory.

10.D.02 Oxygen cylinders and apparatus.

    a. Oxygen cylinders and apparatus shall be kept free from oil, grease, and other flammable or explosive substances and shall not be handled with oily hands or gloves.

    b. Oxygen cylinders and apparatus shall not be used interchangeably with any other gas.

EM 385-1-1
15 Sep 08

10.D.03 Hose and hose connections.

   a. Fuel gas hose and oxygen hose shall be readily distinguishable from each other.

   b. Oxygen and fuel gas hoses shall not be interchangeable. A single hose having more than one gas passage shall not be used.

   c. Hose couplings of the type that can be unlocked or disconnected without a rotary motion are prohibited.

   d. Hose that has been subject to flashback or that shows evidence of severe wear or damage shall be tested to twice the normal pressure to which it is subjected, and in no case less than 300 psi (2068.4-kPa) gauge. Damaged hose and hose connectors, or hose and hose connectors in questionable condition, shall not be used.

   e. When parallel runs of oxygen and fuel gas hose are taped together, not more than 4 out of every 12 in (10 out of every 30.4 cm) shall be covered by tape.

   f. Boxes used for the storage of gas hose shall be ventilated.

   g. Hose connections shall be clamped or otherwise securely fastened in a manner that will withstand, without leakage, twice the pressure to which they are normally subjected in service, but not less than 300 psi (2,068 kPa) gauge.

10.D.04 Torches.

   a. Torches shall be inspected before each use for leaking shutoff valves, hose couplings, and tip connections. Defective torches shall not be used.

EM 385-1-1
15 Sep 08

   b. Hoses shall be purged individually before lighting the torch for the first time each day. Hoses shall not be purged into confined spaces or near ignition sources.

   c. Clogged torch tip openings shall be cleaned with suitable cleaning wires, drills, or other devices designed for such purposes.

   d. Torches shall be lighted by friction lighters or other approved devices, not by matches or from hot work.

10.D.05 Torch valves shall be closed and the gas supply shut off whenever work is suspended.

10.D.06 The torch and hose shall be removed from confined spaces whenever work is suspended.

10.D.07 Protective equipment.

   a. Oxyfuel gas, and other oxygen-fuel gas welding and cutting systems using cylinder-<u>regulator</u>-hose-torch shall be equipped with both a reverse-flow check valve and a flash arrestor, in each hose, at the torch handle <u>or</u> at the regulator.

   b. When oxygen-fuel gas systems are manifolded together the provisions of NFPA 51 shall apply.

10.D.08 Connection of multiple sets of oxyacetylene hoses to a single regulator on a single set of oxyacetylene tanks may only be accomplished by installing a commercially available fitting approved by Compressed Gas Association (CGA) standards and listed by a nationally-recognized testing laboratory. The fitting shall be installed on the output side of the regulator and shall have a built-in shut-off valve and reverse-flow check valve on each branch.

10.D.09 Acetylene regulators shall not be adjusted to permit a discharge greater than 15 psi (103.4 kPa) gauge.

EM 385-1-1
15 Sep 08

10.E ARC WELDING AND CUTTING

10.E.01 Electric welding apparatus shall be installed, maintained, and operated in accordance with the NEC.

10.E.02 Manual electrode holders.

    a. Only manual electrode holders specifically designed for arc welding and cutting of a capacity capable of safely handling the maximum rated current required by the electrodes shall be used.

    b. All current carrying parts passing through the portion of the holder that is gripped by the welder or cutter, and the outer surfaces of the jaws of the holder, shall be fully insulated against the maximum voltage encountered to ground.

10.E.03 <u>Welding</u> cables and connectors.

    a. Cables shall be completely insulated, flexible, capable of handling the maximum current requirements of the work in progress, and in good repair. <u>Cables in need of repair shall not be used.</u>

    b. <u>Welding cables shall be inspected for wear or damage before each use. Cables with damaged insulation or connectors shall be replaced or repaired to achieve the same mechanical strength, insulating quality, electrical conductivity, and water tightness of the original cable</u>. Cables containing splices or repaired insulation within a minimum distance of 10 ft (3 m) from the end of the cable to which the electrode holder is connected shall not be used.

    c. Where it becomes necessary to connect or splice lengths of cable together, insulated connectors of a capacity at least equivalent to that of the cable shall be used. When connections are affected by cable lugs, they shall be securely fastened together to give good electrical contact and the exposed metal parts of the lugs shall be completely insulated. <u>The joining of</u>

lengths of cable shall be accomplished by methods specifically intended for that purpose and connection methods shall provide insulation adequate for the service conditions.

10.E.04 The frames of arc welding and cutting machines shall be grounded either by a third wire in the cable connecting the circuit conductor or by a separate wire that is grounded at the source of the current.

10.E.05 Neither terminal of the welding generator shall be bonded to the frame of the welder.

10.E.06 Pipelines containing gases or flammable liquids or conduits carrying electrical conductors shall not be used for a ground return circuit.

10.E.07 Circuits from welding machines used for other than welding tools shall be grounded.

10.E.08 Welding supply cables shall not be placed near power supply cables or other high-tension wires.

10.E.09 Welding leads shall not be permitted to contact metal parts supporting suspended scaffolds.

10.E.10 Switching equipment for shutting down the welding machine shall be provided on or near the welding machine.

10.E.11 Equipment shall be shut down when the leads are unattended.

10.E.12 Arc welding and cutting operations shall be shielded by noncombustible or flameproof screens to protect employees and other visitors from the direct rays of the arc.

10.E.13 Coiled welding cable shall be spread out before use.

EM 385-1-1
15 Sep 08

10.F GAS METAL ARC WELDING

10.F.01 Chlorinated solvents shall be kept at least 200 ft (61 m) away from the exposed arc, unless shielded. Surfaces prepared with chlorinated solvents shall be dry before welding is permitted on such surfaces.

10.F.02 Persons in the area not protected from the arc by screening shall be protected by filter lenses. When two or more welders are exposed to each other's arc, filter lens goggles shall be worn under welding helmets. Hand shields shall be used to protect the welders against flashes and radiant energy when either the helmet is lifted or the shield is removed.

10.F.03 Welders and other persons who are exposed to radiation shall be protected so that the skin is covered to prevent burns and other damage by ultraviolet rays. Welding helmets and hand shields shall be free of leaks, cracks, openings, and highly reflective surfaces.

10.F.04 When gas metal arc welding is performed on stainless steel, chrome alloy steel, or chrome-coated metal, personnel shall be protected against dangerous concentrations of nitrogen dioxide and other air contaminants such as chromium (VI), by means of an approved local exhaust ventilation system that is capable of reducing and maintaining personal exposures to within permissible limits, or by means of other effective work practice and engineering controls such as the use of an argon-rich (> 75% argon) shielding gas for use in gas metal arc welding (GMAW) or flux cored arc welding (FCAW) operations. Wherever engineering and work practice controls are not sufficient to reduce employee exposures below permissible limits, the employer shall use them to reduce employee exposures to the lowest levels achievable, and shall supplement such methods by the use of respiratory protection that complies with the requirements of this Section and Section 05.

EM 385-1-1
15 SEP 08

SECTION 11

ELECTRICAL

11.A GENERAL

11.A.01 Approval and qualification. The term "Qualified Person", as used in this section, refers to "Qualified Person, Electrical". **> See Appendix Q.**

 a. All electrical wiring and equipment shall be a type listed by a nationally recognized testing laboratory for the specific application for which it is to be used.

 b. All electrical work shall comply with applicable National Electrical Safety Code (NESC), National Electric Code (NEC), OSHA and USCG regulations.

 c. Electrical work shall be performed by Qualified Personnel with verifiable credentials who are familiar with applicable code requirements. Verifiable credentials consist of State, National and/or Local Certifications or Licenses that a Master or Journeyman Electrician may hold, depending on work being performed, and should be identified in the appropriate AHA.

 (1) USACE and/or other Government designated electricians having attained Journeyman Level qualification via completion of USACE/Government-sponsored electrical training programs are considered to be in compliance with this requirement.

 (2) Journeyman/Apprentice ratio shall be in accordance with State, Local and Host Nation requirements applicable to where work is being performed.

11.A.02 Isolation.

 a. Before work is begun, the person in charge shall ascertain by inquiry, by direct observation, or by instruments, whether any part of an electric power circuit (exposed or concealed) is located such that the performance of work could bring any person, tool, or machine into physical or electrical contact with it.

b. Whenever possible, all equipment and circuits to be worked on shall be de-energized before work is started and personnel protected by clearance procedures, lockout/tagout, and grounding. On each machine operated by electric motors, positive means shall be provided for rendering such controls or devices inoperative while repairs or adjustments are being made to the machines they control. *> See Section 12.*

c. Energized work may never be performed without prior authorization. If it is determined that equipment must be worked in an energized condition, an energized work permit shall be submitted to GDA for acceptance. *> See NFPA 70E.* Permits must be prepared in advance and include, as a minimum:

(1) Description of work and location;

(2) Justification for why the work must be performed in an energized condition;

(3) Description of work practices to be followed;

(4) An electrical shock analysis and boundaries (safe working distances);

(5) Arc flash hazard analysis and flash boundary determination;

(6) Necessary PPE to safely perform the task;

(7) Means to restrict access of unqualified persons in work area;

(8) Evidence of completing the job briefing, i.e., safety, tools, PPE or any other hazards and controls.

d. Live parts of wiring or equipment shall be guarded to protect all persons or objects from harm.

e. Transformer banks and high voltage equipment shall be protected from unauthorized access; entrances not under constant observation shall be kept locked; metallic enclosures shall be grounded and signs warning of high voltage and prohibiting unauthorized entrance shall be posted at entrances.

f. Enclosure gates or doors shall swing outward or provide clearance from installed equipment.

11.A.03 Flexible cords.

a. For construction sites, all flexible cords shall be inspected by the user of the cord at least daily.

b. Flexible cord sets used on construction sites or in damp locations shall contain the number of conductors required for the service plus an equipment ground wire. The cords shall be hard usage or extra hard usage as specified in the NEC.

c. Electric wire and flexible cord passing through work areas shall be protected from damage (including that caused by foot traffic, vehicles, sharp corners, protections, and pinching). Flexible cords and cables passing through holes shall be protected by bushings or fittings.

d. Flexible cord shall be used only in continuous lengths without splice or tap. <u>The repair of hard-service cord 14 AWG and larger shall be permitted if conductors are spliced in accordance with NEC</u> (the splices are made by a qualified electrician, the insulation is equal to the cable being spliced, and wire connections are soldered).

e. Patched, oil-soaked, worn, or frayed electric cords or cables shall not be used.

f. Extension cords or cables shall be <u>supported in place at intervals that ensure that they will be protected from physical damage. Support shall be in the form of cable ties, straps or similar type fittings installed so as not to cause damage.</u> They shall not be hung from nails, or suspended by bare wire.

11.A.04 When it is necessary to work on energized lines or equipment, rubber gloves and other protective equipment or hotline tools meeting the provisions of ANSI and ASTM standards shall be used. For work on energized equipment, only tools insulated for the voltage shall be used. **> See Section 05.G.**

11.A.0<u>5</u> <u>The Qualified Person is responsible for determining the number of workers required to perform the job safely and shall identify work hazards and controls in corresponding AHA. Work must be performed with a sufficient number of workers to provide a safe working environment.</u>

11.A.<u>06</u> Switchboxes, receptacle boxes, metal cabinets, enclosures around equipment, and temporary power lines shall be marked to indicate the maximum operating voltage.

11.A.<u>07</u> Insulation mats or platforms of substantial construction and providing good footing shall be placed on floors and on the frames of equipment having exposed live parts so that the operator or persons in the vicinity cannot touch such parts unless standing on the mats, platforms, or insulated floors.

11.A.<u>08</u> Suitable barriers or other means shall be provided to ensure that workspace for electrical equipment cannot be used as a passageway when energized parts of electrical equipment are exposed.

11.A.<u>09</u> When fuses are installed or removed with one or both terminals energized, special tools insulated for the voltage shall be used.

11.A.<u>10</u> Attachment plugs and receptacles.

EM 385-1-1
15 SEP 08

a. Plugs and receptacles shall be kept out of water unless of an approved submersible type.

b. Attachment plugs for use in work areas shall be constructed so that they will endure rough use and shall be equipped with a cord grip to prevent strain on the terminal screws.

c. Attachment plugs and other connectors supplying equipment at more than 300 volts shall be skirted or otherwise designed so that arcs will be confined.

d. When a National Electrical Manufacturers Association (NEMA) standard configuration exists for a particular voltage, amperage, frequency, or type of current, the NEMA standard plug and receptacle shall be used.

11.A.11 Portable hand lamps.

a. Portable hand lamps shall be of molded composition or another type approved for the purpose.

b. Metal-shell, paper-lined lamp holders shall not be used.

c. Hand lamps shall be equipped with a handle and with a substantial guard over the bulb. The guard shall be attached to the lamp holder or the handle.

11.A.12 An AHA and written work procedures must be prepared for unusual or complicated work activities or any activity identified by the Qualified Person. *> See Section 01.*

11.B ARC FLASH

11.B.01 Whenever it is necessary to work on energized parts greater than 50 volts to ground, a risk/hazard analysis/arc flash hazard analysis will be conducted in accordance with NFPA 70E Either Appendices or Tables may be used to conduct analysis. The flash protection boundary, approach distances, hazard/risk

EM 385-1-1
15 SEP 08

category and PPE requirements shall all be identified. This AHA is separate, distinct and in addition to the AHA required in Section 01.

11.B.02 PPE that provides appropriate arc flash protection is required for all personnel working on or near exposed energized electrical equipment operating at 50 volts or more. Identification of required PPE is based on function of hazard/risk category.

11.B.03 PPE garments shall meet and be labeled in accordance with ASTM F1506, *Standard Specification for Flame Resistant Textile Materials for Wearing Apparel for use by Electrical Workers Exposed to Momentary Electric Arc and Related Thermal Hazards.*

11.B.04 Arc flash rated clothing shall be properly worn. Long sleeves must be rolled down and buttoned, shorts are prohibited and trousers shall extend the full length of the leg. Garments with exposed metallic fasteners shall not be worn unless the garments are properly arc rated.

11.B.05 Garments, to include full body safety harnesses, worn over arc flash rated protective clothing must be arc flash rated.

11.B.06 Metal jewelry (i.e., wristbands, watch chains, rings, bracelets, necklaces, body jewelry, piercings, etc) shall not be worn when working on or near electrical equipment.

11.B.07 Clothing that could increase the extent of injuries when exposed to electric arcs or open flames (i.e., acetate, nylon, polyester, rayon or any blend, celluloid or other flammable plastic, shall not be worn. No metal slides or zippers unless they are effectively covered.

11.B.08 Arc Flash signage and labeling must be placed on the energized equipment. Switchboards or panelboards that are likely to be accessed with covers on are required to have a label to warn of potential electrical arc flash hazards and appropriate PPE required.

EM 385-1-1
15 SEP 08

11.C OVERCURRENT PROTECTION, DISCONNECTS, AND SWITCHES

11.C.01 All circuits shall be protected against overload.

a. Overcurrent protection shall be based on the current-carrying capacity of the conductors supplied and the power load being used.

b. No overcurrent device shall be placed in any permanently grounded conductor except where the overcurrent device simultaneously opens all conductors of the circuit or where the device is required by NEC 430 for motor overload protection.

c. Overcurrent protection devices must be readily accessible, clearly labeled, not exposed to physical damage, not placed in the vicinity of easily ignitable materials, and located or shielded such that their operation will not expose employees to injury due to arching or the sudden movement of parts.

d. Circuit breakers shall clearly indicate whether they are in the open (de-energized/off) or closed (energized/open) position.

e. Enclosures containing overcurrent protective devices shall be provided with lockable, close-fitting doors. At least 36 in (91.4 cm) of clearance must be maintained around all sides of the enclosure. On vessels or floating plant where the 36 in clearance is not feasible, sufficient clearance for fully opening the door and/or servicing the electrical enclosure shall be maintained.

11.C.02 Disconnects.

a. Disconnecting means shall be located or shielded so that persons will not be injured when the disconnect is operated.

b. Enclosures for disconnecting means shall be securely fastened to the surface and fitted with covers.

c. <u>Disconnecting means shall be capable of accepting a lock and of being locked in the open position.</u>

11.C.03 Switches.

a. A readily accessible, manually-operated switch shall be provided for each incoming service or supply circuit.

b. Switches shall be of the externally operable type mounted in an enclosure listed for the intended use and installed to minimize the danger of accidental operation.

11.C.04 Switches, fuses, and automatic circuit breakers shall be marked, labeled, or arranged for ready identification of the circuits or equipment that they supply.

11.C.05 Switches, circuit breakers, fuse panels, and motor controllers located out-of-doors or in wet locations shall be in a weatherproof enclosure or cabinet.

11.D GROUNDING

11.D.01 All electrical circuits, <u>equipment and enclosures</u> shall be grounded in accordance with the NEC and the NESC <u>to provide a permanent, continuous and effective path to ground</u> unless otherwise noted in this manual.

a. A ground shall be provided for non-current carrying metallic parts of equipment such as generators <u>(per NEC 250.34, portable and vehicle-mounted generators are exempt from grounding provided conditions of 11.D.01.b and c are met)</u>, electrically powered arc welders, switches, motor controller cases, fuse boxes, distribution cabinets, frames, non-current carrying rails used for travel and motors of electrically operated cranes, electric elevators, metal frames of non-electric elevators to which electric conductors are attached, other electric equipment, and metal enclosures around electric equipment.

EM 385-1-1
15 SEP 08

b. Portable Generators. Portable describes equipment that is easily carried by personnel from one location to another. The frame of a portable generator is not required to be grounded and may serve as the grounding electrode for a system supplied by the generator under the following conditions:

(1) The generator supplies ONLY equipment mounted on the generator, cord-and-plug-connected equipment through receptacles mounted on the generator, or both; and

(2) The non-current-carrying metal parts of the equipment and the equipment grounding conductor terminals of the receptacles are bonded to the generator frame.

c. Vehicle-Mounted Generators. The frame of a vehicle need not be grounded and may serve as the grounding electrode for a system supplied by a generator located on the vehicle under the following conditions:

(1) The frame of the generator is bonded to the vehicle frame;

(2) The generator supplies only equipment located on the vehicle or cord-and-plug-connected equipment through receptacles mounted on the vehicle;

(3) The non-concurrent-carrying metal parts of equipment and the equipment grounding conductor terminals of the receptacles are bonded to the generator frame; and

(4) The system complies with provisions of Section 11.D.01.

d. A system conductor that is required to be grounded by NEC 250.34 shall be bonded to the generator frame where the generator is a component of a separately derived system.

EM 385-1-1
15 SEP 08

e. Portable and semi-portable electrical tools and equipment shall be grounded by a multi-conductor cord having an identified grounding conductor and a multi-contact polarized plug and receptacle.

f. Semi-portable equipment, floodlights, and work lights shall be grounded. The protective ground should be maintained during moving unless supply circuits are de-energized.

g. Tools protected by an approved system of double insulation, or its equivalent, need not be grounded. Double-insulated tools shall be distinctly marked and listed by a nationally-recognized testing laboratory.

11.D.02 Grounding rod and pipe electrodes.

a. Electrodes of rod or pipe shall be free from non-conducting coatings and, if practicable, shall be embedded below permanent moisture levels.

b. Grounding rod and pipe electrodes shall be in unbroken 8-ft (2.4-m) lengths and driven to full depth. Where rock bottom is encountered, the electrode shall be driven at an angle not to exceed 45° from the vertical or shall be buried in a trench that is at least 2.5 ft (0.7 m) deep.

c. A single electrode that does not have a resistance to ground of 25 ohms or less, shall be augmented by one additional electrode spaced no closer than 6 ft (1.8 m) to the first electrode.

d. Electrodes of rods of iron or steel shall be at least 5/8 in (15 mm) diameter. Nonferrous rods, or their equivalent, shall be listed by a nationally-recognized testing laboratory and shall be at least   in (12 mm) diameter.

e. Electrodes of pipe or conduit shall be at least 3/4 in (1.9 cm) trade size. Pipes and conduit of iron or steel shall have the outer surface galvanized or otherwise metal-coated for corrosion control.

f. Grounding electrode systems of permanent facilities shall be in accordance with NEC 250.

11.D.03 Conductors used for bonding or grounding stationary and movable equipment shall be of ample size to carry the anticipated current.

a. When attaching bonding and grounding clamps or clips, a secure and positive metal-to-metal contact shall be made.

b. The ground end shall be attached first. The equipment end shall be attached and removed by insulated tools or other suitable devices.

c. When removing grounds, the grounding device shall be removed from the line or equipment first, using insulated tools or other suitable devices.

d. Bonding and grounding attachments shall be made before systems are activated and shall not be broken until after systems are de-activated.

11.D.04 Grounding circuits shall be checked to ensure that the circuit between the ground and a grounded power conductor has a resistance low enough to permit sufficient current flow to allow the fuse or circuit breaker to interrupt the current.

11.D.05 All receptacle outlets that provide temporary electrical power during construction, remodeling, maintenance, repair, or demolition shall have ground-fault circuit-interrupter (GFCI) protection for personnel.

a. GFCI protection shall be provided on all circuits serving portable electric hand tools or semi-portable electric power tools (such as block/brick saws, table saws, air compressors, welding machines, and drill presses).

EM 385-1-1
15 SEP 08

b. The GFCI device shall be calibrated to trip within the threshold values of 5 ma +/- 1 ma as specified in UL Standard 943. GFCI devices shall be tested before initial use and before use after modification.

c. Receptacle outlets that are not part of the permanent wiring of the building or structure shall be GFCI protected by one of the following means:

(1) A receptacle outlet with integral GFCI protection;

(2) A standard receptacle outlet connected downstream of a receptacle outlet with integral GFCI protection; or

(3) Receptacles protected by a GFCI-type circuit breaker.

d. Receptacle outlets that are part of the permanent wiring of the building or structure and are used for temporary electric power, (including portable generators) shall use a portable GFCI device if the receptacle outlets are not already GFCI protected. The portable GFCI device shall be as near as practicable to the receptacle outlet.

> **_Exception: In industrial facilities only, where conditions of maintenance and supervision ensure that only qualified personnel are involved, an Assured Equipment Grounding Conductor Program (AEGCP, see Appendix D) shall be permitted for only those receptacle outlets used to supply equipment that would create a greater hazard if power was interrupted or having a design that is not compatible with GFCI protection._**

e. Electric tool circuits that are "hard-wired" directly to an electrical source of power shall be GFCI protected by a GFCI-type circuit breaker.

EM 385-1-1
15 SEP 08

f. GFCIs shall be installed in accordance with the NEC. The permanent wiring shall consist of electrical circuits grounded in accordance with the NEC.

g. GFCIs may be sensitive to some equipment (such as concrete vibrators), <u>or unavailable for the voltage and current rating.</u> In these instances, an AEGCP in accordance with Appendix D is acceptable in lieu of GFCIs if the exception is documented on an AHA and contains the following:

(1) The conditions, or need, for the exception; and

(2) Implementation of the requirements of the AEGCP;

(3) The request for the exception, the AHA, and the AEGCP must be submitted and accepted by the GDA prior to implementing the program.

11.E TEMPORARY WIRING AND LIGHTING

11.E.01 A sketch of proposed temporary power distribution systems shall be submitted to the GDA and accepted for use before temporary power is installed. The sketch shall indicate the location, voltages, and means of protection of all circuits, including receptacles, disconnecting means, grounding, GFCIs, and lighting circuits.

11.E.02 Testing.

a. Temporary electrical distribution systems and devices shall be checked and found acceptable for polarity, ground continuity, and ground resistance before initial use and before use after modification. GFCI shall be tested monthly.

b. Ground resistance and circuits shall be measured at the time of installation and shall comply with 11.D.02 and 11.D.04. The measurement shall be recorded and a copy furnished to the GDA.

EM 385-1-1
15 SEP 08

11.E.03 The vertical clearance of temporary wiring for circuits carrying 600 volts or less shall be:

a. 10 ft (3 m) above finished grade, sidewalks, or from any platform;

b. 12 ft (3.8 m) over areas <u>other than public streets, alleys, roads and driveways,</u> subject to vehicular traffic other than truck traffic;

<u>c.</u> 15 ft (4.5 m) over areas other than public streets, alleys, roads and driveways, subject to truck traffic;

<u>d.</u> 18 ft (5.5 m) over public streets, alleys, roads, and driveways.

11.E.04 Wet Locations.

a. <u>USACE personnel and contractors are prohibited from placing electric sump pumps into USACE project bodies of water (lakes, etc.) to support periodic maintenance and/or construction activities. These pumps are not designed to be submerged in locations where people could be present in the water (i.e., recreating, swimming, wading, etc.) and doing so can create an electrical hazard that could result in serious injury or electrocution.</u>

b. Where a receptacle is used in a wet location, it shall be contained in a weatherproof enclosure, the integrity of which is not affected when an attachment plug is inserted.

c. All temporary lighting strings in outdoor or wet locations (such as tunnels, culverts, valve pits, floating plant, etc.) shall consist of lamp sockets and connection plugs permanently molded to the hard service cord insulation.

11.E.05 Wires shall be insulated from their supports.

EM 385-1-1
15 SEP 08

11.E.06 Temporary lighting.

   a. Bulbs attached to temporary lighting strings and extension cords shall be protected by guards unless the bulbs are deeply recessed in a reflector.

   b. Unless designed for suspension, temporary lights shall not be suspended by their electric wire.

   c. Exposed empty light sockets and broken bulbs shall be replaced immediately.

   d. Portable electric lighting used in wet and/or other conductive locations (e.g., drums, tanks, and vessels) shall be operated at 12 volts or less. > *See also 11.H.*

11.E.07 When temporary wiring is used in tanks or other confined spaces, an approved switch, identified and marked, shall be provided at or near the entrance to such spaces for cutting off the current in emergencies.

11.E.08 Non-metallic sheathed cable may be used as allowed by the NEC and as follows:

   a. Along studs, joists, or similar supports closely following the building finish or running boards when 7 ft 8 in (2.3 m) or more above the floor;

   b. When firmly attached to each cabinet, box fitting, or fixture by means of a cable clamp. > *Non-metallic sheathed cable may not be used where precluded by the NEC nor as portable extension cords, lying on the ground subject to any type of traffic, where subject to frequent flexing, or as service entrance cable.*

11.E.09 Temporary lighting circuits shall be separate from electric tool circuits. Receptacle circuits shall be dedicated to either temporary lighting or electric tools and shall be labeled "**LIGHTS ONLY**" or "**TOOLS ONLY**," as applicable.

EM 385-1-1
15 SEP 08

11.F OPERATIONS ADJACENT TO OVERHEAD LINES

11.F.01 Overhead transmission and distribution lines shall be carried on towers and poles that provide safe clearances over roadways and structures.

    a. Clearances shall be adequate for the movement of vehicles and for the operation of construction equipment.

    b. All electric power or distribution lines shall be placed underground in areas where there is extensive use of equipment having the capability to encroach on the clear distances specified in 11.E.03.

    c. Protection of outdoor trolleys and portable cables rated above 600 volts for supplying power to moveable construction equipment such as gantry cranes, mobile cranes, shovels, etc., shall conform to NESC.

11.F.02 Work activity adjacent to overhead lines shall not be initiated until a survey has been made to ascertain the safe clearance from energized lines. *> See 11.A.02.*

11.F.03 Any overhead wire shall be considered energized unless the person owning such line or operating officials of the electrical utility supplying the line certifies that it is not energized and it has been visibly grounded and tested.

11.F.04 Operations adjacent to overhead lines are prohibited unless at least one of the following conditions is satisfied:

    a. Power has been shut off and positive means taken to prevent the lines from being energized.

    b. Equipment, or any part, does not have the capability of coming within the minimum clearance from energized overhead lines as specified in Table 11-1, or the equipment has been positioned and blocked to assure no part, including cables, can

EM 385-1-1
15 SEP 08

come within those clearances; a notice of the minimum required clearance has been posted at the operator's position. <u>Electric line trucks and/or aerial lifts used for working on energized overhead lines must meet the requirements of 1910.269 and Section 11.I.c.</u> In transit with the boom lowered and no load, the equipment clearance shall comply with Table 11-1.

TABLE 11-1

MINIMUM CLEARANCE FROM ENERGIZED OVERHEAD ELECTRIC LINES

(All dimensions are distances from live part to employee)

Voltage (nominal, kV, alternating current)	Minimum rated clearance
Up to 50	10 ft (3 m)
51 – 200	15 ft (4.6 m)
201 – 350	20 ft (6 m)
351 to 500	25 ft (7.6 m)
501 - 650	30 ft (9.1 m)
651 – 800	35 ft (10.7 m)
801 – 950	40 ft (12.2 m)
951 – 1100	45 ft (13.7 m)
Clearance values calculated using: (Initial kV-50kV) x (4 in/10 kV) x (1 ft/12 in) = increased distance (ft) over 10 ft. Add this value to 10 ft to yield minimum rated clearance	

11.F.05 Work activity that could affect or be affected by overhead lines shall not be initiated until coordinated with the appropriate utility officials.

11.F.06 Standard emergency communication procedures shall be established and rehearsed to assure rapid emergency shutdown for all work being conducted on overhead power lines.

EM 385-1-1
15 SEP 08

11.F.07 Floating plant and associated equipment shall not be sited or placed within 20 ft (6 m) of overhead transmission or distribution lines.

11.F.08 Cage boom guards, insulating links, or proximity warning devices may be used on cranes, but such devices shall not alter the requirements of any other regulation of this part, even if such device is required by law or other regulation. Insulating links shall be capable of withstanding a 1 minute dry low frequency dielectric test of 50,000 volts AC.

11.F.09 Induced currents.

    a. Before work near transmitter towers where there is potential for an electrical charge to be induced in equipment or materials, the transmitter shall be de-energized or tests shall be conducted to determine if an electrical charge could be induced.

    b. The following precautions shall be taken to dissipate induced voltages:

    (1) The equipment shall be provided with an electrical ground to the upper rotating structure supporting the boom; and

    (2) Ground jumper cables shall be attached to materials being handled by boom equipment when electrical charge could be induced while working near energized transmitters. Crews shall be provided with nonconductive poles having large alligator clips or other similar protection to attach the ground cable to the load and insulating gloves will be used.

11.G BATTERIES AND BATTERY CHARGING

11.G.01 <u>Storage batteries shall be stored in enclosures with outside vents or in well-ventilated rooms and be so arranged as to prevent the escape of fumes, gases, or electrolyte spray into other areas.</u>

EM 385-1-1
15 SEP 08

11.G.02 <u>Provisions shall be made for sufficient diffusion and ventilation of gases from storage batteries to prevent the accumulation of explosive mixtures</u>.

11.G.03 Battery storage and handling.

   a. Racks and trays shall be substantial and shall be treated to make them resistant to the electrolyte.

   b. Floors shall be of acid resistant construction or protected from accumulation of acid.

   c. Facilities for quick drenching of the eyes and body shall be provided for emergency use within 25 ft (7.6 m) of battery handling areas. *> See Section 06.B.02.b.*

   d. <u>Use only insulated tools in the battery area to prevent accidental shorting across battery connections.</u>

   e. <u>PPE shall be used as prescribed in 11.G.06 and Section 5.</u>

   f. <u>For lead acid batteries, bicarbonate of soda to neutralize any acid spillage (1 lb/gal (0.1 kg/L)of water)</u> shall be provided for flushing and neutralizing spilled electrolyte and for fire protection.

11.G.04 Battery charging.

   a. Battery charging installations shall be located in areas designated for that purpose.

   b. Charging apparatus shall be protected from mechanical damage.

   c. When charging batteries, the vent caps shall be kept in place to avoid spray of electrolyte. Care shall be taken to assure vent caps are functioning.

EM 385-1-1
15 SEP 08

    d. Prior to charging batteries, the electrolyte level shall be checked and adjusted to the proper level if necessary.

11.G.05 Exit from battery area shall remain unobstructed.

11.G.06 PPE. The following shall be available and used fore the safe handling of the battery and protection of personnel:

    a. Safety glasses with side shields and faceshields or goggles;

    b. Acid-resistant rubber gloves;

    c. Protective rubber aprons and safety shoes;

    d. Lifting devices of adequate capacity, when required.

11.H HAZARDOUS (CLASSIFIED) LOCATIONS

11.H.01 Locations of electrical equipment and wiring shall be classified on the properties of the flammable vapors, liquids or gases, or combustible dusts or fibers that may be present and the likelihood that a flammable or combustible concentration or quantity is present. In classifying locations, each room, section, or area shall be classified on an individual basis in accordance with the definitions given in Table 11-2 and NEC Article 500. These hazardous locations within the facility, as designated, shall be documented by the employer.

11.H.02 All equipment, wiring methods, and installations of equipment in hazardous (classified) locations shall be either listed as intrinsically safe, listed for the hazardous location, or demonstrated to be safe for the location.

11.H.03 Only equipment wiring and installation of equipment in hazardous locations shall be permitted in those hazardous (classified) locations.

EM 385-1-1
15 SEP 08

11.H.04 Equipment and wiring listed for the hazardous (classified) location shall be approved not only for the class of location but also for the ignitable or combustible properties of the specific gas, vapor, dust, or fiber that will be present.

    a. This equipment shall be marked to show the class, group, and operating temperature or temperature range for which it is approved.

    b. With the following exceptions, the temperature marking shall not exceed the ignition temperature of the specific gas or vapor to be encountered.

    (1) Equipment of the non-heat producing type (e.g., junction boxes and conduit) and equipment of the heat producing type having a maximum temperature not more than 212 °F (100 °C) need not have a marked operating temperature or temperature range.

    (2) Fixed lighting fixtures marked for use in Class I, Division 2 or Class II, Divison 2 locations need not be marked to indicate the group.

TABLE 11-2

HAZARDOUS (CLASSIFIED) LOCATIONS

Class I	
Gasses, Vapors or Liquids (A, B, C and D)	
Division 1	Division 2
Normally explosive and hazardous	Not normally present in an explosive concentration (but may accidentally exist).
Zone 0 (IEC Stds)	Zone 1 (IEC Stds)
Class II	
Dusts (E, F and G)	
Division 1	Division 2
Ignitable quantity of dust that is normally or may be, in suspension or conductive dust may be present	Dust not normally suspended in an ignitable concentration (but may accidentally exist). Dust layers are present
Class III	
Fibers or Flyings (H)	
Division 1	Division 2
Handled or used in manufacturing	Stored or handled in storage (exclusive of manufacturing).

A - Acetylene
B – Hydrogen, etc
C - Ethyl-ether vapors, ethylene, etc
D – Hydrocarbons, fuels, solvents, etc
E - Metal dust (conductive* and explosive)
F - Carbon dusts (some are conductive* and all are explosive)
G - Flour, starch, grain, Combustible Plastic or Chemical Dusts (explosive)
H – Textiles, woodworking, etc.,(easily ignitable but not likely to be explosive
*Note: Electrically conductive dusts are dusts with a resistivity less than 10^5 OHM-centimeter

EM 385-1-1
15 SEP 08

3) Fixed general-purpose equipment in Class I locations, other than lighting fixtures, that is acceptable for use in Class I, Division 2 locations need not be marked with the class, group, division, or operating temperature.

(4) Fixed dust-tight equipment, other than lighting fixtures, that is acceptable for use in Class II, Division 2, and Class III locations need not be marked with the class, group, division, or operating temperature.

11.H.05 Equipment that is safe for the hazardous (classified) location shall be of a type and design that will provide protection from the hazards arising from the combustibility and flammability of vapors, liquids, gases, dusts, or fibers involved.

11.H.06 Equipment approved for a specific hazardous location shall not be installed or intermixed with equipment approved for another specific hazardous location.

11.H.07 All wiring components and utilization equipment required to be explosion proof (vapor, dust, or fiber tight) shall be maintained in that condition.

   a. There shall be no loose or missing screws, gaskets, threaded connections, or other impairments to this tight condition.

   b. Conduits shall be threaded and made wrench-tight: where it is impractical to make a threaded joint tight, a bonding jumper shall be used.

11.I POWER TRANSMISSION AND DISTRIBUTION

11.I.01 The requirements in this subsection shall apply to the erection of new electric transmission and distribution lines and equipment, and the alteration, conversion, and improvement of existing electric transmission and distribution lines and equipment.

11.I.02 Before starting work, existing conditions shall be evaluated and determined. Such conditions shall include, but not be limited to, location and voltage of energized lines and equipment, conditions of poles, and location of circuits and equipment including power and communication lines and fire alarm circuits.

    a. Electric equipment and lines shall be considered energized until determined to be de-energized by tests, or other means, and grounds applied.

    b. New lines or equipment may be considered de-energized and worked as such where the lines or equipment are grounded or where the hazard of induced voltages is not present and adequate clearances or other means are implemented to prevent contact with energized lines or equipment.

    c. Bare wire communication conductors on power poles or structures shall be treated as energized lines unless protected by insulating materials suitable for the highest voltage that may be accidentally applied to the line.

    d. The operating voltage of equipment and lines shall be determined before working on or near energized parts.

11.I.03 Clearance requirements of either subparagraph a or b below shall be observed.

    a. No employee shall be permitted to approach or take any conductive object without an approved insulating handle closer to exposed energized parts than shown in Table 11-3 (phase to ground) unless:

    (1) The employee is insulated or guarded from the energized part (gloves or gloves with sleeves rated for the voltage involved shall be considered insulation of the employee from the energized part);

EM 385-1-1
15 SEP 08

TABLE 11-3

AC Live Work Minimum Approach Distance

Voltage in kV (phase-to-phase)[1,2]	Distance to Employee			
	Phase-to-ground		Phase-to-phase	
	(m)	(ft-in)	(m)	(ft-in)
0 to 0.050	Not specified		Not specified	
0.051 to 0.300	Avoid contact		Avoid contact	
0.301 to 0.750	0.31	1-0	0.31	1-0
0.751 to 15	0.65	2-2	0.67	2-3
15.1 to 36.0	0.77	2-7	0.86	2-10
36.1 to 46	0.84	2-9	0.96	3-2
46.1 to 72.5	1.00[3]	3-3[3]	1.20	3-11
72.6 to 121	0.95[3]	3-2[3]	1.29	4-3
138 to 145	1.09	3-7	1.50	4-11
161 to 169	1.22	4-0	1.71	5-8
230 to 242	1.59	5-3	2.27	7-6
345 to 362	2.59	8-6	3.80	12-6
500 to 550	3.42	11-3	5.50	18-1
765 to 800	4.53	14-11	7.91	26-0

[1] For single-phase systems use the highest voltage available.
[2] For single-phase lines off three phase systems, use phase-to-phase voltage of the system.
[3] The 46.1 to 72.5 kV phase-to-ground 3-3 (ft-in) distance contains a 1-3 (ft-in) electrical component and a 2-0 (ft-in) inadvertent movement component while the 72.6 to 121 kV phase-to-ground 3-2 (ft-in) distance contains a 2-0 (ft-in) electrical component and a 1-0 (ft-in) inadvertent movement component.

(2) The energized part is insulated or guarded from the employee and any other conductive object at a different potential; or

(3) The employee is isolated, insulated, or guarded from any other conductive object(s), as during live-line, bare-hand work.

b. The minimum phase to ground working distance and minimum clear hot stick distances in Table 11-3 shall not be exceeded. The minimum clear hot stick distance refers to the distance from the hot end of live-line tools to the lineman when performing live-line work. Conductor support tools (such as link sticks, strain carriers, and insulator cradles) may be used provided the clear length of insulation is at least as long as the insulator string or as long as the minimum phase to ground distance in Table 11-3.

11.l.04 When de-energizing lines and equipment operated in excess of 600 volts, and the means of disconnecting from electric energy is not visibly open or visibly tagged and/or locked out, provisions a through g below are required. **> In addition, requirements in Section 12 apply.**

a. The equipment or section of line to be de-energized shall be clearly identified and shall be isolated from all sources of voltage.

b. Notification and assurance from the GDA shall be obtained that:

(1) All switches and disconnects through which electric energy may be supplied to the particular section of line or equipment to be worked have been de-energized;

(2) All switches and disconnects are plainly tagged and/or locked indicating that persons are at work; and

EM 385-1-1
15 SEP 08

(3) All switches and disconnects capable of being rendered inoperable are rendered inoperable.

c. After all designated switches and disconnects have been opened, rendered inoperable, and tagged and/or locked, visual inspections shall be conducted to ensure that equipment or lines are de-energized.

d. Protective grounds shall be applied on the disconnected equipment or lines to be worked on.

e. Guards or barriers shall be erected as necessary to adjacent energized lines.

f. When more than one crew requires the same line or equipment to be de-energized, a prominent tag and/or lock for each crew shall be placed on the line or equipment by the Authorized Individual(s) holding the clearance(s) on said equipment or line.

g. Upon completion of work on de-energized lines or equipment, each Authorized Individual holding a clearance shall determine that all employees in the crew are clear and request a release of the clearance. The protective grounds installed will be removed. Authorized Individual will report to the GDA that all tags and locks protecting the crew may be removed.

11.I.05 When opening or closing a disconnect switch or circuit breaker on a power transmission/distribution line, exposure to potential explosion shall be limited. Safe operating procedures shall be established to minimize the risk of explosion.

11.I.06 When a crew working on a line or equipment can clearly see that the means of disconnecting from electrical energy are visibly open or visibly locked-out, the following provisions are required. > **See Section 12.**

a. Guards or barriers shall be erected as necessary to adjacent energized lines.

b. Upon completion of work on de-energized lines or equipment, each designated person-in-charge shall determine that all employees in the crew are clear that all protective grounds installed by the crew have been removed and shall report to the GDA that all tags and locks protecting the crew may be removed.

11.I.07 Grounding.

a. De-energized conductors and equipment that are to be grounded shall be tested <u>or visually checked by meters or indicators to be de-energized</u>.

b. <u>Requirements as detailed in NEC and NESC for placing and removing protective grounds shall be followed</u>.

c. Grounds shall be placed between the work location and all sources of energy and as close as practicable to the work location, or grounds shall be placed at the work location.

(1) If work is to be performed at more than one location in a line section, the line section must be grounded and short circuited at one location in the line section and the conductor to be worked on shall be grounded at each work location.

(2) The minimum distance in Table 11-3 shall be maintained from ungrounded conductors at the work location.

(3) Where the making of a ground is impractic<u>al</u>, or the conditions resulting from it would be more hazardous than working on the lines or equipment without grounding, the grounds may be omitted and the line or equipment worked as energized.

EM 385-1-1
15 SEP 08

d. Grounds may be temporarily removed only when necessary for test purposes and extreme caution shall be exercised during the test procedures. The lines or equipment from which grounds have been removed shall be considered energized.

e. When grounding electrodes are used, such electrodes shall have a resistance to ground <u>of less than 25 ohms</u> to remove the danger of harm to personnel or permit prompt operation of protective devices (NEC 250).

f. Grounding to tower shall be made with a tower clamp capable of conducting the anticipated fault current.

g. A ground lead, to be attached to either a tower ground or driven ground, shall be capable of conducting the anticipated fault current and shall have a minimum conductance of No. 2 AWG copper.

11.<u>I.08</u> Tools.

a. All hydraulic tools that are used on or around energized lines or equipment shall use non-conducting hoses having adequate strength for the normal operating pressures.

b. All pneumatic tools that are used on or around energized lines or equipment shall have non-conducting hoses of adequate strength for the normal operating pressures and have an accumulator on the compressor to collect moisture.

c. Portable metal or conductive ladders shall not be used near energized lines or equipment except in specialized work such as in high voltage substations where nonconductive ladders might present a greater hazard than conductive ladders. Conductive or metal ladders shall be prominently marked as conductive and all precautions shall be taken when used in specialized work.

d. Tape or rope measures that are metal or contain conductive strands shall not be used when working on or near energized parts.

EM 385-1-1
15 SEP 08

11.I.09 Aerial lift trucks > *See Section 18 and 22.M.*

a. The aerial device manufacturer shall state in the operator's manual and on the instruction plate whether the aerial device is insulating or non-insulating.

b. Aerial lift trucks shall be grounded or barricaded and considered as energized equipment, or the aerial lift truck shall be insulated for the work being performed. Table 11-3 will be legibly printed on a plate of durable non-conductive material and shall be mounted on the bucket or its vicinity so as to be visible to the operator of the boom.

c. Equipment or material shall not be passed between a pole or structure and an aerial lift while an employee working from the basket is within reaching distance of energized conductors or equipment that are not covered with insulating protective equipment.

d. Only qualified electrical workers may operate aerial lift equipment within the restricted approach boundary distances.

11.I.10 With the exception of equipment certified for work on the proper voltage, mechanical equipment shall not be operated closer to any energized line or equipment than the clearances in Table 11-3 unless:

a. An insulated barrier is installed between the energized part and the mechanical equipment;

b. The mechanical equipment is grounded;

c. The mechanical equipment is insulated; or

d. The mechanical equipment is considered as energized.

EM 385-1-1
15 SEP 08

11.I.11 Material handling and storage.

   a. When hauling poles during the hours of darkness, illuminated warning devices shall be attached to the trailing end of the longest pole.

   b. Materials and equipment shall not be stored under energized bus, energized lines, or near energized equipment if it is possible to store them elsewhere. If materials or equipment must be stored under energized lines or near energized equipment, clearance shall be maintained as in Table 11-3 and extraordinary caution shall be exercised in maintaining these clearances when operating equipment or moving materials near such energized equipment.

   c. Tag lines shall be of a non-conducting type when used near energized lines.

11.I.12 Before climbing poles, ladders, scaffolds, or other elevated structures, an inspection shall determine that the structures are capable of sustaining the additional or unbalanced stresses to which they will be subjected. Poles or structures that may be unsafe for climbing shall not be climbed until made safe by guying, bracing, or other means.

11.I.13 Before installing or removing wire or cable, action will be taken as necessary to prevent the failure of poles and other structures.

11.I.14 When setting, moving, or removing poles by cranes, derricks, gin poles, A-frames, or other mechanized equipment near energized lines or equipment, precautions shall be taken to avoid contact with energized lines or equipment, except in bare hand, live-line work, or where barriers or protective devices are used.

11.I.15 Unless using protective equipment for the voltage involved, employees standing on the ground shall avoid contacting equipment or machinery working adjacently to energized lines or equipment.

EM 385-1-1
15 SEP 08

11.I.16 Lifting equipment shall be bonded to an effective ground or it shall be considered energized and barricaded when used near energized equipment or lines.

11.I.17 Pole holes shall not be left unattended or unguarded.

11.I.18 Where necessary to assure the stability of mobile equipment, the location shall be graded and leveled.

11.I.19 When employees are working at two or more levels on a tower, activities shall be conducted such that there is a minimum exposure of employees to falling objects.

11.I.20 Guy lines shall be used to maintain sections or parts of tower sections in position and to reduce the possibility of tipping.

11.I.21 Tower members and sections being assembled shall be adequately supported.

11.I.22 No one shall be permitted under a tower that is in the process of erection or assembly, except as may be required to guide and secure the section being set.

11.I.23 When erecting towers using hoisting equipment adjacent to energized transmission lines, the lines shall be de-energized when practical. If the lines are not de-energized, minimum clearance distances shall be maintained as specified in Table 11-3 and extraordinary caution shall be exercised in maintaining these clearances when operating equipment or moving materials near such energized equipment.

11.I.24 The load line shall not be detached from a tower section until the section is adequately secured.

11.I.25 Except during emergency restoration procedures, tower erection shall be discontinued in high wind or other adverse weather conditions that could make the work hazardous. When work is conducted under such conditions, the AHA and the means for their control shall be delineated in an AHA.

11.I.26 Before stringing operations, a briefing shall be held to discuss the following:

    a. The plan of operation;

    b. The type of equipment to be used;

    c. Grounding devices and procedures to be followed;

    d. Crossover methods to be employed; and

    e. Clearance authorizations that are required.

11.I.27 When there is a possibility of a de-energized conductor being installed or removed coming into accidental contact with an energized circuit or receiving a dangerous induced voltage buildup, the conductor being installed or removed shall be grounded or provisions made to insulate or isolate the employee.

11.I.28 If an existing line is de-energized, proper clearance authorization shall be secured and the line grounded on both sides of the crossover or the wire being strung or removed shall be considered and worked as energized.

11.I.29 When crossing over energized conductors in excess of 600 volts, ropes, nets or guard structures shall be installed unless provision is made to isolate or insulate the worker or the energized conductor. Where practical the automatic re-closing feature of the circuit-interrupting device shall be made inoperative. In addition, the line being strung shall be grounded on either side of the crossover or considered and worked as energized.

11.I.30 Conductors being strung or removed shall be kept under positive control by tension reels, guard structures, tie lines, or other means to prevent accidental contact with energized circuits.

EM 385-1-1
15 SEP 08

11.I.31 Guard structure members shall be sound, of adequate dimension and strength, and adequately supported.

11.I.32 Catch-off anchors, rigging, and hoists shall be of ample capacity to prevent loss of the lines.

11.I.33 Reel handling equipment, including pulling and braking machines, shall have ample capacity, operate smoothly, and be leveled and aligned in accordance with the manufacturer's operating instructions.

11.I.34 The manufacturer's load rating shall not be exceeded for stringing lines, pulling lines, sock connections, and all load-bearing hardware and accessories.

11.I.35 Pulling lines and accessories shall be inspected regularly and replaced or repaired when damaged or when dependability may be doubtful.

11.I.36 Conductor grips shall not be used on wire rope unless designed for this application.

11.I.37 Employees shall not be permitted under overhead operations or on cross-arms while a conductor or pulling line is being pulled (in motion).

11.I.38 A transmission clipping crew shall have a minimum of two structures clipped between the crew and the conductor being sagged. When working on bare conductors, clipping and tying crews shall work between grounds at all times; the grounds shall remain intact until the conductors are clipped in, except on dead end structures.

11.I.39 Except during emergency restoration procedures, work from structures shall be discontinued when adverse weather (such as high wind or ice on structures) makes the work hazardous. Stringing and clipping operations shall be discontinued during an electrical storm in the vicinity.

EM 385-1-1
15 SEP 08

11.I.40 Reliable communications between the reel tender and pulling rig operator shall be provided.

11.I.41 Each pull shall be snubbed or dead ended at both ends before subsequent pulls.

11.I.42 Before stringing parallel to an existing energized transmission line, a competent determination shall be made to ascertain whether dangerous induced voltage buildups will occur, particularly during switching and ground fault conditions. When there is a possibility that such dangerous induced voltage may exist, the employer shall comply with the provisions of 11.I.42 through 11.I.49 in addition to the provisions of 11.I.25 through 11.I.40 unless the line is worked as energized.

11.I.43 When stringing adjacent to energized lines, the tension stringing method or other methods that preclude unintentional contact between the lines being pulled and any person shall be used.

11.I.44 All pulling and tensioning equipment shall be isolated, insulated, or grounded.

11.I.45 A ground shall be installed between the tensioning reel setup and the first structure to ground each bare conductor, sub-conductor, and overhead ground conductor during stringing operations.

11.I.46 During stringing operations, each bare conductor, sub-conductor, and overhead ground conductor shall be grounded at the first tower adjacent to both the tensioning and pulling setup and in increments so that no point is more than 2 miles (mi) (3.2 km) from a ground.

   a. The grounds shall be left in place until conductor installation is complete.

   b. Such grounds shall be removed as the last phase of aerial cleanup.

EM 385-1-1
15 SEP 08

    c. Except moveable-type grounds, the grounds shall be placed and removed with a hot stick.

11.I.47 Conductors, sub-conductors, and overhead ground conductors shall be grounded at all dead-end or catch-off points.

11.I.48 A ground shall be located at each side and within 10 ft (3 m) of working areas where conductors, sub-conductors, or overhead ground conductors are being spliced at ground level. The two ends to be spliced shall be bonded to each other. Splicing should be carried out on either an insulated platform or a conductive metallic grounding mat bonded to both grounds. The grounding mat should be roped off and an insulated walkway provided for access to the mat.

11.I.49 All conductors, sub-conductors, and overhead ground conductors shall be bonded to any isolated tower where it may be necessary to complete work on the transmission line.

    a. Work on dead-end towers shall require grounding on all de-energized lines.

    b. Grounds may be removed as soon as the work is completed provided the line is not left open-circuited at the isolated tower at which work is being completed.

11.I.50 When performing work from the structure, clipping crews and all others working on conductors, sub-conductors, or overhead ground conductors shall be protected by individual grounds installed at every workstation.

11.I.51 Before using the live-line bare-hand technique on energized high-voltage conductors or parts, a check shall be made of:

    a. The voltage rating of the circuit on which the work is to be performed;

b. The clearances to ground of lines and other energized parts of which work is to be performed; and

c. The voltage limitations of the aerial-lift equipment intended to be used.

11.I.52 Only tools and equipment designed, tested, and intended for live-line bare-hand work shall be used, and such tools and equipment shall be kept clean and dry.

11.I.53 All work shall be personally supervised by a person trained and qualified to perform live-line bare-hand work.

11.I.54 The automatic re-closing feature of circuit interrupting devices shall be made inoperative where practical before working on any energized line or equipment.

11.I.55 Work shall not be performed during electrical storms or when electrical storms are imminent.

11.I.56 A conductive bucket liner or other suitable conductive device shall be provided for bonding the insulated aerial device to the energized line or equipment.

   a. The employee shall be connected to the bucket liner by conductive shoes, leg clips, or other suitable means; climbers shall not be worn while performing work from an aerial lift.

   b. Where necessary, electrostatic shielding for the voltage being worked or conductive clothing shall be provided.

11.I.57 Before the boom is elevated, the outriggers on the aerial truck shall be extended and adjusted to stabilize the truck. The body of the truck shall be bonded to an effective ground or barricaded and considered as energized equipment.

11.I.58 Before moving an aerial lift into the work position, all controls (ground level and bucket) shall be checked and tested to determine that they are in proper working condition.

11.I.59 Electrical insulating components and systems of aerial devices that are rated and used as an insulating device shall be, after a thorough inspection of their condition and cleanliness, tested for compliance with their rating.

    a. Tests shall be conducted in accordance with the manufacturer's recommendations.

    b. Tests shall be conducted only by qualified persons who are knowledgeable of the hazards.

11.I.60 All aerial lifts to be used for live-line bare-hand work shall have dual controls (ground level and basket).

    a. The basket controls shall be within easy reach of the employee in the basket. If a two-basket lift is used, access to the controls shall be within easy reach from either basket.

    b. The ground level controls shall be located near the base of the boom and will permit override operation of equipment at any time.

    c. Except in case of an emergency, ground level lift control shall not be operated unless permission has been obtained from the employee in the lift.

11.I.61 Before an employee contacts the energized part to be worked on, the conductive bucket liner shall be bonded to the energized conductor by a positive connection that shall remain attached to the energized conductor until the work on the energized circuit is completed.

11.I.62 The minimum clearances for live-line bare-hand work shall be as specified in Table 11-3.

a. These minimum clearances shall be maintained from all grounded objects and from lines and equipment at a different potential than that to which the insulated aerial device is bonded, unless such grounded objects or other lines and equipment are covered by insulated guards.

b. These distances shall be maintained when approaching, leaving, and when bonded to the energized circuit.

c. When approaching, leaving, or bonding to an energized circuit, the minimum distances in Table 11-3 shall be maintained among all parts of the insulated boom assembly and any grounded parts (including the lower arm or portions of the truck).

d. When positioning the bucket alongside an energized bushing or insulator string, the minimum line-to-ground clearances of Table 11-3 must be maintained among all parts of the bucket and the grounded end of the bushing or insulator string.

e. A minimum clearance table (as in Table 11-3) shall be printed on a plate of durable nonconductive material and mounted in the bucket or in its vicinity so as to be visible to the boom operator.

f. Only insulated measuring sticks shall be used to verify clearance distances.

11.I.63 Handlines between buckets, booms, and the ground are prohibited.

a. Conductive materials more than 36 in (1 m) long shall NOT be placed in the bucket, except for appropriate length jumpers, armor rods, and tools.

b. Non-conductive handlines may be used from line to ground when not supported from the bucket.

EM 385-1-1
15 SEP 08

11.I.64 The bucket and boom shall not be over- stressed by attempting to lift or support weights in excess of the manufacturer's rating.

11.J UNDERGROUND ELECTRICAL INSTALLATIONS

11.J.01 Guarding underground openings.

    a. Warning signs and rigid barricades shall be promptly placed when covers of manholes, handholes, or vaults are removed.

    b. When an employee enters an underground opening the opening shall be protected with a barricade, temporary cover, or other guard appropriate for the hazard.

    c. Underground opening guards and warning signs shall be lighted at night.

11.J.02 Maintenance holes and unvented vaults shall be treated as, and subjected to the requirements of, confined spaces. **> See Section 34.**

11.J.03 Smoking shall be prohibited in maintenance holes and vaults.

11.J.04 When open flames must be used in manholes, extra precautions shall be taken to provide ventilation.

11.J.05 Before using open flames in maintenance holes or vaults, the holes/vaults shall be tested and found safe or cleared of any combustible gases or liquids.

11.J.06 When underground facilities are exposed (electric, gas, water, telephone, etc., or cables other than the one being worked on), they shall be protected to avoid damage.

EM 385-1-1
15 SEP 08

11.J.07 Before cutting into a cable or opening a splice, the cable shall be identified and verified to be the proper cable and de-energized.

11.J.08 When working on buried cable or on cable in manholes, metallic sheath continuity shall be maintained by bonding across the opening or by equivalent means.

11.K WORK IN ENERGIZED SUBSTATIONS

11.K.01 When working in an energized substation, authorization shall be obtained from the GDA before work is begun.

11.K.02 When work is to be done in an energized substation, the following shall be determined:

   a. What facilities are energized, and

   b. What protective equipment and precautions are necessary for the safety of personnel.

11.K.03 Clearance requirements per Section 11.I.03 shall be followed.

11.K.04 Only qualified employees shall perform work on or adjacent to energized control panels. > *See Section 11.A.01, 11.A.05.*

11.K.05 Precautions shall be taken to prevent accidental operation of relays or other protective devices due to jarring, vibration, or improper wiring.

11.K.06 Use of vehicles, gin poles, cranes, and other equipment in unguarded high voltage equipment areas shall at all times be controlled by qualified employees.

EM 385-1-1
15 SEP 08

11.K.07 All mobile cranes and derricks shall be effectively grounded when being moved or operated near energized lines or equipment or the equipment shall be considered energized.

11.K.08 When a substation fence must be expanded or removed, a temporary fence affording similar protection, when the site is unattended, shall be provided. Adequate interconnection with ground shall be maintained between temporary fence and permanent fence.

11.K.09 All gates to all unattended substations shall be locked except when work is in progress.

11.K.10 When switching gang switches, visual inspection shall be made to ensure all insulators and the switch handle ground are in good condition. Insulating gloves must be worn when operating switch handles.

11.L COMMUNICATION FACILITIES

11.L.01 Employees shall not look into an open wave guide or antenna that is connected to an energized electromagnetic source.

11.L.02 If the electromagnetic radiation level within an accessible area exceeds the levels given in Section 06.F, the area shall be posted with appropriate signs.

11.L.03 When an employee works in an area where the electromagnetic radiation could exceed the levels given in Section 06.F, measures shall be taken to ensure that the employee's exposure is not greater than that permitted.

EM 385-1-1
15 Sep 08

SECTION 12

CONTROL OF HAZARDOUS ENERGY

12.A GENERAL

12.A.01 This Section shall apply to contractor-managed Hazardous Energy Control Programs (HECP) only, as well as all requirements of 1910.147, ANSI Z244.1, and ANSI A10.44. When a site is controlled by a contractor and USACE employees are affected by contractor-managed HECP (e.g., QA's on construction sites, etc.), they shall comply with the contractor's HECP.

12.A.02 USACE-owned/operated facilities that involved hazardous energy shall comply with ER 385-1-31, the applicable regional HECP and any local supplements.

12.A.03 When contractor work involving hazardous energy will be performed at or on a USACE-operated facility, the following coordination must occur:

a. The GDA and the Contractor shall fully coordinate all control activities with one another throughout the planning and implementation of these activities. Each shall inform the other of their HECPs and Hazardous Energy Control (HEC) procedures, ensure that their own personnel understand and comply with rules and restrictions of the procedures agreed upon to be used for the job, and ensure that their employees affected by the hazardous energy control activity are notified when the procedural steps outlined in the HECP are to be initiated.

b. When Contractors are planning the use of HEC procedures, they shall submit their HECP to the GDA for acceptance. Implementation of HEC procedures shall not be initiated until the HECP has been accepted by the GDA. The Prime Contractor, as the Controlling Contractor, is also responsible for the HEC procedures of all their sub-contractors.

EM 385-1-1
15 Sep 08

12.A.04 Systems with energy isolating devices that are capable of being locked out shall be locked out. If an energy isolating device is not capable of being locked out, the HEC procedures shall use tagout providing full personnel protection. **> See 12.A.11.c.**

12.A.05 Locks must always be used when the clearance involves equipment that is accessible by the public.

12.A.06 All equipment shall be covered by a safe clearance (or lockout/tagout procedures) and all energy sources shall be controlled before performing service or maintenance on equipment in which the unexpected energizing, startup, or release of stored energy could occur and cause any of the following: Personal injury, property damage, loss of content, loss of protection, loss of capacity, or harm to the environment.

12.A.07 A preparatory meeting and inspection with the GDA and Contractor personnel shall be conducted to insure that all affected employees understand the energy hazards and the procedures for their control. This meeting/inspection shall be documented.

    a. Employees shall be trained and tested prior to working on Corps' Facilities where the Corps' HECP is in use to ensure that they are knowledgeable of the procedures. Contractors shall ensure that all of their employees and sub-contractors are knowledgeable of their HECPs.

    b. When HEC procedures affect both USACE and Contractors, USACE and Contractor clearance holders will participate in the preparatory inspection, verifying that equipment has been properly cleared and that locks and tags have been placed as appropriate.

12.A.08 Lockout and tagout shall be performed only by Authorized employees.

12.A.09 All employees affected by the lockout/tagout shall be notified, before and upon completion of, the application and removal of locks or tags.

EM 385-1-1
15 Sep 08

12.A.10 Coordination (Shift/Schedule Change). Provisions shall be made to ensure the continuity of lockout/tagout protection during shift or personnel change.

12.A.<u>11</u> Locks and tags.

   a. Systems with energy isolating devices that are capable of being locked out <u>shall be locked out.</u>

   b. Locks must always be used when the clearance involves equipment that is accessible by the public.

   <u>c.</u> If an energy-isolating device is not capable of being locked out, the HEC procedures shall use tagout providing full personnel protection as follows:

   (1) All tagout requirements of this regulation and of the HEC procedures shall be complied with;

   (2) The tag shall be attached to the same location, if possible, that the lock would have been attached. If this is not possible then the tag shall be attached as close a safely possible to the device and in a position that will be immediately obvious to anyone attempting to operate the device; AND

   (3) Additional means (e.g., placement of the tag in a manner that inhibits operation of the energy isolating device, removal of an isolating circuit mechanism, blocking of a control switch, opening of an extra disconnecting device, removal of a valve handle to reduce the likelihood of inadvertent energizing, etc.) shall be employed to provide a level of protection commensurate with that provided by a locks.

12.A.<u>12</u> Hazardous Energy Control <u>Program (HECP)</u>

   a. <u>HEC</u> procedures shall be developed in the <u>HECP</u>.

b. The HECP shall clearly and specifically outline the scope, purpose, authorization, responsibilities, rules, and techniques to be used for the control of hazardous energy, including, but not limited to, the following:

(1) A statement of the intended use of the procedure;

(2) Means of coordinating and communicating HEC activities;

(3) Procedural steps and responsibilities for shutting down, isolating, blocking, and securing systems to control hazardous energy;

(4) Procedural steps and responsibilities for the placement, removal, and transfer of lockout and tagout devices;

(5) Procedural steps, responsibilities and a means of accounting for placing and removing personal protective grounds;

(6) Procedural steps, responsibilities and requirements for testing the system to verify the effectiveness of isolation and lockout and tagout devices;

(7) Procedural steps and responsibilities for transfer of clearances when and if necessary;

(8) Procedural steps and responsibilities for Multi-Shift Safe Clearances;

(9) A description of any emergencies that may occur during system lockout/tagout and procedures for safely responding to those emergencies; and

(10) The means to enforce compliance with the procedures.

12.B TRAINING

12.B.01 Training shall be provided to ensure that the purpose and function of the HEC procedures are understood by employees and that employees possess the knowledge and skills required for the safe application, usage, and removal of HEC devices.

    a. Each Authorized Employee shall receive training in the recognition of hazardous energy sources, the type and magnitude of energy available in the workplace, and the methods and means for energy isolation and control.

    b. Each Affected employee shall be instructed in the purpose and use of the HEC procedures.

    c. All incidental personnel shall be informed of the procedures and prohibitions relating to restarting or reenergizing systems which are locked or tagged out.

    d. When tagout systems are used (only when lockout is not possible), employees shall be trained in the limitations of tags.

12.B.02 Employees shall be retrained in HEC procedures whenever:

    a. There is a change in their job assignments, a change in systems or processes that present a new energy control hazard, or a change in HEC procedures; or

    b. Periodic inspection reveals, or there is reason to suspect the presence of, inadequacies in or deviations from the employee's knowledge or use of HEC procedures.

12.B.03 The supervisor shall certify and document all training and retraining. Certification shall contain such information as the names of employees trained; the time, date, and location of training; the name of the trainer, etc.

12.C PERIODIC INSPECTIONS

12.C.01 Daily inspections shall be conducted to ensure that all requirements of the HEC procedures are being followed.

12.C.02 Periodic Inspections shall be documented and shall specify the system where the HEC procedures were inspected, the date of the inspection, the names of employees performing and included in the inspections, and any deficiencies in complying with the HEC procedures.

12.D LOCKS AND TAGS

12.D.01 Locks and tags shall:

    a. Be capable of withstanding the environment that they are exposed to for the maximum period of time the exposure is expected, and

    b. Indicate the identity of the employee applying the device.

12.D.02 Locks shall, in addition to the requirements of 12.D.01, be substantial enough to prevent removal without the use of excessive force or unusual techniques (such as with the use of bolt cutters).

12.D.03 Tags shall, in addition to the requirements of 12.D.01, meet all of the following requirements:

    a. Have a standardized (within a project) print and format;

    b. Be constructed and printed so that exposure to weather conditions, ultraviolet (UV) light, wet or damp locations, or corrosive environments will not cause the tag to deteriorate or the message to become illegible;

    c. Be attached by means that are: Non-reusable; Substantial enough to prevent inadvertent or accidental removal; Attachable by hand; Self-locking; Non-releasable, with a minimum

EM 385-1-1
15 Sep 08

unlocking strength of no less than 50 lb (22.6 kg); and have the basic characteristics of being at least equivalent to a one-piece, all-environment-tolerant nylon cable tie; and

d. Warn against the hazardous condition resulting from system energization and include a legend such as **"DANGER - DO NOT START, OPEN, CLOSE, ENERGIZE, OPERATE,"** etc.

12.E APPLICATION AND REMOVAL OF LOCKS AND TAGS

12.E.01 The authorized employee shall ensure that all energy isolating devices needed to control energy to or within the system are identified and that the system is shut down, isolated, blocked and secured in accordance with HEP procedures.

12.E.02 Any system operated by a remotely controlled source will be completely isolated such that it cannot be operated by that or any other source.

12.E.03 The authorized employee shall affix locks and/or tags to each energy isolating device in accordance with the HEC procedures.

12.E.04 In areas with public access, not under strict control of personnel involved with the HEC activities, locks or other positive controls must be installed on the isolation devices.

12.E.05 Personal Protective Grounds. Following the application of locks or tags to energy isolating devices, all potentially hazardous stored or residual energy shall be relieved, disconnected, restrained, discharged, or otherwise rendered safe.

a. Protective grounds shall be identified and accounted for in some manner, as identified in the Contractor's HECP and procedures.

b. The authorized employee (or his designee) is responsible for ensuring the control of residual energy and for placing and removing personal protective grounds in accordance with the Contractor's HECP and procedures.

12.E.06 When there is a possibility of re-accumulation of stored energy to a hazardous level, verification of isolation shall be continued until the energy control procedure is complete.

12.E.07 Before starting work on systems that have been locked/tagged out, the authorized individual shall verify that isolation and de-energization of the system have successfully been accomplished.

12.E.08 When tags only must be used (the use of locks is not possible), employees shall be instructed in the following requirements and limitations of tags.

> a. Tags must be legible and understood by all authorized and affected employees and incidental personnel.
>
> b. Tags and their means of attachment must be made of materials that will withstand the environments encountered in the workplace.
>
> c. Tags shall be securely attached to energy isolating devices so that they cannot become inadvertently or accidentally detached during use.
>
> d. Tags shall not be removed without authorization of the authorized employee and shall never be bypassed, ignored, or otherwise defeated.
>
> e. Tags are essentially warning devices affixed to energy isolating devices and do not provide the physical protection that is provided by a lock; tags may evoke a false sense of security.

12.E.09 Before locks or tags are removed and energy restored to the system, the authorized individual shall ensure that the following actions have been taken:

EM 385-1-1
15 Sep 08

a. The work area has been inspected and all nonessential items (e.g., tools and materials) have been removed from the system, the system components are operationally intact, and all employees have been safely positioned or removed from the area; and

b. All affected individuals have been notified that the <u>locks or tags</u> are about to be removed.

12.E.10 With the exception of the following conditions, each <u>lock and/or tag</u> shall be removed from each energy-isolating device by the authorized individual or systems operator who applied the device. When this employee is not available, the device(s) may be removed by another individual appointed by, and under the direction of the <u>Contractor Project Manager or Contractor designated authority</u>, provided that the following procedures are complied with:

a. The Contractor ensures that the individual appointed to remove locks and/or tags is knowledgeable of the scope and procedures of the safe clearance.

b. This individual and the requirements for transferring removal authority to him<u>/her</u> from the authorized individual are listed in the hazardous energy control plan.

c. Verification by the <u>Contractor</u> that the authorized employee who applied the device is not at the facility.

d. The <u>Contractor</u> designated authority makes all reasonable efforts to contact the authorized employee to inform him that the locks and/or tags are to be removed; <u>and if a group clearance is involved, then an attempt must be made to have all affected persons sign off on the clearance or they must be contacted by phone. If contact cannot be made, then the lift may be made only after all necessary precautions are taken.</u>

EM 385-1-1
15 Sep 08

e. The authorized employee, upon returning, must be immediately notified of the lift prior to resuming their work.

EM 385-1-1
15 Sep 08

SECTION 13

HAND AND POWER TOOLS

13.A GENERAL

13.A.01 Power tools shall be of a manufacture listed by a nationally recognized testing laboratory for the specific application for which they are to be used.

13.A.02 Use, inspection, and maintenance.

> a. Hand and power tools shall be used, inspected, and maintained in accordance with the manufacturer's instructions and recommendations and shall be used only for the purpose for which designed. A copy of the manufacturer's instructions and recommendations shall be maintained with the tools.
>
> b. Hand and power tools shall be inspected, tested, and determined to be in safe operating condition before use. Continued periodic inspections shall be made to assure safe operating condition and proper maintenance.
>
> c. Hand and power tools shall be in good repair and with all required safety devices installed and properly adjusted. Tools having defects that will impair their strength or render them unsafe shall be removed from service.

13.A.03 Guarding.

> a. Power tools designed to accommodate guards shall be equipped with such guards. All guards must be functional.
>
> b. Reciprocating, rotating, and moving parts of equipment shall be guarded if exposed to contact by employees or otherwise create a hazard.

EM 385-1-1
15 Sep 08

13.A.04 When work is being performed overhead, tools not in use shall be secured or placed in holders.

13.A.05 Throwing tools or materials from one location to another or from one person to another, or dropping them to lower levels, shall not be permitted.

13.A.06 Only non-sparking tools shall be used in locations where sources of ignition may cause a fire or explosion.

13.A.07 Tools requiring heat treating or redressing shall be tempered, formed, dressed, and sharpened by personnel who are experienced in these operations.

13.A.08 The use of cranks on hand-powered winches or hoists is prohibited unless the hoists or winches are provided with positive self-locking dogs. Hand wheels with exposed spokes, projecting pins, or knobs shall not be used.

13.A.09 Hydraulic fluid used in powered tools shall retain its operating characteristics at the most extreme temperatures to which it will be exposed. **> For underground use, see 26.D.07.**

13.A.10 Manufacturers' safe operating pressures for hydraulic hoses, valves, pipes, filters and other fittings shall not be exceeded.

13.A.11 All hydraulic or pneumatic tools that are used on or around energized lines or equipment shall have non-conducting hoses of adequate strength for the normal operating pressures.

13.A.12 When fuel-powered tools are used in confined or enclosed spaces, the requirements for concentrations of toxic gases as outlined in Sections 5 and 34 of this manual, shall apply.

13.A.13 Clothing.

    a. PPE shall be used as outlined in Sections 5 of this manual.

EM 385-1-1
15 Sep 08

b. Loose and frayed clothing, loose long hair, dangling jewelry (including dangling earrings, chains, and wrist watches) shall not be worn while working with any power tool.

13.A.14 See Section 11.D for grounding requirements.

13.A.15 The electrical power control shall be provided on each machine/power tool to make it possible for the operator to cut off the power for the machine/power tool without leaving the point of operation.

13.A.16 Where injury to the operator may result if motors were to restart after power failures, provisions shall be made to prevent machines/power tools from automatically restarting upon restoration of power.

13.A.17 Floor- and bench-mounted power tools shall be anchored or securely clamped to a firm foundation. Anchoring or securing shall be sufficient to withstand lateral or vertical movement.

13.B GRINDING AND ABRASIVE MACHINERY

13.B.01 With the exception of the following, abrasive wheels shall be used only on machines provided with safety guards: **> See ANSI B74.2 for descriptions of abrasive wheel types.**

　　a. Wheels used for internal work while within the work being ground;

　　b. Mounted wheels, 2 in (5 cm) and smaller in diameter, used in portable operations;

　　c. Types 16, 17, 18, 18R, and 19 cones and plugs and threaded hole pot balls where the work offers protection or where the size does not exceed 3 in (7.6 cm) in diameter by 5 in (12.7 cm) long;

EM 385-1-1
15 Sep 08

    d. Type 1 wheels not larger than 2 in (5 cm) in diameter and not more than   in (1.2 cm) thick, operated at peripheral speeds less than 1800 surface-feet per minute (ft/min) (9.1 surface-m/s) when mounted in mandrels driven by portable drills;

    e. Type 1 reinforced wheels not more than 3 in (7.6 mm) in diameter and   in (6 mm) in thickness, operating at peripheral speeds not exceeding 9500 surface-ft/min (48.3 surface-m/s), if safety glasses and face shield protection are worn.

13.B.02 Tongue guards on bench/stand grinders shall be adjustable to within   in (6 mm) of the constantly decreasing diameter of the wheel at the upper opening.

13.B.03 Grinders shall be supplied with power sufficient to maintain the spindle speed at safe levels under all conditions of normal operation.

13.B.04 Work or tool rests shall not be adjusted while the grinding wheel is in motion.

13.B.05 Work/tool rests on power grinders shall not be more than 1/8 in (3 mm) distance from the wheel.

13.B.06 Abrasive wheels shall be closely inspected and ring-tested before mounting. Cracked or damaged grinding wheels shall be destroyed.

13.B.07 Grinding wheels shall not be operated in excess of their rated safe speed.

13.B.08 Floor stand and bench-mounted abrasive wheels used for external grinding shall be provided with safety guards (protective hoods).

    a. The maximum angular exposure of the grinding wheel periphery and sides shall be not more than 90°, except that when work requires contact with the wheel below the horizontal

EM 385-1-1
15 Sep 08

plane of the spindle the angular exposure shall not exceed 125°; in either case, the exposure shall begin not more than 65° above the horizontal plane of the spindle.

b. Safety guards shall be strong enough to withstand the effect of a bursting wheel.

13.C POWER SAWS AND WOODWORKING MACHINERY

13.C.01 Woodworking machinery shall be operated and maintained in accordance with ANSI 01.1.

13.C.0<u>2</u> Guarding.

a. Circular saws shall be equipped with guards that automatically and completely enclose the cutting edges, splitters, and anti kickback devices.

b. Portable power-driven circular saws shall be equipped with guards above and below the base plate or shoe.

<u>(1)</u> The upper and lower guards shall cover the saw to the depth of the teeth, except for the minimum arc required to permit the base to be tilted for bevel cuts and for the minimum arc required to allow proper retraction and contact with the work, respectively.

<u>(2)</u> When the tool is withdrawn from the work, the lower guard shall automatically and instantly return to the covering position.

c. Blades of planers and jointers shall be fully guarded and have cylindrical heads with throats in the cylinder.

d. Band saw blades shall be fully enclosed except at the point of operation.

13.C.0<u>3</u> Automatic feeding devices shall be installed on machines whenever possible. Feeder attachments shall have the feed rolls or

EM 385-1-1
15 Sep 08

other moving parts covered or guarded so as to protect the operator from hazardous points.

13.C.04 The operating speed shall be permanently marked on circular saws more than 20 in (50.8 cm) in diameter or operating at over 10,000 peripheral ft/minute (min) (50.8 peripheral m/s).

    a. Any saw so marked shall not be operated at a speed other than that marked on the blade.

    b. When a marked saw is re-tensioned for a different speed, the marking shall be corrected to show the new speed.

13.C.05 Radial arm power saws shall be equipped with an automatic brake.

13.C.06 The table of radial arm or swing saws shall extend beyond the leading edge of the saw blade.

13.C.07 Radial arm power saws shall be installed in such a manner that the cutting head will return to the starting position when released by the operator. All swing cutoff and radial saws or similar machines that are drawn across a table shall be equipped with limit stops to prevent the leading edge of the tool from traveling beyond the edge of the table.

13.C.08 Each hand-fed crosscut table saw and each hand-fed circular ripsaw shall have a spreader to prevent the material from squeezing the saw or being thrown back on the operator.

13.C.09 Operating procedures.

    a. Band saws and other machinery requiring warm-up for safe operation shall be permitted to warm up before being put into operation whenever the temperature is below 45 °F (7 °C).

    b. A push-stick, block, or other safe means shall be used on all operations close to high-speed cutting edges.

EM 385-1-1
15 Sep 08

c. The use of cracked, bent, or otherwise defective parts such as saw blades, cutters, or knives is prohibited.

d. A brush shall be provided for the removal of sawdust, chips, and shavings on all woodworking machinery.

e. Power saws shall not be left running unattended.

13.D PNEUMATIC TOOLS

13.D.01 Safety clips or retainers shall be installed and maintained on pneumatic impact tools to prevent dies and tools from being accidentally expelled from the barrel.

13.D.02 Pressure shall be shut off and exhausted from the line before disconnecting the line from any tool or connection.

13.D.03 Safety lashing shall be provided at connections between tool and hose and at all quick makeup type connections.

13.D.04 Hoses shall not be used for hoisting or lowering tools.

13.D.05 Airless spray guns of the type which atomize paints and fluids at high pressures (1,000 lb (453.5 kg) or more) shall be equipped with automatic or visible manual safety devices that will prevent pulling of the trigger to prevent release of the paint or fluid until the safety device is manually released. In lieu of the above, a diffuser nut that will prevent high-pressure velocity release while the nozzle tip is removed plus a nozzle tip guard that will prevent the tip from coming into contact with the operator, or other equivalent protection may be provided.

13.D.06 Impact wrenches shall be provided with a locking device for retaining the socket.

13.E EXPLOSIVE-ACTUATED TOOLS

13.E.01 Explosive-actuated (powder-actuated) tools shall meet the design requirements of ANSI A10.3.

13.E.02 Only qualified operators shall operate explosive-actuated tools. A qualified operator is one who has:

> a. Been trained by an authorized instructor (one who has been trained, authorized, and provided an authorized instructor's card by the tool manufacturer or by an authorized representative of the tool manufacturer);
>
> b. Passed a written examination provided by the manufacturer of the tool; and
>
> c. Possesses a qualified operator's card supplied by the manufacturer and issued and signed by both the instructor and the operator.

13.E.03 Each tool shall be provided with the following:

> a. A lockable container with the words **"POWDER-ACTUATED TOOL"** in plain sight on the outside and a notice reading **"WARNING - POWDER-ACTUATED TOOL TO BE USED ONLY BY A QUALIFIED OPERATOR AND KEPT UNDER LOCK AND KEY WHEN NOT IN USE"** on the inside;
>
> b. Operator's instruction and service manual;
>
> c. Power load and fastener charts;
>
> d. Tool inspection record; and
>
> e. Service tools and accessories.

13.E.04 Inspection and testing.

EM 385-1-1
15 Sep 08

a. Daily inspection, cleaning, and testing shall be performed as recommended by the manufacturer.

b. Explosive-actuated tools shall be tested, in accordance with the manufacturer's recommended procedure, each day before loading to see that safety devices are in proper working condition.

c. Explosive-actuated tools shall be inspected, thoroughly cleaned, and tested after each 1,000 fastenings.

13.E.05 Explosive-actuated tools and the charges shall be secured at all times to prevent unauthorized possession or use.

13.E.06 Explosive-actuated tools shall not be loaded until just before the intended firing time. Neither loaded nor empty tools are to be pointed at any employees. Hands shall be kept clear of the open barrel end.

13.E.07 The use of explosive-actuated tools is prohibited in explosive or flammable atmospheres.

13.E.08 Fasteners shall not be driven:

a. Into soft or easily penetrable materials unless they are backed by a material that will prevent the fastener from passing through to the other side;

b. Into very hard or brittle material, such as cast iron, hardened steel, glazed or hollow tile, glass block, brick, or rock;

c. Into concrete unless the material thickness is at least three times the penetration of the fastener shank; or

d. Into spalled concrete.

13.E.09 The tool operator shall wear safety goggles or other face and eye protection.

13.F CHAIN SAWS

13.F.01 Chain saws shall have an automatic chain brake or kickback device.

13.F.02 The idle speed shall be adjusted so that the chain does not move when the engine is idling.

13.F.03 Operators will wear proper PPE. Eye, ear, hand, foot (safety shoes), and leg protection are required as a minimum.

13.F.04 Chain saws will not be fueled while running, while hot, or near an open flame. Saws will not be started within 10 ft (3 m) of a fuel container.

13.F.05 The operator will hold the saw with both hands during all cutting operations.

13.F.06 A chain saw must never be used to cut above the operators' shoulder height.

13.F.07 See Section 31 for tree maintenance and removal requirements.

13.G ABRASIVE BLASTING EQUIPMENT

13.G.01 Hose and hose connections shall be designed to prevent build up of static electricity.

13.G.02 Connections and nozzles shall be designed to prevent accidental disengagement. All connections shall be equipped with safety lashings. > *See 20.A.16, 20.A.17.*

13.G.03 Nozzle attachments shall be of metal and fit on the outside of the hose. A deadman-type control device shall be provided at the nozzle to cut off the flow if the operator looses control of hose. A support shall be provided on which the nozzle may be mounted when it is not in use.

EM 385-1-1
15 Sep 08

13.G.04 Additional requirements on abrasive blasting are in Sections 5 and 6.

13. H POWER-DRIVEN NAILERS AND STAPLERS

13.H.01 This section applies to hand-held electric, combustion or pneumatically driven nailers, staplers, and other similar equipment (heretofore referred to as "nailers" in this section) which operate by ejecting a fastener into the material to be fastened when a trigger, lever, or other manual device is actuated. This does not apply to common spring-loaded "staple guns".

13.H.02 Nailers shall have a safety device on the muzzle to prevent the tool from ejecting fasteners unless the muzzle is in contact with the work surface. The contact trip device or trigger shall not be secured in an "on" position.

13.H.03 Nailers shall be operated in a way to minimize the danger to others and the operator from ricochets, air-firing, and firing through materials being fastened.

> a. Except when used for attaching sheet goods (sheathing, sub-flooring, plywood, etc.) or roofing products, nailers shall be operated with a sequential trigger system that requires the surface contact trip device to be depressed before the firing trigger can be activated and that limits ejection to one nail per trigger pull before resetting.

> b. When used for sheet goods and roofing materials, nailers may be operated in the contact trip mode (bump or bounce-nailing) only as allowed by the manufacturer. This mode may only be used when the operator has secure footing, such as on a work platform, floor or deck, and shall not be used when the operator is on a ladder, beam, or similar situations where the operator's balance and/ or reach may be unstable.

BLANK

EM 385-1-1
15 Sep 08

SECTION 14

MATERIAL HANDLING, STORAGE, AND DISPOSAL

14.A MATERIAL HANDLING

14.A.01 Employees shall be trained in and shall use safe lifting techniques.

14.A.02 Requirements for PPE are covered in Section 5.

14.A.03 Material handling devices shall be available for the material handling needs of an activity.

14.A.04 Whenever heavy or bulky material is to be moved, the material handling needs shall be evaluated in terms of weight, size, distance, and path of movement. The following hierarchy shall be followed in selecting a means for material handling:

   a. Elimination of material handling needs by engineering;

   b. Movement by mechanical device (e.g., lift truck, overhead crane, or conveyor);

   c. Movement by manual means with handling aid (e.g., dollie or cart); or

   d. Movement using safe lifting techniques. **> Reference NIOSH, Work Practices Guide for Manual Lifting.**

14.A.05 Materials will not be moved over or suspended above personnel unless positive precautions have been taken to protect the personnel from falling objects.

14.A.06 Where the movement of materials may be hazardous to persons, taglines or other devices shall be used to control the loads

EM 385-1-1
15 Sep 08

being handled by hoisting equipment. These devices shall be nonconductive when used near energized lines.

14.B MATERIAL STORAGE

14.B.01 All material in bags, containers, bundles, or stored in tiers shall be stacked, blocked, interlocked, and limited in height so that it is stable and secured against sliding or collapse.

    a. Material shall be stacked as low as practical and in no case higher than 20 ft (6 m) unless otherwise specified in this Section.

    b. Storage of flammable and combustible materials is covered in Section 9.

    c. Storage of hazardous and toxic agents is covered in Section 6.

14.B.02 Material stored inside buildings under construction shall not be placed within 6 ft (1.8 m) of any hoistway or floor opening, nor within 10 ft (3 m) of an exterior wall that does not extend above the material stored.

14.B.03 Accessways shall be kept clear.

14.B.04 Unauthorized persons shall be prohibited from entering storage areas. All persons shall be in a safe position while materials are being loaded or unloaded from railroad cars, trucks, or barges.

14.B.05 Material shall not be stored on scaffolds or runways in excess of needs for normal placement operations or in excess of safe load limits.

14.B.06 Noncompatible materials shall be segregated in storage.

14.B.07 Storage of lumber.

EM 385-1-1
15 Sep 08

a. Storage of lumber during construction shall be in sections containing a maximum of 1 million board feet with at least a 10 ft (3 m) clearance from buildings.

b. Lumber shall be supported on stable sills and shall be stacked level, stable, and self-supporting.

c. Reusable lumber shall have all nails withdrawn before it is stacked for storage.

d. Lumber piles shall not exceed 20 ft (6 m) in height; lumber to be handled manually shall not be stacked more than 16 ft (4.8 m) high.

14.B.08 Storage of bagged materials.

a. Bagged materials shall be stacked by stepping back the layers and cross-keying the bags at least every 10 bags high.

b. Bags of cement and lime shall not be stacked more than 10 high without setback, except when restrained by walls of appropriate strength.

c. The bags around the outside of the stack shall be placed with the mouths of the bags facing the center of the stack.

d. During unstacking, the top of the stack shall be kept nearly level and the necessary setback maintained.

14.B.09 Storage of brick.

a. Brick shall be stacked on an even, solid surface.

b. Bricks stacks shall not be more than 7 ft (2.1 m) high. when stacked loose brick reaches a height of 4 ft (1.2 m), it shall be tapered back 2 in (5 cm) in every 1 ft (0.3 m) of height above the 4 ft (1.2 m) level.

c. Unitized brick (brick securely gathered into large standard packages and fastened with straps) shall not be stacked more than three units high.

14.B.10 Storage of floor, wall, and partition block.

a. Blocks shall be stacked in tiers on solid, level surfaces.

b. When masonry blocks are stacked higher than 6 ft (1.8 m), the stack shall be tapered back one-half block per tier above the 6 ft level.

14.B.11 Storage of reinforcing and structural steel.

a. Reinforcing steel shall be stored in orderly piles away from walkways and roadways.

b. Structural steel shall be securely piled to prevent members sliding off or the pile toppling over.

14.B.12 Storage of cylindrical material.

a. Structural steel, poles, pipe, bar stock, and other cylindrical materials, unless racked, shall be stacked and blocked so as to prevent spreading or tilting.

b. Pipe, unless racked, shall not be stacked higher than 5 ft (1.5 m).

c. Either a pyramid or battened stack shall be used.

d. Where a battened stack is used, the outside pile or pole shall be securely chocked. Battened stacks shall be tapered back at least one pile or pole in each tier.

e. Unloading of round material shall be done so that no person is required to be on the unloading side of the carrier after the tie wires have been cut or during the unlocking of the stakes.

EM 385-1-1
15 Sep 08

14.C HOUSEKEEPING

14.C.01 Work areas and means of access shall be maintained safe and orderly.

    a. Sufficient personnel and equipment shall be provided to ensure compliance with all housekeeping requirements.

    b. Work areas shall be inspected daily for adequate housekeeping and findings <u>shall be</u> recorded on daily inspection reports.

    c. Work will not be allowed in those areas that do not comply with the requirements of this Section.

14.C.02 All stairways, passageways, gangways, and accessways shall be kept free of materials, supplies, and obstructions at all times.

14.C.03 Loose or light material shall not be stored or left on roofs or floors that are not closed in, unless it is safely secured.

14.C.04 Tools, materials, extension cords, hoses, or debris shall not cause tripping or other hazards.

14.C.05 Tools, materials, and equipment subject to displacement or falling shall be adequately secured.

14.C.06 Empty bags having contained lime, cement, and other dust-producing material shall be removed periodically as specified by the GDA.

14.C.07 Form and scrap lumber and debris shall be cleared from work areas and accessways in and around building storage yards and other structures.

14.C.08 Protruding nails in scrap boards, planks, and timbers shall be removed, hammered in, or bent over flush with the wood.

EM 385-1-1
15 Sep 08

14.C.09 Storage and construction sites shall be kept free from the accumulation of combustible materials.

   a. Weeds and grass shall be kept down.

   b. A regular procedure shall be established for the cleanup of the areas as specified by the GDA.

   c. Rubbish, brush, long grass, or other combustible material shall be kept from areas where flammable and combustible liquids are stored, handled, or processed.

14.C.10 Accumulation of liquids, particularly flammable and combustible liquids, on floors, walls, etc., is prohibited. All spills of flammable and combustible liquids shall be cleaned up immediately.

14.D DEBRIS NETS

14.D.01 When used with personnel safety nets, debris nets shall be secured on top of the personnel safety net but shall not compromise the design, construction or performance of the personnel nets.

14.D.02 A competent person shall determine and document the size, weight and height of fall of anticipated debris. The debris netting shall have a mesh of the size and strength sufficient to contain the expected debris without penetration when properly supported.

14.D.03 Materials, scraps, equipment, tools and debris that have fallen into the net shall be removed as soon as possible from the net and at lest before the next work shift.

14.D.04 Nets and debris shall be protected from sparks and hot slag resulting from welding and cutting operations.

14.D.05 Inspection of debris nets.

EM 385-1-1
15 Sep 08

a. Debris nets shall be inspected by a competent person in accordance with the manufacturer's recommendations.

b. Inspections shall be conducted after installation, at least weekly thereafter, and following any alteration, repair or any occurrence that could affect the integrity of the net system. Inspections shall be documented and maintained on site.

c. Defective nets shall not be used; defective components shall be removed from service.

d. When welding or cutting operations occur above the nets, frequency of inspections shall be increased in proportion to the potential for damage to the nets.

14.E MATERIAL DISPOSAL

14.E.01 Waste material and rubbish shall be placed in containers or, if appropriate, in piles.

14.E.02 Waste materials and rubbish shall not be thrown down from a height of more than 6 ft (1.8 m), unless the following are complied with:

a. The materials or rubbish are dropped through an enclosed chute constructed of wood or equivalent material. Chutes for debris shall be enclosed, except for openings equipped with closures at or about floor level for the insertion of materials. The openings shall not exceed 4 ft (1.2 m) in height measured along the wall of the chute. Openings shall be kept closed when not in use.

b. When debris cannot be handled by chutes, the area into which the material is dropped shall be enclosed with barricades not less than 42 in (1.1) in height. Barricades shall be positioned to keep personnel from all debris landing areas. Signs warning of the hazard of falling material shall be posted at all debris landing areas and at each level exposed to falling debris.

14.E.03 See Section 9 for burning requirements.

14.E.04 Separate covered, self-closing, nonflammable/non-reactive containers shall be provided for the collection of garbage, oily, flammable, and dangerous wastes.

   a. The containers shall be labeled with a description of the contents.

   b. The contents shall be properly disposed of daily.

14.E.05 Hazardous material waste (i.e., vehicle and equipment oils and lubricants, containers and drums for solvents, adhesives, etc.) shall be collected, stored, and disposed of in accordance with Federal, State, and local requirements.

EM 385-1-1
15 Sep 08

SECTION 15

RIGGING

15.A GENERAL

15.A.01 Inspection and use.

a. Rigging equipment shall be inspected as specified by the manufacturer, by a Competent Person, before use on each shift and as necessary during its use to ensure that it is safe.

b. Defective rigging shall be removed from service.

c. The use and maintenance of rigging equipment shall be in accordance with recommendations of the rigging manufacturer and the equipment manufacturer. Rigging equipment shall not be loaded in excess of its recommended safe working load.

d. Rigging equipment, when not in use, shall be removed from the immediate work area and properly stored and maintained in a safe condition.

15.A.02 Hoist rope shall not be wrapped around the load.

15.A.03 Running lines located within 6 ft - 6 in (1.9 m) of the ground or working level shall be guarded or the area restricted by physical barriers to preclude injury or injury from broken lines.

15.A.04 All eye splices shall be made in an approved manner. Rope thimbles of proper size shall be fitted in the eye, except that in slings the use of thimbles shall be optional.

15.A.05 When hoisting loads, a positive latching device shall be used to secure the load and rigging (i.e., self-closing safety latches, hook with a spring-loaded gate, an alloy anchor type shackle with a bolt, nut and retaining pin).

EM 385-1-1
15 Sep 08

15.A.06 Hooks, shackles, rings, pad eyes, and other fittings that show excessive wear or that have been bent, twisted, or otherwise damaged shall be removed from service.

15.A.07 Custom designed grabs, hooks, clamps, or other lifting accessories (i.e., equalizing beams, lifting or spreader beams, etc.) for such units as modular panels, prefabricated structures, and similar materials shall be marked to indicate the safe working loads and shall be proof-tested before use, to 125% of their rated load.

15.B PERSONNEL QUALIFICATIONS

15.B.01 Any worker acting in the capacity of Rigging Lift Supervisor shall meet the requirements of this section.

15.B.02 Any worker engaged in the duties and the performance of rigging shall be a **Qualified Rigger** and as such, shall meet the following requirements:

   a. Be at least 18 years of age;

   b. Be able to communicate effectively with the crane operator, the lift supervisor, flagman and affected employees on site;

   c. Have basic knowledge and understanding of equipment-operating characteristics, capabilities, and limitations.

15.B.03 In addition, Qualified Riggers and Lift Supervisors shall be able to demonstrate knowledge and proficiency to appropriate management personnel in the following;

   a. Personnel roles and responsibilities;

   b. Site preparation (terrain, environment);

   c. Rigging equipment and materials;

   d. Safe Operating procedures;

e. Principles of safe rigging;

f. Environmental hazards (overhead interferences);

g. Rigging the load, handling the load, common causes of crane-related accidents.

15.C MULTIPLE LIFT RIGGING (MLR)

15.C.01 USACE allows multiple lift rigging practices for the purpose of erecting/placing structural steel ONLY. Strict compliance with this section and 1926.753 Subpart R shall be mandated.

15.C.02 A Multiple Lift **is considered a critical lift** and requires a carefully detailed, written critical lift plan per Section 16.H. In addition, all details and requirements of this section are required to be addressed in the Critical Lift Plan to include, as a minimum: identifying all multi-lift hazards on the job site, beam list; determining load capacity; determining weight of a member; proper crane hand signals; safety rules for Multi-lift rigging; seven- foot rule; wind/environmental limits; safe route; power line issues; crane requirements; marking centerlines; use of tag line; qualifications and/or certifications of the operator(s) and rigger(s) to be performing these operations; rigging equipment: wire rope slings, hooks & shackles; clean lay-down area; cribbing; storage/staging; personal protective equipment.

15.C.03 A multiple lift may only be performed if the following criteria are met:

a. A MLR assembly is used;

b. A maximum of five members are hoisted per lift;

c. Only beams and similar structural members are lifted;

d. All employees engaged in MLR shall be trained in the following:

(1) The nature of the hazards associated with multiple lifts;

(2) The proper procedures and equipment to perform multiple lifts required in this section and as per 1926.753(e).

e. All loads shall be rigged by a qualified rigger per 15.B;

f. No crane is permitted to be used for a multiple lift where such use is contrary to the manufacturer's specifications and limitations;

g. Components of the MLR assembly shall be specifically designed and assembled with a maximum capacity for total assembly and for each individual attachment point. This capacity, certified by the manufacturer or a qualified rigger, shall be based on the manufacturer's specifications with a 5:1 safety factor for all components.

h. The total load shall not exceed:

(1) The rated capacity of the hoisting equipment specified in the hoisting equipment load charts;

(2) The rigging capacity specified in the rigging rating chart.

i. The MLR assembly shall be rigged with members:

(1) Attached at their center of gravity and maintained reasonably level;

(2) Rigged from the top down; and

(3) Rigged at least 7 feet (2.1 m) apart.

EM 385-1-1
15 Sep 08

j. The members on the MLR assembly shall be set from the bottom up.

k. Controlled load lowering shall be used whenever the load is over the connectors.

15.D WIRE ROPE

15.D.01 Wire rope must be inspected, maintained and replaced per 16.D.12

15.D.02 Wire rope removed from service due to defects shall be cut up or plainly marked as unfit for further use as rigging.

15.D.03 Wire rope clips attached with U-bolts shall have the U-bolts on the unloaded (dead) or short end of the rope. The clip nuts shall be retightened immediately after initial load carrying use and at frequent intervals thereafter. *> See Figure 15-1 and Table 15-1.*

15.D.04 When a wedge socket fastening is used, the unloaded (dead) or short end of the wire rope shall be looped back and secured to itself by a clip or have a separate piece of equal size wire rope attached with a clip or be properly secured to an extended wedge. The clip shall not be attached to the load (live) end. *> See Figure 15-2.*

FIGURE 15-1

Wire Rope Clip Spacing
(Not to be used for slings)

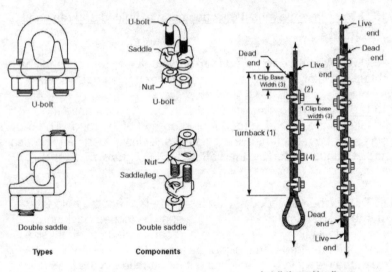

Installation and Loading

GENERAL NOTE: Correct number of clips for wire rope size shall be used.
NOTES:
(1) correct turnback length should be used
(2) correct orientation of saddle on live end shall be observed
(3) correct spacing of clips should be used
(4) correct torque on nuts shall be applied

EM 385-1-1
15 Sep 08

FIGURE 15-2

WIRE ROPE CLIP ORIENTATION
(NOT TO BE USED FOR SLINGS)

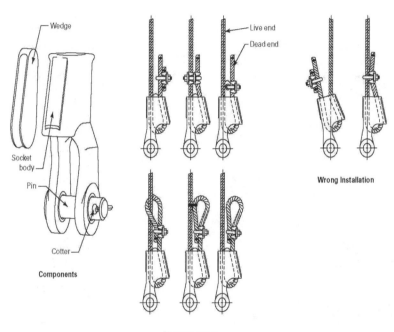

TABLE 15-1

NUMBER OF CLIPS AND THE PROPER TORQUE NECESSARY TO ASSEMBLE WIRE ROPE EYE LOOP CONNECTIONS WITH A PROBABLE EFFICIENCY NOT MORE THAN 80%

Rope diameter (in/cm)	Nominal size of clips (in/cm)	Number of clips	Torque to be applied to nuts of clips (ft-lb/N-m)
5/16 (0.7)	3/8 (0.9)	3	25 (33.9)
3/8 (0.9)	3/8 (0.9)	3	25 (33.9)
7/16 (1.0)	1/2 (1.2)	4	40 (54.3)
1/2 (1.2)	1/2 (1.2)	4	40 (54.3)
5/8 (1.5)	5/8 (1.5)	4	65 (88.2)
3/4 (1.9)	3/4 (1.9)	5	100 (135.7)
7/8 (2.2)	1 (2.5)	5	165 (223.9)
1 (2.5)	1 (2.5)	6	165 (223.9)
1 1/4 (3.1)	1 1/4 (3.1)	7	250 (339.3)
1 3/8 (3.4)	1 1/2 (3.8)	7	375 (508.9)
1 1/2 (3.8)	1 1/2 (3.8)	8	375 (508.9)
1 3/4 (4.3)	1 3/4 (4.3)	8	560 (760.0)

The spacing of clips should be 6 times the diameter of the wire rope. Thimbles shall be used if wire rope is to be spliced.

EM 385-1-1
15 Sep 08

15.D.05 Protruding ends of strands in splices on slings and bridles shall be covered or blunted.

15.D.06 Fabricated slings with eyes or endless loop slings using wire rope clips for hoisting material or lifting are prohibited except where the application precludes the use of prefabricated slings. All slings fabricated using wire rope clips shall be designed by a RPE for the specific application.

15.D.07 Except for eye splices in the ends of wires and for endless wire rope slings, wire rope used in hoisting, lowering, or pulling loads shall consist of one continuous piece without knot or splice.

    a. An eye splice made in any wire rope shall have not less than five full tucks (this requirement shall not preclude the use of another form of splice or connection that can be shown to be as efficient and that is not otherwise prohibited).

    b. Wire rope shall not be secured by knots except on haul back lines on scrapers.

15.D.08 Eyes in wire rope bridles, slings, or bull wires shall not be formed by wire rope clips or knots.

15.D.09 Wire rope clips shall not be used to splice rope.

15.E CHAIN

15.E.01 Only alloyed chain shall be used in rigging.

15.E.02 Chain shall be inspected before initial use and weekly thereafter. Inspect chains on an individual link basis. Chains shall be cleaned before they are inspected, as dirt and grease can hide nicks and cracks.

    a. Wear: Replacement shall be as scheduled in Table 15-2.

EM 385-1-1
15 Sep 08

b. Stretch: Compare the chain with its rated length or with a new length of chain. If the length is increased 3%, the chain must be thoroughly inspected. If the length is increased by 5% or more, the chain shall be replaced.

c. Deformed links: Deformed (twisted or bent) links, or any chain in which a link assembly does not hinge freely with the adjoining link.

d. Cuts, gouges, or nicks: If the depth of the cut or gouge exceeds the value shown in Table 15-2, the assembly shall be replaced.

e. Cracks: Cracks and other visible damage that causes doubt as to the strength of the chain.

TABLE 15-2

ALLOWABLE CHAIN WEAR

Nominal Chain Size	Maximum allowable wear of diameter
9/32 in (0.7 cm)	0.037 in (.09 cm)
3/8 in (0.9 cm)	0.052 in (.13 cm)
1/2 in (1.3 cm)	0.069 in (.18 cm)
5/8 in (1.5 cm)	0.084 in (.21 cm)
3/4 in (1.9 cm)	0.105 in (.27 cm)
7/8 in (2.1 cm)	0.116 in (.29 cm)
1 in (2.5 cm)	0.137 in (.35 cm)
1-1/4 in (3.1 cm)	0.169 in (.43 cm)

EM 385-1-1
15 Sep 08

15.E.03 When used with alloy steel chains, hooks, rings, oblong links, pear-shaped links, welded or mechanical coupling links, or other attachments shall have a rated capacity at least equal to that of the chain.

15.E.04 Job or shop hooks and links, makeshift fasteners formed from bolts and rods, and other similar attachments shall not be used.

15.F FIBER ROPE (NATURAL AND SYNTHETIC)

15.F.01 Fiber rope shall be inspected by a competent person for the following:

    a. Broken or cut fibers, either internally or externally.

    b. Cuts, gouges, abrasions; seriously or abnormally worn fibers.

    c. Powdered fiber or particles of broken fiber inside the rope between the strands.

    d. Variations in size or roundness of strands.

    e. Discoloration or rotting; weakened or brittle fibers.

    f. Excessive pitting or corrosion, or cracked, distorted, or broken fittings.

    g. Kinks.

    h. Melting or charring of the rope.

    i. Other visible damage that causes doubt as to the strength of the rope.

15.F.02 Fiber rope shall not be used if it is frozen or if it has been subjected to acids or excessive heat.

EM 385-1-1
15 Sep 08

15.F.03 Fiber rope shall be protected from abrasion by padding where it is fastened or drawn over square corners or sharp or rough surfaces.

15.F.04 All splices in rope slings provided by the employer shall be made in accordance with fiber rope manufacturer's recommendations.

15.F.05 Eye splices.

   a. In manila rope, eye splices shall contain at least three full tucks and short splices shall contain at least six full tucks (three on each side of the centerline of the splice).

   b. In layed synthetic fiber rope, eye splices shall contain at least four full tucks and short splices shall contain at least eight full tucks (four on each side of the centerline of the splice).

15.F.06 Strand end tails shall not be trimmed short (flush with the surface of the rope) immediately adjacent to the full tucks: this applies to both eye and short splices and all types of fiber rope.

   a. For fiber ropes less than 1 in (2.5 cm) diameter, the tails shall project at least six rope diameters beyond the last full tuck.

   b. For fiber ropes 1 in (2.5 cm) diameter and larger, the tails shall project at least 6 in (15.2 cm) beyond the last full tuck.

15.F.07 In applications where the projecting tails may be objectionable, the tails shall be tapered and spliced into the body of the rope using at least two additional tucks (which will require a tail length of approximately six rope diameters beyond the last full tuck).

15.F.08 For all eye splices, the eye shall be sufficiently large to provide an included angle of not greater than 60° at the splice when the eye is placed over the load or support.

EM 385-1-1
15 Sep 08

15.F.09 Knots shall not be used in lieu of splices.

15.G SLINGS All slings shall be in accordance with ASME B30.9.

15.G.01 Slings and their fittings and fastenings, shall be inspected before use on each shift and as necessary during use.

a. Metal Mesh Slings shall be inspected for the following:

(1) Broken weld or brazed joint along the sling edge.

(2) Broken wire in any part of the mesh.

(3) Reduction in wire diameter of 25% due to abrasion or 15% due to corrosion.

(4) Lack of flexibility due to distortion of the mesh.

(5) Distortion of the choker fitting so that the depth of the slot is increased by more than 10%.

(6) Distortion of either end fitting so the width of the eye opening is decreased by more than 10%.

(7) A 15% reduction of the original cross-sectional area of metal at any point around the hook opening of end fitting.

(8) Excessive pitting or corrosion of fittings; broken or cracked fittings; distortion of either end fitting out of its plane.

(9) Other visible damage that causes doubt as to the strength of the sling.

b. Synthetic Webbing Slings shall be inspected for the following:

(1) Acid or caustic burns.

EM 385-1-1
15 Sep 08

(2) Melting or charring of any part of the sling.

(3) Snags, holes, tears, or cuts.

(4) Broken or worn stitches.

(5) Excessive abrasive wear.

(6) Knots in any part of the sling.

(7) Wear or elongation exceeding the amount recommended by the manufacturer.

(8) Excessive pitting or corrosion, or cracked, distorted, or broken fittings.

(9) Other visible damage that causes doubt as to the strength of the sling.

15.G.02 Protection shall be provided between the sling and sharp unyielding surfaces of the load to be lifted.

15.G.03 The use of slings will be such that the entire load is positively secured.

15.G.04 Lengths.

    a. Wire rope slings shall have a minimum length of clear wire rope equal to ten times the rope diameter between each end fitting or eye splice.

    b. Braided slings shall have a minimum clear length of braided body equal to forty times the diameter of component ropes between each end fitting or eye splice.

15.G.05 Welded alloy steel chain slings shall have affixed durable permanent identification stating size, grade, rated capacity, and sling manufacturer.

EM 385-1-1
15 Sep 08

15.G.06 Wire rope slings shall have affixed a durable permanent identification tag stating the diameter, rated load, lifting capacity in vertical, choker, basket configuration, and date placed in service.

15.G.07 The employer shall have each synthetic rope sling, metal mesh sling, synthetic web sling, or roundsling marked or coded to show name or trademark of the manufacturer, rated capacities for the type of hitch, and type of material.

15.H RIGGING HARDWARE

15.H.01 Drums, sheaves, and pulleys shall be smooth and free of surface defects that may damage rigging. All rigging hardware shall be inspected for defects prior to use:

> a. Hooks that have been opened more than 15% of the normal throat opening (measured at the narrowest point) or twisted more than 10% from the plane of the unbent hook.
>
> b. Deformed master links and coupling links.
>
> c. Assemblies with cracked hooks or other end fittings.
>
> d. Excessive pitting or corrosion, or distorted or broken fittings.
>
> e. Other visible damage that causes doubt as to the strength of the attachment.

15.H.02 The ratio between the diameter of the rigging and the drum, block, sheave, or pulley tread diameter shall be such that the rigging will adjust itself to the bend without excessive wear, deformation, or damage.

15.H.03 In no case will the safe diameters of drums, blocks, sheaves, or pulleys be reduced in replacement of such items unless compensating changes are made in terms of the rigging used and the safe loading limits.

EM 385-1-1
15 Sep 08

15.H.04 Drums, sheaves, or pulleys having eccentric bores, cracked hubs, spokes, or flanges shall be removed from service.

15.H.05 Connections, fittings, fastenings, and attachments used with rigging shall be of good quality, of proper size and strength, and shall be installed in accordance with recommendations of the manufacturer.

15.H.06 Shackles. > See ASME B30.26.

   a. Only marked shackles (marked by manufacturer with name or trademark of manufacturer, rated load and size) shall be used. Shackles shall be maintained by the user so as to be legible throughout the life of the shackle.

   b. Each new shackle pin shall be marked by manufacturer to show name or trademark of manufacturer and grade, material type or load rating.

   c. Shackles shall be inspected visually by the use (or other designated person) and at least annually to determine condition is safe for use.

   d. Repairs and/or modifications may only be as specified by the manufacturer or Qualified Person. Replacement parts, like pins, shall meet or exceed the original manufacturer's specifications.

   e. Shackles shall not be eccentrically loaded (apply load to center of bow), shock loaded, nor shall they be loaded in excess of rated capacity.

   f. Multiple sling legs shall not be applied to the shackle pin.

15.H.07 Hooks. > See ASME B30.10. See Figure 15-3.

   a. The manufacturer's recommendations shall be followed in determining the safe working loads of the various sizes and types of specific and identifiable hooks. Any hook for which the

EM 385-1-1
15 Sep 08

manufacturer's recommendations are not available shall be tested to twice the intended safe working load before it is put into use. The employer shall maintain a record of the dates and results of such tests.

b. Open hooks are prohibited in rigging used to hoist loads.

c. Hoisting hooks rated at 10 tons (9,072 kg) or larger shall be provided with a means for safe handling.

d. Miscellaneous-type hooks (i.e., grab hooks, foundry hooks, sorting hooks and choker hooks) may be used as long as they are used, inspected and maintained in accordance with Manufacturer's recommended use.

15.H.08 Drums.

a. Drums shall have sufficient rope capacity with recommended rope size and reeving to perform all hoisting and lowering functions.

b. At least three full wraps (not layers) of rope shall remain on the drum at all times.

c. The drum end of the rope shall be anchored by a clamp securely attached to the drum with an arrangement approved by the manufacturer.

d. Grooved drums shall have the correct groove pitch for the diameter of the rope. The depth of the groove shall be correct for the diameter of the rope.

(1) The flanges on grooved drums shall project beyond the last layer of rope a distance of either 2 in (5 cm) or twice the diameter of the rope, whichever is greater.

(2) The flanges on ungrooved drums shall project beyond the last layer of rope a distance of either 2 1/2 in (6.3 cm) or twice the diameter of the rope, whichever is greater.

EM 385-1-1
15 Sep 08

FIGURE 15-3

HOOKS

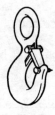

SELF-CLOSING TIPLOCK LATCH (EYE HOOK)

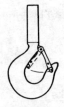

SELF-CLOSING TIPLOCK LATCH (SHANK HOOK)

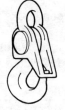

SELF-CLOSING BAIL (EYE HOOK)

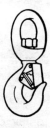

SELF-CLOSING FLAPPER LATCH LAMINATED PLATE HOOK

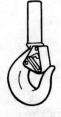

SELF-CLOSING FLAPPER LATCH (SHANK HOOK)

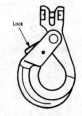

SELF-LOCKING CLEVIS HOOK (CLOSED)

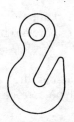

EYE GRAB HOOK

EM 385-1-1
15 Sep 08

15.H.09 Sheaves.

a. Sheaves shall be compatible with the size of rope used, as specified by the manufacturer.

b. Sheaves shall be inspected to ensure they are of correct size, properly aligned, lubricated, and in good condition.

c. When rope is subject to riding or jumping off a sheave, the sheave shall be equipped with cable-keepers.

15.H.10 Eyebolts, Eye Nuts, Swivel Hoist Rings and Turnbuckles.

a. Use of this equipment shall be in accordance with ASME B30.26.

b. Rated load shall be in accordance with the manufacturer's recommendation.

c. Each turnbuckle, eye nut and eyebolt shall be marked with name or trademark of manufacturer, size or rated load and grade (for alloy eyebolts). In addition, each swivel hoist ring must also be marked to show torque value. Markings shall remain legible.

d. This equipment shall be inspected visually before each use by the user (or other designated person) and at least annually to determine condition is safe for use.

e. Turnbuckles shall not be side loaded and shall be rigged and secured to prevent unscrewing during the lift.

f. Eyebolts shall be tightened and secured against rotation during the lift. Eye bolts shall only be loaded in the plain of the eye and shall not be loaded at angles of less than 45° to the horizontal.

g. Shoulderless eye bolts shall not be loaded at an angle.

BLANK

SECTION 16

CRANES AND HOISTING EQUIPMENT

16.A GENERAL

16.A.01 Unless otherwise specified, the requirements of this Section are applicable to all cranes and hoisting equipment, to include, but not limited to, articulating cranes (knuckle-boom cranes), floating cranes, cranes on barges, locomotive cranes, mobile cranes (i.e., wheel-mounted, rough-terrain, all-terrain, commercial truck-mounted and boom truck cranes, etc.), multi-purpose machines when configured to hoist and lower by means of a winch or hook and horizontally move a suspended load, industrial cranes, dedicated pile drivers, service/mechanic trucks with a hoisting device, cranes on a monorail, tower cranes (i.e., fixed jib/hammerhead boom, luffing boom and self-erecting), pedestal cranes, portal cranes, overhead and gantry cranes, straddle cranes, side-boom tractors, all derricks, hydraulic excavators and other such equipment when used with chains, slings or other rigging to lift suspended loads, and variations of such equipment.

16.A.02 Before any crane or hoisting equipment is placed in use, it shall be inspected and tested and certified in writing by a competent person to be in accordance with the manufacturer's recommendations and the requirements of this manual. **> See 16.D, E and F.**

16.A.03 The employer shall comply with all manufacturer's instructions, procedures and recommendations applicable to the operational functions of equipment, including its use with attachments. The safe operating speeds or loads shall not be exceeded. When they are not available, the employer shall develop and ensure compliance with all procedures necessary for the safe operation of the equipment and attachments.

    a. Procedures for the operational controls must be developed by a qualified person.

b. Procedures related to the capacity of the equipment must be developed and signed by a Registered Professional Engineer (RPE) familiar with the equipment.

16.A.04 When the manufacturer's instructions or recommendations are more stringent than the requirements of this manual, the manufacturer's instructions or recommendations shall apply.

16.A.05 The use of electronic equipment for entertainment purposes while operating equipment is prohibited.

16.A.06 Mechanized equipment shall be shut down before and during fueling operations. Closed systems, with an automatic shut-off that will prevent spillage if connections are broken, may be used to fuel diesel powered equipment left running.

16.A.07 Inspections or determinations of road and shoulder conditions and structures shall be made in advance to assure that clearances and load capacities are safe for the passage or placing of any mechanized equipment.

16.A.08 Equipment requirements, as applicable to the type equipment.

   a. An operable fuel gage;

   b. An operable audible warning device (horn);

   c. Adequate rearview mirror or mirrors;

   d. Non-slip surfaces on steps;

   e. A power-operated starting device;

   f. Seats or equal protection must be provided for the operator and all personnel required to be in/on equipment;

   g. Whenever visibility conditions warrant additional light, all vehicles, or combinations of vehicles, in use shall be equipped with at least two headlights and two taillights in operable condition;

h. Glass in windshields, windows, and doors shall be safety glass. Cracked or broken glass shall be replaced;

i. One (minimum) dry chemical or CO fire extinguisher with a minimum rating of 10B:C installed in the cab or at the machinery housing;

j. All self-propelled equipment, whether moving alone or in combination, shall be equipped with a backup alarm. **> See 18.B.01.**

16.A.09 Rollover protective structures (ROPS) as required by the manufacturer must be in place and maintained.

16.A.10 The manufacturer's specifications and operating manuals for hydraulic equipment and attachments utilizing quick connect/disconnect systems shall be followed. After completing a switch in attachments, the equipment operator shall take the actions necessary to ensure the quick connect/disconnect system is positively engaged.

16.A.11 All guarding and safety devices shall be provided, used and maintained:

a. All belts, gears, shafts, pulleys, sprockets, spindles, drums, flywheels, chains, or other reciprocating, rotating, or moving parts of equipment shall be guarded when exposed to contact by persons or when they otherwise create a hazard.

b. All hot surfaces of equipment, including exhaust pipes or other lines, shall be guarded or insulated to prevent injury and fire.

c. Platforms, foot walks, steps, handholds, guardrails, and toe boards shall be designed, constructed, and installed on

EM 385-1-1
15 Sep 08

machinery and equipment to provide safe footing and access ways.

d. Equipment shall be provided with suitable working surfaces of platforms, guardrails, and hand grabs when attendants or other employees are required to ride for operating purposes outside the operator's cab or compartment. Platforms and steps shall be of nonskid materials.

16.A.12 Work Area Control. When there are accessible areas in which the equipment's rotating superstructure (permanently or temporarily mounted) poses a risk of striking and injuring an employee or pinching/crushing an employee against another part of the equipment or another object, employees shall be prevented from entering these areas (i.e., communication or risk, placement/maintenance of control or warning lines, railings or barriers).

16.A.13 The controls of excavators or similar equipment with folding booms or lift arms shall not be operated from a ground position unless so designed.

16.A.14 Personnel shall not work in, pass under, or ride in the buckets or booms of excavators in operation.

16.A.15 Maintenance/repairs of cranes and hoisting equipment.

a. Maintenance, including preventive maintenance, and repairs shall be performed in accordance with the manufacturer's recommendations. Records of maintenance and repairs conducted during the life of a contract shall be made available upon request of the GDA.

b. Replacement parts or repairs shall have at least the original design factor; replacement parts for load bearing and other critical parts shall be obtained from the original manufacturer, (if possible) or certified by a registered engineer knowledgeable in cranes.

c. All equipment shall be shut down and positive means taken to prevent its operation while repairs or manual lubrications are being done. Equipment designed to be serviced while running are exempt from this requirement. **> See Section 12.**

d. All repairs shall be made at a location that will protect repair personnel from traffic.

e. Cranes, hoisting equipment, or parts thereof that are suspended or held apart by slings, hoists, or jacks also shall be substantially blocked or cribbed before personnel are permitted to work underneath or between them.

16.A.16 Parking.

a. Whenever equipment is parked, the parking brake shall be set.

b. Equipment parked on an incline shall have the wheels chocked or track mechanisms blocked and the parking brake set.

c. All equipment left unattended at night, adjacent to a highway in normal use or adjacent to construction areas where work is in progress, shall have lights or reflectors, or barricades equipped with lights or reflectors, to identify the location of the equipment.

16.B PERSONNEL QUALIFICATIONS

16.B.01 Cranes and hoisting equipment shall be operated only by designated qualified personnel. Proof of qualification shall be in writing. In addition to fully qualified crane and hoisting equipment operators, the following personnel may be designated to operate cranes and hoisting equipment under limited conditions (may not perform critical lifts).

a. Trainees under the direct supervision of the designated operator of the crane or hoist;

EM 385-1-1
15 Sep 08

    b. Maintenance personnel who have completed all operator qualification requirements. Operation is limited only to those functions necessary to perform maintenance or verify performance of a crane or hoist;

    c. Inspectors who have completed all operator qualification requirements. Operation is limited only to functions necessary to accomplish inspection.

16.B.02 Crane Operator Requirements - General (excluding vehicle mounted, rotating aerial devices (i.e., bucket trucks), see Section 22.M; excluding hydraulic excavating equipment. **> See Section 16.S**).

    a. Crane Operators shall be able to communicate effectively with the lift supervisor, rigger(s), flagmen and other affected employees on site.

    b. Prior to the start of work, documentation of operator qualifications shall be provided to the GDA.

    c. Qualification for all crane operators shall be by written examination and practical operational testing.

    d. All crane operators shall have knowledge of USACE crane safety requirements and manufacturer requirements and recommendations provided in the crane operator manual.

    e. Crane operators shall demonstrate their ability to read, write and comprehend in the language of the crane manufacturer's operation and maintenance instruction materials, exhibit arithmetic skills and load/capacity chart usage and use written manufacturer procedures applicable to the class/type of equipment for which certification is being sought.

16.B.03 Crane Operator Qualifications and/or Certifications. Crane operators shall possess at least one of the following licenses or certifications:

EM 385-1-1
15 Sep 08

a. Option 1. A current certification by an accredited (a nationally recognized accrediting agency) crane/derrick operator testing organization. The organization shall:

(1) Administer written and practical tests that assess operator applicants regarding necessary knowledge and skills;

(2) Provide different levels of certification based on equipment capacity and type;

(3) Have procedures for operators to re-apply and be retested in event operator applicant fails a test or is decertified;

(4) Have testing procedures for recertification;

(5) Have accreditation reviewed by the nationally recognized accrediting agency at least every 3 years;

(6) A certification issued under this option is portable and is valid for 5 years from issuance.

b. Option 2. Qualification by a professional source that qualifies crane operators (e.g., independent testing and qualifying company, a union, or a qualified consultant who can be an in-house resource) as long as the program is an audited employer program. Employer's qualification of its employee shall meet the following:

(1) Administer written and practical tests that assess operator applicants regarding necessary knowledge and skills. These tests shall be either developed by an accredited crane/derrick operator testing organization (see Option 1 above) OR approved by an examiner in accordance with the following:

(a) The examiner is certified to evaluate such tests by an accredited crane/derrick operator testing organization (see Option 1 above);

EM 385-1-1
15 Sep 08

(b) The approval shall be based on the examiner's determination that the tests meet nationally recognized test development criteria and are valid and reliable in assessing the operator applicant's knowledge and skill needed;

(2) The employer program shall be audited within 3 months of the beginning of the program and every 3 years thereafter;

(3) The employer program shall have testing procedures for recertification;

(4) Any significant deficiencies identified by the examiner shall be corrected prior to further qualification of any operators;

(5) Records of audits shall be retained for 3 years and made available to the GDA upon request;

(6) A qualification under this option is non-portable and is valid for 5 years from date of issuance.

c. Option 3. Qualification by the U.S. Military. Operator is considered valid if he has a current operator qualification issued by the U.S. military for operation of the equipment. Qualification meets operator qualification requirements of this section for operation of equipment only within the jurisdiction of the government entity and is valid for the period stipulated but no longer than 5 years from issuance.

d. Option 4. Licensing by a Government Entity. An examiner that issues operator licenses for operating equipment is considered a government accredited crane/derrick operator examiner if the following criteria are met:

(1) The requirements for obtaining the license include an assessment by written and practical tests of the operator applicant regarding knowledge and skills, as applicable to the specific type of equipment the individual will operate.

EM 385-1-1
15 Sep 08

(2) The testing meets industry recognized criteria for written testing materials, practical examinations, test administration, grading, facilities/equipment and personnel. Testing shall include:

(a) The controls and operational/performance characteristics;

(b) Responsibilities of operator, rigger, signalpersons, and lift supervisor;

(c) Knowledge of USACE crane safety requirements and the crane operator manual;

(d) Ability to determine the crane configuration, determine size and shape of loads, and the crane's applicable capacity using the load chart;

(e) Use and limitations of crane safety devices and operator aids;

(f) Inspection, testing, and maintenance requirements;

(g) Suitability of ground and surface to handle expected loads;

(h) Identification of site hazards and site access conditions;

(i) Outrigger and matting requirements (as applicable);

(j) Crane set-up, assembly, dismantling, and demobilization procedures;

(k) Requirements for clearance from power sources, procedures for preventing contact and responding to contact with said sources;

(l) Signaling and communication procedures;

(m) Factors that reduce rated capacity; and

EM 385-1-1
15 Sep 08

(n) Emergency control skills.

(3) The government authority that oversees the examiners has determined that the requirements for Option 4 licensing have been met.

(4) The examiner has testing procedures for recertification designed to ensure that the operator continues to meet the technical knowledge and skills requirements.

(5) A license issued by an examiner that meets the requirements of this Option:

(a) Meets operator qualification requirements of this section for operation of equipment only within the jurisdiction of the government entity.

(b) Is valid for the period stipulated but no longer than 5 years from issuance.

16.B.04 USACE Examiner Qualifications. It is recommended that each USACE Command select in-house crane examiners and that the individuals be designated in writing.

    a. Examiners shall be trained and licensed or certified by a commercial qualifying/certifying organization.

    b. Examiners will examine, qualify and certify the Command's crane operators based on criteria in this section.

    c. For Commands with few crane operators, where an in-house examiner would not be cost effective, operators should be examined, qualified or certified by a commercial qualifying/certifying organization.

16.B.05 Operator Practical Examination Requirements. Crane operators shall pass a practical operational test that demonstrates the following:

EM 385-1-1
15 Sep 08

a. Ability to rrecognize, from visual and audible observation, the items listed in 16.D.08 for shift inspections;

b. Ability to establish a stable foundation and leveling the crane;

c. Operating skills - Raising, lowering, extending, retracting, and swinging the boom, raising and lowering the load line;

d. Attaching the load, holding the load, and moving the load;

e. Reading and applying load, boom angle, and other indicator devices;

f. Maneuvering skills; and

g. Applying safe shut-down and securing procedures.

16.B.06 Operator Physical Qualifications/Examination. All crane/derrick operators shall be physically qualified to operate the equipment. Physical examinations for operators are required to be conducted every 2 years and any time a condition is observed that may impact the safe operation of a crane. Written proof, signed by a physician stating that the crane operator has had a physical examination and meets the medical requirements set forth below shall be submitted to the GDA for acceptance prior to allowing an operator to operate a crane.

a. Crane operators shall have a current physician's certification, dated within the past 2 years, that states the operator meets the following physical qualifications:

(1) Vision of at least 20/30 Snellen in one eye and 20/50 in the other, with or without corrective lenses;

(2) Normal depth perception and field of vision;

(3) Ability to distinguish colors, regardless of position;

EM 385-1-1
15 Sep 08

(4) Adequate hearing, with or without hearing aid, for the specific operation;

(5) Sufficient strength, endurance, agility, coordination, manual dexterity, and speed of reaction to meet the demands of equipment operation;

(6) No tendencies to dizziness or similar undesirable characteristics; and

(7) Has a negative result for substance abuse test.

b. Evidence of physical defects, emotional instability that could render a hazard to the operator, others, or safe operation of the crane, or evidence that the operator is subject to seizures or loss of physical control shall be sufficient reason for disqualification. In such cases, specialized medical tests may be required to evaluate these conditions and determine their impact.

c. All crane/derrick operators shall participate in a drug testing program and have a negative result for a substance abuse test. The level of testing will be in accordance with standard practices for industry or by the agencies random drug testing program. This test will be confirmed by a recognized laboratory service.

16.B.07 Signal Person Qualifications

a. The employer shall insure that the signal person is qualified either by a third party qualified evaluator or the employer's qualified evaluator.

b. The qualification means that the evaluator has assessed the individual's capabilities and knowledge and has determined that the individual meets the following qualification requirements:

EM 385-1-1
15 Sep 08

(1) Know and understand the type of signals used (radio, cell, hand, etc). If hand signals are used, the signal person must know and understand the Standard Method for hand signals.

(2) Be competent in the application of the type of signals used.

(3) Have a basic understanding of crane operation and limitations, including crane dynamics involved in swinging and stopping loads and boom deflection from hoisting loads.

(4) Demonstrate that he/she meets the requirements above through a practical test.

16.C. CLASSIFICATION OF EQUIPMENT AND TRAINING OF OPERATORS (FOR USACE-OWNED AND -OPERATED CRANES AND HOISTS ONLY)

16.C.01 Designated personnel must be qualified to operate a particular type of crane or hoist (i.e., mobile, tower, overhead, etc.) and the training provided shall be applicable to that type of crane or hoist. The three classifications of cranes and hoisting equipment and their associated training requirements are identified here. All exams shall meet the applicable parts of Option 4, based on type of equipment.

a. Class I: Class I cranes are mobile and locomotive cranes, hammerhead, portal, tower, derricks (post or stiff leg), floating or barge mounted cranes/derricks, overhead, gantry, bridge, underhung, monorail:

(1) Class I crane operators may perform critical lifts, preventive maintenance and inspections as required on specific equipment as trained:

(2) Training must be, as a minimum:

(a) Initial: 24-hour training with written and practical/operational examinations;

EM 385-1-1
15 Sep 08

(b) Annual: 8-hour refresher training, to include practical/operational examination.

b. Class II: Class II cranes are overhead, bridge and gantry cranes, underhung, monorail, pedestal and wall-mounted jib cranes, and similar.

(1) Class II crane operators may perform only routine lifts in the performance of their duties, preventive maintenance and inspection as required on specific equipment as trained. Class II crane operators may not perform critical lifts with this equipment.

(2) Class II training, must be, as a minimum:

(a) Initial: 8-hour training with written and practical/operational examinations;

(b) Annual: 1-hour refresher training, to include practical/operational examination.

c. Class IIIA Hoisting Equipment: greater than 10 tons (>10T rated capacity), and shop equipment used for lifting or lowering a freely suspended (unguided) loads.

(1) Class IIIA operators are qualified to operate, perform preventive maintenance and inspection of this equipment as required.

(2) Class IIIA training, must be on the specific type(s) of hoist operated and be, as a minimum:

(a) Initial: 4-hour training with written (as applicable, see 16.B.03.d) and practical/operational examinations;

(b) Annual: 1-hour refresher training, to include practical/operational examination.

EM 385-1-1
15 Sep 08

d. Class IIIB Hoisting Equipment: up to and including 10 tons (</= 10T rated capacity), and shop equipment used for lifting or lowering a freely suspended (unguided) loads.

(1) Class IIIB operators are qualified to operate, perform preventive maintenance and inspection of this equipment as required.

(2) Class IIIB training must be on the safe operation and use of the hoist and be, as a minimum:

(a) Initial: 1-hour training with written (as applicable, see 16.B.03.d) and practical/operational examinations;

(b) Annual: 1-hour refresher training, to include practical/operational examination.

16.C.02 Prior to re-issuance of qualification, crane and hoisting equipment operators must have attended applicable training (initial and annual) and passed the written and operational examination requirements specified above.

16.C.03 Each USACE activity or operating project will maintain a current list of operators, complete crane and hoisting equipment training records for each operator, and a list of equipment that each operator is qualified to operate.

16.D INSPECTION CRITERIA for CRANES and HOISTING EQUIPMENT

16.D.01 Inspections of cranes and hoisting equipment shall be in accordance with this section, applicable ASME standards, OSHA regulations and the manufacturer's recommendations.

16.D.02 Records of crane and hoisting equipment tests and inspections shall be maintained onsite. Contractors shall make these records readily available upon request and, when submitted, they shall become part of the official project file.

EM 385-1-1
15 Sep 08

16.D.03 Contractor shall provide the GDA 24-hours notice in advance of any crane or hoisting equipment entering the site (prior to inspection/tests) so that observation of the Contractor's inspection process and spot checks may be conducted.

16.D.04 Whenever any crane and/or hoisting equipment is found to be unsafe, or whenever a deficiency that affects the safe operation of a crane and/or hoisting equipment is observed, the affected equipment shall be immediately taken out of service and its use prohibited until unsafe conditions have been corrected.

16.D.05 Cranes and derricks in regular service. Inspection procedures for cranes/derricks in regular service are divided into three general classifications based on the intervals at which inspections shall be performed. The intervals depend on the nature of critical components of the crane and the degree of their exposure to wear, deterioration, or malfunction. The three general classifications are Periodic, Start-up, and Frequent, with respect to intervals between inspections as defined.

16.D.06 Inspection Frequency. Required inspection frequency shall be as per Table 16-1.

16.D.07 Initial Inspections. Prior to use, all new, re-assembled, modified or altered cranes, derricks or hoisting equipment (as applicable) that have had modifications or additions which affect the safe operation of the equipment (i.e., involving a safety device, operator aid, critical part of a control system, power plant, braking system, load-sustaining structural components, load hook or in-use operating mechanism) or capacity shall be inspected by a qualified person.

   a. Any deficiencies shall be carefully examined and a determination made as to whether they constitute a hazard.

   b. The inspection shall include functional testing.

EM 385-1-1
15 Sep 08

16.D.08 Start-Up Inspections (Pre-Operational, Each shift). Before every crane or derrick operation (at beginning of each shift) or following a change of operator, a competent person shall visually inspect the items listed below. If any deficiency is identified, an immediate determination shall be made by the competent person as to whether the deficiency constitutes a safety hazard. If it does, the equipment shall be properly removed from service (i.e., a tag shall be placed in a conspicuous location on the crane or hoisting equipment indicating that it shall not be operated and that the tag shall remain in its attached location until it is demonstrated to the individual deadlining the crane or hoisting equipment that it is safe to operate. When required, lockout procedures shall be used as well. *> See Sections 8 and 12.* If any deficiency in safety device/operational aids is identified, the action identified in Section 16.E shall be taken prior to using the equipment.

a. Control mechanisms for proper operation;

b. Brake actions to ensure brakes are functioning normally and that there is no slippage, excessive play, or binding. Exercise brakes to assure they are dry;

c. Control mechanisms for excessive wear of components and contamination by lubricants or other foreign matter;

d. Operator aids and other safety devices for proper functioning and accuracy of settings;

e. Chords and lacing for damage, bent members, cracked welds, etc.;

f. Hydraulic and pneumatic systems for deterioration or leakage - with particular emphasis given to those that flex during normal operation;

g. Hooks and latches for deformation, chemical damage, cracks, and wear;

EM 385-1-1
15 Sep 08

h. Rope for proper spooling onto the drum(s) and sheave(s) and rope reeving for compliance with crane or derrick manufacturer's specifications;

i. Electrical apparatus for proper functioning, signs of excessive deterioration, dirt, and moisture accumulation;

j. Tires (when in use) for recommended inflation pressure and condition;

k. Ground conditions around the equipment for proper support, including ground settling under and around outriggers and supporting foundations, ground water accumulation, or similar conditions;

l. Hydraulic system for proper fluid level;

m. The equipment for level position, both shift and after each move and setup;

n. Operator cab windows for significant cracks, breaks or other deficiencies that would hamper the operator's view;

o. Safety devices and operational aids for proper operation;

p. Wedges and supports for looseness or dislocation (climbing tower cranes);

EM 385-1-1
15 Sep 08

TABLE 16-1

CRANE & DERRICK INSPECTION FREQUENCY

When to inspect	Type of Inspection
Prior to initial use - all new cranes [a]	Initial inspection
Prior to use - all altered cranes [b]	Initial inspection
Prior to initial use on a USACE project [c]	Periodic inspection
Monthly after initial use on a USACE project	Periodic inspection
Prior to every operation (shift)	Start-up inspection
Before using a crane that is not in use on a regular basis and that has been idle for more than 1 month, but less than 6 months [d]	Frequent inspection
Before using a crane that is not in use on a regular basis and that has been idle for more than 6 months [d]	Periodic inspection
Standby cranes, at least semi-annually [e]	Frequent inspection
Standby cranes, prior to use [f]	Frequent inspection

Notes:
(a) Performed by the manufacturer.
(b) "Altered" is defined as any change to the original manufacturer's design configuration, that is, replacement of weight handling equipment parts and components.
(c) Initial use refers to (1) the first time the USACE takes possession of and assembles a crane, or (2) whenever a Contractor brings a crane onto a job site and assembles the crane.
(d) This requirement is in addition to the requirement for a periodic inspection.
(e) Standby cranes are those cranes that are not used on a regular basis but are available - on a standby basis - for emergencies (e.g., emergency operations & maintenance (O&M) work); requirements for frequent inspections of standby cranes are in addition to the requirement for a periodic inspection.
(f) In addition to the semi-annual frequent inspection, a frequent inspection shall be conducted prior to use

EM 385-1-1
15 Sep 08

q. Braces and guys supporting crane masts for safe condition and proper tension; anchor bolt base connections for tightness or retention of preload; wedges and supports of climbing cranes for tightness and proper positioning;

r. For derricks, inspect all chords and lacing, tension in guys, plump of the mast, and derrick mast fittings and connections for compliance with manufacturer's recommendations;

s. Barge or pontoon ballast compartments for proper ballast; deck loads for proper securing; chain lockers, storage, fuel compartments, and battening of hatches; firefighting and lifesaving equipment in place and functional; hull void compartments sounded for leakage (floating cranes and derricks); and

t. Wire rope per 16.D.12.

16.D.09 Frequent Inspections (Monthly intervals). Each month the equipment is in service, it shall be inspected according to the criteria in 16.D.08 for pre-operational/shift inspection.

a. The items checks, the results of the inspection, the name and signature of the person who conducted the inspection and the date shall all be documented. Documentation shall be retained for a minimum 3 months or the life of the contract.

b. Equipment shall not be used until an inspection performed under this paragraph demonstrates that no corrective action is required.

16.D.10 Periodic Inspections/Comprehensive (at least annually or as recommended by the manufacturer). This inspection shall include functional testing to determine that the equipment as configured in the inspection is functioning properly.

a. If any deficiency is identified, an immediate determination shall be made by the qualified person as to whether the

EM 385-1-1
15 Sep 08

deficiency constitutes a safety hazard. If so, then the equipment shall be removed from service until it has been corrected. If not yet a safety hazard, the qualified person may determine that the employer shall monitor the deficiency in the monthly inspections.

b. The comprehensive inspection must be documents and shall include:items checked and results of inspection, name and signature of the person who conducted the inspection and the date and this documentation must be retained until at least the next annual/comprehensive inspection occurs, or 12 months, whichever is longer.

c. The following, in addition to those items required by a pre-operational inspection in 16.D.08 above, shall be inspected by a qualified person:

(1) Equipment structure – to include boom and, if equipped, the jib;

(2) Bolts, rivets, and other fasteners for tightness, corrosion;

(3) Welds for cracks;

(4) Proper tension (torque) of high strength (traction) bolts used in connections and at the slewing bearing;

(5) Power plants for performance and compliance with safety requirements;

(6) Drive components such as pins, bearings, wheels, shafts, gears, sheaves, drums, rollers, locking and clamping devices, sprockets, drive chains or belts, bumpers, and stops for absence of wearing, cracks, corrosion, or distortion;

(7) All crane function operating mechanisms for proper operation, proper adjustment, and the absence of unusual sounds;

(8) Travel, steering, holding, braking, and locking mechanisms for proper functioning and absence of excessive wear or damage;

(9) Hydraulic, pneumatic and other pressurized hoses, fittings and tubing for leaks, deformation or other signs of failure/impending failure, abrasion or scrubbing;

(10) Hydraulic and pneumatic pumps and motors for performance indicators (noises, vibration low operating speed, excessive heating of the fluid, low pressure, etc.), loose bolts or fasteners, seals and joints between pump sections for leaks, Tires for damage or excessive wear;

(11) Hydraulic and pneumatic valves (Spools – sticking, Leaks, Valve housing cracks, Relief valves – failure to reach correct pressure);

(12) Hydraulic and pneumatic cylinders for: drifting; rod seals and welded joints for leaks; cylinder rods for scores, nicks or dents; barrel for significant dents; rod eyes and connecting joints for looseness and deformity;

(13) Brake and clutch system parts, linings, pawls, and ratchets for excessive wear;

(14) Wire rope per 16.D.12;

(15) Sheaves and drums for cracks or significant wear;

(16) Crane operator aids and safety devices and indicating devices for proper operation, to include accuracy;

(17) A means to verify the proper setup of the boom stops and functioning of the boom hoist disengaging device. This test will be conducted before initiating the operational test required by 16.F;

(18) Motion limiting devices for proper operation with the crane unloaded (each motion should be inched into its limiting device to run in at slow speed with care exercised) and load limiting devices for proper operation and accuracy of settings;

(19) Safety and function labels for legibility and replacement;

(20) For floating plant, inspect ballast compartments for proper ballast; deck loads for proper securing; safety of chain lockers, storage, fuel compartments; battening of hatches; hull void compartments sounded for leakage; tie-downs for barge-mounted land cranes for wear, corrosion, and tightness; cleats, bitts, chocks, fenders, capstans, ladders, stanchions for corrosion, wear, deterioration, and deformation; take four corner draft readings;

(21) Outrigger pads/floats and slider pads for excessive wear and cracks;

(22) Electrical components and wiring for cracked or split insulation and loose or corroded terminations;

(23) Operator seat – missing or unusable;

(24) Originally equipped steps, ladders, handrails, guards – missing; OR

(25) Steps, ladders, handrails, guards in unusable or unsafe condition.

16.D.11 Inspection of cranes, derricks and other hoisting equipment not in regular use shall be inspected as follows:

(a) Frequent (Monthly) Inspection Criteria (see 16.D.09) – Cranes or hoisting equipment that have been idle for a period of one month or more, but less than one year;

EM 385-1-1
15 Sep 08

(b) Periodic (Annual/Comprehensive) Inspection Criteria (see 16.D.10) – Cranes or hoisting equipment that have been idle for a period of one year or more;

(c) Cranes or hoisting equipment that are exposed to adverse environmental conditions shall be inspected more frequently, as determined by a qualified person (of GDA or the Contractor) with the concurrence of GDA.

16.D.12 Wire Rope Inspection, Maintenance and Replacement.

a. A competent person shall perform this inspection for each shift, visually inspecting all running ropes and counterweight ropes and load trolley ropes, if provided. Visual inspection shall concentrate on identifying apparent deficiencies in wire rope as categorized below. Opening of wire rope or booming down is not required as part of this inspection.

b. Category I. Apparent deficiencies in this category include the following:

(1) Distortion of wire rope structure such as kinking, crushing, unstranding, birdcaging, main strand displacement, core failure or protrusion between the outer strands;

(2) General corrosion;

(3) Electric arc (from a source other than power lines) or heat damage;

(4) Severely corroded or broken wires at end connections; severely corroded, cracked bent, worn, or improperly applied end connections.

c. Category II. Apparent deficiencies in this category include the following:

(1) Number, distribution and type of visible broken wires are as per Table 16-2;

(2) A diameter reduction of more than 5% from nominal diameter due to loss of core support, internal or external corrosion, or wear of outside wires.

d. Category III. Apparent deficiencies in this category include the following:

(1) Core failure or protrusion in rotation resistant ropes;

(2) Electrical contact with a power line; OR

(3) A broken strand (care shall be taken when inspecting rotation resistant ropes because of their susceptibility to damage from misuse and potential for deterioration when used on equipment with limited design parameters).

e. Critical Review Items. Particular attention should be given to:

(1) Rotation resistant wire rope in use;

(2) Boom hoist ropes and sections of rope subject to rapid deterioration such as at flange points, crossover points, and repetitive pickup points on drums;

(3) Sections in contact with saddles, equalizer sheaves, or other sheaves where rope travel is limited;

(4) Sections of the rope at or near terminal ends where corroded or broken wires may protrude; AND

(5) Sections subject to reverse bends and sections normally hidden during routine visual inspections, such as parts passing over outer sheaves.

EM 385-1-1
15 Sep 08

f. Removal from Service.

(1) If a Category I deficiency is identified, an immediate determination shall be made by the competent person as to whether the deficiency constitutes a safety hazard. If so, operations involving the use of the wire rope in question shall be prohibited until:

(a) The wire rope is replaced; OR

(b) If the deficiency (other than power line contact) is localized and the problem is corrected by severing the wire rope in two; the undamaged portion may continue to be used. Joining lengths of wore rope by splicing is prohibited. Repair of wire rope that contacted an energized power line is also prohibited.

(2) If a Category II deficiency is identified, one of the following actions must occur:

(a) Employer shall consider the deficiency to constitute a safety hazard where it meets the wire rope manufacturer's established criterion for removal from service or meets a different criterion that the wire rope manufacturer has approved in writing for that specific wire rope. If the deficiency is considered a safety hazard, operations involving use of the wire rope shall be prohibited until the wire rope is either replaced OR the damage is removed in accordance with 16.D.12.f(1)(b), OR

(b) Institute alternative measures. The wire rope may continue to be used if the employer ensures that the following measures are implemented:

(i) A qualified person assesses the deficiency in light of the load and other conditions of use and determines it is safe to continue to sue the wire rope as long as the conditions established under this paragraph are met;

EM 385-1-1
15 Sep 08

(ii) A qualified person establishes the parameters for the use of the equipment with the deficiency, including a reduced maximum rated load;

(iii) A qualified person establishes a specific number of broken wires, strands or diameter reduction that, when reached, will require3 the equipment to be taken out of service until the wire rope is replaced or the damage is removed in accordance with 16.D.12.f(1)(b);

(iv) a qualified person sets a time limit, not to exceed 30 days from the date the deficiency is first identified, by which the wire rope must be replaced, or the damage removed in accordance with 16.D.12.f(1)(b).

(3) If a Category III deficiency is identified, operations involving the use of the wire rope in question shall be prohibited until:

(a) The wire rope is replaced; OR

(b) If the deficiency (other than power line contact) is localized, the problem is corrected by severing the wire rope in two; the undamaged portion may continue to be used. Joining lengths of wore rope by splicing is prohibited. Repair of wire rope that contacted an energized power line is also prohibited.

TABLE 16-2

Wire Rope Removal and Replacement Criteria

Standard	Equipment		# OF BROKEN WIRES IN RUNNING ROPES			# OF BROKEN WIRES IN STANDING ROPES	
			In one rope lay	In one strand	At end connection	In one rope lay	At end connection
ASME/B30.2	Overhead & gantry cranes		12**	4	N/S	Not Specified	
ASME/B30.4	Portal, tower, & pillar cranes		6**	3	2	3	2
ASME/B30.5	Mobile & locomotive cranes	Running ropes	6**	3	2	3	2
		Rotation-resistant ropes	2 randomly distributed broken wires in 6 rope dia. or 4 randomly distributed broken wires in 30 rope dia. **				
ASME/B30.6	Derricks		6**	3	2	3	2
ASME/B30.7	Base-mount drum hoists		6**	3	2	3	2
ASME/B30.8	Floating cranes and derricks		6**	3	2	3	2
ASME/B30.16	Overhead hoists		12**	4	N/S	Not Specified	
ANSI/A10.4	Personnel hoists		6**	3	2	2**	2
ANSI/A10.5	Material hoists		6**	Not Specified		Not Specified	

EM 385-1-1
15 Sep 08

16.E SAFETY DEVICES AND OPERATIONAL AIDS. Safety devices and operational aids shall not be used as a substitute for the exercise of professional judgment by the operator.

16.E.01 Safety Devices. The following safety devices are required on all cranes and derricks covered by Section 16 unless otherwise specified.

a. Crane level indicator.

(1) The equipment shall have a crane level indicator that is either built into the equipment or is available on the equipment.

(2) If a built-in crane level indicator is not working properly, is shall be tagged-out or removed.

(3) This requirement does not apply to portal cranes, derricks, floating cranes/derricks and crane/derricks on barges, pontoons, vessels or other means of flotation.

b. Boom stops, except for derricks and hydraulic booms.

c. Jib stobs (if jib is attached), except for derricks.

d. Equipment with foot pedal brakes shall have locks, except for portal floating cranes.

e. Hydraulic outrigger jacks shall have an integral holding device (check valve).

f. Equipment on rails shall have rail clamps and rail stops, except for portal cranes.

16.E.02 Proper Operation of Safety Devices. Operations shall not begin unless the safety devices listed above are in proper working order. If a safety device stops working properly during operations, the operator shall safely stop operations. Operations shall not resume until the device is again working properly. Alternative measures are not permitted to be used.

16.E.03 Operational Aids.

a. The devices listed here as "operational aids" are required on all cranes and derricks covered by Section 16 unless otherwise specified.

b. Operations shall not begin unless the listed operational aids are in proper working order except where the employer meets the specified temporary alternative measures. More protective alternative measures specified by the crane/derrick manufacturer, if any, shall be followed.

c. If a listed operational aid stops working properly during operations, the operator shall safely stop operations until the temporary alternative measures are implemented or the device is again working properly. If a replacement part is not longer available, the use of a substitute device that performs the same type of function is permitted and is not considered a modification.

d. Category I operational aids and alternative measures. Operational aids listed in this paragraph that are not working properly shall be repaired not later than 7 days after the deficiency occurs. EXCEPTION: If the employer documents that it has ordered the necessary parts within 7 days of the occurrence of the deficiency, the repair shall be completed within 7 days of receipt of the parts.

(1) Boom hoist limiting device. TEMPORARY alternative measures (use at least one):

(a) Use a boom angle indicator;

(b) Clearly mark the boom hoist cable, in a visible location to the operator, at a point that will give the operator sufficient time to stop the hoist to keep the boom within the minimum allowable

EM 385-1-1
15 Sep 08

radius. In addition, install mirrors or remote video cameras and displays if necessary for the operator to see the mark;

(c) Clearly mark the boom hoist cable, in a visible location to the spotter, at a point that will give the spotter sufficient time to signal the operator and have the operator stop the hoist to keep the boom within the minimum allowable radius.

(2) Luffing jib limiting device.

(a) Equipment with a luffing jib shall have a luffing jib limiting device.

(b) Temporary alternative measures are the same as in 16.E.03.d.(1)(a) except to limit the movement of the luffing jib.

(3) Anti two-blocking device (A2B). Anti-two blocking devices shall be installed at all points of two-blocking.

(a) All cranes and derricks shall be equipped with A2B/Hoist-limit device that will disengage the function that is causing the two-blocking or an A2B damage prevention feature (except as noted). They shall be tested and certified functional by a competent person prior to operating the crane.

(b) Lattice boom cranes. Lattice boom cranes shall be equipped with an A2B device to stop the load hoisting and boom-down functions before the load block or load contacts the boom tip.

EXCEPTION 1 – Duty Cycle: Lattice boom cranes that are used exclusively for duty cycle operations are exempt from A2B equipment requirements. When a lattice boom crane engaged in duty cycle work is required to make a non-duty cycle lift (for example, to lift a piece of equipment), it will be exempt from the A2B equipment requirements if the following procedures are implemented:

EM 385-1-1
15 Sep 08

- An international orange colored warning device (flag, tape or ball) is properly secured to the hoist line at a distance of 8 ft to 10 ft (2.4 m to 3m) above the rigging;

- The signal person acts as a spotter to alert the crane operator with a "STOP" signal when the warning device approaches the boom tip and the crane operator ceases hoisting functions when alerted of this;

- While the non-duty cycle lift is underway the signal person shall not stand under the load, shall have no duties other than as a signal person, an shall comply with the signaling requirements of this manual.

EXCEPTION 2 – Lattice boom cranes with manually operated friction brakes: Lattice boom crane and hoisting equipment with manually activated friction brakes, A2B warning devices may be used in lieu of A2B prevention devices.

(c) Telescopic boom cranes.

(i) Telescopic boom cranes shall be equipped with an A2B device to stop the load hoisting function before the load block or load contacts the boom tip and to prevent damage to the hoist rope or other machine components when extending the boom.

(ii) Telescopic boom cranes that are used exclusively for duty cycle operations shall be equipped with a two-blocking damage prevention feature or warning device to prevent damage to the hoist rope or other machine components when extending the boom.

(d) Floating cranes. Floating cranes may use an A2B alarm system in lieu of a disengaging device unless they are hoisting personnel.

(e) Other cranes used in duty cycle operations, to include clamshell (grapple), magnet, drop ball, container handling,

EM 385-1-1
15 Sep 08

concrete bucket, pile driving and extracting operations, drilled shaft operations (except telescopic boom cranes, see 16.E.03.d(3)(c)(2)), are exempt from the requirements for A2B devices.

(f) Temporary alternative measure: clearly mark the cable (so that it can be easily seen by the operator) at a point that will give the operator sufficient time to stop the hoist to prevent two-blocking and use a spotter when extending the boom.

e. Category II operational aids and alternative measures. Operational aids listed in this paragraph that are not working properly shall be repaired not later than 30 days after the deficiency occurs. EXCEPTION: If the employer documents that it has ordered the necessary parts within 7 days of the occurrence of the deficiency, and the parts are not received in time to complete the repair in 30 days, the repair shall be completed within 7 days of receipt of the parts.

(1) Boom angle or radius indicator. The equipment (except articulating boom cranes) shall have a boom angle or radius indicator readable from the operator's station. Temporary alternative measures: radii or boom angle shall be determined by measuring the radii or boom angle with a measuring device. Calibration and testing of indicators will be performed in accordance with the manufacturer's recommendations.

(2) Jib angle indicator (if equipment has luffing jib). Temporary alternative measures: radii or jib angle shall be determined by ascertaining the main boom angle and then measuring the radii or jib angle with a measuring device.

(3) Boom length indicator if the equipment has a telescopic boom, except where the load rating is independent of the boom length. Temporary alternative measures: one of the following methods shall be used:

(a) Mark the boom with measured marks to calculate boom length;

EM 385-1-1
15 Sep 08

(b) Calculate boom length from boom angle and radius measurements; OR

(c) Measure the boom with a measuring device.

(4) Load weighing and similar devices. Equipment, other than derricks, shall have at least one of the following: load weighing device, load moment indicator (LMI), rated capacity indicator or rated capacity limiter. Temporary alternative measures: The weight of the load shall be determined from a reliable source (i.e., load manufacturer), by a reliable calculation method (i.e., calculating a steel beam from measured dimensions and a known per foot weight), or by other equally reliable means. This information shall be provided to the operator prior to the lift.

EXCEPTION: When cranes are used in duty cycle operations they are exempt from the requirements for load indicating devices and LMI devices.

(5) Hoist drum rotation indicator if the drum is not visible from the operator's station. Temporary alternative measures: mark the drum. In addition, install mirrors or remote video cameras and displays if necessary for the operator to see the mark.

(6) Outrigger position (horizontal beam extension) sensor/monitor if the equipment has outriggers (required on equipment manufactured after January 1, 2008). Temporary alternative measure: the operator shall verify that the position of the outriggers is correct (in accordance with manufacturer's procedures) before beginning operations requiring outrigger deployment.

16.F TESTING

16.F.01 Written reports of tests, showing test procedures and confirming the adequacy of repairs or alterations, shall be

EM 385-1-1
15 Sep 08

maintained with the crane and hoisting equipment or at the on-site project office.

16.F.02 Operational Testing.

a. A qualified person shall conduct operational tests in accordance with ANSI/ASME and the manufacturer's recommendations. If the manufacturer has no procedures, reference Appendix I for procedures. At the minimum, operational testing shall meet the requirements listed below.

(1) Before initial use of a crane or hoisting equipment after a load   bearing or load controlling part or component, brake, travel component, or clutch (to include securing devices, skids and barges for floating cranes) has been altered, replaced, or repaired;

(2) Every time a crane or hoisting equipment(s) is reconfigured or re-assembled after disassembly (to include booms);

(3) Every time a crane and/or hoisting equipment is brought onto a USACE project; and

(4) Every year during periodic inspection.

b. Operational testing after the replacement of wire rope is not required.

16.F.03 Load Testing.

a. Load tests shall be performed in accordance with ANSI/ASME and the manufacturer's recommendations by, or under the direction of, a qualified person. If the manufacturer has no procedures, a Registered Professional Engineer familiar with the type of equipment involved must approve procedures and frequency of testing using as a minimum, Appendix I for procedures and taking into account age of equipment, history of use, testing and inspection, anticipated future use, and other such factors.

b. Test loads shall be made at 110% of the anticipated load for the specified configuration, not to exceed 100% of the manufacturer's load rating at the configuration of the test, except for manufacturer testing of new crane and hoisting equipment, which shall be conducted in accordance with the ANSI/ASME standards B30.1 through B30.17 as appropriate for the crane and hoisting equipment.

c. Load testing shall be performed:

(1) Before initial use of crane or hoisting equipment in which a load bearing or load controlling part or component, brake, travel component, or clutch has been altered, replaced, or repaired.

(2) Every time the crane or hoisting equipment is reconfigured or reassembled after disassembly (to include booms); and

(3) When the manufacturer requires load testing.

(a) The employer shall specifically research, identify and document manufacturer required load-testing frequency for each USACE-owned/operated and/or Contractor-owned/operated crane or hoisting equipment and maintain and/or provide this information to the GDA;

(b) Under conditions (1) and (2) above, a selective load test (testing only those components that have or may have been affected by the alteration, replacement, or repaired) may be performed;

(c) The replacement of the rope is specifically excluded from this requirement. However, a functional test of the crane or hoisting equipment under a normal operating load shall be made prior to putting the crane back in service.

d. The manufacturer's specifications and limitations applicable to the operation of any crane and hoisting equipment shall be followed. At no time shall a crane or hoisting equipment be

EM 385-1-1
15 Sep 08

loaded in excess of the manufacturer's rating, except overhead and gantry cranes in accordance with ANSI/ASME B30.2. Loads shall not exceed 125% of the rated load for test purposes or planned engineered lifts for overhead and gantry cranes.
> See 16.H, Critical Lifts.

(1) Where manufacturer's specifications are not available, the limitations assigned to the equipment shall be based on the determinations of a registered engineer competent in this field, and such determinations will be documented and recorded.

(2) Attachments used with crane and hoisting equipment shall not exceed the capacity, rating, or scope recommended by the manufacturer.

e. Written reports that show test procedures and confirm the adequacy of repairs or alterations shall be maintained and provided upon request.

16.G OPERATION

16.G.01 All cranes and hoisting equipment shall have the following documents with them (in the cab, if applicable) at all times they are to be operated:

a. A copy of the operating manual developed by the manufacturer for the specific make and model of the crane or hoist.

(1) When not available from a manufacturer, a qualified person shall establish the ratings and operating limitations (load charts), recommended operating speeds, special hazard warnings, instructions and operators manual, maintenance, testing, and inspection requirements that apply during the use.

(2) Where load capacities are available only in electronic form: in the event of a failure which makes the load capacities inaccessible, the operator must immediately cease operations

EM 385-1-1
15 Sep 08

or follow safe shut-down procedures until the load capacities (in electronic or other form) are available.

b. A copy of the load-rating chart (separate or included in the operating manual), shall include:

(1) The crane/hoist make and model, serial number, and year of manufacturer;

(2) Load ratings for all operating configurations, including optional equipment;

(3) Recommended reeving for the hoist line; and

(4) Operating limits in windy or cold weather conditions.

c. A durable load chart with legible letters and figures shall be fixed at a location visible to the operator while seated at the control station;

d. The crane log book shall be used to record operating hours and all crane inspections, tests, maintenance, and repair. The log shall be updated daily as the crane is used and shall be signed by the operator and supervisor. Service mechanics shall sign the log after conducting maintenance or repairs on the crane.

e. All inspections, test, maintenance and repairs for hoisting equipment shall be maintained in the log, the O&M records or equivalent for that piece of equipment.

16.G.02 No modifications or additions that affect the capacity or safe operation of cranes or hoisting equipment shall be made without the manufacturer's written approval.

a. If such modifications or changes are made, the capacity, operation, and maintenance instruction plates, tags, or decals shall be changed accordingly.

EM 385-1-1
15 Sep 08

b. In no case shall the original safety factor of the equipment be reduced.

16.G.03 Hoisting wire ropes shall be installed in accordance with ANSI/ASME standards and the equipment manufacturer's recommendations.

a. Overhead and gantry cranes shall have at least two full wraps of wire rope on the drums at all times.

b. All other cranes shall have at least three full wraps (not layers) of wire rope on the drums at all times.

c. The drum end of the wire rope shall be anchored to the drum by an arrangement specified by the crane manufacturer.

16.G.04 Responsibilities.

a. The responsibilities of the operator shall include, but are not limited to the following requirements:

(1) The operator shall not engage in any activity that will divert his attention while operating the equipment;

(2) The operator shall not leave the controls while a load is suspended;

(3) Before leaving the crane or hoisting equipment unattended, the operator shall:

(a) Land any load, bucket, lifting magnet, or other device;

(b) Disengage the master clutch;

(c) Set travel, swing, boom brakes, and other locking devices;

(d) Put the controls in the "OFF" or neutral position;

EM 385-1-1
15 Sep 08

(e) Secure the equipment against accidental travel; and

(f) Stop the engine.

(g) Exception: When crane operation is frequently interrupted during a shift and the operator must leave the crane. Under these circumstances, the engine may remain running and the following conditions (including those in paragraphs (a) thru (e) above) shall apply:

(i) The operator shall remain adjacent to the equipment and is not engaged in any other duties;

(ii) The competent person determines that it is safe to do so and implements measures necessary to restrain the boom hoist and telescoping, load, swing and outrigger functions;

(iii) The crane shall be located within an area protected from unauthorized entry.

(4) The operator shall respond to signals from the person who is directing the lift or an appointed signal person. When a signal person is not used in the crane operation, the operator shall ensure he has full view of the load and the load travel paths at all times the load is rigged to the crane and hoisting equipment;

(5) Each operator is responsible for those operations under his direct control. Whenever there is a concern as to safety, the operator shall have the authority to stop and refuse to handle loads until a qualified person has determined that safety has been assured.

b. The operator, qualified lift supervisor and rigger shall jointly ensure that:

(1) The crane is level and, where necessary, blocked;

EM 385-1-1
15 Sep 08

(2) The load is well secured and balanced in the sling or lifting device before it is lifted more than a few inches;

(3) The lift and swing path is clear of obstructions and adequate clearance is maintained from electrical sources per Table 16-3; and

(4) All persons are clear of the swing radius of the counterweight.

c. When two or more cranes (tandem lift is a critical lift) are used to lift one load, the lift supervisor shall be responsible for the following:

(1) Analyzing the operation and instruct all personnel involved in the proper positioning, rigging of the load, and the movements to be made;

(2) Making determinations as necessary to reduce crane ratings, load position, boom location, ground support, and speed of movement, which are required to safely make the lift;

(3) Ensuring that dedicated personnel are present and equipment is functioning properly. All personnel involved with the crane operation shall understand the communication systems and their responsibilities.

16.G.05 Communications.

a. A standard signal system shall be used on all cranes and hoisting equipment (by hand, voice, audible or comparable signals). Manual (hand) signals may be used when the distance between the operator and signal person is not more than 100 ft (30.4 m). If using hand signals, Standard Method must be used per Figure 16-

(1) Radio, telephone, or a visual and audible electrically-operated system shall be used when the distance between

EM 385-1-1
15 Sep 08

operator and signal person is more than 100 ft or when they cannot see each other.

b. A signal person must be used in the following situations:

(1) When the point of operation, load travel, area near or at load placement, is not in full view of the operator;

(2) When the equipment is traveling and the view in the direction of travel is obstructed;

(3) Due to site specific safety concerns, either the operator or the person handling the load determines that it is necessary.

c. During crane operations requirement signals, the ability to transmit signals between the operator and signal person shall be maintained. If that ability is interrupted at any time, the operator shall safely stop operations requiring signals until it is reestablished and a proper signal is given and understood.

d. Only one person gives signals to a crane/derrick operator at a time unless an emergency stop signal is given (which may be given by anyone and must be obeyed by the operator).

16.G.06 Riding on loads, hooks, hammers, buckets, material hoists, or other hoisting equipment not meant for personnel handling is prohibited.

EM 385-1-1
15 Sep 08

FIGURE 16-1

CRANE HAND SIGNALS

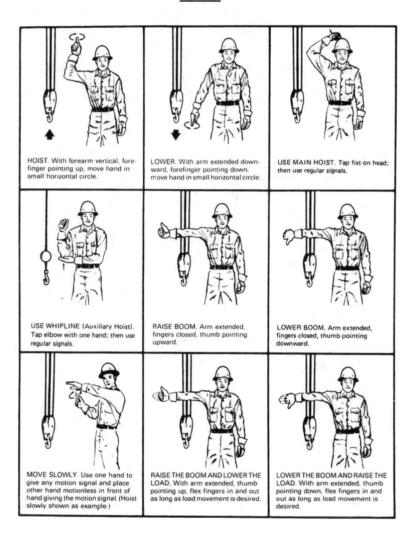

FIGURE 16-1 (Continued)

CRANE HAND SIGNALS

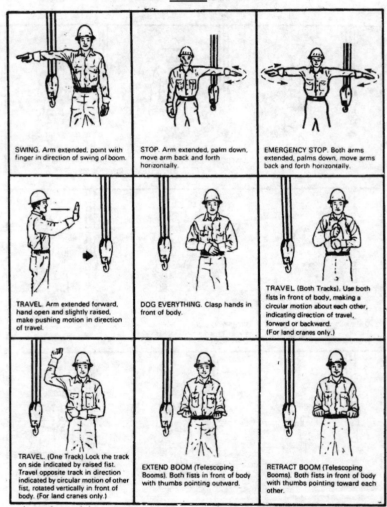

EM 385-1-1
15 Sep 08

FIGURE 16-1 (Continued)

CRANE HAND SIGNALS

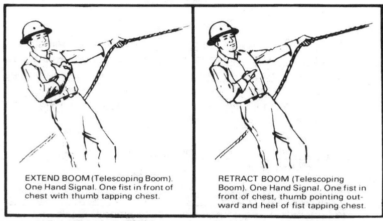

EXTEND BOOM (Telescoping Boom). One Hand Signal. One fist in front of chest with thumb tapping chest.

RETRACT BOOM (Telescoping Boom). One Hand Signal. One fist in front of chest, thumb pointing outward and heel of fist tapping chest.

NOTE: Crane signals taken from ANSI/ASME B30 series standards with permission of ASME.

16.G.07 When practical and when their use does not create a hazard, tag lines shall be used to control loads.

16.G.08 Whenever a slack line condition occurs, the proper seating of the rope in the sheaves and on the drum shall be checked prior to further operations.

16.G.09 Clearances.

a. Power line clearance. The employer must identify the work zone for the crane in question (work zone is the area 360 degrees around the crane, up to the crane's maximum working radius). A determination shall be made if any part of the crane, load line or load (to include rigging and lifting accessories), if operated up to the crane's maximum working radius in the work

EM 385-1-1
15 Sep 08

zone, could get within 20 ft (6 m) of the power line. If possible, one of the following options must be met:

(1) De-energize and ground. Confirm from the utility owner/operator that the line has been de-energized and visibly grounded at the worksite;

(2) Table 16-3, Minimum approach distances. Determine the line's voltage and the minimum approach distance permitted by Table 16-3 and insure that no part of the crane, load line or load (including rigging and lifting accessories) while operating up to the crane's maximum working radius in the work zone, gets within the minimum approach distance;

(3) Permanently installed overhead and gantry cranes clearances shall be in accordance with NFPA 70;

(4) Operations below power lines. No part of a crane, load line or load (including rigging and lifting accessories) is allowed below a power line unless it has been confirmed that the utility owner/operator has de-energized and visibly grounded the power line at the work site;

(5) It shall be assumed that all power lines are energized unless the utility owner/operator confirms that the power line has been and will continue to be de-energized and visibly grounded at the worksite.

b. Physical clearances.

(1) Adequate clearance shall be maintained between moving and rotating structures of the crane and hoisting equipment and fixed objects to allow the passage of employees without harm. The minimum adequate clearance is 24 in (61 cm).

(2) Accessible areas within the swing radius of the rear of the crane and hoisting equipment's rotating superstructure, either permanently or temporarily mounted, shall be barricaded to

prevent an employee from being struck or crushed by the crane and hoisting equipment.

(3) No employee shall be permitted to work under any suspended loads. Exception: Where workers are engaged in the initial connection of steel or employees are unhooking the load.

16.H CRITICAL LIFTS

16.H.01 When using cranes or hoists, the following are identified as critical lifts requiring detailed planning and additional or unusual safety precautions. Critical lifts are defined as:

a. Lifts involving hazardous materials (e.g., explosives, highly volatile substances);

b. Hoisting personnel with a crane or hoist;

c. Lifts made with more than one crane;

d. Lifts where the center of gravity could change;

TABLE 16-3

MINIMUM CLEARANCE FROM ENERGIZED OVERHEAD ELECTRIC LINES

(All dimensions are distances from live part to employee)

Voltage (nominal, kV, alternating current)	Minimum rated clearance
Up to 50	10 ft (3 m)
51 – 200	15 ft (4.6 m)
201 – 350	20 ft (6 m)
351 to 500	25 ft (7.6 m)
501 - 650	30 ft (9.1 m)
651 – 800	35 ft (10.7 m)
801 – 950	40 ft (12.2 m)
951 – 1100	45 ft (13.7 m)
Clearance values calculated using: (Initial kV-50kV) x (4 in/10 kV) x (1 ft/12 in) = increased distance (ft) over 10 ft. Add this value to 10 ft to yield minimum rated clearance	

e. Lifts the operator believes should be considered critical;

f. Lifts made when the load weight is 75% of the rated capacity of the crane load chart or more (not applicable to gantry, overhead or bridge cranes);

g. Lifts without the use of outriggers using rubber tire load charts;

h. Lifts using more than one hoist on the same crane or trolleys;

i. Lifts involving non-routine or technically difficult rigging arrangement (to include lifts involving Multiple Lift Rigging;

EM 385-1-1
15 Sep 08

j. Lifts involving submerged loads (EXCEPTION: lifts that were engineered to travel in guided slots throughout the lift and have fixed rigging and/or lifting beams, i.e., intake gates, roller gates, tailgates/logs,);

k. Lifts out of the operator's view; **EXCEPTION: if hand signals via a signal person in view of the operator or radio communications are available and in use, load does not exceed two tons AND is determined a routine lift by the lift supervisor.**

16.H.02 Critical lift plans. Before making a critical lift, a critical lift plan shall be developed:

a. By a qualified person and shall include the crane operator, lift supervisor, and the rigger and signed by all involved personnel prior to the lift;

b. For a series of lifts on one project or job, as long as the cranes, personnel, type loads and configuration do not differ;

c. And documented with a copy provided to the GDA prior to the lift(s) being made;

d. And shall include, as a minimum:

(1) The specific make and model of the cranes, the line, boom, and swing speeds;

(2) The exact size and weight of the load to be lifted and all crane and rigging components that add to the weight. The manufacturer's maximum load limits for the entire range of the lift, as listed in the load charts, shall also be specified;

(3) The plan shall specify the lift geometry and procedures, including the crane position, height of the lift, the load radius, and the boom length and angle, for the entire range of the lift;

(4) Site drawing shall be included to identify placement/location(s) of crane, adjacent equipment and/or facilities, etc.;

(5) The plan shall designate the crane operator, lift supervisor and rigger and include their qualifications;

(6) The plan will include a rigging plan that shows the lift points and describes rigging procedures and hardware requirements;

(7) The plan will describe the ground conditions, outrigger or crawler track requirements, and, if necessary, the design of mats, necessary to achieve a level, stable foundation of sufficient bearing capacity for the lift;

(8) For floating crane or derricks, the plan shall describe the operating base (platform) condition and any potential maximum list / trim;

(9) The plan will list environmental conditions under which lift operations are to be stopped;

(10) The plan will specify coordination and communication requirements for the lift operation;

(11) For tandem or tailing crane lifts, identify the requirements for an equalizer beam if applicable.

16.I ENVIRONMENTAL CONSIDERATIONS

16.I.01 Projects shall have adequate means for monitoring local weather conditions, including a wind-indicating device

16.I.02 Cranes shall not be operated when wind speeds at the site attain the maximum wind velocity recommendations of the manufacturer. At winds greater than 20 mph (9 m/s), the operator, rigger, and lift supervisor shall cease all crane operations, evaluate conditions and determine if the lift shall proceed. The

EM 385-1-1
15 Sep 08

determination to proceed or not shall be documented in the crane operator's logbook.

16.I.03 When a local storm warning has been issued, the competent person shall determine whether it is necessary to implement manufacturer recommendations for securing the equipment.

16.I.04 Operations performed during weather conditions that produce icing of the crane and hoisting equipment structure or reduced visibility shall be performed at reduced functional speeds and with signaling means appropriate to the situation.

16.I.05 When conditions are such that lightning is observed all crane and hoisting equipment operations shall cease. A period of 30 minutes between subsequent observations shall be observed prior to resuming work.

16.I.06 For night operations, lighting adequate to illuminate the working areas while not interfering with the operator's vision shall be provided. **> See Section 7.**

16.J LATTICE, HYDRAULIC, CRAWLER-, TRUCK-, WHEEL-, AND RINGER-MOUNTED CRANES

16.J.01 For required operator aids and indicating devices, see Section 16.E.03.

16.J.02 Boom assembly and disassembly. This operation shall be covered in the AHA and Competent Person shall be identified.

> a. The manufacturer's boom assembly and disassembly procedures shall be reviewed by the team before starting the assembly or disassembly. The Competent Person shall be present during assembly/disassembly operations.

> b. When removing pins or bolts from a boom, workers shall stay out from under the boom. Sections shall be blocked or otherwise secured to prevent them from falling.

16.J.03 Outriggers.

a. Anytime outriggers are required to be used, they shall be extended or deployed per the crane manufacturer's load/capacity chart specifications and set to remove the machine weight from the wheels at all settings, except for locomotive cranes.

b. When partially extended outriggers are used, the following requirements, shall be met:

(1) Crane operation with partially extended outriggers shall only be undertaken if approved by the crane manufacturer;

(2) Outriggers shall be set at equal positions that correspond to the load/capacity charts supplied by the manufacturer for those positions. Only the load chart(s) corresponding to the outrigger positions shall be used for operation;

(3) When situations arise where outriggers must be set at unequal positions that correspond to the load/capacity charts corresponding with the individual quadrants of operation. The manufacturer or qualified person shall be consulted to determine if the capacity reductions, special operating procedures, or limitations are required;

c. When outrigger floats are used, they shall be securely attached to the outriggers.

d. Blocking under outriggers floats shall meet the following requirements:

(1) Sufficient strength to prevent crushing, bending, or shear failure;

(2) Such thickness, width, and length as to completely support the float, transmit the load to the supporting surface, and

EM 385-1-1
15 Sep 08

prevent shifting, toppling, or excessive settlement under load; and

(3) Use of blocking only under the outer bearing surface of the extended outrigger beam floats.

16.J.04 Unless the manufacturer has specified an on-rubber rating, mobile cranes shall not pick or swing loads over the side of the crane unless the outriggers are down and fully extended.

16.J.05 Unless recommended against by the manufacturer, crane booms shall be lowered to ground level or secured against displacement by wind loads or other outside forces when not in use. If the manufacturer recommends against this practice, the manufacturer's recommended practice shall be followed.

16.J.06 When pick and carry operations occur (Rough Terrain Crane's), the boom must be centered over the front of the crane, the mechanical swing lock engaged, and the load restrained from swinging.

16.K PORTAL, TOWER, AND PILLAR CRANES

16.K.01 All load bearing foundations, supports, and rail tracks shall be constructed or installed as determined by a Registered Professional Engineer with knowledge in this area, in accordance with the crane manufacturer's recommendations.

16.K.02 Cranes shall be erected/dismantled in accordance with the manufacturer's recommendations, (or if manufacturer procedures are not available, in accordance with procedures developed by a Registered Professional Engineer with knowledge in this area).

a. When erected/dismantled, written instructions by the manufacturer and/or Registered Professional Engineer and a list of the weights of each component shall be kept at the site.

b. Erection and dismantling shall be performed under the supervision of a qualified person.

EM 385-1-1
15 Sep 08

c. An AHA shall be developed and procedures established before the erection/dismantling work commences to insure site-specific needs are considered. The analysis will include:

(1) The location of the crane in relation to other tower cranes, adjacent buildings or towers, overhead power and communication lines, underground utilities;

(2) Foundation design and construction requirements; and

(3) When the tower is erected within a structure, clearances between the tower and the structure and bracing and wedging requirements.

d. Wind velocity at the site at the time of erection/dismantling shall be a consideration as a limiting factor that could require suspending the erection/dismantling operation and shall be as determined by the manufactured or if this data is not available, by a qualified person.

e. Before crane components are erected, they shall be visually inspected for damage. Dented, bent, torn, gouged or otherwise damaged members shall not be erected.

f. Initially and after each climb, the crane shall be plumbed and then held in the plumbed condition by wedges or other means. Cranes shall be plumbed to a tolerance of 1:500 (1 in:40 ft; 2.4 cm:12 m) unless the manufacturer specifies otherwise.

16.K.03 Pre-operation tests shall be performed when cranes are erected and after each climbing operation, before placing the crane in service. All functional motions, motion limiting devices and brakes shall be properly tested for operation in accordance with the manufacturer's recommended procedures and ANSI/ASME B30.3 or B30.4, as applicable:

a. Crane supports;

b. Brakes and clutches, limit and overload switches, and locking and safety devices; and

c. Load hoisting and lowering, boom hoisting and lowering, and swing motion mechanisms and procedures.

16.K.04 Climbing Procedures. Prior to and during, all climbing procedures (to include inside and top climbing), the employer shall:

a. Comply with all manufacturer prohibitions;

b. Have a registered professional engineer verify that the host structure is strong enough to sustain the forces imposed through the braces, brace anchorages and supporting floors;

c. Ensure that no part of the climbing procedure takes place when wind velocity at the crane superstructure exceeds the limit set by the manufacturer or a qualified person, or 20 mph (9 m/s) at the crane superstructure if no such limit has been set. The characteristics of the gusts should be considered for their effect on the climbing operation; and

d. The operator of a hammerhead tower crane shall be present during climbing or telescoping operations.

16.K.05 Safety devices and operational aids. Operations shall not begin unless the safety devices and operational aids are in place and in proper working order. In addition to those listed in 16.E.03, the following shall be provided:

a. Rail clamps, if used, shall have slack between the point of attachment to the rail and the end fastened to the crane. Rail clamps shall not be used as a means of restraining tipping of a crane display magnitude of load on the hook;

b. Hydraulic system pressure limiting device;

EM 385-1-1
15 Sep 08

    c. The following brakes, which shall automatically set in the event of pressure loss or power failure, are required: hoist brake on all hoists, swing brake, trolley brake, rail travel brake;

    d. Deadman control or forced neutral return control (hand) levers;

    e. Emergency stop switch at the operator's station;

    f. Trolley travel limiting device prevents trolley from running into the trolley end stops;

    g. Ambient wind velocity device. This device shall be mounted at or near the top of the crane. A velocity readout shall be provided at the operator's station in the cab, and a visible or audible alarm shall be triggered in the cab and at remote control stations when a preset wind velocity has been exceeded;

    h. Hoist line pull limiting device (limits lifted load).

16.K.06 Multiple tower crane jobsites. On jobsites where more than one fixed jib (hammerhead) tower crane is installed, the cranes shall be located such that no crane may come in contact with the structure of another crane. Cranes are permitted to pass over one another.

16.K.07 Weathervaning. Tower cranes required to weathervane when out-of-service shall be installed with clearance for boom (jib) and supersutructure to swing through a full 360 degree arc without striking any fixed object or other weathervaning crane. The boom shall be taken in the attitude dictated by its wind area balance. Nonweathervaning boom (jibs) shall be taken in the least favorable attitude. Traveling cranes shall also resist design wind level induced sliding.

16.L FLOATING CRANES/DERRICKS, CRANE BARGES, AND AUXILIARY SHIPBOARD MOUNTED CRANES

16.L.01 The requirements in this section are supplemental requirements for floating cranes/derricks, land cranes/derricks on barges, pontoons, vessels or other means of flotation and auxiliary shipboard mounted cranes, unless otherwise specified.

16.L.02 The load rating of a floating crane/derrick shall be the maximum working loads at various radii as determined by the manufacturer or qualified person considering list and trim for each installation. The load rating shall specifically reflect the: design standard; machine trim; machine list; and dynamic/environmental loadings anticipated for the operational envelope of the floating crane or auxiliary shipboard crane. A Naval Architectural Analysis shall be performed to determine these parameters that shall be used in generating the load rating.

   a. The load rating is dependent upon the structural competence of the crane, rope strength, hoist capacity, structural attachment to the floating platform, and stability and freeboard of the floating platform.

   b. When deck loads are to be carried while lifting, the situation shall be analyzed for modified ratings.

   c. When mounted on barges or pontoons, the rated loads and radii of land cranes shall be modified as recommended by the manufacturer or qualified person. The modification shall be evaluated by the qualified person specific to the flotation device/platform being used.

   d. Load charts shall be posted in the cab or at the operator's station (if no cab). All other procedures applicable to the operation of the equipment (instructions and operators manual, recommended operating speeds, etc.) shall be readily available on board.

   e. Load charts shall, at a minimum, identify the following:

(1) Naval Architect Notes:

(a) Draft limits (with deck cargo considered);

(b) Vessel motion limits ;

(c) Vessel and crane list/trim limits, and

(d) Vessel condition (e.g., dry bilges, watertight integrity, etc.).

(2) Crane manufacturer Notes, or reference to them.

(3) Safe Working Load Chart with:

(a) Mode of operation;

(b) Environmental limits;

(c) Capacity (net or gross);

(d) Load, boom elevation, radius (with list/trim considered), and

(e) Crane configuration, to include boom length, amount of counterweight, parts of wire, and block size.

16.L.03 Floating cranes/derricks. All floating cranes/ derricks intended for permanent attachment to a barge, pontoon or other means of flotation shall be designed in accordance with the requirements of 46 CFR 173.005 through 173.025.

a. Load Charts.

(1) The manufacturer load charts applicable to operations on water shall not be exceeded. When using these charts, the employer shall comply with all parameters and limitations (dynamic, environmental, etc.) applicable to the use of these charts.

EM 385-1-1
15 Sep 08

(2) The load charts shall take into consideration a minimum wind speed of 40 mph (18 m/s).

b. Maximum Operating list or trim. Unless the crane manufacturer recommends a lesser value, maximum operating list or trim shall comply with requirements below:

(1) Cranes designed for marine use (barge or pontoon mounting) by permanent attachment, with a rated capacity of up to 25 tons (22,680 kg) shall have a maximum allowable list or trim of 5°;

(2) Cranes designed for marine use (barge or pontoon mounting) by permanent attachment, with a rated capacity of greater than 25 tons (22,680 kg) shall have a maximum allowable list or trim of 7°, although 5° is recommended;

(3) Derricks, designed for marine use (barge or pontoon mounting) by permanent attachment, of any capacity shall have a maximum allowable list or trim of 10°;

c. Stability. The equipment shall be made stable with the following maximum allowable freeboard requirements:

(1) Operated at rated capacity, 60 mph (100 kph) wind, 2 ft (0.6 m) minimum freeboard;

(2) Operated at rated capacity plus 25%, 60 mph (100 kph) wind, 1 ft (0.3 m) minimum freeboard;

(3) Operated at high boom, no load, 60 mph (100 kph) wind, 2 ft (0.6 m) minimum freeboard;

(4) For backward stability of the boom - high boom, no load, full back list (least stable condition), 90 mph (145.8 kph) wind.

d. If the equipment is employer-made, it shall not be used unless the employer has documents demonstrating that the load charts and applicable parameters for use meet the requirements of paragraphs 16.L.03.a, b and c. Such documents shall be signed by a marine engineer or a registered professional engineer who is a qualified person with respect to the design of this type of equipment (including the means of flotation).

16.L.04 Land cranes/derricks mounted on barges, pontoons or other means of flotation.

a. The rated capacity of the equipment (load charts) applicable for use on land shall be reduced by the equipment manufacturer, or a qualified person who has expertise with respect to both land crane/derrick capacity and the stability of vessels/flotation devices.

b. Load Charts. The rated capacity of the equipment for use on land shall be reduced to:

(1) Account for increased loading from list, trim, wave action and wind;

(2) Be applicable to a specified location(s) on the specific barge, pontoons, vessel or other means of flotation that will be used, under the expected environmental conditions;

(3) Insure that the maximum allowable list and trim for the land crane/derrick shall not exceed the amount specified by the crane/derrick manufacturer or if not specified, the amount specified by the qualified person;

(4) Maximum allowable list and trim for the barge, pontoon, or other means of flotation shall not exceed the amount necessary to ensure:

(a) All deck surfaces of the barge, pontoon or flotation device shall be above the water;

EM 385-1-1
15 Sep 08

(b) The entire bottom area of the barge, pontoon or flotation device shall be submerged; AND

(c) The maximum allowable list or trim shall not exceed the least of the following: 5°, the maximum specified by the crane/derrick manufacturer or if not specified, the amount specified by the qualified person.

c. Physical attachment.

(1) Derricks shall be secured to the deck to transmit the loading to the barge or pontoon.

(2) Cranes shall be blocked or secured to prevent shifting.

(3) The crane shall be allowed to travel on the barge for repositioning only. If traveling is required while lifting the load, this lift shall be deemed a critical lift and a critical lift plan is required. It must include a Naval Architectural Analysis to determine these parameters. A marine engineer or registered professional engineer familiar with floating crane design shall perform this analysis. In addition, the manufacturer's recommendations shall be followed.

16.L.05 When loads approach the maximum rating of the crane or derrick, the person responsible for the job shall ascertain that the weight of the load has been determined within +/- 10% before it is lifted.

16.L.06 Safety devices and Operational Aids. In addition to those required by section 16.E.03, the following are required:

a. Pontoon, barge, vessel or flotation device list and trim device: Shall be located in the cab or at the operator's station (if there is no cab) as a means for the operator to visually determine the list and trim;

b. Wind speed and direction indicator: within clear view of the operator's station;

EM 385-1-1
15 Sep 08

> c. Anti two-block device: only when hoisting personnel or hoisting over an occupied cofferdam or shaft.

16.L.07 Principal walking surfaces shall be of a skid-resistant type.

16.L.08 In addition to inspection of the crane/derrick per 16.D, inspection of the barge, pontoons, vessel or other means of flotation used to support a land crane/derrick by a competent person is required:

> a. Each shift - the means used to secure/attach the equipment to the vessel/flotation device shall be inspected for proper condition, to include wear, corrosion, loose or missing fasteners, defective welds and (where applicable) insufficient tension.
>
> b. Monthly. In addition to 16.L.08.a, The vessel/means of flotation used shall be inspected for the following:
>
> (1) Taking on water;
>
> (2) Deckload for proper securing;
>
> 3) Chain lockers, storage, fuel compartments and battening of hatches for serviceability as a water-tight appliance;
>
> (4) Firefighting and lifesaving equipment in place and functional.
>
> c. If any deficiency is identified, an immediate determination shall be made by a qualified person as to whether the deficiency constitutes a hazard. If so, the vessel/flotation device shall be removed from service until it has been corrected.

16.L.09 Operations.

> a. Operators shall monitor the wire lead from the boom tip carefully to ensure that limits on off-lead and side-lead identified in the load chart are not exceeded.

EM 385-1-1
15 Sep 08

b. Operators shall monitor environmental criteria for compliance with the criteria set forth in the load chart.

c. Operators should be aware that safety devices such as LLD(s) and LMI(s) do not offer protection against loads generated by relative motions between a floating crane and a fixed object to be lifted.

d. Whenever practical, crane use during buoy tending shall be limited to lifting the freely suspended buoy clear of the water onto the vessel.

e. Bilges shall be kept as dry as possible to eliminate the adverse effect of free surface (sloshing liquid).

16.L.10 All lifts must be planned to avoid procedures that could result in configurations where the operator cannot maintain safe control of the lift. (A plan, in this case, might be a quick discussion with the deck crew, and a verification of the proposed operation.) Lifts shall reflect floating operational parameters such as: anticipated values for wire leads, unknown load for extractions, and upper limits on crane force.

16.L.11 Mobile Auxiliary Cranes. For mobile auxiliary cranes used on deck of a floating crane/derrick, the requirement for physical attachment does not apply when the following can demonstrate the following requirements have been met:

a. A marine engineer or registered professional engineer familiar with floating crane/derrick design develops and signs a written plan for the use of the mobile auxiliary crane.

b. The plan shall be designed so that the requirements for safe location of equipment will be met despite the position, travel, operation, and lack of physical attachment of the mobile auxiliary crane.

c. The plan shall specify the areas of the deck where the mobile auxiliary crane is permitted to be positioned, travel and operate

EM 385-1-1
15 Sep 08

and the parameters or limitations of such movements and operation.

d. The deck shall be marked to identify the permitted areas for positioning, travel and operation.

e. The plan shall specify the dynamic and environmental conditions that must be present for the use of the plan.

f. If the dynamic and environmental conditions are exceeded, the mobile auxiliary crane shall be physically attached or corralled.

16.L.12 Anchor handling barge/vessel.

a. An anchor handling barge/vessel may be used for anchor handling, low lifting of loads such as anchor buoys/weights, dredge pipe, submerged pipeline, pontoons, and other loads provided they do not exceed the load rating of the anchor barge/vessel. If used for any other lifting application, the work platform will be considered a floating derrick and all other requirements of Section 16 apply. Anchor barge/vessels shall also comply with the following:

(1) All deck surfaces of the pontoon or barge shall be above the water;

(2) Means for limiting the applied load, such as mechanical means or marking the draft of the barge corresponding to the rated load, shall be provided. Calculations shall be available and the barge shall be tested to verify rated load;

(3) A ratchet and pawl shall be provided for releasing the load from the hoisting machinery brake;

(4) An operating manual/procedure shall be available for use by the operator. The operator shall be trained in the anchor handling barge systems operation.

EM 385-1-1
15 Sep 08

b. If additional external load is superimposed above that which can be hoisted with the onboard hoisting machinery, then a chain stopper shall be used to remove the external load from the A-frame and hoist machinery.

16.M OVERHEAD AND GANTRY CRANES

16.M.01 The requirements in this section are supplemental requirements for overhead and gantry cranes whether permanently installed in a facility or not and includes overhead/bridge cranes, semi gantry, cantilever gantry, wall cranes, storage bridge cranes, and others having the same fundamental characteristics whether it travels on tracks, wheels or other means (unless otherwise specified).

16.M.02 All load bearing foundations, anchorages, runways, and rail tracks shall be constructed or installed in accordance with the crane manufacturer's recommendations and ANSI/ASME B30.2 or B30.17, as applicable.

16.M.03 The rated load of the crane shall be plainly marked on each side of the crane.

   a. If the crane has more than one hoisting unit, each hoist shall have its rated load marked on it or its load block.

   b. Markings on the bridge, trolley, and load block shall be legible from the ground or floor.

16.M.04 Clearance shall be maintained between the crane, any structure or object, and any parallel running cranes and cranes operating at different elevations.

16.M.05 Contacts with runway stops or other cranes shall be made with extreme caution. The operator shall do so with particular care for the safety of persons on or below the crane, and only after making certain that any persons on the other cranes are aware of what is being done.

EM 385-1-1
15 Sep 08

16.M.06 Operators of outdoor cranes shall secure them when leaving.

16.M.07 When the wind-indicating alarm of a cab-operated outdoor crane sounds, crane operations shall be discontinued and the crane shall be prepared and stored for excessive wind conditions.

16.N MONORAILS AND UNDERHUNG CRANES

16.N.01 Crane runways, monorail tracks, track supports, and track control devices shall be constructed or installed in accordance with the crane manufacturer's recommendations and ANSI/ASME B30.11.

16.N.02 The rated load of the crane shall be plainly marked on each side of the crane.

   a. If the crane has more than one hoisting unit, each hoist shall have its rated load marked on it or its load block.

   b. Markings on the bridge, trolley, and load block shall be legible from the ground or floor.

16.O DERRICKS

16.O.01 For permanent fixed locations, the following load anchoring data shall be provided to the GDA. For non-permanent installations, this data shall be determined by a qualified person.

   a. Guy derricks.

   (1) Maximum horizontal and vertical forces when handling rated loads with the particular guy slope and spacing stipulated for the application, and

EM 385-1-1
15 Sep 08

(2) Maximum horizontal and vertical forces at the guy when handling rated loads with the particular guy slope and spacing stipulated for the application.

b. Stiffleg derricks.

(1) Maximum horizontal and vertical forces at the mast base when handling rated loads with the particular stiffleg slope and spacing stipulated for the application, and

(2) Maximum horizontal and vertical forces at the stifflegs when handling rated loads with the particular stiffleg arrangement stipulated for the application.

16.O.02 Derrick booms, load hoists, and swinger mechanisms shall be suitable for the derrick work intended and shall be anchored to prevent displacement from imposed loads.

16.O.03 When rotating a derrick, sudden starts and stops shall be avoided and rotational speed shall be such that the load does not swing out beyond the radius at which it can be controlled. A tagline shall be used.

16.O.04 Boom and hoisting rope systems shall not be twisted.

16.O.05 Ropes shall not be handled on a winch head without the knowledge of the operator. When a winch head is being used, the operator shall be within reach of the power unit controls.

16.O.06 When securing the boom, dogs or other positive holding mechanisms on the hoist shall be engaged.

16.O.07 When not in use the derrick boom shall be either:

a. Laid down;

b. Secured to a stationary member as nearly under the head as possible by attachment of a sling to the load block;

EM 385-1-1
15 Sep 08

> c. Lifted to a vertical position and secured to the mast (for guy derricks); or
>
> d. Secured against a stiffleg (for stiffleg derricks).

16.P HANDLING LOADS SUSPENDED FROM ROTORCRAFT

16.P.01 Helicopter cranes shall comply with regulations of the Federal Aviation Administration (FAA).

16.P.02 Before each day's operation, a briefing shall be conducted to set forth the plan of operation for the pilot and ground personnel.

16.P.03 Loads shall be properly slung.

> a. Tag lines shall be of a length that will not permit their being drawn up into rotors.
>
> b. Pressed sleeve, swedged eyes, or equivalent means shall be used for all freely suspended loads to prevent hand splices from spinning open or wire clamps from loosening.

16.P.04 All electrically operated cargo hooks shall have the electrical activating device so designed and installed as to prevent inadvertent operation.

> a. In addition, these cargo hooks shall be equipped with an emergency mechanical control for releasing the load.
>
> b. The hooks shall be tested prior to each day's operation to determine that the release functions properly, both electrically and mechanically.

16.P.05 PPE for employees receiving the load shall consist of eye protection and hard hats secured by chinstraps.

16.P.06 Loose-fitting clothing likely to flap in the downwash, and be snagged on the hoist line, shall not be worn.

EM 385-1-1
15 Sep 08

16.P.07 Every practical precaution shall be taken to provide for the protection of the employees from flying objects in the rotor downwash. All loose gear within 100 ft (30.4 m) of the place of lifting or depositing the load, and all other areas susceptible to rotor downwash, shall be secured or removed.

16.P.08 The helicopter pilot shall be responsible for the size, weight, and manner in which loads are connected to the helicopter. If, for any reason, the helicopter pilot believes the lift cannot be made safely, the lift shall not be made.

16.P.09 When employees are required to work under hovering craft, safe access shall be provided for employees to reach the hoist line hook and engage or disengage cargo slings. Employees shall not work under hovering craft except to hook, unhook, or position loads.

16.P.10 Static charge on the suspended load shall be dissipated with a grounding device before ground personnel touch the suspended load, or protective rubber gloves shall be worn by all ground personnel touching the suspended load.

16.P.11 The weight of an external load shall not exceed the rated capacity.

16.P.12 Hoist wires or other gear, except for pulling lines or conductors that are allowed to "pay out" from a container or roll off a reel, shall not be attached to any fixed ground structure or be allowed to foul on any fixed structures.

16.P.13 When visibility is reduced by dust or other conditions, ground personnel shall exercise special caution to keep clear of main and stabilizing rotors. Precautions shall also be taken to eliminate reduced visibility.

16.P.14 No unauthorized person shall be allowed to approach within 50 ft (15.2 m) of the helicopter when the rotor blades are turning.

16.P.15 Whenever approaching or leaving a helicopter with blades rotating, all employees shall remain in full view of the pilot and keep in a crouched position. Employees shall avoid the area from the cockpit or cabin rearward unless authorized by the helicopter pilot to work there.

16.P.16 There shall be constant reliable communication between the pilot and a designated employee of the ground crew who acts as a signal person during loading and unloading. This signal person shall be distinctly recognizable from other ground personnel. **> See Figure 16-2**

16.P.17 Good housekeeping shall be maintained in all helicopter loading and unloading areas.

16.Q MATERIAL HOISTS

16.Q.01 Material hoists shall be designed to raise and lower materials during construction, alteration, or demolition. It is not applicable to the temporary use of permanently installed elevators as material hoists. They shall be constructed and installed in accordance with the requirements of ANSI A10.5.

16.Q.02 Material hoist towers, masts, guy or braces, counterweights, drive machinery supports, sheave supports, platforms, supporting structures, and accessories shall be designed by a licensed engineer.

16.Q.03 Hoist towers shall be erected and dismantled only under the direct supervision of a qualified individual.

16.Q.04 A copy of the hoist operating manual shall be available at all times it is operated.

EM 385-1-1
15 Sep 08

FIGURE 16-2

HELICOPTER HAND SIGNALS

Arms crossed in front of body and pointing down

Land

Right hand behind back, left hand pointing up

Takeoff

Hands above arm, palms out using a noticeable shoving motion

Move Rearward

Combination of arm and hand movement in a collecting motion pulling toward body

Move Forward

Right arm extended horizontally, left arm sweeps upward to position overhead

Move Left

Left arm extended horizontally, right arm sweeps upward to position over head

Move Right

Arms extended, palms up, arms sweeping up

Move Upward

Arms extended, palms down, arms sweeping down

Move Downward

The signal "hold" is executed by placing arms over head with clenched fists

Hold-Hover

Left arm held down away from body right arm cuts across left arm in a slashing movement from above

Release Sling Load

EM 385-1-1
15 Sep 08

16.Q.05 Material hoists and hoist tower systems shall be inspected in accordance with the manufacturer's recommendations.

a. Prior to initial use and each time after the tower is extended, all parts of the tower or mast, cage, bucket, boom, platform, hoisting machine, guy, and other equipment shall be inspected by a qualified person to ensure compliance with the manufacturer's inspection guidelines and ANSI A10.5.

b. Prior to initial use on a USACE project, and monthly thereafter, a periodic inspection shall be conducted by a qualified person. Periodic inspections shall cover those items specified by the manufacturer.

c. A GDA shall be notified at least 24 hours prior to any of the above inspections and may wish to accompany the contractor's inspector.

d. Pre-operational inspections (start-up procedures) shall be conducted by the operator prior to every operation (shift) of the hoist.

16.Q.06 Before a hoist is placed in service and every 4 months thereafter, a car-arresting-device test shall be performed.

a. For rope-supported cars, the test shall be conducted in the following manner:

(1) Pull a loop in the lifting rope and attach the test rope to each side of the loop above the bucket or platform;

(2) Raise the platform or bucket to allow the load to be supported by the test rope; and

(3) Cut the test rope to allow the load to fall and activate the car-arresting device.

EM 385-1-1
15 Sep 08

b. For car suspension other than rope supported, the test shall be conducted by creating an over speed condition of the car.

c. Structural components shall be inspected for damage after the test and before the hoist is placed in operation again.

16.Q.07 Maintenance and repairs.

a. Replacement parts for load bearing or critical components shall be either obtained from or certified by the equipment manufacturer.

b. Maintenance and repairs shall be conducted in accordance with the manufacturer's procedures.

16.Q.08 Landings and runways.

a. Landing platforms and runways that connect the hoist way or tower to a structure shall be designed and constructed to sustain the maximum intended load without failure.

b. Floors or platforms that may become slippery shall have slip-resistant surfaces.

c. When workers may be exposed to falling objects, overhead protection, composed of 2-in (5-cm) planking or the equivalent, shall be provided.

d. A barricade shall be provided at the open ends of each landing. The barricade shall extend a minimum distance of 6 ft (1.8 m) laterally along the outer edge of the landing from each side of the hoist way, shall extend from the floor a distance of at least 3 ft (0.9 m), and shall be of #19 US gauge wire or the equivalent, with openings not exceeding 0.5 in (1.2 cm).

e. All hoist way entrances shall be protected by substantial gates or bars that shall guard the full width of the landing entrance. Gates shall be not less than 66 in (167.6 cm) in

EM 385-1-1
15 Sep 08

height, with a maximum under clearance of 2 in (5 cm), and shall be located not more than 4 in (10 cm) from the hoist way line. Gates of grille, lattice, or other open work shall have openings of not more than 2 in (5 cm).

f. Material shall not be stored on landing platforms or runways.

16.Q.09 Whenever a slack line condition occurs, the proper seating of the rope in the sheaves and on the drum shall be checked prior to further operations.

16.Q.10 Riding on material hoists or other hoisting equipment not meant for personnel handling is prohibited.

16.Q.11 While hoisting equipment is in operation, the operator shall not perform any other work and shall not leave his/her position at the controls until the load has been safely landed or returned to ground level.

16.Q.12 Not more than one cage or bucket shall be operated at the same time by any one hoisting machine or operator.

16.Q.13 Operating rules shall be established and posted at the operator's station of the hoist. Such rules shall include signal system and allowable line speed for various loads. Rules and notices shall be posted on the car frame or crosshead in a conspicuous location, including the statement **"NO RIDERS ALLOWED."**

16.Q.14 Air-powered hoists shall be connected to an air supply of sufficient capacity and pressure to safely operate the hoist. Pneumatic hoses shall be secured by some positive means to prevent accidental disconnection.

16.R PILE DRIVERS

16.R.01 Other cranes used in duty cycle operations, to include pile driving and extracting operations (except telescopic boom cranes),

EM 385-1-1
15 Sep 08

are exempt from the requirements for A2B devices. > *See 16.E.03.d.(3)*

16.R.02 Guy, outriggers, thrust outs, counter-balances, or rail clamps shall be provided to maintain stability of pile-driver rigs.

16.R.03   Pile-driver leads.

  a. Swinging (hanging) leads.

  (1) Swinging (hanging) leads shall have fixed ladders.

  (2) Employees shall be prohibited from remaining on leads or ladders while pile is being driven.

  b. Fixed leads.

  (1) Fixed pile-driver leads shall be provided with decked landings having guard rails, intermediate rails, and toe boards. Fixed ladders or stairs shall be provided for access to landings and head blocks.

  (2) Fixed leads shall be provided with rings or attachment points so that workers exposed to falls of 6 ft (1.8 m) or greater may attach their safety harnesses to the leads.

  c. Landings or leads shall not be used for storage of any kind.

  d. Pile-driver leads shall have stop blocks to prevent the hammer from being raised against the head block.

  e. A blocking device, capable of supporting the weight of the hammer, shall be provided for placement in the leads under the hammer at all times while employees are working under the hammer.

  f. Leads shall be free of projections or snags to minimize line damage and personnel safety hazards.

16.R.04 Dogs, on pile-driver hoist drums, that automatically disengage when the load is relieved or the drum is rotated shall be prohibited.

16.R.05 Guards shall be provided across the top of the head block to prevent wire from jumping out of the sheaves.

16.R.06 All hose connections to pile-driver hammers, pile ejectors, or jet pipes shall be securely attached with an adequate length of at least ___ in (0.6-cm) alloy steel chain, having 3,250 lb (1,500 kg) working load limit, or equal strength wire, to prevent whipping if the joint is broken.

16.R.07 Steam/hydraulic line controls shall consist of two shutoff valves, one of which shall be a quick-acting lever type within easy reach of the hammer operator.

16.R.08 Floating pile drivers.

    a. The width of hulls of floating pile drivers shall not be less than 45% of the height of the lead above the water.

    b. The operating deck of floating pile drivers shall be so guarded as to prevent piles that are being hoisted into driving position from swinging in over the deck.

16.R.09 Hoisting and moving pile.

    a. All employees shall be kept clear when piling is being hoisted into the leads.

    b. Hoisting of steel piling shall be done by use of a closed shackle or other positive attachment that will prevent accidental disengagement.

    c. Taglines shall be used for controlling unguided piles and free hanging (flying) hammers.

EM 385-1-1
15 Sep 08

d. Hammers shall be lowered to the bottom of the leads while the pile driver is being moved.

16.R.10 When driving jacked piles, all access pits shall be provided with ladders and bulk headed curbs to prevent material from falling into the pit.

16.R.11 When it is necessary to cut off the tops of driven piles, pile-driving operations shall be suspended except where the cutting operations are located at least twice the length of the longest pile from the driver.

16.R.12 Pile extraction.

a. If piling cannot be pulled without exceeding the load rating of equipment, a pile extractor shall be used.

b. When pulling piling, the crane shall be equipped with LID devices (unless the load can be calculated and is within the load rating chart of the crane) and the booms shall not be raised more than 60° above the horizontal. (This requirement does not apply to vibrating-type pulling devices.)

c. Piling shall not be pulled by tipping the crane, releasing the load brake momentarily, and catching the load before the crane has settled.

16.S HYDRAULIC EXCAVATORS, WHEEL/TRACK/BACKHOE LOADERS USED TO TRANSPORT OR HOIST LOADS WITH RIGGING

16.S.01 Hydraulic excavating equipment shall not be used to hoist personnel. The riding of personnel on loads, hooks, hammers, buckets or any other hydraulic excavating equipment attachment is prohibited.

EM 385-1-1
15 Sep 08

16.S.02 Hydraulic excavating equipment may only be used to transport or hoist loads if allowed by the equipment manufacturer. > *See Figure 16-3*

16.S.03 When hydraulic excavating equipment is to be used to transport or hoist loads utilizing hooks, eyes, slings, chains, or other rigging the following requirements shall apply:

a. Operations involving the use of hydraulic excavating equipment and rigging to transport or hoist loads require different operator skills and considerations than the standard excavating operations routinely performed with hydraulic excavating equipment. An AHA specific to the transporting or hoisting operation shall be prepared. The AHA shall include, but not be limited to:

(1) Written proof of qualifications of equipment operators, riggers, and others involved in the transporting and hoisting operations;

(2) Performance of the operational test described in 16.F;

(3) Proper operating procedures in accordance with the equipment manufacturer's operating manual;

(4) Proper use and on site availability of manufacturer's load rating capacities or charts;

(5) Proper use of rigging, including positive latching devices to secure the load and rigging;

(6) Inspection of rigging;

(7) Use of tag lines to control the load;

(8) Adequate communications;

EM 385-1-1
15 Sep 08

(9) Establishment of a sufficient swing radius (equipment, rigging and load) and

(10) Stability of surfaces beneath the hydraulic excavating equipment.

b. An operational test with the selected hydraulic excavating equipment will be performed in the presence of the GDA.

(1) The operational test shall consist of a demonstration that the test load and selected rigging can be safely lifted, maneuvered, controlled, stopped, and landed.

(2) The operational test shall be representative of the complete cycle of the proposed transporting or hoisting operation, including configuration, orientation and positioning of the excavating equipment and the use of identical rigging.

(3) The test load shall be equivalent to the maximum anticipated load, but shall not exceed 100% of the manufacturer's load rating capacity for the excavating equipment as configured. Written documentation of the performance of the operational test outlining test procedures and results shall be maintained at the on-site project office.

c. All rigging and rigging operations shall comply with the requirements of Section 15. Hooks, eyes, slings, chains or other rigging shall not be attached to or hung from the teeth of a bucket during the transporting or hoisting of a load by hydraulic excavating equipment.

d. After the completion and acceptance of an operational test described in 16.F, if repairs, major maintenance or reconfiguration are required to be performed on the hydraulic excavating equipment or attachments, another operational test as described in 16.F shall be performed to demonstrate that the completed repairs are satisfactory and that the test load and selected rigging can be safely lifted, maneuvered, controlled, stopped, and landed.

EM 385-1-1
15 Sep 08

16.S.04 Loads shall be lifted the minimum height necessary to clear the ground or other obstacles and carried as low as possible when the equipment is traveling.

16.S.05 Loads shall not be lifted over personnel.

16.S.06 Adequate clearances shall be maintained from electrical sources.

FIGURE 16-3

HYDRAULIC EXCAVATING EQUIPMENT USED TO TRANSPORT OR HOIST LOADS

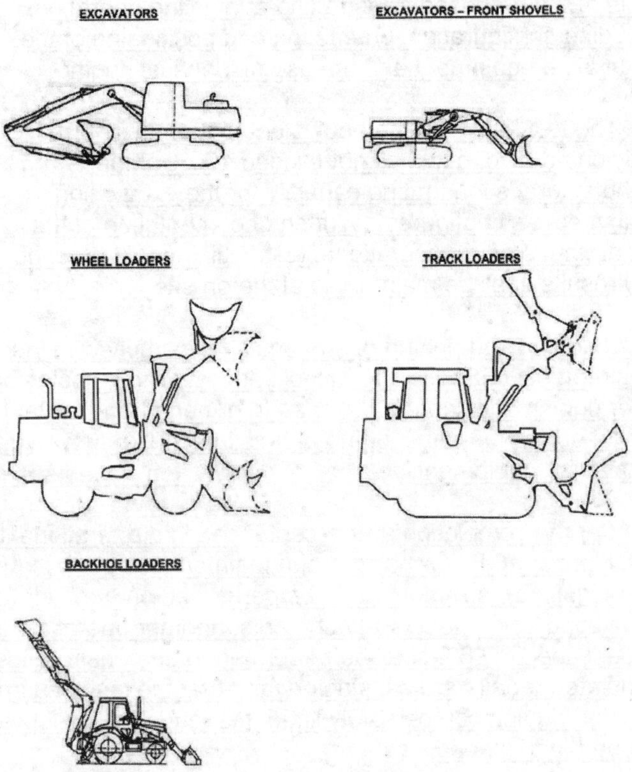

EXCAVATORS

EXCAVATORS – FRONT SHOVELS

WHEEL LOADERS

TRACK LOADERS

BACKHOE LOADERS

EM 385-1-1
15 Sep 08

16.T CRANE-SUPPORTED PERSONNEL (WORK) PLATFORMS

16.T.01 Crane supported personnel platforms are prohibited, except when the erection, use, and dismantling of conventional means of reaching a work site, such as a personnel hoist, ladder, stairway, aerial lift, elevating work platform or scaffold would be more hazardous or is not possible because of structural design or worksite conditions.

16.T.02 If a crane supported work platform is determined to be the only safe method of access, the operation shall be deemed a critical lift (per Section 16.H) and meet the following requirements:

   a. The person responsible for the lift shall perform an AHA and attest to the need for the operation in writing.

   b. The responsible person shall sign the AHA and submit it to the GDA for acceptance.

   c. Personnel shall not be hoisted until the GDA has accepted the AHA.

   d. Crane supported work platforms may be used for routine access of employees to underground construction via a shaft.

16.T.03. The work platform and suspension system shall be designed and certified by a Registered Professional Engineer with knowledge in this area.

   a. The work platform (excluding fall protection systems) shall be capable of supporting, without failure, its own weight and at least five times the maximum intended load. Criteria for fall protection systems are contained in Sections 21 and 16.T.10.

   b. The suspension system shall be designed to minimize tipping of the platform due to movement of the employees on the work platform.

EM 385-1-1
15 Sep 08

    c. The system used to connect the work platform to the equipment shall allow the platform to remain within 10 degrees of leel, regardless of boom angle.

    d. All welding of the work platform and its components shall be performed by a Certified Welder familiar with the weld grades, types, and material specified in the platform design.

16.T.04 Crane supported work platforms shall meet the following requirements:

    a. The scaffold shall be of metal or metal frame construction with a standard guardrail system and shall be enclosed at least from the toeboard to mid-rail with either solid construction material or expanded metal having openings no greater than ___ inch (1.2 cm).

    b. A grab rail shall be installed inside the entire perimeter of the personnel platform.

    c. Access gates, if installed, shall not swing outward and shall be equipped with a device to prevent accidental opening.

    d. Headroom shall be provided which allows employees to stand upright in the platform.

    e. In addition to the use of hardhats, employees shall be protected by overhead protection on the personnel platform when the employee(s) are exposed to falling objects.

    f. The platform shall be conspicuously posted with a plate or other permanent marking that indicates the weight of the platform and its rated load capacity or maximum intended load.

16.T.05 Rigging.

    a. When a wire rope bridle is used to connect the work platform to the load line, each bridle leg shall be connected to a master

EM 385-1-1
15 Sep 08

link or shackle in such a manner to ensure that the load is evenly distributed among the bridle legs.

b. The hook connection to the platform rigging shall be of a type that can be closed and locked to eliminate the hook throat opening and shall be closed and locked when attached. Alternately, an alloy anchor type shackle with a bolt, nut, and retaining pin, in place OR of the screw type, with the screw pin secured from accidental removal may be used.

c. Wire rope and rigging hardware and hooks shall be capable of supporting, without failure, at least five times the maximum intended load.

d. Where rotation-resistant rope is used the slings shall be capable of supporting without failure at least ten times the maximum intended load.

e. Rope sling suspension systems with mechanically spliced flemish eyes, if used, shall be designed with thimbles in all eyes.

f. Bridles and associated rigging for attaching the platform to the hoist line shall be used only for the platform and the employees, their tools and the materials necessary to do the work and shall not be used for any other purpose when not hoisting personnel.

16.T.06 Work Practices.

a. Before employees enter or exit a hoisted personnel platform that is not landed, the platform shall be secured to the structure, unless securing to the structure creates an unsafe condition.

b. The rated load capacity of the platform shall not be exceeded.

c. The number of employees occupying the work platform shall not exceed the number required for the work to be performed.

EM 385-1-1
15 Sep 08

d. Work platforms shall be used only for employees, their tools and the materials necessary to do their work. Work platforms shall not be used to hoist only materials or tools when not hoisting personnel.

e. Materials and tools for use during a personnel lift shall be secured to prevent displacement. They shall be evenly distributed within the confines of the platform while it is suspended.

f. No lifts shall be made on another of the crane's or derrick's loadlines while personnel are suspended on a platform.

g. Employees (except a designated signal personal) shall keep all parts of the body inside the platform during raising, lowering, and positioning.

h. A competent person shall observe the operations while personnel are working from the crane supported work platform.

i. Environmental conditions.

(1) Wind. When wind speed (sustained or gusts) exceeds 20 mph (9 m/s) at the work platform, a qualified person shall determine if, in light of the wind conditions, if it is safe to lift personnel. If not, the lifting operation shall be terminated.

(2) Other weather and environmental conditions. A qualified person shall determine if, in light of indications of dangerous weather conditions, or other impending or existing danger, it is safe to lift personnel. If not, the lifting operation shall be terminated.

j. Employees being hoisted shall remain in the continuous sight of, and in direct communication with, the crane operator or signal person. In situations where direct visual contact with the operator is not possible and the use of a signal person would create a greater hazard for that person, direct communication by

EM 385-1-1
15 Sep 08

radio shall be maintained at all times. The crane operator shall bring all operations to an immediate stop if radio communications are lost.

k. Taglines shall be used to help control the work platform unless the competent person determines that their use creates an unsafe condition.

l. The crane or derrick operator shall remain at the controls at all times with the engine crane running whenever the platform is occupied.

m. Hoisting personnel within 20 ft (6 m) of a power line that is up to 350 kV and hoisting personnel within 50 ft (15.2 m) of a power line that is over 350 kV is prohibited, except for Power Transmission and Distribution Work.

16.T.07 Operational Criteria

a. Hoisting of the personnel platform shall be in a slow, controlled, cautious manner with no sudden movements.

b. Load lines shall be capable of supporting, without failure, at least 7 times the maximum intended load, except where rotation resistant rope is used the lines shall be capable of supporting, without failure, at least 10 times the maximum intended load. The required design factor is achieved by taking the current safety factor of 3.5 and applying the 50% de-rating of the crane capacity.

c. The crane shall be uniformly level within 1% of level grade and located on firm footing. Cranes equipped with outriggers shall have them all fully deployed to load chart criteria following manufacturer's specifications, as applicable, when hoisting personnel.

d. The total weight of the loaded personnel platform and related rigging shall not exceed 50% of the rated capacity for the radius and configuration of the crane or derrick.

e. Only cranes with power-operated up and down boom hoists and load lines shall be used to support work platforms. The use of machines having live booms is prohibited. Platforms shall be lowered under power and not by the brake.

f. Only cranes with an A2B device that prevents contact between the load block or overhaul ball and the boom tip, or a system that deactivates the hoisting action before damage occurs shall be used.

g. Cranes with variable angle booms shall be equipped with a boom angle indicator readily visible to the operator.

h. Cranes with telescoping booms shall be equipped with a device to indicate clearly to the operator, at all times, the boom's extended length, or an accurate determination of the load radius to be used during the lift shall be made prior to hoisting personnel.

i. The load line hoist drum shall have a system or device on the power train, other than the load hoist brake, that regulates the lowering rate of speed of the hoist mechanism (controlled lowering). Free fall is prohibited.

16.T.08 Trial Meeting, Lift and Inspection.

a. Prior to every trial lift, the crane or derrick operator, signal person, employees to be lifted, and the competent person shall attend a pre-lift meeting to review the applicable parts of this manual, the AHA, and the details of this particular lift.

b. A trial lift with the unoccupied work platform loaded at least to the anticipated lift weight shall be made from the ground level, or any other location where employees will enter the platform, to each location at which the work platform is to be hoisted and positioned.

c. The trial lift shall be made immediately prior to placing personnel on the platform and shall be repeated prior to hoisting employees after the crane is moved and set up at new location or returned to a previously used location, and when the lift route is changed unless the competent person determines that the route change is not significant.

d. The operator shall determine that all systems, controls, and safety devices are activated and functioning properly; that no interferences exist; and that all configurations necessary to reach those work locations will allow the operator to remain under the 50% limit of the crane's rated capacity.

e. Materials and tools to be used during the actual lift may be loaded in the platform (evenly distributed and secured) for the trial lift.

f. After the trial lift and just prior to hoisting employees, the platform shall be hoisted a few inches and inspected to ensure that it is secure and properly balanced.

g. A visual inspection of the crane, derrick, rigging, work platform, and the crane or derrick support base shall be conducted by a competent person immediately after the trial lift to determine whether the testing has exposed any defect or produced any adverse effect upon any component or structure.

h. Any defects found during inspection which create a safety hazard shall be corrected before hoisting personnel.

i. If the load rope goes slack, the hoisting system shall be re-inspected to ensure that all ropes are properly seated on drums and sheaves.

EM 385-1-1
15 Sep 08

16.T.09 Proof Testing

a. At each job site, prior to hoisting employees on the work platform, and after any report or modification, the platform and rigging shall be proof tested to 125% of the platform's rated capacity by holding it in a suspended position for 5 minutes with the proof test load evenly distributed on the platform (this may be done concurrently with the trial lift).

b. After proof testing, a competent person shall inspect the platform and rigging. Personnel hoisting shall not be conducted until the proof testing requirements are satisfied.

16.T.10 Personnel Fall Protection.

a. For work over water, see section 21.N for fall protection and PFD requirements. Lifesaving equipment and safety skiffs meeting the requirements of this manual shall be available.

b. When NOT working over water, all employees occupying the work platform shall use a properly anchored personal fall protection (arrest or restraint) system. The system shall be attached to a structural member within the platform.

(1) The attachment points to which personal fall arrest or restraint systems are attached on the platform must meet the anchorage requirements in Section 21.

(2) Depending on the type of work to be done and the height of the work platform above a lower surface, all workers shall wear a full-body harness as part of a fall arrest or fall restraint system. The competent person for fall protection on-site will assess each situation and determine which system would best fit the current work requirement and be in accordance with the crane manufacturer's instructions and recommendations. Particular attention should be paid to anchor points and capacities.

EM 385-1-1
15 Sep 08

(3) Workers working from the platform suspended from a crane are permitted to be tied off to the lower load block or overhaul ball. An AHA shall be developed to details on how work will be safely performed. AHA must be submitted to the GDA for acceptance.

16.T.11 Employees shall not be hoisted unless the following conditions are determined to exist:

a. The load test and proof test requirements are satisfied;

b. Hoist ropes are free of kinks;

c. Multiple part lines are not twisted around one another,

d. The primary attachment is centered over the platform, and

e. The hoisting system is inspected if the load rope is slack to ensure all ropes are properly seated on drums and in sheaves.

16.T.12 Traveling.

a. Hoisting of personnel while the crane is traveling is prohibited, except for:

(1) Portal, tower, and locomotive cranes; or

(2) Where it is demonstrated and documented that there is no less hazardous way to perform the work.

b. If the requirements above (16.T.12.a) are satisfied, the following safeguards shall be implemented while cranes travel with hoisted personnel:

(1) Crane travel shall be restricted to a fixed track or runway;

(2) Travel shall be limited to the load radius of the boom used during the lift;

(3) The boom must be parallel to the direction of travel;

(4) A completed trial run shall be performed to test the route of travel before employees are allowed to occupy the platform (this trial run may be performed when the trial lift required by this manual is performed.

EM 385-1-1
15 Sep 08

BLANK

BLANK

EM 385-1-1
15 Sep 08

SECTION 17

CONVEYORS

17.A GENERAL

17.A.01 Conveyor systems shall be constructed and installed in accordance with the manufacturer's recommendations.

17.A.02 Inspection, maintenance, and repair.

>   a. Inspection, maintenance, and repairs shall be performed in accordance with the manufacturer's recommendations by qualified personnel. <u>The entire system shall be visually inspected daily before start up</u>.

>   b. No maintenance shall be performed when a conveyor is in operation except for the following:

>   (1) If lubrication is to be done while the conveyor is in motion, lubrication points shall be easily accessible and safe for lubrication. Only trained personnel who are aware of the hazards of the conveyor in motion shall be allowed to lubricate a conveyor that is operating; and

>   (2) When adjustments or maintenance is required while the conveyor is in operation, only trained personnel who are aware of the hazards shall be permitted to make the adjustment or maintenance.

>   c. <u>Control of Hazardous Energy Procedures</u> shall be used.
>   **> See Section 12.**

>   d. Safe access shall be provided to permit inspection, lubrication, repair, and maintenance activities.

17.A.03 Safety devices.

a. On all conveyors where reversing or runaway are potential hazards or the effects of gravity create a potential for hazardous uncontrolled lowering, anti-runaway devices, brakes, backstops, or other safeguards shall be installed to protect persons from injury and property from damage.

b. Conveyor systems shall be equipped with a time-delay audible and visual warning signal to be sounded immediately before starting of the conveyor. **> On overland conveyors systems, the devices shall be required only at the transfer, loading, and discharge points and those points where personnel are normally stationed.**

c. All conveyors shall be equipped with emergency stopping devices along their full length.

d. Safety devices shall be arranged to operate in such a manner that if power failure or a failure of the device occurs a hazardous condition would not result. The safety devices shall be designed to prevent the conveyor from restarting until the safety device is manually reset.

17.A.04 All exposed moving machinery parts that present a hazard shall be mechanically or electrically guarded or guarded by location.

a. Nip and shear points shall be guarded.

b. Take-up mechanisms may be guarded as an entity by placing standard railings or fencing, and warning signs, around the area in lieu of guarding each nip and shear point.

c. In the case of a trolley conveyor when mechanical or electrical guarding would render the conveyor unusable, prominent and legible warnings shall be posted in the area or on the equipment and, where feasible, areas barricaded or lines marked on the ground to indicate the hazard area.

d. Guards shall be provided at points where personnel could contact cables, chains, belts, and runaways of exposed bucket conveyors.

e. Unless guarded by location, those sections of chain conveyors that cannot be enclosed without impairing the function shall be provided with warning signs or personnel barriers.

f. Trolley conveyors shall be provided with spill guards, pan guards, or the equivalent if there is a potential for material to fall off the conveyor and endanger personnel or equipment.

g. At transfer, loading, and discharge points, unconfined and uncontrolled free fall of material that may result from flooding, ricocheting, overloading, trajectory, leakage, or a combination thereof, shall be prevented if the material would create a hazard to personnel. > **In the absence of a guard specifically erected to protect personnel, warnings shall be provided to restrict unauthorized personnel from entering such hazardous areas**.

h. At all points along the conveyor, except at points where loads are removed from or placed on a conveyor or where a conveyor discharges to or receives material from another conveyor, provisions shall be made to eliminate the possibility of loads or material being dislodged from the conveyor.

i. The build-up of excess material shall be removed from all points along the conveyor.

17.A.05 Access.

a. Crossovers or underpasses with safeguards shall be provided for passage over or under all conveyors: crossing over or under conveyors is prohibited except where safe passageways are provided.

b. Whenever conveyors pass adjacent to, or over, work areas, roadways, highways, railroads, or other public passageways, protective guards shall be installed. The guards shall be designed to catch and hold any load or material that may fall off or become dislodged from the system.

c. Where conveyors are operated in tunnels, pits, and similar enclosures, ample room shall be provided to allow safe accessway and operating space for all personnel.

17.A.06 Emergency stop devices.

a. Unless the design, construction, and operation of a conveyor is clearly non-hazardous to personnel, emergency stop buttons, pull cords, limit switches, or similar emergency devices shall be provided at the following locations for remotely or automatically controlled conveyors or conveyors where operator stations are not manned or are beyond voice and visual contact from drive areas:

(1) Loading arms;

(2) Transfer points; and

(3) Other potentially hazardous locations on the conveyor path not guarded by location or guards.

b. All emergency stop devices shall be easily identifiable and readily accessible.

c. Emergency stop devices shall act directly on the control of the conveyor concerned and shall not depend on the stopping of any other equipment. If a multi-conveyor system, the emergency stop shall stop all conveyors that are tied together.

d. Emergency stop devices shall be installed so that they cannot be overridden from other locations.

EM 385-1-1
15 Sep 08

17.A.07 Gates and switches.

   a. Power-positioned gate and switch sections shall be provided with devices that will prevent these sections from falling in case of power failure.

   b. Means shall be provided on all gates and switch sections to prevent conveyed material from discharging into the open area created by lifting of the gate or switch.

17.A.08 Counterweights.

   a. When counterweights are supported by belts, cables, chains, or similar means, the weights shall be confined in an enclosure to prevent the presence of personnel beneath the counterweight, or the arrangement shall provide a means to restrain the falling weight in case of failure of the normal counterweight support.

   b. When counterweights are attached to lever arms they shall be securely fastened.

17.A.09 When two or more conveying systems are interfaced, special attention shall be given to the interfaced area to ensure the presence of adequate guarding and safety devices.

17.A.10 Conveyor controls shall be arranged so that in case of an emergency stop, manual reset or restart is required at the location where the emergency stop was initiated to resume conveyor operations.

17.A.11 Control stations shall be arranged and located so that the operation of the equipment is visible from them.

17.A.12 Controls shall be clearly marked or labeled to indicate the function controlled.

17.A.13 Hoppers and chutes.

a. All openings to the hopper and chutes shall be guarded to prevent persons from accidentally stepping into them. If guards are not practical, warning signs shall be posted.

b. Dump hoppers having the hopper flush with the floor and which by their use cannot be guarded shall be equipped with grating having a maximum opening of 4 in (10 cm) and heavy enough to withstand any load which may be imposed on it. If the openings in the grating are larger or if no grating is provided, temporary railing shall be placed around ground level hoppers when dumping operation are not in progress. During dumping operation, warning signs shall be placed in conspicuous locations warning personnel of an open pit.

17.A.14 Mobile conveyors.

a. Mobile conveyors shall be provided with brakes or other position locking devices for each degree of motion where movement would present a hazard.

b. Mobile conveyors shall be designed to be stationary against runaway and stable against overturning under normal conditions of operation.

c. When an operator is required on a mobile conveyor, a platform or cab shall be provided for his/her protection.

17.A.15 Portable conveyors.

a. The raising and lowering mechanism for the boom of a portable conveyor shall be provided with a safety device that will hold the boom at any rated angle of inclination.

b. Portable conveyors shall be stable so that the conveyor will not topple when used with the manufacturer's rating and in a manner in which it was intended or when being moved.

EM 385-1-1
15 Sep 08

17.A.16 Screw Conveyors.

   a. Screw conveyors shall not be operated unless the conveyor housing completely encloses the conveyor moving elements and power transmission guards are in place, except that if the conveyor must have an open housing as a condition of use, the entire conveyor shall then be guarded by railing, fence, or by location.

   b. Feed openings for shovel, front-end loader, or other manual or mechanical equipment shall be constructed in such a way that the conveyor screw is covered by grating. If the nature of the material is such that grating cannot be used, then the exposed section of the conveyor shall be guarded by a railing and warning signs shall be posted.

17.B OPERATION

17.B.01 Conveyor equipment shall be used to convey only those materials for which it was designed and within the rated capacities and speeds.

17.B.02 Flight and apron conveyors shall be "jogged" or hand run through at least one complete revolution at installation to check design clearances prior to running under automatic power.

17.B.03 A conveyor that could cause injury when started shall not be started until all personnel in the area are alerted by a signal or by a designated person that the conveyor is about to start.

17.A.04 When a conveyor that could cause injury when started is automatically controlled or must be controlled from a remote location, an audible warning device shall be provided. The device shall be clearly audible at all points along the conveyor where personnel may be present.

   a. The warning device shall be activated by the controller device that starts the conveyor and shall continue for a period of time before the conveyor starts. A flashing light or similar visual warning shall be used with the audible device.

b. If a conveyor system is not exposed to the public, and if function of the system would be seriously hindered or adversely affected by the required time delay or where the intent of the warning may be misinterpreted, clear, concise, and legible warning signs shall be provided and indicate that the system may be started at any time, that danger exists, and that personnel must keep clear. These warnings signs shall be provided along the conveyor at areas that are not guarded or protected by their location.

17.B.05 Before restarting a conveyor that has been stopped because of an emergency, an inspection of the conveyor shall be conducted and the cause of the emergency stop determined.

17.B.06 Only trained personnel shall be permitted to operate a conveyor. Training shall include instruction in operation under normal conditions and in emergencies.

17.B.07 The area around loading and unloading points shall be kept clear of obstructions that could create a hazard.

17.B.08 Riding on conveyors is prohibited.

17.B.09 Personnel working with or near a conveyor shall be:

a. Instructed as to the location and operation of pertinent stopping devices; and

b. Alerted of the potential hazard of entanglement in conveyors caused by such items as loose clothing and jewelry and long hair.

17.B.10 Only trained personnel shall track a conveyor belt that must be done while the conveyor is operating.

EM 385-1-1
15 Sep 08

17.B.11 Applying a belt dressing or other foreign material to a rotating drive pulley or conveyor belt shall be avoided.

17.B.12 Flight and apron conveyors handling sticky materials that tend to build up shall be cleaned as often as required for safe operation.

BLANK

EM 385-1-1
15 Sep 08

SECTION 18

MOTOR VEHICLES, MACHINERY AND MECHANIZED EQUIPMENT, ALL TERRAIN VEHICLES, UTILITY VEHICLES, AND SPECIALTY VEHICLES

18.A GENERAL

18.A.01 The requirements in this Section apply to the operations of all motor vehicles, machinery and mechanized equipment, all terrain vehicles (ATV's), utility vehicles (UV's), and other specialty vehicles. Operators must also comply with State and Host Nation regulations as applicable to the above listed equipment.

18.A.02 Every person operating a motor vehicle shall possess, at all times while operating such vehicle, a license/permit valid for the equipment being operated. Licensing requirements will be as per Service regulation for military personnel and State regulations for civilian personnel, to include contractors. The operator must present the license/permit to the GDA upon request. Failure to do so will result in the immediate prohibition of the operator to operate motor vehicles.

> ***USACE equipment/vehicle operators: In lieu of a license/permit, an operator equipment qualification record (OF 346) shall be maintained on file for all USACE vehicle/equipment operators.***

18.A.03 Inspections, tests, maintenance, and repairs.

   a. Inspections, tests, maintenance, and repairs shall be conducted by a qualified person in accordance with the manufacturer's recommendations.

   b. Before initial use, vehicles not otherwise inspected by State or local authorities, shall be inspected by a qualified mechanic

EM 385-1-1
15 Sep 08

and found in safe operating condition <u>and in compliance with all required published vehicle safety standards.</u> The inspection shall be documented and available for inspection on the work site. > ***This is a one-time inspection.***

c. When dump trucks are brought onto a USACE job site, they shall be inspected and found in compliance with the requirements of this Section before they are placed in service. This inspection shall be documented on a checklist.

d. All vehicles shall be inspected on a scheduled maintenance program.

e. Prior to each use, but not more often than daily, motor vehicles shall be checked by the operator to assure that the following parts, equipment, and accessories are in safe operating condition and free of apparent damage that could cause failure while in use:

(1) Service brakes, including trailer brake connections;

(2) Parking system (hand brake);

(3) Emergency stopping system (brakes);

(4) Tires;

(5) Horns;

(6) Steering mechanism;

(7) Coupling devices;

(8) Seat belts;

EM 385-1-1
15 Sep 08

(9) Operating controls;

(10) Safety devices (e.g., backup alarms and lights, fire extinguishers, first-aid kits, etc.); and

(11) Accessories including lights, reflectors, windshield wipers, and defrosters where such equipment is necessary.

f. Inspection, test, repair, and maintenance records shall be maintained at the site available on request to the GDA.

18.A.04 Vehicles not meeting safe operating conditions shall be immediately removed from service, its use prohibited until unsafe conditions have been corrected, and re-inspected before being placed in service again.

18.A.05 Whenever visibility conditions warrant additional light, all vehicles, or combinations of vehicles, in use shall be equipped with:

a. Two headlights, one on each side in the front;

b. At least two red taillights and one red or amber stoplight on each side of the rear;

c. Directional signal lights (both front and back); and

d. Three emergency flares, reflective markers, or equivalent portable warning device.

18.B GUARDING AND SAFETY DEVICES

18.B.01 Reverse signal (backup) alarm.

a. All self-propelled construction and industrial equipment, whether moving alone or in combination, shall be equipped with a backup alarm.

EM 385-1-1
15 Sep 08

> *Equipment designed and operated so that the operator is always facing the direction of motion does not require a backup alarm.*

b. Backup alarms shall be audible and sufficiently distinct to be heard <u>above the surrounding noise level</u>.

c. Alarms shall operate automatically upon commencement of backward motion. Alarms may be continuous or intermittent (not to exceed 3-second intervals) and shall operate during the entire backward movement.

d. Backup alarms shall be in addition to requirements for signal persons.

e. <u>Commercial cargo vehicles such as pick-up trucks, utility cargo/tool trucks, and flat bed cargo trucks intended for use on public highways with a normally clear view through the rear window are not required to have backup alarms. If the view to the rear is temporarily obstructed by a load or permanently blocked by a utility/tool box body or other modification, then a signal person/observer to back up must be used or a backup alarm must be installed.</u>

f. <u>The removal or disabling of any backup alarm is strictly prohibited.</u>

<u>18.B</u>.02 A warning device or signal person shall be provided where there is danger to persons from moving equipment, swinging loads, buckets, booms or similar.

<u>18.B</u>.03 Guarding.

a. All belts, gears, shafts, pulleys, sprockets, spindles, drums, flywheels, chains, or other reciprocating, rotating, or moving parts of equipment shall be guarded when exposed to contact by persons or when they otherwise create a hazard.

EM 385-1-1
15 Sep 08

b. All hot surfaces of equipment, including exhaust pipes or other lines, shall be guarded or insulated to prevent injury and fire.

c. All equipment having a charging skip shall be provided with guards on both sides and open end of the skip area to prevent persons from walking under the skip while it is elevated.

d. Platforms, foot walks, steps, handholds, guardrails, and toe boards shall be designed, constructed, and installed on machinery and equipment to provide safe footing and access ways.

e. Equipment shall be provided with suitable working surfaces of platforms, guardrails, and hand grabs when attendants or other employees are required to ride for operating purposes outside the operator's cab or compartment. Platforms and steps shall be of nonskid material.

f. Substantial overhead protection shall be provided for the operators of forklifts and similar material handling equipment.

18.B.04 Brake systems.

a. All vehicles, except trailers having a gross weight of 5,000 lb (2,268 kg) or less, shall be equipped with service brakes and manually-operated parking brakes.

b. Service and parking brakes shall be adequate to control the movement of, to stop, and to hold the vehicle under all conditions of service.

c. Service brakes on trailers and semi-trailers shall be controlled from the driver's seat of the prime mover.

d. Braking systems on every combination of vehicles shall be so designed as to be in approximate synchronization on all wheels and develop the required braking effort on the rear-most wheels first. The design shall also provide for application of the brakes by the driver of the prime mover from the cab. Exceptions to this are vehicles in tow by <u>an</u> approved tow bar hitch.

18.B.05 Fuel tanks shall be located in a manner that will not allow spills or overflows to run onto engine, exhaust, or electrical equipment.

18.B.06 Exhaust or discharges from equipment shall be so directed that they do not endanger persons or obstruct the view of the operator.

18.B.07 A safety tire rack, cage, or equivalent protection shall be provided and used when inflating, mounting, or dismounting tires installed on split rims, or rims equipped with locking rings of similar devices. **> See 18.G.21.**

18.B.08 No guard, safety appliance, or device shall be removed from machinery or equipment, or made ineffective, except for making immediate repairs, lubrications, or adjustments, and then only after the power has been shut off. All guards and devices shall be replaced immediately after completion of repairs and adjustments and before power is turned on.

18.B.09 Seatbelts and anchorages meeting the requirements of 49 CFR 571 shall be installed and worn in all motor vehicles (installation and usage on buses is optional). Two-piece seat belts and anchorages for construction equipment shall comply with applicable Federal specifications or Society of Automotive Engineers (SAE) Standard J386.

18.B.10 All high lift PITs shall be equipped with overhead guards that meet the structural requirements defined in paragraph 4.21 of ANSI/ASME B56.1.

18.B.11 Suitable protection against the elements, falling or flying objects, swinging loads, and similar hazards shall be provided for

EM 385-1-1
15 Sep 08

operators of all machinery or equipment. Glass used in windshields or cabs shall be safety glass.

18.B.12 Falling object protective structures (FOPS).

   a. All bulldozers, tractors, or similar equipment used in clearing operations shall be provided with guards, canopies, or grills to protect the operator from falling and flying objects as appropriate to the nature of the clearing operations.

   b. FOPS for other construction, industrial, and grounds-keeping equipment will be furnished when the operator is exposed to falling object hazards.

   c. FOPS will be certified by the manufacturer or a licensed engineer as complying with the applicable recommended practices of SAE Standards J231 and J1043.

18.B.13 Rollover protective structures (ROPS).

   a. In addition to the requirements of 18.B.09 and 18.B.11, seat belts and ROPS shall be installed on:

   (1) Crawler and rubber-tire tractors including dozers, push and pull tractors, winch tractors, and mowers;

   (2) Off-the-highway self-propelled pneumatic-tire earth movers such as trucks, pans, scrapers, bottom dumps, and end dumps;

   (3) Motor graders;

   (4) Water tank trucks having a tank height less than the cab; and

   (5) Other self-propelled construction equipment such as front-end loaders, backhoes, rollers, and compactors.

   b. ROPS are not required on:

(1) Trucks designed for hauling on public highways;

(2) Crane-mounted dragline backhoes;

(3) Sections of rollers and compactors of the tandem steel-wheeled and self-propelled pneumatic tired type that do not have an operator's station;

(4) Self-propelled, rubber-tired lawn and garden tractors and side boom pipe laying tractors operated solely on flat terrain (maximum 10° slope; 20° slope permitted when off-loading from a truck) not exposed to rollover hazards; and

(5) Cranes, draglines, or equipment on which the operator's cab and boom rotate as a unit.

c. ROPS may be removed from certain types of equipment when the work cannot be performed with the ROPS in place and when ROPS removal is justified and delineated in an AHA and accepted in writing by the GDA.

d. The operating authority shall furnish proof from the manufacturer or certification from a licensed engineer that the ROPS complies with applicable SAE Standards (i.e., J167, J1040, J1042, J1084, and J1194).

e. ROPS shall also be acceptable if they meet the criteria of any State that has a Department of Labor approved OSHA program or meets Water and Power Resources Service requirements.

f. The following information permanently affixed to the ROPS is acceptable in lieu of a written certification:

(1) Manufacturer's or fabricator's name and address;

(2) ROPS model number, if any; and

EM 385-1-1
15 Sep 08

(3) Machine make, model, or series number that the structure is designed to fit.

g. Field welding on ROPS shall be performed by welders who are certified by the contractor as qualified in accordance with ANSI/AWS D1.1, Naval Sea Systems Command (NAVSEA) S9074-AQ-GIB-010/248, or the equivalent.

18.B.14 All points requiring lubrication during operation shall have fittings so located or guarded to be accessible without hazardous exposure.

18.B.15 All machinery or equipment and material hoists operating on rails, tracks, or trolleys shall have positive stops or limiting devices either on the equipment, rails, tracks, or trolleys to prevent overrunning safe limits.

18.B.16 Under the following circumstances, long-bed end-dump trailers used in off-road hauling should be equipped with a roll-over warning device. The device should have a continuous monitoring display at the operator station to give the operator a quick and easily read indicator and audible warning of an unsafe condition.

    a. The material being dumped is subject to being stuck or caught in the trailer rather than exiting the bed freely, and

    b. The dumpsite cannot be maintained in a nominally level condition (lateral slope less than $1° - 2°$).

18.C OPERATING RULES

18.C.01 GENERAL. <u>For the purpose of this paragraph, a USACE motor vehicle is any vehicle (government-owned; POV or Rental Car if being used while on-duty in lieu of government-owned vehicle) used to transport Government employees.</u>

    a. Operators of USACE motor vehicles and operators of Contractor motor vehicles being used on USACE projects may

EM 385-1-1
15 Sep 08

only use cellular telephones with hands-free devices while the vehicle is in motion. Prior to using a hand-held cellular phone, drivers shall find a safe place to bring their vehicle to a stop. Text messaging is strictly prohibited while operating motor vehicles. This requirement does NOT preclude passenger(s) from using cellular phones while the vehicle is in motion.

b. The use of any other portable headphones, earphones, or other listening devices (except for hands–free cellular phones) while operating USACE motor vehicles or contractor motor vehicles (being used on USACE projects) is prohibited. **> See AR 190-5.**

c. Operators of USACE motor vehicles (whether government or contractor personnel) being used on USACE projects shall not eat, drink, or smoke while the vehicle is in motion.

d. GPS Systems. GPS systems shall be mounted within the vehicle so that they do not create sight hazards for the operator. Programming of dashboard GPS systems while driving is prohibited. The use of non-mounted GPS systems may only be used by the vehicle operator while the vehicle is in a stopped position.

18.C.02 The principles of defensive driving shall be practiced. All USACE personnel who operate any motor vehicle while on-duty or TDY are to complete Defensive Driver Training initially and every four years thereafter.

18.C.03 Seat belts shall be installed and worn per 18.B.09. Buses are exempt from this requirement.

18.C.04 At all times, the operator must have the vehicle under control and be able to bring it to a complete stop within a safe stopping distance.

18.C.05 Vehicles may not be driven at speeds greater than the posted speed limit, with due regard for weather, traffic, intersections, width and character of the roadway, type of motor vehicle, and any other existing condition.

18.C.06 Headlights shall be lighted from sunset to sunrise, during fog, smoke, rain, or other unfavorable atmospheric conditions, and at any other time when there is not sufficient light for the vehicle to be seen or the operator to see on the highway at a distance of 500 ft (150.4 m), unless local regulations prohibit.

18.C.07 Vehicles shall not be driven on a downgrade with gears in neutral or clutch disengaged.

18.C.08 Railroad crossings and drawbridges.

a. Upon approaching a railroad crossing or drawbridge, vehicles shall be driven at such a speed as to permit stopping before reaching the nearest track or the edge of the draw bridge and shall proceed only if the course is clear.

b. Vehicles transporting 15 or more persons, explosives, or flammable or toxic substances shall stop at railroad crossings and drawbridges and shall not proceed until the course is clear, except at a railroad crossing or drawbridge protected by a traffic officer or a traffic signal giving a positive indication for approaching vehicles to proceed.

18.C.09 Vehicles shall not be stopped, parked, or left standing on any road, or adjacent thereto, or in any area in a manner as to endanger the vehicle, other vehicles, or personnel using or passing that road or area.

18.C.10 Vehicles shall not be left unattended until the motor has been shut off, the key removed (unless local regulations prohibit), parking brake set, and gear engaged in low, reverse, or park. If stopped on a hill or grade, front wheels shall be turned or hooked into the curb or the wheels securely chocked.

18.C.11 Vehicles carrying loads that project beyond the sides or rear of the vehicle shall carry a red flag, not less than 144 in^2 (929

EM 385-1-1
15 Sep 08

cm^2), at or near the end of the projection. At night or when atmospheric conditions restrict visibility, a warning light shall be used in lieu of the red flag. Drivers will assure the load does not obscure vehicle lights and/or reflectors.

18.C.12 Employees shall not be permitted to get between a towed vehicle and towing vehicle except when hooking or unhooking.

18.C.13 No vehicle or combination of vehicles hauling unusually heavy loads or equipment shall be moved until the driver has been provided with the required permits, the correct weights of the vehicles and load, and a designated route to be followed.

18.C.14 When backing or maneuvering, operators will take the applicable precautions outlined in 08.C.04. If a signal person or spotter is not used, operators will walk behind their vehicle to view the area for possible hazards before backing their vehicle.

18.C.15 When a bus, truck, or truck-trailer combination is parked or disabled on a highway or the adjacent shoulder, <u>yellow flashing lights and other traffic warning devices (cones, flags, signs, etc) per 49 CFR 571.5 shall be used during the daytime and reflector, flares, electric lights or other effective means of identification shall be displayed at night.</u>

18.C.16 Loading vehicles.

    a. Drivers of trucks and similar vehicles shall leave the cab while the vehicle is being loaded when they are exposed to danger from suspended loads or overhead loading equipment, unless the cab is adequately protected.

    b. Vehicles shall not be loaded in a manner that obscures the driver's view ahead or to either side or which interferes with the safe operation of the vehicle.

    c. The load on every vehicle shall be distributed, chocked, tied down, or secured. Loads shall be covered when there is a hazard of flying/falling dirt, rock, debris, or material. Tail gates

EM 385-1-1
15 Sep 08

shall not be removed without implementing a positive means to prevent material from falling out of the back of the vehicle and may be done only with the acceptance of the GDA.

18.C.17 Maintenance Vehicles. All maintenance vehicles that are used at USACE recreational areas (or projects) shall be provided with two 28 in (0.7 m) day glow/high-visibility orange traffic cones. Vehicle operators that operate maintenance vehicles in USACE recreational areas shall place a cone in front and behind the vehicle when parked, remove and place in vehicle prior to departure.

18.D TRANSPORTATION OF PERSONNEL

18.D.01 The number of passengers in passenger-type vehicles shall not exceed the number that can be seated.

18.D.02 Trucks used to transport personnel shall be equipped with a securely anchored seating arrangement, a rear end gate, and guardrail. Steps or ladders, for mounting and dismounting, shall be provided.

18.D.03 All tools and equipment shall be guarded, stowed, and secured when transported with personnel.

18.D.04 No person will be permitted to ride with arms or legs outside of a vehicle body, in a standing position on the body, on running boards, seated on side fenders, cabs, cab shields, bed of the truck, or on the load.

18.D.05 All vehicles transporting personnel during cold or inclement weather shall be enclosed. Passengers shall be protected from inclement weather elements.

18.D.06 Explosives, flammable materials (excepting normal fuel supply), or toxic substances may not be transported in vehicles carrying personnel.

EM 385-1-1
15 Sep 08

18.D.07 Vehicles transporting personnel shall not be moved until the driver has ascertained that all persons are seated and the guardrails and rear end gates are in place or doors closed.

18.D.08 Getting on or off any vehicle while it is in motion is prohibited.

18.D.09 All motor vehicles shall be shut down prior to and during fueling operations. **> See _18.G.09._**

18.E MOTOR VEHICLES (FOR PUBLIC ROADWAY USE)

18.E.01 For the purposes of the section, a motor vehicle is defined as a sedan, van, SUV, truck, motorcycle, or other mode of conveyance intended for use on public roadways. This includes construction equipment that is driven on public highways. Other types of equipment such as machinery and mechanized equipment, all terrain vehicles, utility vehicles and other specialty vehicles are addressed later in this section.

18.E.02 Every motor vehicle shall have:

   a. An operable speedometer;

   b. An operable fuel gage;

   c. An operable audible warning device (horn);

   d. An adequate rearview mirror or mirrors;

   e. A power-operated starting device;

   f. A windshield equipped with an adequate windshield wiper;

   g. An operable defrosting and defogging device;

   h. Non-slip surfaces on steps; and

i. Cabs, cab shields, and other protection to protect the driver from the elements and falling or shifting materials;

NOTE: Items f through i do not apply to motorcycles. Gloves, a DOT approved motorcycle helmet with full-face shield or goggles, sturdy footwear, long sleeved shirt or jacket, long trousers, full fingered gloves, and high-visibility garments (bright color for day and retroreflective for night), shall be worn at all times while operating or riding as a passenger on motorcycles.

18.E.03 Glass in windshields, windows, and doors shall be safety glass. Any cracked or broken glass shall be replaced.

18.E.04 All buses, trucks, and combinations of vehicles with a carrying capacity of 1.5 tons (1,360.8 kg) or over, when operated on public highways, shall be equipped with emergency equipment required by State laws but not less than:

   a. One red flag not less than 12 in^2 (77.4 cm^2) with standard and three reflective markers that shall be available for immediate use in case of emergency stops;

   b. Two wheel chocks for each vehicle or each unit of a combination of vehicles;

   c. At least one 2A:10B:C fire extinguisher (at least two properly rated fire extinguishers are required for flammable cargoes).

18.E.05 All rubber-tired motor vehicles shall be equipped with fenders, and tires shall not extend beyond fenders. Mud flaps may be used in lieu of fenders whenever motor vehicle equipment is not designed for fenders.

18.F TRAILERS.

18.F.01 All towing devices used on any combinations of vehicles shall be structurally adequate for the weight drawn and shall be properly mounted.

18.F.02 A locking device or double safety system shall be provided on every fifth wheel mechanism and tow bar arrangement to prevent the accidental separation of towed and towing vehicles.

18.F.03 Every trailer shall be coupled with safety chains or cables to the towing vehicle. Such chain or cable shall prevent the separation of the vehicles in case of tow bar failure.

18.F.04 Trailers equipped with power brakes shall be equipped with a breakaway device that effectively locks-up the brakes in the event the trailer separates from the towing vehicle.

18.G MACHINERY AND MECHANIZED EQUIPMENT

18.G.01 For the purposes of the section, machinery and mechanized equipment is defined as equipment intended for use on construction sites or industrial sites and not intended for operations on public highways. Equipment such as dump trucks, cargo trucks, and other vehicles that may also travel on public roadways must also meet the requirements of 18.E above.

18.G.02 Before any machinery or mechanized equipment is placed in use, it shall be inspected and tested in accordance with the manufacturer's recommendations and requirements of this manual and shall be certified in writing by a competent person to meet the manufacturer's recommendations and requirements of this manual.

   a. The Contractor shall keep records of tests and inspections. These records shall be made available in a timely manner upon request of the GDA and, when submitted, shall become part of the official project file.

EM 385-1-1
15 Sep 08

b. All safety deficiencies noted during the inspection shall be corrected prior to the equipment being placed in service at the project.

c. Re-inspection. Subsequent re-inspections will be conducted at least annually thereafter. Anytime the machinery or mechanized equipment is removed and subsequently returned to the project (other than equipment removed for routine off-site operations as part of the project), it shall be re-inspected and recertified prior to use.

d. The Contractor shall provide the GDA ample notice in advance of any equipment entering the site so that he/she may observe the Contractor's inspection process and so that spot checks may be conducted.

18.G.03 No modifications or additions that affect the capacity or safe operation of machinery or equipment shall be made without the manufacturer's written approval.

a. If such modifications or changes are made, the capacity, operation, and maintenance instruction plates, tags, or decals shall be changed accordingly.

b. In no case shall the original safety factor of the equipment be reduced.

18.G.04 Daily/shift inspections and tests.

a. All machinery and equipment shall be inspected daily (when in use) to ensure safe operating conditions. The employer shall designate competent persons to conduct the daily inspections and tests.

b. Tests shall be made at the beginning of each shift during which the equipment is to be used to determine that the brakes and operating systems are in proper working condition and that all required safety devices are in place and functional.

18.G.05 Whenever any machinery or equipment is found to be unsafe, or whenever a deficiency that affects the safe operation of equipment is observed, the equipment shall be immediately taken out of service and its use prohibited until unsafe conditions have been corrected.

>   a. A tag indicating that the equipment shall not be operated, and that the tag shall not be removed, shall be placed in a conspicuous location on the equipment. **> See Section 8.** Where required, lockout procedures shall be used. **> See Section 12**.

>   b. The tag shall remain in its attached location until it is demonstrated to the individual deadlining the equipment that it is safe to operate.

>   c. When corrections are complete, the machinery or equipment shall be retested and re-inspected before being returned to service.

18.G.06 Machinery and mechanized equipment shall be operated only by designated qualified personnel.

>   a. Machinery or equipment shall not be operated in a manner that will endanger persons or property nor shall the safe operating speeds or loads be exceeded.

>   b. Getting off or on any equipment while it is in motion is prohibited.

>   c. Machinery and equipment shall be operated in accordance with the manufacturer's instructions and recommendations.

>   d. The use of headphones for entertainment purposes (e.g., AM/FM radio or cassette) while operating equipment is prohibited.

EM 385-1-1
15 Sep 08

e. USACE in-house equipment licensing examiners must be qualified to operate the equipment on which they are qualifying others (bulldozers, tractors, backhoes, etc.).

(1) These examiners may not license themselves, but instead, must be licensed by another qualified examiner.

(2) All licensing/qualification of equipment operators by examiners must include, at a minimum, requirements of this section, the manufacturer's instructions and recommendations as well as observation of a practical operating examination on the equipment.

18.G.07 When the manufacturer's instructions or recommendations are more stringent than the requirements of this manual, the manufacturer's instructions or recommendations shall apply.

18.G.08 Inspections or determinations of road and shoulder conditions and structures shall be made in advance to assure that clearances and load capacities are safe for the passage or placing of any machinery or equipment.

18.G.09 Equipment requirements.

a. An operable fuel gage;

b. An operable audible warning device (horn);

c. Adequate rearview mirror or mirrors;

d. Non-slip surfaces on steps;

e. A power-operated starting device;

f. Seats or equal protection must be provided for each person required to ride on equipment;

g. Whenever visibility conditions warrant additional light, all vehicles, or combinations of vehicles, in use shall be equipped

EM 385-1-1
15 Sep 08

<u>with at least two headlights and two taillights in operable condition;</u>

h. All equipment with windshields shall be equipped with powered wipers. Vehicles that operate under conditions that cause fogging or frosting of windshields shall be equipped with operable defogging or defrosting devices. <u>Glass in windshields, windows, and doors shall be safety glass. Cracked or broken glass shall be replaced;</u>

i. Mobile equipment, operating within an off-highway job site not open to public traffic, shall have a service brake system and a parking brake system capable of stopping and holding the equipment while fully loaded on the grade of operation. In addition, it is recommended that heavy-duty hauling equipment have an emergency brake system that will automatically stop the equipment upon failure of the service brake system. This emergency brake system should be manually operable from the driver's position.

18.G.10 Mechanized equipment shall be shut down before and during fueling operations. Closed systems, with an automatic shut-off that will prevent spillage if connections are broken, may be used to fuel diesel powered equipment left running.

18.G.11 Bulldozer and scraper blades, end-loader buckets, dump bodies, and similar equipment shall be either fully lowered or blocked when being repaired or when not in use. All controls shall be in a neutral position, with the engines stopped and brakes set, unless work being performed on the machine requires otherwise.

18.G.12 Stationary machinery and equipment shall be placed on a firm foundation and secured before being operated.

18.G.13 All mobile equipment and the areas in which they are operated shall be adequately illuminated while work is in progress.

EM 385-1-1
15 Sep 08

18.G.14 Equipment powered by an internal combustion engine will not be operated in or near an enclosed area unless adequate ventilation is provided to ensure the equipment does not generate a hazardous atmosphere.

18.G.15 All vehicles that will be parked or are moving slower than normal traffic on haul roads shall have a yellow flashing light or four-way flashers visible from all directions.

18.G.16 No one shall be permitted in the truck cab during loading operations except the driver, and then only if the truck has a cab protector. > *See also 18.C.16.a.*

18.G.17 All machinery or equipment operating on rails, tracks, or trolleys (except railroad equipment) shall be provided with substantial track scrapers or track clearers (effective in both directions) on each wheel or set of wheels.

18.G.18 Steering or spinner knobs shall not be attached to the steering wheel unless the steering mechanism prevents road reactions from causing the steering handwheel to spin. When permitted, the steering knob shall be mounted within the periphery of the wheel.

18.G.19 Safeguards, i.e., bumpers, railings, tracks, etc., shall be provided to prevent machinery and equipment operating on a floating plant from going into the water.

18.G.20 The controls of loaders, excavators, or similar equipment with folding booms or lift arms shall not be operated from a ground position unless so designed.

18.G.21 Personnel shall not work in, pass under, or ride in the buckets or booms of loaders in operation.

18.G.22 Tire service vehicles shall be operated so that the operator will be clear of tires and rims when hoisting operations are being performed. Tires large enough to require hoisting equipment will be secured from movement by continued support of the hoisting

equipment unless bolted to the vehicle hub or otherwise restrained.
> *Also see 18.B.07.*

<u>18.G.23</u> Each bulldozer, scraper, dragline, crane, motor grader, front-end loader, mechanical shovel, backhoe, and other similar equipment shall be equipped with at least one dry chemical or CO_2 fire extinguisher with a minimum rating of 10-B:C.

<u>18.G.24</u> Fill hatches on water haul vehicles shall be secured or the opening reduced to a maximum of 8 in (20.3 cm).

18.G.25 Maintenance and repairs.

   a. Maintenance, including preventive maintenance, and repairs shall be in accordance with the manufacturer's recommendations and shall be documented. Records of maintenance and repairs conducted during the life of a contract shall be made available upon request of the GDA.

   b. All machinery or equipment shall be shut down and positive means taken to prevent its operation while repairs or manual lubrications are being done. Equipment designed to be serviced while running are exempt from this requirement.

   c. All repairs on machinery or equipment shall be made at a location that will protect repair personnel from traffic.

   d. Heavy machinery, equipment, or parts thereof that are suspended or held apart by slings, hoist, or jacks also shall be substantially blocked or cribbed before personnel are permitted to work underneath or between them.

<u>18.G.26 Dump trucks.</u>

   a. <u>All dump trucks shall be equipped with a physical holding device to prevent accidental lowering of the body while maintenance or inspection work is being done.</u>

EM 385-1-1
15 Sep 08

b. <u>All hoist levers shall be secured to prevent accidental starting or tripping of the mechanism.</u>

c. <u>All off-highway end-dump trucks shall be equipped with a means (plainly visible from the operator's position while looking ahead) to determine whether the dump box is lowered.</u>

d. <u>Trip handles for tailgates on all dump trucks shall be arranged to keep the operator in the clear.</u>

18.G.27 Parking.

a. Whenever equipment is parked, the parking brake shall be set.

b. Equipment parked on an incline shall have the wheels chocked or track mechanisms blocked and the parking brake set.

c. All equipment left unattended at night, adjacent to a highway in normal use or adjacent to construction areas where work is in progress, shall have lights or reflectors, or barricades equipped with lights or reflectors, to identify the location of the equipment.

18.G.28 Towing.

a. All towing devices used on any combination of equipment shall be structurally adequate for the weight drawn and securely mounted.

b. Persons shall not be permitted to get between a towing vehicle and the piece of towed equipment until both have been completely stopped with all brakes set and wheels chocked on both vehicle and equipment.

18.G.29 Powered Industrial Trucks (PITs)/Forklifts. All PITs shall meet the requirements of design, construction, stability, inspection, testing, maintenance, and operation (as defined in ANSI/ASME B56.1).

a. All PITs, lift trucks, stackers, and similar equipment shall have the rated capacity posted on the vehicle so as to be clearly visible to the operator. When the manufacturer provides auxiliary removable counterweights, corresponding alternate rated capacities also shall be clearly shown on the vehicle. The ratings shall not be exceeded.

b. Only trained and authorized operators shall be permitted to operate a PIT.

(1) Training must be both classroom and practical operation and in accordance with OSHA Standard 29 CFR 1910.178. It must be on the same type of truck the student uses on the job.

(2) The employer must certify that the operator has been trained and evaluated as required by the standard. The certification shall include the name of the operator, the date of the training, the date of the evaluation, and the identity of the person(s) performing the training or evaluation. Refresher training shall be provided as indicated by the standard.

c. When a PIT is left unattended, load engaging means shall be fully lowered, controls shall be neutralized, power shall be shut off, and brakes shall be set. Wheels shall be blocked if the truck is parked on an incline.

d. An overhead guard shall be used as protection against falling objects. It should be noted that an overhead guard is intended to offer protection from the impact of small packages, boxes, bagged material, etc., representative of the job application, but not to withstand the impact of a falling capacity load.

e. Dock board or bridge plates shall be properly secured before they are driven over. Dock board or bridge plates shall be driven over carefully and slowly and their rated capacity shall never be exceeded.

EM 385-1-1
15 Sep 08

f. Under all travel conditions the PIT shall be operated at a speed that will permit it to be brought to a stop in a safe manner.

g. On all grades the load and load engaging means shall be tilted back if applicable, and raised only as far as necessary to clear the road surface.

h. When ascending or descending grades in excess of 10%, loaded PITs shall be driven with the load upgrade.

18.H DRILLING EQUIPMENT

18.H.01 Applicability. The requirements of this section are in addition to other requirements identified in Section 18 and are applicable to rock, soil, and concrete drilling operations.

18.H.02 Drilling equipment shall be operated only by qualified (by training and experience) personnel who are authorized by their respective employer to operate subject equipment. The drilling equipment shall be operated, inspected, and maintained as specified in the manufacturer's operating manual. A copy of the manual will be available at the job site.

18.H.03 Prior to bringing earth drilling equipment on the job site, a survey shall be conducted to identify overhead electrical hazards and potential ground hazards, such as contact with unexploded ordnance, hazardous agents in the soil, or underground utilities.

a. The location of any overhead or ground hazards shall be identified on a site layout plan.

b. The findings of this survey and the controls for all potential hazards shall become a part of the AHA.

18.H.04 The AHA for an earth drilling activity will not be accepted unless:

a. It contains a copy of the MSDS for the drilling fluids, if required;

b. It meets the requirements of 01.A.13; and

c. It indicates that the site layout plan specified in 18.H.03 will become a part of the analysis, and will be covered at the preparatory inspection (pre-activity safety briefing), when the plan has been completed.

18.H.05 Training.

a. Members of drilling crews shall be trained in:

(1) The operation, inspection, and maintenance of the equipment;

(2) The safety features and procedures to be used during operation, inspection, and maintenance of the equipment; and

(3) Overhead electrical line and underground hazards.

b. This training will be based on the equipment operating manual and the AHA.

18.H.06 Drilling equipment shall be equipped with two easily accessible emergency shutdown devices, one for the operator and one for the helper.

18.H.07 Clearance from electrical sources shall be as specified in Table 11-1

a. Drilling equipment shall be posted with signs warning the operator of electrical hazards.

b. The equipment operator shall assure proper clearance before moving equipment. Clearance shall be monitored by a spotter or by an electrical proximity warning device.

18.H.08 Moving equipment.

a. Before drilling equipment is moved, the travel route shall be surveyed for overhead and terrain hazards, particularly overhead electrical hazards.

b. Earth drilling equipment shall not be transported with the mast up. The exception is movement of the equipment required in drilling a series of holes, such as in blasting, if the following conditions are satisfied:

(1) Movement is over level, smooth terrain;

(2) The path of travel has been inspected for stability and the absence of holes, other ground hazards, and electrical hazards;

(3) The travel distance is limited to short, safe distances; <u>and</u>

(4) <u>Travel with mast up may only be performed according to manufacturer's recommendations and/or specification.</u>

18.H.09 Equipment set-up.

a. Equipment shall be set-up on stable ground and maintained level. Cribbing shall be used when necessary.

b. Outriggers shall be extended per the manufacturer's specifications.

c. When drilling equipment is operated in areas with the potential for classification as a confined space, the requirements of <u>34.A</u> shall be followed.

18.H.10 <u>When drilling equipment is parked or disabled on a highway or the adjacent shoulder, yellow flashing lights and other traffic warning devices (cones, flags, signs, etc) per 49 CFR 571.5 shall be used during the daytime and reflector, flares, electric lights or other effective means of identification shall be displayed at night.</u>

18.H.11 Equipment operation.

a. Weather conditions shall be monitored. Operations shall cease during electrical storms or when electrical storms are imminent. **> See *06.I.01.***

b. Drill crewmembers shall not wear loose clothing, jewelry, or equipment that might become caught in moving machinery.

c. Auger guides shall be used on hard surfaces. (If impractical due to type of drill rig being used (fullsize and/or crane-mount), a risk assessment shall be performed by a qualified person, and documented in the AHA as to why this requirement is not practical. Identification of additional precautions and/or controls shall be identified to insure an equal level of safety is being accomplished).

d. The operator shall verbally alert employees and visually ensure employees are clear from dangerous parts of equipment before starting or engaging equipment.

e. The discharge of drilling fluids shall be channeled away from the work area to prevent the ponding of water.

f. Hoists shall be used only for their designed intent and shall not be loaded beyond their rated capacity. Steps shall be taken to prevent two-blocking of hoists.

g. The equipment manufacturer's procedures shall be followed if rope becomes caught in, or objects get pulled into, a cathead.

h. Drill rods shall not be run or rotated through rod slipping devices. No more than 1 ft (0.3 m) of drill rod column shall be hoisted above the top of the drill mast. Drill rod tool joints shall not be made up, tightened, or loosened while the rod column is supported by a rod-slipping device.

EM 385-1-1
15 Sep 08

i. Dust shall be controlled. When there is potential for silica exposure, the requirements contained in Section 06.M shall be implemented.

j. Augers shall be cleaned only when the rotating mechanism is in neutral and the auger stopped. Long-handled shovels shall be used to move cutting from the auger.

k. Open boreholes shall be capped and flagged. Open excavations shall be barricaded.

l. Means (e.g., guard around the auger; barricade around the perimeter of the auger; electronic brake activated by a presence-sensing device) shall be provided to guard against employee contact with the auger.

m. The use of side-feed swivel collars on drill rods are restricted to those collars that are retained by either a manufacturer-designed stabilizer or a stabilizer approved by a professional engineer.

18.I ALL TERRAIN VEHICLES (ATVS)

18.I.01 ATVs are vehicles intended for off-road use that travel on four low pressure tires with a seat designed to be straddled by the operator.

> Utility Vehicles are designed to perform off-road utility tasks such as passenger and cargo transportation and are described separately in Section 18.J. (e.g., Rangers, Rhino, M-Gators, Gators, and Mules).

18.I.02 Every ATV operator shall have completed a nationally-recognized accredited ATV training course (such as provided by the Specialty Vehicles Institute of America or by in-house resources that have been certified as trainers by an accredited organization) prior to operation of the vehicle.

a. The operator must pass an operating skills test prior to being allowed to operate an ATV. Proof of completion of this training shall be made available to the GDA upon request.

b. <u>The in-house trainer, certified by an accredited organization, must perform at least 1 training session every 3 years to maintain certification. If the accrediting agency requires the trainer to return for refresher training to maintain certification, this shall be in addition to the 1 training session taught every 3 years.</u>

18.I.03 All ATVs shall be equipped with:

a. <u>An adequate audible warning device (horn) at the operator's station in operable condition (if determined necessary for the work being performed); and</u>

b. <u>Brake lights in operable condition (regardless of light conditions).</u>

18.I.04 Whenever visibility conditions warrant the need for additional light, all vehicles or combinations of vehicles in use, shall be equipped with at least two headlights and two taillights in operable condition.

18.I.05 The manufacturer's recommended payload/passenger limitations shall not be exceeded at any time.

18.I.06 Gloves and a DOT-approved motorcycle helmet with full-face shield or goggles shall be worn at all times while operating ATVs. <u>When required for operators, passengers shall wear an approved motorcycle helmet with full-face shield or goggles.</u>

18.I.07 <u>ATVs will not be driven on public roadways except to cross the roadway, and may only be driven on public roadways at designated crossing points or with a road guard (no paved road use unless allowed by the manufacturer).</u>

18.I.08 Only ATVs with four or more wheels may be used.

EM 385-1-1
15 Sep 08

18.I.09 A copy of the operator's manual will be kept on the vehicle and protected from the elements (if practicable).

18.I.10 Tires shall be inflated to the pressures recommended by the manufacturer.

18.I.11 ATVs shall be equipped with mufflers.

18.I.12 All ATVs shall be equipped with spark arresters.

18.J UTILITY VEHICLES

18.J.01 For the purposes of the section, utility vehicles are defined as specialty vehicles designed to perform off-road utility tasks such as passenger and cargo transportation (e.g., Rangers, Rhino, M-Gators, Gators, Mules, etc.).

18.J.02 Utility vehicle operators shall be trained.

   a. They must be familiar with the use of all controls and understand proper moving, stopping, turning and other operating characteristics of the vehicle.

   b. Operators must review all training materials provided by the manufacturer for the specific vehicles, and training should be in accordance with appropriate manufacturer recommendations. At a minimum, training shall be documented and shall address:

   (1) Basic riding tips from the manufacturer's published literature for each vehicle;

   (2) Reading terrain;

   (3) Climbing hilly terrain;

   (4) Descending a hill;

   (5) Traversing a slope;

EM 385-1-1
15 Sep 08

(6) Riding through water;

(7) Cargo carriers and accessories;

(8) Loading and unloading;

(9) Troubleshooting;

(10) Proper preventative maintenance, i.e., oil levels, tire pressure requirements and scheduled maintenance requirements according to the manufacturer's guidelines.

18.J.03 A copy of the operator's manual shall be kept on the vehicle at all times and protected from the elements.

18.J.04 Utility vehicles shall be equipped with:

   a. An adequate audible warning device (horn), in operable condition, at the operator's station; and

   b. Brake lights in operable condition regardless of light conditions..

18.J.05 Whenever visibility conditions warrant additional light, all vehicles, or combinations of vehicles, in use shall be equipped with at least two headlights and two taillights in operable condition, a yellow flashing light or equivalent.

18.J.06 Occupancy in utility vehicles is limited to manufacturer designated seating that has built-in seatbelts. Passengers may not ride in the vehicles back cargo area unless the vehicle is otherwise equipped.

> **When used for emergency response, medical litters may be placed in the back cargo area but must be secured as described in 18.J.08.**

EM 385-1-1
15 Sep 08

18.J.07 The manufacturer's recommended load carrying capacity, personnel capacity, or maximum safe vehicle speed shall not be exceeded at any time.

18.J.08 Cargo items will be secured as necessary to prevent movement/tipping. All loads over 50 lb (22.7 kg)(to include medical litters) must be securely strapped to cargo tie-downs in the rear and to the cargo shelf in the front.

18.J.09 Manufacturer-installed safety equipment will be maintained in working order and used in compliance with the requirement of this regulation and in accordance with manufacturer's recommendations.

18.J.10 Seat belts and anchorages meeting the requirements of 49 CFR Part 571 (DOT, Federal Motor Vehicle Safety Standards) shall be installed in all utility vehicles and will be worn by operators and passengers.

18.J.11 Operators and passengers shall wear goggles at all times when a utility vehicle, not equipped with a windshield, is in motion.

18.J.12 Utility vehicles will not normally be driven on public roadways except to cross the roadway, and will only be driven on a public roadway at designated crossing points or with a road guard.

18.J.13 Utility vehicles that are allowed to operate outside a controlled work area and/or on public roads will meet the minimum vehicle safety standards in accordance with 49 CFR 571.5, to include ROPs, seatbelts, and placement of "Slow Moving Vehicle" emblems where required.

18.J.14 When not equipped with ROPS, operators and passengers of utility vehicles will wear approved head protection (helmet) that at a minimum conforms to DOT 218 standards or equivalent and protective goggles or face shield.

18.K SPECIALTY VEHICLES

18.K.01 For the purposes of the section, specialty vehicles are defined as all other vehicles not meeting any of the definitions above and may include burden or personnel carriers or custom vehicles (i.e., Taylor-Dunn/Cushman), golf carts, Segway HT, and snow machines, etc.).

18.K.02 A driver qualification and training program specific to the specialty vehicle shall be established.

18.K.03 An AHA/SOP that includes at a minimum, the safe operations, limits of operational work areas, required PPE and vehicle safety equipment requirements shall be established for the use of all specialty vehicles.

18.J.04 Whenever visibility conditions warrant additional light, all vehicles, or combinations of vehicles, in use shall be equipped with at least one headlight and one taillight in operable condition.

18.K.05 The manufacturer's recommended load carrying capacity, personnel capacity, and maximum safe vehicle speed shall not be exceeded at any time.

18.K.06 Specialty vehicles shall not be used for other than their manufactured purpose. Manufacturer-installed safety equipment will be maintained in working order and used in compliance with the requirement of this regulation and in accordance with manufacturer's recommendations.

18.K.07 Cargo items will be secured as necessary to prevent movement/tipping.

18.K.08 Specialty vehicles shall not be operated on unimproved surfaces.

18.K.09 For Segway HT, the minimum head protection standard is an approved bicycle helmet.

EM 385-1-1
15 Sep 08

18.K.10 A snow machine is any vehicle designed to travel over ice and snow using mechanical propulsion in conjunction with skis, belts, cleats, or low-pressure tires.

   a. All state and local laws and regulations shall be observed. Snow machines may be used on public roadways only where authorized by state and local regulations or in an emergency.

   b. Operator training for snow machines will include:

(1) Hand signals;

(2) Riding positions;

(3) Towing of a sled;

(4) Surface conditions and types (e.g. snow, ice, tundra, etc.);

(5) Proper apparel while riding;

(6) Dangers to avoid.

   c. The following minimum equipment is required on all snow machines:

(1) Brakes that will work under normal driving conditions and when loading;

(2) A throttle in which, when released by hand, will return engine speed to idle, close the carburetor, and disengage the clutch;

(3) A rear snowflap to deflect material or objects thrown by the track;

(4) A protective shield over all moving parts;

(5) Reflectors on the sides or side cowling (must meet Society of Automotive Engineers Standards);

EM 385-1-1
15 Sep 08

(6) A rigid drawbar that is no longer than 10 ft (30 m) when towing;

d. When working from snow machines, two machines are the minimum (the buddy system). When working more than five miles from support base, a support vehicle such as a snowcat or other track vehicle will be used to support the operation.

e. Passengers are not authorized on personal snow machines (snowmobiles) except in case of an emergency (i.e., a broken-down machine).

EM 385-1-1
15 Sep 08

SECTION 19

FLOATING PLANT AND MARINE ACTIVITIES

19.A GENERAL

19.A.01 Floating plant inspection and certification.

a. All floating plant regulated by the USCG shall have <u>required USCG documentation that is current before</u> being placed in service. A copy shall be posted in a public area on board the vessel. A copy of any USCG Form 835 issued to the vessel in the preceding year shall be available to the GDA and a copy shall be on board the vessel.

b. All dredges and quarter boats not subject to USCG inspection and certification or not having a current ABS classification shall be inspected in the working mode annually by a marine surveyor accredited by the National Association of Marine Surveyors (NAMS) or the Society of Accredited Marine Surveyors (SAMS) and having at least 5 years experience in commercial marine plant and equipment.

<u>(1)</u> All other plant shall be inspected before being placed in use and at least annually by a qualified person.

<u>(2)</u> The inspection shall be documented, a copy of the most recent inspection report shall be posted in a public area on board the vessel, and a copy shall be furnished to the GDA upon request.

<u>(3)</u> The inspection shall be appropriate for the intended use of the plant and shall, as a minimum, evaluate structural condition and compliance with NFPA 302.

<u>c</u>. Periodic inspections and tests shall assure that a safe operating condition is maintained.

d. Records of inspections shall be maintained at the site and shall be available to the GDA.

e. Floating plant found in an unsafe condition shall be taken out of service and its use prohibited until unsafe conditions have been corrected.

19.A.02 Personnel qualifications.

a. Officers and crew shall be in possession of a current, valid USCG license, which shall be posted in a public area on board the vessel, or correctly endorsed document as required by the USCG.

b. Government operators shall be licensed or certified in accordance with the requirements outlined in ER 385-1-91. A qualified individual designated as the USACE Command's marine licensing official will perform licensing and certification. in accordance with the requirements of ER 385-1-91.

c. Officers and crew of government floating plant shall be licensed and/or documented by the USCG when the plant is subject to one or more of the following criteria:

(1) The vessel is inspected and certified by USCG in accordance with EP 1130-2-500, Appendix L;

(2) The vessel is normally engaged in or near a channel or fairway in operations that restrict or affect navigation of other vessels and is required by law to be equipped with radio-telephones of the 156-162 band frequency; or

(3) Floating plant is engaged in the transfer of oil or hazardous material in bulk.

d. A USCG Radar Observers endorsement on licenses is required for Operators of Uninspected Towing Vessels and Masters and Pilots on radar-equipped vessels 26 ft (7.9 m) or

EM 385-1-1
15 Sep 08

more in length. Endorsements must be issued from a USCG-approved training facility.

e. Individuals shall not be scheduled to work more than 12 hours in any 24-hour period. Work schedules shall consider fatigue factors and optimize continuous periods available for uninterrupted sleep. The employee is responsible for reporting to work properly rested and fit for duty.

(1) All personnel shall be scheduled to receive a minimum of 8 hours rest in any 24-hour period. When quarters are provided immediately adjacent to or aboard the work site, these hours of rest may be divided into no more than two periods, one of which must be at least 6 continuous hours in length. All cases exclude travel time.

(2) Rest periods may be interrupted in case of emergency, drill, or other overriding operational necessity.

(3) Due to events listed in paragraph (2), the total minimum daily 8 hours of rest may be reduced to not less than 6 consecutive hours as long as no reduction extends beyond 2 days and not less than 56 hours of rest are provided in each 7-day period.

19.A.03 Severe weather precautions.

a. Where floating plant may be endangered by severe weather (including sudden and locally severe weather, storms, high winds, hurricanes, and floods) plans shall be made for removing or securing plant and evacuation of personnel in emergencies. **> See 06.I.01.** This plan shall be part of the AHA and shall include at least the following:

(1) A description of the types of severe weather hazards the plant may potentially be exposed to and the steps that will be taken to guard against the hazards;

(2) The time frame for implementing the plan (using as a reference the number of hours remaining for the storm to reach the work site if it continues at the predicted speed and direction), including the estimated time to move the plant to safe harbor after movement is started;

(3) The name and location of the safe location(s);

(4) The name of the vessel(s), type, capacity, speed, and availability that will be used to move any non-self-propelled plant;

(5) River/tide gage readings at which floating plant must be moved away from dams, river structures, etc., to safe areas;

(6) Method for securing equipment if not moved.

b. Extended movement of floating plant and tow shall be preceded by an evaluation of weather reports and conditions by a responsible person to ascertain that safe movement of the plant and tow can be accomplished.

c. Work or task orders shall be preceded by an evaluation of weather reports and conditions by a responsible person to ascertain that safe working conditions exist and safe refuge of personnel is assured.

d. USCG approved PFD (Types I, II, III, or V) shall be worn by all personnel on decks exposed to severe weather, regardless of other safety devices used. <u>USCG-approved Type V automatic inflatable PFDs rated for commercial use may be worn by workers on USACE sites per 05.H.02.</u>

e. A sufficient number of vessels of adequate size and horsepower, each designed, outfitted, and equipped for towing service, shall be available at all times to move both self- and non-self-propelled plant against tides, current, and winds during severe weather conditions.

EM 385-1-1
15 Sep 08

f. Contractors working in an exposed marine location shall monitor the National Oceanic and Atmospheric Administration (NOAA) marine weather broadcasts and use other commercial weather forecasting services as may be available.

g. The floating plant shall be capable of withstanding whatever sea conditions may be experienced in the work area during the time period the work is being performed (i.e., seaworthiness, or good "sea keeping" qualities).

19.A.04 Emergency planning.

a. Plans shall be prepared for response to marine emergencies such as fire, sinking, flooding, severe weather, man overboard, hazardous materiel incidents, etc. (Fire: USCG-approved fire plans meet this requirement.) **> See 01.E.**

b. A station bill, setting forth the special duties and the duty station of each crewmember for various emergencies, shall be prepared and posted in conspicuous locations throughout the vessel.

c. Each crewmember shall be given a written description of, and shall become familiar with, his/her emergency duties and shall become familiar with the vessel's emergency signals.

d. "Abandon ship/boat" and "person overboard" procedures shall include instructions for mustering personnel.

e. On all floating plant that have a regular crew or on which people are quartered, the following drills shall be held at least monthly during each shift (unless the vessel is required, under USCG regulations, to be drilled more frequently): abandon ship/boat drills, fire drills, and person overboard or rescue drills.

(1) The first set of drills shall be conducted within 24 hours of the vessel's occupancy or commencement of work.

EM 385-1-1
15 Sep 08

(2) Where crews are employed or quartered at night, every fourth set of drills shall be at night; the first set of night drills shall be conducted within the first 2 weeks of the vessel's occupancy.

(3) Drills shall include, where appropriate, how to handle a pump shell or pipe rupture or failure within the hull (proper shutdown procedures, system containment, etc.) and how to handle leaks or failures of the hull or portions of it (what compartments to secure, how to handle power losses, pulling spuds to move to shallow water, etc.).

f. Person overboard or rescue drills shall be held at least monthly at boat yards, locks, dams, and other locations where marine rescue equipment is required.

g. Emergency lighting and power systems shall be operated and inspected at least monthly to ensure proper operation.

(1) Internal combustion engine driven emergency generators shall be operated under load for at least 2 hours each month.

(2) Storage batteries for emergency lighting and power systems shall be tested at least once every 2 months.

h. A record of all drills and emergency system checks, including any deficiencies noted in equipment and corrective action taken, shall be made in the station log.

19.A.05 Equipment requirements.

a. Fenders shall be provided to prevent damage and sparking and to provide safe areas for workers exposed to pinching situations caused by floating equipment.

b. Axes or other emergency cutting equipment shall be sharp and provided in accessible positions on all towing vessels for use such as freeing lines. On other floating plant (i.e., work barges, and floating cranes) emergency cutting equipment shall be provided in accessible positions.

c. Signal devices shall be provided on all vessels to give signals required by the navigation rules applicable to the waters on which the vessel is operated.

d. All controls requiring operation in cases of emergency (i.e., boiler stops, safety valves, power switches, fuel valves, alarms, and fire extinguishing systems) shall be located so that they are protected against accidental operation but are readily accessible in an emergency.

e. Electric lights used on or around gasoline and oil barges or other marine locations where a fire or explosion hazard exists shall be explosion-proof or approved as intrinsically safe.

f. General alarm systems shall be installed and maintained on all floating plant where it is possible for either a passenger or crewman to be out of sight or hearing from any other person.

(1) Where general alarm systems are used they shall be operated from the primary electrical system with standby batteries on trickle charge that will automatically furnish the required energy during an electrical-system failure.

(2) A sufficient number of signaling devices shall be placed on each deck so that they can be distinctly heard/seen above the normal background noise at any point on the deck.

(3) All signaling devices shall be so interconnected that actuation can occur from at least one strategic point on each deck.

g. Smoke alarms are required for all living quarters of floating plant; smoke alarms, if wired, should use the same electrical system as that of the electrical alarms.

EM 385-1-1
15 Sep 08

h. For floating plant with internal combustion engines, marine quality listed CO monitors shall be installed and maintained in all enclosed occupied spaces (crew quarters, pilot houses, etc.).

i. All doors shall be capable of being opened from either side and provided with positive means to secure them in both the open and closed position.

j. Escape hatches and emergency exits shall be marked on both sides with letters, at least 1 in (2.5 cm) high, stating **"EMERGENCY EXIT - KEEP CLEAR."**

k. Each prime mover (engine, turbine, motor) driving a dredge pump shall be capable of being stopped by controls remote from the prime mover locations.

l. Shore power receptacles shall have a grounding conductor to prevent potential difference between the shore and the vessel.

m. All 120-, 208-, and 240-volt systems in toilet/shower spaces, galley, machinery spaces, weather deck, exterior, or within 3 ft (0.9 m) of any sink shall be grounded and fitted with GFCI protection.

(1) Cord connected equipment used in any of the above areas shall be connected to an outlet with GFCI protection.

(2) Ground-fault protected receptacles shall be conspicuously marked **"GFCI PROTECTED"**.

n. Where appropriate, vessels should have watertight compartments readily identified and properly maintained in a watertight condition (i.e., sealable doors in place and fully functional). Penetrations shall be maintained in a watertight condition.

o. All reciprocating, rotating and moving parts of winch gears and other equipment shall be properly guarded.

EM 385-1-1
15 Sep 08

19.A.06 Fuel systems and fuel transfers. The provisions of the Oil Pollution Act of 1990, as amended, shall apply to floating plant operations as applicable.

  a. Gauge glasses or try cocks shall not be installed on fuel tanks or lines unless they meet the requirements of 46 CFR 58.50-10.

  b. A shutoff valve shall be installed at the fuel tank connection: arrangement shall be made for operating this valve from outside the compartment in which the tank is located and from outside the engine compartment and outside the house bulkheads at or above the weather deck of the vessel.

  c. A shutoff valve shall be installed at the engine end of the fuel line unless the length of the supply pipe is 6 ft (1.8 m) or less.

  d. All carburetors on gasoline engines shall be equipped with a backfire trap or flame arrestor.

  e. All carburetors, except down-draft type, shall be provided with a drip pan, with flame screen, that is continuously emptied by suction from the intake manifold or by a waste tank.

  f. Fuel and lubricant containers and tanks shall be diked, curbed or controlled by other means complying with USCG requirements to contain the tank contents in case of leakage in accordance with 46 CFR 98.30-15, and 33 CFR 155.320.

  g. Fuel oil transfers for floating plant shall be in accordance with the provisions of USCG regulations, 33 CFR 155, and/or 33 CFR 156. For uninspected vessels, USCG regulations in 33 CFR 156.120 and 33 CFR 155.320 for fuel coupling devices and fuel oil discharge containment apply.

  h. All decks, overheads, and bulkheads, serving as fuel oil tank boundaries shall indicate the tank boundary with contrasting paint and be labeled **"FUEL OIL TANK-NO HOT WORK"**.

19.A.07 Safe practices.

a. Obstructing cables/lines that cross waterways between floating plant or between plant and mooring shall be clearly marked.

b. On floating plant where people are quartered, one person shall be on watch at all times to guard against fire and provide watch person service. In lieu of a watch person, an automatic fire detection and fire and emergency warning system(s) may be used.

c. Provisions shall be made to prevent accumulation of fuel and grease on floors and decks and in bilges.

d. Swimming shall be prohibited for personnel on floating plant and other marine locations, except certified divers in the performance of their duties, unless necessary to prevent injury or loss of life.

e. A person in the water shall be considered as a person overboard and appropriate action shall be taken.

f. When barriers or blanks are installed in piping systems as a lock-out procedure, positive means (such as protruding handles) shall be used to easily recognize their presence. Barriers shall be marked (including name of installer, name of inspector, and date of installation) and accounted for prior to installation and subsequent to removal.

g. Deck loading will be limited to safe capacity. Loads will be secured and holdbacks or rings will be provided to secure loose equipment during rough weather.

h. Deck openings and other fall hazards not addressed by 19.C shall be protected in accordance with Section 21.

i. Safeguards such as barriers, curbs, or other structures shall be provided to prevent front-end loaders, bulldozers, trucks,

EM 385-1-1
15 Sep 08

backhoes, track hoes, and similar operating equipment on floating equipment from falling into the water. <u>Whenever this equipment is operating on deck, deck surfaces of floating plant shall remain above water and the entire bottom area of a floating plant shall remain submerged</u>

j. Projection and tripping hazards shall be removed, identified with warning signs, or distinctly marked with safety yellow.

<u>k.</u> Deck cargo carried on fuel barges shall be placed on dunnage.

l. When two or more pieces of floating plant are being used as one unit, they shall be securely fastened together to prevent openings between them or the openings shall be covered or guarded.

<u>m. When three or more floating plant are configured for stationary work, a competent person shall identify any openings between decks of stationary vessels or vessels and other structures that create fully enclosed water areas (duck ponds) into which personnel can fall. If such openings are detected, means shall be taken to protect personnel from the hazard.</u>

<u>(1) When practical, duck pond protection will consist of guardrails, nets or other physical barriers to prevent employees from falling into the openings.</u>

<u>(2) When physical barriers are not practical, ladders and life rings shall be installed in each enclosed water area to allow personnel to self-rescue. Ladders may be a rigid type or Jacob's ladder, and must be securely anchored to the vessel or structure. Life rings shall have a sufficient length of rope to allow them to float on the water surface and the rope shall be securely anchored to the vessel. The number and placement of ladders and life rings shall be sufficient so that the maximum swimming distance to them is no more than 25 feet. Ladders and life rings may be retracted during reconfiguration or movement of plant.</u>

EM 385-1-1
15 Sep 08

n. Anchor points shall be clearly identified and shall be inspected prior to applying a load or putting cables under tension. Anchor points not structurally sound shall be cut out, removed, and/or welded over to preclude usage. Visual checks and "all clear" warnings shall be made prior to tensioning cables.

o. Provisions shall be made to protect persons being transported by water from the elements.

p. Plant fleeting areas will be designated in which all idle plant shall be moored. Such areas shall have warning buoys, signs, and lights in prominent locations.

q. The Contractor or, for Government-conducted operations, the GDA, shall provide information to the local USCG Office identifying the marine activity and hazards.

r. Open or pelican hooks may be used for lifting anchor buoys.

s. Mechanical means such as securing pins shall be used to hold spuds safely in place before transiting from one site to another.

19.A.08 Work Inside Confined and Enclosed Spaces in Ships and Vessels. **> See *Section 34.B***

19.A.09 When there is a potential for marine activities to interfere with or damage utilities or other structures, including those underwater, a survey shall be conducted to identify the utilities or structures in the work area, analyze the potential for interference or damage, and recommend steps to be taken to prevent the interference or damage.

19.A.10 Ventilation.

a. Motor vessels or boats powered by internal combustion engines having electric spark ignition systems or having auxiliary engines of this type in cabins, compartments, or confined spaces shall be equipped with an exhaust fan(s) for ventilating engine space and bilges.

b. At least two ventilators fitted with fans capable of ventilating each machinery space and fuel tank compartment, including bilges, shall be provided to remove any flammable or explosive gases, except those vessels constructed with the greater portions of the bilges open or exposed to the natural atmosphere at all times. **> Note this requirement does not apply to diesel engines.**

c. Other compartment spaces within a vessel, not covered in this Section, may be naturally vented.

d. Living spaces, including the galley, shall be adequately ventilated in a manner suitable to the purpose of the space.

e. For launches and motorboats having diesel power plants not equipped with fans, ventilating shall be by natural draft through permanently open inlet and outlet ducts extending into the bilges. Inlet and exhaust ducts shall be equipped with cowls or exhaust heads.

f. For launches, motorboats (survey boats), and skiffs having deck-mounted internal combustion engines (such as generators, jigger pumps) and not equipped with fans, exhaust piping shall be located away from personnel spaces to minimize CO infiltration in the work space.

g. Vent and ventilator requirements.

(1) Fans shall be rated for Class I hazardous locations and located as remotely from potential explosive areas as practical. **> See 11.H.**

(2) The vent intake shall extend to within 1 ft (0.3 m) of the bottom of the compartment.

(3) Means shall be provided for stopping fans in ventilation systems serving machinery components and for closing doorways, ventilators, chases, and annular spaces around tunnels and other openings from outside these spaces in case of fire.

h. Engines shall not be started until the engine space and bilges have been ventilated to remove fuel vapor.

19.A.11 The most current, pertinent information published by the USCG regarding aids to navigation shall be maintained aboard self-propelled vessels 26 ft (7.9 m) or more in length.

19.B ACCESS

19.B.01 General.

a. Means of access shall be properly secured, guarded, and maintained free of slipping and tripping hazards **> See Sections 21, 24 and 19.C.**

b. Non-slip surfaces shall be provided on working decks, stair treads, ship ladders, platforms, catwalks, and walkways, particularly on the weather side of doorways opening on deck.

c. Double rung or flat tread type Jacob's ladders shall be used only when no safer form of access is practical. When in use, they shall hang without slack and be properly secured.

d. Vertical ladders shall comply with ASTM F1166-95a.

19.B.02 Access to/from vessels.

a. Safe means for boarding or leaving a floating plant shall be provided and guarded to prevent persons from falling or slipping thereon. Walking on rip-rap should be avoided where practical.

EM 385-1-1
15 Sep 08

b. A stairway, ladder, ramp, gangway, personnel <u>hoist or other safe means of access</u> shall be provided at personnel points of access with breaks of 19 in (48.2 cm) or more in elevation.

c. Ramps for access of equipment and vehicles to or between vessels shall be of adequate strength, be provided with sideboards, and be well maintained.

d. Gangways and ramps shall be:

(1) Secured at one end by at least one point on each side with lines or chains to prevent overturning;

(2) Supported at the other end in such a manner <u>to carry them and their normal load during use</u> in the event they slide off their supports;

(3) Placed at an angle no greater than that recommended by the manufacturer; and

(4) Provided with a standard guardrail (toe boards are optional depending on their usefulness and the hazard involved).

19.B.03 Access on vessels.

a. Vertical access shall be provided between various decks by means of stairs, ramps, or vertical ladders installed in accordance with ASTM F1166.

b. Employees shall not be permitted to pass fore and aft, over, or around deck loads unless there is a safe passage.

c. If cargo or materials are stored on deck of barges, scows, floats, etc., the outboard edge shall not be used as a passageway unless at least 2 ft (0.6 m) of clearance is maintained.

EM 385-1-1
15 Sep 08

d. Vessel loads shall be limited so that access and passageways in use will remain above the waterline. Decks and passageways shall not be used for access if submerged or subject to constant breaking waves, except in an emergency.

19.B.04 Emergency access.

a. Vessels, except those easily boarded from the water, shall be equipped with:

(1) At least one portable or permanent ladder of sufficient length to allow a person to self-rescue by boarding the ladder from the water, and

(2) Other methods or means designed to assist in the rescue of an incapacitated person overboard.

b. Two means of escape shall be provided for normal work, assembly, sleeping, and messing areas on floating plants.

c. Means of access shall be maintained as safe and functional.

19.B.05 Access on floating pipelines.

a. Floating pipelines used as access ways shall be equipped with a walkway and handrail on at least one side.

b. Walkways shall be at least 20 in (50.8 cm) wide and anchored to the pipeline.

c. PFDs must be worn at all times by anyone on pipelines > *See 05.J.*

d. When walkways and handrails are not provided (i.e., the pipeline is not intended for access), the pipeline shall be barricaded at both ends to prevent access by any person.

EM 385-1-1
15 Sep 08

19.C MARINE FALL PROTECTION SYSTEMS

19.C.01 On decks or work surfaces 6 ft (1.8 m) or more above the main deck or 6 ft or more above adjacent vessel decks, docks, or other hard surfaces, Railing Type A or Type B, as described in Section 19.E., or bulwarks, coamings, or other structures meeting the height and strength requirements of these railing systems shall be provided except as excluded in 19.C.03 and 19.C.04.

19.C.02 Deck edge toe boards not less than 3.5 in (8.75 cm) high for Type A and 2 in (5 cm) high for Type B railings shall be provided when the railings are used for fall protection. Toe boards shall meet the strength requirements in Section 21.B.02.d. Scuppers and/ or drainage holes may be installed as needed as long as the top edge of the toeboard is intact and the strength requirements are retained.

19.C.03 Personal Fall Protection Systems meeting the requirements of Section 21.C. may be used when railing systems are not installed.

19.C.04 Railing Systems and Personal Fall Protection Systems are not considered feasible on the main deck of vessels that perform duty cycle material loading and unloading operations from barges, scows or other vessels alongside.

19.D MAIN DECK PERIMETER PROTECTION

> ***NOTE: Existing main deck perimeter protection shall be retrofitted as needed to meet the design and construction parameters of this standard not later than March 2010.***

>***NOTE: New vessels built or purchased for USACE use shall meet these requirements upon delivery or prior to first use.***

19.D.01 Main deck perimeter protection systems are intended to provide protection against falling overboard. Main deck perimeter protection is required on all manned vessels, except where excluded in Section 19.D.05. Unmanned vessels do not require

EM 385-1-1
15 Sep 08

perimeter protection, however, fall protection shall be provided where the vessel configuration and operation exposes personnel to falls onto a hard surface from vertical distances greater than 6 ft (1.8 m). The design parameters for the different types of main deck railing systems listed in this section are in Section 19.E unless otherwise noted.

    a. Manned vessels are vessels that operate with crews, or quartered personnel, or that have work areas that are occupied by assigned personnel during normal work activities.

    b. Unmanned vessels are typically those that carry cargo such as materials, supplies, equipment, or liquids, and do not have personnel on board except during loading and unloading and during short term operations such as tie-down, inspections, etc.

19.D.02 Manned vessels over 26 ft (7.9 m) in length operating in unprotected or partially protected waters (as defined in 46 CFR) shall have Type B Railings provided around the deck edge, except where excluded in Section 19.D.05.

19.D.03 Manned vessels over 26 ft (7.9 m) in length operating in rivers or protected waters shall have Type B or Type C Railings provided around the deck edge, except where excluded in Section 19.D.05.

19.D.04 Type D Grab rails shall be provided on all manned vessels in the following instances:

    a. On deckhouses or other similar permanent structures more than 48 in (1.23m) from deck edge rail systems;

    b. On deck houses or similar permanent structures that are within 8 ft (2.46m) of the deck edge in areas where the deck edge rail has been omitted or may be temporarily removed in accordance with 19.D.05.

19.D.05 The following are main deck areas where perimeter protection may be omitted or temporarily removed:

EM 385-1-1
15 Sep 08

> a. Deck perimeter rails may be omitted from deck work areas specifically intended for line handling, working over the side of the vessel, load handling operations and designated boarding areas. Railings in these areas may obstruct work or access and present additional hazards such as pinch points against railings. Such deck edge areas may include those for line handling, fleeting scows, mooring vessels, towing, pile driving activities, and handling or placing of construction materials and equipment pipelines, and anchors.
>
> b. Deck Perimeter rails may be omitted from main deck areas where the overall walkway width is less than 24 in (0.6 m) between deck structures/permanent equipment and the deck edge.
>
> c. Removable perimeter rail sections may be installed in areas where activities such as working over the side of the vessel or loading operations are not normally performed. These rails shall be maintained in place when vessel operations do not include activity in these areas or during periods of tie-up or inactivity.

19.D.06 When deck-edge perimeter protection is not present, standard operating procedures, AHAs, or other documents shall be developed to address the hazards involved. These documents shall be reviewed by all crew during initial orientation and at regular intervals afterward. The following operational procedures shall be followed:

> a. PFD's must be worn by personnel in areas where deck perimeter protection is not present. Such areas may be used by crew to transit or access areas of the boat, but when doing so, all other requirements of this section must be met. Areas where railings are removed shall be blocked off from access by a suitable barrier, or shall be clearly marked as PFD- required areas by signage, deck markings, or other means;

EM 385-1-1
15 Sep 08

b. Continuous sight and verbal/radio contact shall be maintained between personnel in the non-protected deck perimeter areas and the vessel operator or a designated crew member who is in sight and verbal/radio contact with the operator, and who will monitor the workers in the area;

c. A safety skiff or equivalent rescue vessel shall be readily available
throughout the duration of these activities in accordance with 05.K.

19.D.07 Small boats with length 26 ft (7.9 m) or less shall be provided with integrated combinations of two or more of the below listed items to provide continuous perimeter protection around the vessel: Cockpits; Coamings; Handholds; Toe Rails; Life Rails; Deck Rails; Stern Rails and Bow Rails. The installations shall be in accordance with either ABYC Standards or ISO Standard 15085, as demonstrated by a Manufacturer's certificate, label or other documentation.

19.E MARINE RAILING TYPES

19.E.01 Allowable types of railings on vessels (A, B, C, & D) are identified below. Specific requirements for the vessel types and areas where each may be used are delineated in sections 19.G and 19.H. See Appendix U for illustrations of each.

19.E.02 Railing Type A: Two-Tier Rigid Fall Protection Rail. This railing is comprised of rigid vertical stanchions and two rigid horizontal tiers in accordance with section 21.E.01. Minimum top rail height is 42 in +/- 3 in (106.6 cm +/- 7.6 cm) and the lower horizontal tier is at half height.

19.E.03 Railing Type B: Three-Tier Marine Rigid or Tensioned Railing. This railing is comprised of rigid vertical stanchions and three rigid or tensioned horizontal tiers. The following parameters apply:

EM 385-1-1
15 Sep 08

a. Clear spacing between tiers shall be no greater than 9 in (22.8 cm), 15 in (38 cm) and 15 in (38 cm) respectively. The 9 in space is closest to the deck surface. Minimum height from deck to the top tier may not be less than 39 in (99 cm).

b. The 9 in, 15 in, and 15 in tier spacing above may not be exceeded.

c. The bottom tier may be omitted in way of deck fittings or in order to facilitate line handling. The space resulting from the removed lower tier may not extend more than 2 ft (60.8 cm) beyond either side of the deck fitting.

d. Vertical stanchions may be pipe or structural sections. Horizontal tiers may be constructed from rigid (pipe or structural sections) or non-rigid (wire rope or chain) components, or from combinations of these components. Non-rigid tiers must be tensioned with turnbuckles or similar components.

e. Railings may be either fixed or removable in sections. All vertical stanchions must be adequate to withstand a 200 lbs (60.9 kg) load applied horizontally at the top of the stanchion. Stanchion spacing may not exceed 8 ft (2.4 m).

f. Pipe or structural section rail components shall be sized appropriately to meet the performance criteria of 21.E.01.

g. Chain or wire rope together with all connecting fittings shall have minimum breaking strength of 4,000 lbs (1814.3 kg).

h. Chain or wire rope horizontal tiers shall be tensioned so that:

(1) There is no slack,

EM 385-1-1
15 Sep 08

(2) Sag does not exceed 1/4 in (.625 cm) at any point between stanchions, and

(3) The lowest point from deck to the top of the upper rail may not be less than 39 in at any point between the stanchions. Tensioned railing tiers shall not deflect more than 1 in (2.5 cm) under a load of 200 lbs (60.9 kg).

i. Solid bulwarks or coamings providing equal perimeter protection to a height of 39 in (99 cm) may also be provided. Bulwarks may be constructed of structural plate and shapes. Bulwarks must meet all strength/deflection/open spacing requirements presented above for railings.

19.E.04 Railing Type C: Non-Tensioned Railings and Flexible or Swing-Away Railings shall consist of rigid vertical stanchions with horizontal non-tensioned chain, wire rope or rigid tiers that clip to the verticals.

a. Non-Tensioned Railings shall consist of horizontal tiers constructed from chain, wire rope, pipe or structural sections or combinations of these components. Vertical stanchions shall be pipe or structural sections. Vertical support spacing shall not exceed 8 ft (2.4 m).

b. Flexible or Swing-Away Rails shall consist of chain or wire rope tensioned vertical support lines with non-tensioned chain, wire rope or clip-on rigid horizontal tiers. Vertical support line spacing shall not exceed 6 ft (1.8 m).

c. Pipe or structural section rail components shall be sized appropriately to meet the performance criteria of 21.E.01. Chain or wire rope together with all connecting fittings shall have minimum breaking strength of 4,000 lbs (1800 kg).

d. For Non-Tensioned Railings and Flexible or Swing-Away Railings, sag of horizontal tiers shall not exceed 3 in (10 cm) between vertical
supports.

EM 385-1-1
15 Sep 08

e. Non-Tensioned Railings and Flexible or Swing-Away Railings shall be configured with four or more horizontal tiers. The number of horizontal tiers shall be sufficient to meet the following requirements:

(1) Effective clear spacing between the deck and bottom tier shall be no greater than 9 in (22.8 cm).

(2) Effective clear spacing between all tiers above the bottom tier shall be no greater than 15 in (38.1 cm).

(3) Effective minimum height from deck to the top tier may not be less than 39 in (99 cm).

f. The effective tier spacing identified above includes the effect of the increased spacing associated with sag in the tiers, applied either up or down. Clear spacing measurements shall be made with the railing tiers spread to form the largest opening.

g. Railing height is reduced by the amount of sag in the tiers. Railing minimum height shall be measured at the lowest point in the rail.

h. The bottom tier may be omitted in way of deck fittings or in order to facilitate line handling. The space caused by the removed lower tier may not extend more than 2 ft (60.8 cm) beyond either side of the deck fitting.

i. The top tier may not deflect to a height less than 39 in (99 cm) above the deck under a force of 200 lbs (60.9 kg), applied vertically. In addition, the top tier may not deflect more than 12 in (30.4 cm) horizontally under a force of 200 lbs applied horizontally.

j. Tensioning springs in the vertical support lines, if provided, must be of the compression with drawbar type.

EM 385-1-1
15 Sep 08

19.E.05 Railing Type D: Grab Rails are railing sections mounted to deckhouse sides or to the sides of other permanent structures.

   a. Grab rail height shall match the height of the deck top rail/tier. Where there is no top rail near the grab rail, grab rail height shall be 39 in (99cm).

   b. Grab rail strength shall be adequate to withstand a 200 lb (60.9 kg) load applied in any direction.

   c. Grab rails shall be sized dimensionally comparable to 1.5 in (3.8 cm) pipe. Clear distance between the rail and house side may not be less than 3 in (7.6 cm).

19.F LAUNCHES, MOTORBOATS, AND SKIFFS

19.F.01 Crew requirements.

   a. In the following circumstances a qualified employee shall be assigned to assist with deck duties:

   (1) When extended trips including overnight trips are made from the work site;

   (2) When conditions of navigation make it hazardous for an operator to leave the wheel while underway;

   (3) When operations being performed, other than tying-in, require the handling of lines;

   (4) When operating at night or during inclement weather; or

   (5) When towing;

   (6) While a vessel is transporting crew or passengers.

   b. A qualified employee is any individual who has established, to the satisfaction of the operator of the vessel, that he/she is physically and mentally capable of adequately performing the deck duties to which he/she may be assigned.

19.F.02 Personnel and cargo requirements.

   a. The maximum number of personnel and weight that can safely be transported shall be posted on all launches, motorboats, and skiffs. The number of personnel (including crew) shall not exceed the number of PFDs aboard.

   b. Each boat shall have sufficient room, freeboard, and stability to safely carry the cargo and number of persons allowed with consideration given to the weather and water conditions in which it will be operated.

   c. Launches, motorboats and skiffs less than 20 ft (6 m) in length shall meet 33 CFR 183 requiring level floatation after flooding or swamping.

   d. All open cabin launches or motorboats shall be equipped with "kill (dead man) switches".

19.F.03 Fire protection.

   a. The minimum number and rating of fire extinguishers that shall be carried on all launches and motorboats, including outboards, are shown in Table 19-1:

TABLE 19-1

FIRE EXTINGUISHER REQUIREMENTS FOR LAUNCHES/MOTORBOATS

LENGTH	EXTINGUISHER
Less than 26 ft (7.9 m)	One 1-A:10-B:C
26 ft (7.9 m) or more	Two 1-A:10-B:C

    b. All launches and motorboats having gasoline or liquid petroleum gas power plants or equipment in cabins, compartments, or confined spaces shall be equipped with a built-in automatic CO^2 fire extinguishing system meeting the requirements of 46 CFR 25.30-15.

19.F.04 Float Plans. Float plans shall be prepared by the operator of a launch or motorboat when engaged in surveying, patrolling, or inspection activities that are remote and are expected to take longer than 4 hours or when the operator is traveling alone. The plan shall be filed with the boat operator's supervisor and shall contain the following, as a minimum:

    a. Vessel information (make/model or local identifier);

    b. Personnel on-board;

    c. Activity to be performed;

    d. Expected time of departure, route, and time of return;

    e. Means of communication (adequate means of communication shall be provided).

EM 385-1-1
15 Sep 08

19.F.05 All motorboat operators shall complete and document the following training:

a. A boating safety course meeting the criteria of the USCG Auxiliary, National Association of Safe Boating Law Administrators (NASBLA), or equivalent;

b. Motorboat handling training, based on the type of boats they will operate, provided by qualified instructors (in-house or other). Operators must pass a written and operational test;

c. Current USCG licensed personnel are exempt from the boating safety training, but they shall complete the written exam and operational test;

d. Government employees shall complete a USACE-approved 24-hour initial boating safety course and refresher as prescribed in ER 385-1-91.

19.G DREDGING

19.G.01 Prior to repair or maintenance on the pump, suction or discharge lines below the water line, or within the hull, the ladder (or drag arm) shall be raised (above the waterline) and positively secured. This provision is in addition to the normal securing of hoisting machinery. Blank or block plates shall also be set in suction or discharge lines as appropriate.

19.G.02 Dredge pipelines that are floating or supported on trestles shall display appropriate lights at night and in periods of restricted visibility in accordance with USCG regulations and 33 CFR 88.15.

19.G.03 Submerged and floating dredge pipeline.

a. Submerged pipeline and any anchor securing the pipeline shall rest on the channel bottom where a pipeline crosses a navigation channel. The depth of the submerged pipeline will be provided to the USCG for publication.

(1) Whenever buoyant or semi-buoyant pipeline is used, the dredge operator will assure that the pipeline remains fully submerged and on the bottom. Whenever it is necessary to raise the pipeline, proper clearances shall be made and maintained and the entire length of the pipeline will be adequately marked.

(2) Submerged pipelines shall be marked in accordance with local USCG requirements and as approved by the GDA.

(a) Unless otherwise specified by the USCG, submerged pipelines are considered to require special marks and shall have a USCG-approved flashing yellow light.

(b) Indicators, such as signs or buoys, that state **"DANGER SUBMERGED PIPELINE"** will be placed at the beginning and end of the pipeline. In addition, indicators are required beginning in areas which reduce the charted depth by more than 10%, and, as a minimum, every 1000 ft (304.8 m) to clearly warn of the pipeline length and course.

(c) If barges or other vessels are used to anchor the beginning and/or end of the submerged pipeline, they shall be lighted in accordance with 33 CFR 88.13.

(d) Within a navigation channel, each end of the pipeline shall be identified with a regulatory marker buoy.

(e) Lengths of submerged pipeline located outside of the navigation channel, which reduce the charted depth by more than 10 percent, will be identified with high visibility buoys marked with 360 degree visibility retro-reflective tape, such as orange neoprene buoys, placed at an interval not to exceed 500 ft (152.4 m) to clearly show the pipeline length and course.

(3) Routine inspections of the submerged pipe shall be conducted to ensure anchorage.

EM 385-1-1
15 Sep 08

(4) All anchors and related material shall be removed when the submerged pipe is removed.

b. Floating pipeline is any pipeline that is not anchored on the channel bottom. Floating pipeline, including rubber discharge hoses, shall be clearly marked in accordance with 33 CFR 88.15.

c. Pipelines shall not be permitted to fluctuate between the water surface and the channel bottom or lie partially submerged.

19.G.04 Dredges shall be designed so that a failure or rupture of any of the dredge pump components, including dredge pipe, shall not cause the dredge to sink. Data or plans supporting this capability must be available to the GDA upon request.

19.G.05 Mobilization, demobilization, and relocation of dredges, support barges, support tenders, tugs, and heavy equipment shall be by qualified persons under the direct supervision of a responsible individual.

19.G.06 Hopper dredges shall offer a safe means and process to load and unload personnel.

19.G.07 Any dredge that has a dredge pump below the waterline shall have a bilge alarm or shutdown interface.

19.G.08 Covers of "stone boxes" shall be secured with at least two positive means when the boxes are working under positive pressure.

19.G.09 Dredge disposal sites.

a. Drinking water. An adequate supply of drinking water shall be provided at all dredge disposal sites. Cool water shall be provided during hot weather. Portable drinking dispensers shall comply with Section 2 of this manual.

b. Toilet facilities. Toilet facilities shall be provided in accordance with and meet the requirements of Section 2 of this manual.

c. Medical and first-aid requirements. All disposal area watchmen shall be certified in first aid and CPR in accordance with 03.A.02. At least one 16-unit first-aid kit complying with ANSI Z308.1 shall be provided onsite at all times. The first-aid kit shall be protected from the environment.

19.H SCOWS AND BARGES

19.H.01 Scows dumping in open ocean waters should be equipped with remote opening devices to preclude the transfer of personnel between the vessels.

19.H.02 A safe means for transferring personnel between the towing vessels and scow shall be provided in accordance with 19.B.02.

19.H.03 The Contractor shall identify general and site-specific adverse weather and sea conditions (e.g., currents) under which the towing of scows or cargo barges is prohibited.

19.H.04 All barges and scows that are used as deck cargo barges shall comply with 46 CFR 174.010 through 174.020 for intact stability of deck cargo barges.

19.H.05 Personal fall protection devices or other fall protection as listed in Section 21 and 19.C shall be used on all scows and open barges to prevent personnel transiting between the stern and bow of the vessel from falling into the hopper or falling off the side of the vessel to structures (e.g., dock, vessels) located 6 ft (1.8 m) or more below.

EM 385-1-1
15 Sep 08

19.I NAVIGATION LOCKS AND VESSEL LOCKING

19.I.01 Smoking, open flames, or other ignition sources shall be prohibited on lock structures within 50 ft (15.2 m) of vessels containing hazardous cargos of flammable or other hazardous materials ("Red Flag" vessels) during approach and lockage.

> a. When construction, maintenance, and other non-navigational related activities are taking place on or adjacent to the lock structure, the Lock Master will relay information to supervisory personnel in these activities regarding the approach and passage of Red Flag vessels.
>
> b. The Lock Master or Work Crew supervisor may suspend hot work at their discretion during the approach and passage of Red Flag vessels.
>
> c. Prior to the start of work on these activities, the Work Crew Supervisor will establish safe zones that maintain at least the minimum 50 ft (15.2 m) required distance between Red Flag vessels and sources of ignition such as hot work and smoking areas.
>
> (1) The minimum distance shall be calculated vertically and horizontally throughout a lock chamber when the chamber is pumped out for maintenance.
>
> (2) These zones shall be marked, barricaded, or otherwise designated so personnel can easily distinguish them.
>
> (3) The location of and restricted activities within these zones shall be included in the activity AHA and discussed with workers prior to start of work.

19.I.02 Pleasure and commercial recreational craft shall not be locked through a lock chamber with Red Flag vessels.

19.I.03 Lockage Of Red Flag Vessels.

EM 385-1-1
15 Sep 08

a. Simultaneous lockage of two Red Flag Vessels or tows or simultaneous lockage of another vessel or tow carrying non-dangerous cargoes and vessel or tow carrying dangerous cargoes, shall not be permitted when river traffic in the approach to a lock is light.

b. When the river approach to a lock is congested, simultaneous lockage of the aforementioned vessels or tows, other than pleasure craft, shall be permitted provided:

(1) The first vessel or tow entering and the last vessel or tow exiting are secured before the other enters or leaves;

(2) Any vessel or tow carrying dangerous cargoes is not leaking; and

(3) All masters involved have agreed to the joint use of the lock chamber.

19.I.04 Vessels with flammable or highly hazardous cargo will be passed separately from all other vessels. Hazardous materials are described in 49 CFR 171; flammable materials are defined in the National Fire Code of the NFPA.

EM 385-1-1
15 Sep 08

SECTION 20

PRESSURIZED EQUIPMENT AND SYSTEMS

20.A GENERAL

20.A.01 Inspections and tests - general.

a. Pressurized equipment and systems shall be inspected and performance tested before being placed in service and after any repair or modification.

b. Unless State or local codes specify more frequent inspection, temporary or portable pressurized equipment and systems shall be inspected at intervals of not more than 6 months and permanent installations shall be inspected at least annually.

c. Inspections of pressure vessels prior to being placed in service shall be in accordance with the ASME "*Boiler and Pressure Vessel Code*". In-service inspections of pressure vessels shall be in accordance with the National Board of Boiler and Pressure Vessel Inspectors (NBBI), "*National Board Inspection Code*."

d. Inspections and tests will be performed by personnel qualified in accordance with the ASME Code or the NBBI.

20.A.02 Hydrostatic testing.

a. Unless otherwise specified by State or local codes, hydrostatic testing of unfired pressured vessels shall be performed:

(1) When vessels are installed;

(2) When vessels are placed in service after lay-up;

(3) After any repairs or modifications;

EM 385-1-1
15 Sep 08

(4) Every 3 years, (starting at the time of installation);

(5) If the vessel shows any rust or other deterioration; or

(6) When conditions found during inspections warrant tests.

b. The following unfired vessels are exempt from this requirement:

(1) Vessels designed for a maximum allowable pressure not exceeding 15 psi (103.4 kPa);

(2) Vessels having an internal volume of 5 ft^3 (0.14 m^3) or less and a maximum pressure of 100 psi (689.4 kPa);

(3) Compression tanks containing water under pressure not exceeding 100 psi (689.4 kPa) and temperatures not exceeding 200 °F (93.3 °C);

(4) Compression tanks containing water and fitted with a permanent air charging line subject to pressures not exceeding 15 psi (103.4 kPa) and temperatures not exceeding 200 °F (93.3 °C);

(5) Fire extinguishers - **> See Section 9**.

(6) For vessels with inspection doors (such as oil-filled (governor) pressure tanks), hydrostatic tests need only be given to repaired, modified, or deteriorated tanks. Inspections to determine deterioration will be made every
2 years for external condition and every 4 years for internal condition.

20.A.03 Records of the inspections and tests shall be available for review on request. A certificate shall be posted near the vessel controls prior to operation of the equipment.

EM 385-1-1
15 Sep 08

20.A.04 Tests for structural integrity or leaks using pressurized gases, such as air, are prohibited, except for testing of bulk petroleum, oil, and lubricant (POL) storage tanks under API standards.

20.A.05 Any pressurized equipment or system found to be in an unsafe operating condition shall be tagged **"UNSAFE PRESSURIZED SYSTEM - DO NOT USE"** at the controls and its use shall be prohibited until the unsafe conditions have been corrected.

20.A.06 Pressurized equipment and systems shall be operated and maintained only by qualified, designated personnel.

20.A.07 The normal operating pressure of pressurized equipment and systems shall not exceed the design pressure.

20.A.08 No safety appliance or device shall be removed or made ineffective, except for making immediate repairs or adjustments, and then only after the pressure has been relieved and the power shut off using proper lockout/tagout procedures. *> See Section 12.*

20.A.09 Repairs or adjustments to equipment or systems under pressure require a written safe clearance procedure.

20.A.10 The discharge from safety valves, relief valves, and blowoffs shall be located so that it is not a hazard to personnel.

20.A.11 Master valves and controls shall be either located or equipped to permit operation from the floor level or they shall be provided with safe access.

20.A.12 A pressure gauge shall be provided on all pressurized equipment and systems.

20.A.13 Safety and relief valves shall be provided on all pressurized equipment and systems.

EM 385-1-1
15 Sep 08

a. A safety relief valve setting not more than 10% over working pressure is recommended. In no case shall the safety relief valve setting be higher than the maximum allowable pressure of the receiver or the system.

b. No valve shall be placed between the pressure vessel or generating equipment and a safety or relief valve or between the safety or relief valve and the atmosphere.

c. Adjustments and settings of safety relief valves must be made by a qualified mechanic with equipment designed for valve adjustment. Valves shall be sealed after adjustment.

d. In the event that the pressure registers above the maximum allowable working pressure on the gauge without the safety or relief valve operating, the pressure gauge shall be checked immediately. If such check indicates that the safety or relief valve is inoperative, the equipment shall be removed from service until the safety or relief valve has been adjusted or replaced.

20.A.14 Piping shall meet requirements of the AMSE B31.

20.A.15 Pressurized manual equipment, subject to whipping or rotation if released, shall be provided with an automatic shut-off or control of the dead-man type.

20.A.16 Except where automatic shutoff values are used, safety lashings or suitable double action locking devices shall be used at connections to machines of high pressure hose lines and between high pressure hose lines.

20.A.17 If connections of high pressure hoses are secured with a safety lashing:

a. Safety lashings shall consist of two metal hose clamps connected by a flexible lacing: the metal hose clamps shall be attached to the hose ends separate from the quick makeup connection;

b. The flexible lacing shall be suitably strong cables, chains, or wires. Wires or pins through the quick makeup connection are not acceptable for use as safety lashings.

20.A.18 All pressurized cylinders, actuating booms, outriggers, or other load supporting appliances shall be equipped with pilot check valves, holding valves, or positive mechanical locks to prevent movement in case of failure in the pressure system. Replacement of pressure system fittings shall be with new parts equivalent to the manufacturer's standards.

20.B COMPRESSED AIR AND GAS SYSTEMS

20.B.01 Standards.

a. Air receivers shall be constructed in accordance with the ASME "*Code for Unfired Pressure Vessels.*"

b. All safety valves used shall be constructed, installed, tested, and maintained in accordance with the ASME "*Code for Unfired Pressure Vessels.*"

20.B.02 Access and guarding.

a. Compressors and related equipment shall be located to provide safe access to all parts of the equipment for operation, maintenance, and repairs.

b. Safety appliances, such as valves, indicating devices, and controlling devices, shall be constructed, located, and installed so that they cannot be readily rendered inoperative by any means, including the elements.

20.B.03 Air hose, pipes, valves, filters, and other fittings shall be pressure rated by the manufacturer and this pressure shall not be exceeded. Defective hose shall be removed from service.

20.B.04 Hose shall not be laid over ladders, steps, scaffolds, or walkways to create a tripping hazard.

20.B.05 Compressed air for cleaning.

> a. The use of compressed air for blowing dirt from hands, face, or clothing is prohibited.

> b. Compressed air shall not be used for other cleaning purposes except where reduced to less than 30 psi (206.8 kPa) and then only with effective chip guarding and PPE <u>(face shield and safety glasses)</u>. This 30 psi (<u>206.8</u> kPa) requirement does not apply for concrete forms, mill scale, and similar cleaning purposes.

20.B.06 When used on tools and equipment such as track drills, all airlines exceeding 0.5 in (1.2 cm) inside diameter shall have a safety device at the source of supply or branch line to reduce pressure in case of hose failure.

20.B.07 Governors.

> a. A speed governor, independent of the unloaders, shall be installed on all air compressors except those driven by electrical induction or electrical synchronized motors.

> b. If the air compressor is engine or turbine driven, an auxiliary control to the governor shall be installed to prevent racing when the unloader operates.

20.B.08 Every air compressor shall automatically stop its air-compressing operation before the discharge pressure exceeds the maximum working pressure allowable on the weakest portion of the system.

EM 385-1-1
15 Sep 08

a. If this automatic mechanism is electrically operated, the actuating device shall be so designed and constructed that the electrical contact or contacts cannot lock or fuse in a position that will cause the compressor to continue its operation.

b. An air bypass and alarm may be used as an alternative.

20.B.09 Provision shall be made to exclude flammable materials and toxic gases, vapors, or dusts from the compressor and compressor intake and to prevent steam, water, or waste being blown or drawn into a compressor intake.

20.B.10 No valve shall be installed in the air intake pipe to an air compressor with an atmospheric intake.

20.B.11 The air discharge piping from the compressor to the air receiver shall be at least as large as the discharge opening on the air compressor.

20.B.12 A stop valve shall be installed between the air receiver and each piece of stationary utilization equipment at a point convenient to the operator, and a stop valve shall be installed at each outlet to which an air hose may be attached.

20.B.13 If a stop valve is installed between the compressor and the receiver, spring-loaded safety valves shall be installed between the air compressor and the stop valve.

a. The capacity of safety valves shall be sufficient to limit pressure in the air discharge piping to 10% above the working pressure of the piping.

b. Stop valves <u>should be</u> of the gate type. If a globe valve is used, it shall be installed so that the pressure is under the seat and that the valve will not trap condensation.

20.B.14 Provision shall be made in compressed air and gas systems for expansion and contraction and to counteract pulsation and vibration.

20.B.15 Piping shall be equipped with traps or other means for removing liquid from the lines.

20.B.16 Air discharge piping shall be installed to eliminate possible oil pockets.

20.B.17 Installation and location of air receivers.

> a. Air receivers shall be installed so that all drains, hand holes, and manholes are accessible.
>
> b. Air receivers should be supported with sufficient clearance to permit a complete external inspection and to avoid corrosion of external surfaces.
>
> c. An air receiver shall not be buried underground or located in an inaccessible place.
>
> d. The receiver should be located to keep the discharge pipe as short as possible.
>
> e. The receiver should be located in a cool place to facilitate condensation of moisture and oil vapors.

20.B.18 A drain valve shall be installed at the lowest point of every air receiver for the removal of accumulated oil and water.

20.B.19 Automatic traps may be installed in addition to drain valves.

20.B.20 The drain valve on the air receiver shall be opened and the receiver drained often enough to prevent the accumulation of excessive liquid in the receiver.

20.B.21 No tool change or repair work shall be done until the stop valve in the air line supplying the equipment is closed.

20.B.22 Soapy water or any suitable non-toxic, non-inflammable solution may be used for cleaning the system.

20.B.23 Hose and hose connections used for conducting compressed air to utilization equipment shall be designed for the pressure and service to which they are subjected.

20.C BOILERS AND SYSTEMS

20.C.01 Provisions of the ASME *"Boiler and Pressure Vessel Code"* shall apply in the construction, operation, maintenance, and inspection of steam boilers and pressure vessels.

20.C.02 Inspection.

> a. Inspections shall be made to assure that all safety devices affecting operation of the firing equipment are installed in such a location that they cannot be isolated from the heat source by the closing of a valve.
>
> b. Boilers that have undergone major structural repairs or that have been relocated during the 12 calendar months for which certification has been made shall be reinspected and a new certificate posted before being put into operation.

20.C.03 When any boiler is being placed in service or restored to service after repairs to control circuits or safety devices, an operator shall be in constant attendance until controls have functioned through several cycles <u>or for a period of 24 hours whichever is greater. A report of the operating test shall be provided to the GDA and include the following specific information: time, date, and duration of test; water pressure at boiler; boiler make, type, and serial number; design pressure and rated capacity; gas pressure at burner; flue gas temperature at boiler outlet; and</u>

EM 385-1-1
15 Sep 08

the surface temperature of the boiler jacket. All indicating instruments shall be read at half-hour intervals.

20.C.04 Fusible plugs shall be provided on all boilers, other than those of the water tube type.

    a. <u>Replacement of fusible plugs shall coincide with the inspections recommended by the ASME *Boiler and Pressure Vessel Code.*</u>

    b. When necessary to <u>replace</u> fusible plugs between inspections, a written report covering the circumstances and giving make and heat number of plugs removed and inserted shall be forwarded to the responsible boiler inspector.

20.C.05 All boilers shall be equipped with water columns, gauge glass, and try cocks approved by a nationally-recognized testing laboratory.

    a. Gauge glasses and water columns shall be guarded.

    b. When shutoffs are used on the connections to a water column, they shall be approved locking or sealing type.

20.C.06 All boilers shall be equipped with blowoff cocks or valves approved by a nationally-recognized testing laboratory. The blowoff line shall be arranged so that leakage can be observed by the operator.

20.D COMPRESSED GAS CYLINDERS

20.D.01 Compressed gas cylinders shall be visually inspected in accordance with 49 CFR 171 through 179, CGA C6, and CGA C8.

20.D.02 All Government-owned cylinders shall be color coded and the gas contained identified by name in accordance with Military Standard (MIL-STD) 101B.

EM 385-1-1
15 Sep 08

20.D.03 Storage. **> *See also 20.D.10.***

a. Cylinders shall be stored in well-ventilated locations.

b. Cylinders containing the same gas shall be stored in a segregated group. Empty cylinders shall be labeled as empty and stored in the same manner.

c. Cylinders in storage shall be separated from flammable or combustible liquids and from easily ignitable materials (such as wood, paper, packaging materials, oil, and grease) by at least 40 ft (12 m) or by a fire resistive partition having at least a 1-hour rating.

d. Cylinders containing oxygen or oxidizing gases shall be separated from cylinders in storage containing fuel gases by at least 20 ft (6 m) or by a fire resistive partition having at least a 1-hour rating.

e. Areas containing hazardous gas in storage shall be appropriately placarded.

20.D.04 Smoking shall be prohibited wherever cylinders are stored, handled, or used.

20.D.05 Cylinders shall be protected from physical damage, electric current, and extremes of temperature. The temperature of cylinders shall not be allowed to exceed 125 °F (51.7 °C).

20.D.06 Cylinders containing oxygen and acetylene (or other fuel gas) shall not be taken into confined spaces.

20.D.07 Cylinder valves and valve caps.

a. Cylinder valves shall be closed when cylinders are in storage, in transit, not in use, or empty.

EM 385-1-1
15 Sep 08

    b. Cylinder valve caps shall be in place when cylinders are in storage, in transit, or whenever the regulator is not in place.

20.D.08 All compressed gas cylinders in service shall be secured in substantial fixed or portable racks or hand trucks.

20.D.09 Compressed gas cylinders transported by crane, hoist, or derrick shall be securely transported in cradles, nets, or skip pans, and never directly by slings, chains, or magnets.

20.D.10 Compressed gas cylinders shall be secured in an upright position at all times, except when being hoisted (except acetylene cylinders shall never be laid horizontal). Horizontal storage configurations approved for transportation are permitted for cylinders other than acetylene.

20.D.11 Valve wrench or wheel shall be in operating position when cylinder is in use.

    a. Valves shall be opened slowly.

    b. Quick closing valves on fuel gas cylinders shall not be opened more than 1 1/2 turns.

20.D.12 Cylinders shall be used only for their designed purpose of containing a specific compressed gas.

20.D.13 Cylinders shall be refilled only by qualified persons.

20.D.14 Cylinders shall be handled in a manner that will not weaken or damage the cylinder or valve.

<u>20.D.15 If the movement can be accomplished safely, leaking cylinders shall be moved to an isolated location out of doors, the valve shall be cracked and the gas shall be allowed to escape slowly.</u>

EM 385-1-1
15 Sep 08

a. Personnel and all sources of ignition shall be kept <u>at least 100 ft (30 m) away.</u>

b. <u>Instrumentation should be used to assure protection of personnel from health and flammability hazards.</u>

<u>c.</u> The cylinder shall be tagged "**DEFECTIVE**," <u>after the gas has escaped.</u>

20.D.16 Cylinders containing different gases shall not be bled simultaneously in close proximity of each other.

20.D.17 Bleeding of cylinders containing toxic gases shall be accomplished <u>in accordance with environmental regulations, and in accordance with a government accepted APP and AHA specifically addressing the bleeding of compressed gas cylinders, and</u> only under the direct supervision of qualified personnel.

20.D.18 Oxygen cylinders and fittings shall be kept away from oil or grease.

a. Cylinders, cylinder valves, couplings, regulators, hose, and apparatus shall be kept free from oil or greasy substance and shall not be handled with oily hands or gloves.

b. Oxygen shall not be directed at oily surfaces, greasy cloths, or within a fuel oil or other storage tank or vessel.

20.D.19 Oxygen and fuel gas pressure regulators, including their related gauges, shall be in proper working order while in use.

BLANK

EM 385-1-1
15 Sep 08

SECTION 21

FALL PROTECTION

21.A GENERAL. The fall protection threshold height requirement is 6 ft (1.8 m) for ALL WORK covered by this manual, unless specified differently below, whether performed by Government or Contractor work forces, to include steel erection activities, systems-engineered activities (prefabricated) metal buildings, residential (wood) construction and scaffolding work.

> ***NOTE: Floating plant and vessels are excluded from these requirements except where specifically cited in Sections 19.D and 19.E.***

21.A.01 Workers exposed to fall hazards shall be protected from falling to a lower level by the use of standard guardrail as defined in 21.E.01.b, work platforms, temporary floors, safety nets, engineered fall protection systems, personal fall arrest systems, or the equivalent, in the following situations:

a. On access ways (excluding ladders), work platforms, or walking/working surfaces from which workers may fall 6 ft (1.8 m) or more;

b. For access ways or work platforms over water, machinery, or dangerous operations;

c. When installing or removing sheet piles, h-piles, cofferdams, or other interlocking materials from which workers may fall 6 ft (1.8 m) or more. > ***NOTE: The use of sheet pile stirrups as a fall protection method is prohibited;***

d. Whenever workers are exposed to falls from unprotected sides or edges; fixed ladders over 20 ft (6 m) in height; roof or floor openings; holes and skylights; unstable surfaces; leading

EM 385-1-1
15 Sep 08

edge work, excavations; scaffolds; formwork; work platforms, rebar assembly, steel erection and engineered metal buildings;
> *For Steel Erection activities, when connectors are working at same connecting point, they shall connect one end of the structural member before going out to connect the other end. Whenever possible, the connectors shall straddle the beam instead of walking along the top flange. Connectors shall remain 100% tied off.*

e. Where there is a possibility of a fall from any height onto dangerous equipment, into a hazardous environment, or onto an impalement hazard.

f. For all USACE-owned/operated permanent facilities with open-sided floors or platforms 4 ft (1.2m) or more above adjacent floor or ground level, see Section 24.A.01.d.

21.A.02 The order of control measures (the hierarchy of controls) to abate fall hazards or to select and use a fall protection method to protect workers performing work at heights shall be:

a. Elimination: Remove the hazard from work areas or change task, process, controls or other means to eliminate the need to work at heights and subsequent exposure to fall hazards (i.e. build roof trusses on ground level and then lift into place or design change by lowering a meter or valve at high locations to a worker's level);

b. Prevention (traditional or same-level barrier): isolate and separate fall hazards from work areas by erecting same level barriers such as guardrails, walls, covers or parapets;

c. Work platforms (movable or stationary): Use scaffolds, scissors lifts or aerial lift equipment to facilitate access to work location and to protect workers from falling when performing work at high locations;

d. Personal Protective Systems and Equipment: Use of fall protection systems, including restraint, positioning or personal

EM 385-1-1
15 Sep 08

fall arrest, (i.e., requiring the use of full body harness, lanyard, and lifeline);

e. Administrative Controls: Introduce new work practices that reduce the risk of falling from heights, or to warn a person to avoid approaching a fall hazard (i.e. warning systems, warning lines, audible alarms, signs or training of workers to recognize specific fall hazards).

21.A.03 When using stilts, or raised platforms, workstands or floors above a walking/working surface that exposes workers to a fall of 6 ft (1.8 m) or more in areas protected by guardrails, the height of the guardrail must be raised accordingly to maintain a protective height of 42 in (107 cm) above the stilt, raised platform, workstand or floor height.

21.A.04 When conducting inspection, investigation or assessment work during construction activities, fall protection is required for employees exposed to fall hazards.

21.B TRAINING.

21.B.01 Each worker who might be exposed to fall hazards from heights and using fall protection equipment shall be trained by a Competent Person for fall protection, who is qualified in delivering fall protection training to the workers in the safe use of fall protection systems/equipment and the recognition of fall hazards related to their use, including:

a. The nature of fall hazards in the work area;

b. The correct procedures for erecting, using, dismantling, maintaining, and storing fall protection equipment;

c. The application limits, free fall distance, total fall distance and clearance requirements of fall protection systems and equipment;

d. Rescue equipment and procedures;

EM 385-1-1
15 Sep 08

   e. Hands-on training and practical demonstrations;

   f. All applicable requirements from this Section.

21.B.02 Retraining shall be provided, as necessary, for workers to maintain an understanding of these subjects.

21.B.03 The employer shall verify worker training by a written certification record identifying the worker trained, the dates of the training, and the signature of the trainer and trainee.

21.C FALL PROTECTION PROGRAM.

21.C.01 If Contractor has personnel working at heights, exposed to fall hazards and using fall protection equipment, he shall develop a Site-Specific Fall Protection and Prevention Plan and submit it to the GDA for acceptance as part of their APP. The plan shall describe, in detail, the specific practices, equipment and methods used to protect workers from falling to lower level. This plan shall be updated as conditions change, at least every six months and shall include:

   a. Duties and responsibilities. Identify Competent and Qualified Persons for fall protection and their responsibilities and qualifications;

   b. Description of the project or task performed;

   c. Training requirements to include the safe use of fall protection equipment;

   d. Anticipated hazards and fall hazard prevention and control;

   e. Rescue plan and procedures;

   f. Design of anchorages/fall arrest and horizontal lifeline systems:

EM 385-1-1
15 Sep 08

(1) It is realized that the provision of fall protection for the first person up for establishing anchorages ONLY would be difficult. In this situation, fall protection may not be required. After anchorages are installed, fall protection is required.

(2) The contractor shall identify all locations where anchorages need to be established, and detail in the Plan/AHA how work will be performed safely.

g. Inspection, maintenance and storage of fall protection equipment;

h. Incident investigation procedures;

i. Evaluation of program effectiveness and,

j. Inspection and oversight methods employed.

21.C.02 Each USACE-owned facility shall develop a written fall protection program if they have personnel working at heights, exposed to fall hazards and using fall protection equipment. The facility shall conduct a fall hazard survey, prepare survey report at existing buildings or structures, and comply with the program elements and requirements as identified.

21.D CONTROLLED ACCESS ZONES. The use of Controlled Access Zone as a fall protection method is prohibited.

21.E FALL PROTECTION SYSTEMS.

21.E.01 Standard Guardrail Systems.

a. For marine and floating plant guardrail systems, see Sections 19.D and 19.E.

b. A standard guardrail shall consist of:

EM 385-1-1
15 Sep 08

(1) Toprails, midrails, and posts, and shall have a vertical height of 42 +/- 3 in (106.6 +/- 7.6 cm) from the upper surface of the toprail to the floor, platform, runway, or ramp level.

(2) Midrails shall be erected halfway between the toprails and the floor, platform, runway, or ramp.

(3) The ends of the toprails and midrails shall not overhang the terminal posts except where such overhang does not create a projection hazard.

(4) Toe boards shall be provided on all open sides/ends at locations where persons are required or permitted to pass or work under the elevated platform or where needed to prevent persons and material from falling from the elevated platform.

c. Strength requirements: toprails and midrails shall be designed to meet the following requirements:

(1) Toprail shall be capable of withstanding, without failure, a force of at least 200 lb (0.9 kN) applied within 2 in (5 cm) of the top edge, in any outward or downward direction, at any point along the top edge;

(2) When the force described in (1), above, is applied in a downward direction, the top edge of the top rail shall not deflect more than 3 in (7.6 cm) nor to a height less than 39 in (99 cm) above the walking/working level;

(3) Midrails, screens, mesh, intermediate vertical members, solid panels, and equivalent structural members shall be capable of withstanding, without failure, a force of at least 150 lb (666 N) applied in any downward or outward direction at any point along the midrail or other member;

(4) Guardrail systems shall be so surfaced as to prevent injury to a worker from punctures or lacerations and to prevent snagging of clothing.

EM 385-1-1
15 Sep 08

d. Minimum construction materials for standard guardrail components. The following are the minimum requirements used for designing guardrail systems. The employer is responsible for designing a complete system and assembling these components in accordance with 21.E.01.

> ***Synthetic or natural fiber ropes shall not be used as toprails or midrails.***

> ***Wood railing components shall be minimum 1,500 lb-ft/square inch fiber (stress grade) construction grade lumber.***

(1) Wood railings:

(a) Toprails: Constructed of at least 2-in x 4-in (5-cm x 10-cm) lumber;

(b) Midrails: Constructed of at least 1-in x 6-in (2.5-cm x 15.2-cm) lumber; and,

(c) Posts: Constructed of at least 2-in x 4-in (5-cm x 10-cm) lumber spaced not to exceed 8 ft (2.4 m) on centers.

(2) Pipe railings:

(a) Toprails and midrails: At least 1.5 in (3.8 cm) nominal diameter (schedule 40 steel pipe); and

(b) Posts: At least 1   in (3.8 cm) nominal diameter (schedule 40 steel pipe) spaced not more than 8 ft (2.4 m) on centers.

(3) Structural steel railings:

(a) Toprails and midrails: At least 2-in x 2-in x 3/8 in (5 cm x 5 cm x .9 cm) angles; and,

EM 385-1-1
15 Sep 08

(b) Posts: At least 2-in x 2-in x 3/8-in (5 cm x 5 cm x .9 cm) angles spaced not more than 8 ft (2.4 m) on centers.

(4) Steel Cable (Wire Rope) railings:

(a) Toprail and midrail: -in (6.25 mm) steel cable, flagged every 6 ft (1.8 m) with high visibility material, may be used if tension is maintained to provide not more than 3 in (7.5 cm) deflection, in any direction from the center line, under a 200 lb (0.89 kN) load;

(b) Support posts shall be located to insure proper tension is maintained;

(c) Perimeter safety cables shall meet the criteria and requirements for guardrail systems. If the perimeter safety cables are used by the workers as a method of attaching a lanyard to the cables they shall meet the requirements of Horizontal Lifeline System (see 21.H.05(c)(5)(b)).

e. Toe boards (Used to protect those below from falling objects).

(1) Toe boards shall be 3 in (8.75 cm) in vertical height and shall be constructed from 1-in x 4-in (2.5-cm x 10.1-cm) lumber or the equivalent.

(2) Toe boards shall be securely fastened in place and have not more than 1/4 in (0.6 cm) clearance above floor level.

(3) Toe boards shall be made of any substantial material, either solid or with openings not greater than 1 in (2.5 cm) in greatest dimension.

(4) Where material is piled to such a height that a standard toe board does not provide protection, paneling or screening from floor to toprail or midrail shall be provided.

EM 385-1-1
15 Sep 08

(5) Toe boards shall be able to withstand, without failure, a force of 50 lbs (0.22 kN) applied in any outward or downward direction at any point along the toe board.

21.E.02 Guardrails receiving heavy stresses from workers trucking or handling materials shall be provided additional strength by using heavier stock, closer spacing of posts, bracing, or by other means.

21.E.03 When guardrails are used at hoisting areas, a minimum of 4 ft (1.2 m) of guardrail shall be erected on each side of the access point through which materials are hoisted.

21.E.04 A gate or removable guardrail section may be used as long as it meets the standard guardrail height 42 +/- 3 in (106.6 +/- 7.6 cm) and is secured across the opening between the guardrail sections when hoisting operations are not taking place.

21.E.05 When guardrails are used at bitumen pipe outlets on roofs, a minimum of 4 ft (1.2 m) of guardrail shall be erected on each side of the pipe.

21.F COVERS.

21.F.01 Install covers on any hole 2 in (5.1cm) or more in its least dimension on walking/working surfaces such as floors, roofs or other openings.

21.F.02 Covers shall be capable of supporting, without failure, at least twice the weight of the worker, equipment and material combined.

21.F.03 Covers shall be secured when installed, clearly marked with the word "HOLE", "COVER" or "Danger, Roof Opening-Do Not Remove" or color-coded or equivalent methods (e.g., red or orange "X"). Workers must be made aware of the meaning for color coding and equivalent methods.

EM 385-1-1
15 Sep 08

21.G SAFETY NET SYSTEM (for fall protection).

> ***Debris nets are addressed in Section 14.C Housekeeping.***

21.G.01 Safety nets shall be installed as close under the work surfaces as practical but in no case more than 25 ft (7.6 m) below such work surface. Nets shall be hung with sufficient clearance to prevent contact with the surfaces or structures below. Such clearance shall be determined by impact load testing. When nets are used on bridges, multi story buildings or structures, the potential fall area from the walking/working surface to the net shall be unobstructed.

    a. The maximum size of the mesh openings shall not exceed 36 in^2 (230 cm^2), nor be longer than 6 in (15 cm) on any side.

    b. The border rope or webbing shall have a minimum breaking strength of 5,000 lb (22.2 kN).

21.G.02 Nets shall extend outward from the outermost projection of the work surface as shown in Table 21-1:

TABLE 21-1

SAFETY NET DISTANCES

Vertical Distance From Working Level To Horizontal Plane Of Net	Minimum Required Horizontal Distance Of Outer Edge Of Net From Edge Of Working Surface
Up to 5 feet (up to 1.5 m)	8 feet (2.5 m)
5 feet up to 10 feet (1.5 m up to 3.1 m)	10 feet (3.1 m)
more than 10 feet (more than 3.1 m)	13 feet (4 m)

EM 385-1-1
15 Sep 08

21.G.03 Operations requiring safety net protection shall not be undertaken until the net(s) is in place and has been tested without failure.

    a. Safety nets and safety net installations shall be tested in the suspended position immediately after installation under the supervision of Qualified Person and in the presence of the GDA and before being used as a fall protection system; whenever relocated, after major repair; and when left at one location, at not more than 6 month intervals.

    b. The test shall consist of dropping into the net a 400 lb (180 kg) bag of sand, not more than 30 in+/- 2 in (76.2 cm +/- 5 cm) in diameter, at least 42 in (106.6 cm) above the highest working/walking surface at which workers are exposed to fall hazards. Means must be taken to ensure the weight can be safely retrieved after the test is conducted.

21.G.04 Shackles and hooks used in safety net installations shall be made of forged steel.

21.G.05 When used with safety nets, debris nets shall be secured on top of the safety net but shall not compromise the design, construction, or performance of the safety nets.

21.G.06 Materials, scrap pieces, equipment, and tools that have fallen into the safety net shall be removed as soon as possible and at least before the next work shift. Safety nets shall be protected from sparks and hot slag resulting from welding and cutting operations.

21.G.07 Inspection of safety nets.

    a. Safety nets shall be inspected by a Competent Person in accordance with the manufacturer's recommendations.

    b. Inspections shall be conducted immediately after installation, at least weekly thereafter, and following any alteration, repair, or

EM 385-1-1
15 Sep 08

any occurrence that could affect the integrity of the net system. Inspections shall be documented.

c. If any welding or cutting operations occur above the net(s), noncombustible barriers shall be provided. The frequency of inspections shall be increased in proportion to the potential for damage to the nets.

d. Defective nets shall not be used. Defective components shall be removed from service and replaced.

21.H PERSONAL FALL PROTECTION SYSTEMS

21.H.01 Personal fall protection equipment and systems (to include fall arrest, positioning and restraint) shall be used when a person is working at heights and exposed to a fall hazard.

21.H.02 Inspection of personal Fall Protection Equipment. Personal fall protection equipment shall be inspected by the end user prior to each use to determine that it is in a safe working condition. A Competent Person for fall protection shall inspect the equipment at least once semi-annually and whenever equipment is subjected to a fall or impacted. Inspection by the Competent Person shall be documented. Defective or damaged equipment shall be immediately removed from service and replaced. Inspection criteria shall include:

a. Harnesses, lanyards, straps and ropes: Check all components for cuts, wear, tears, damaged threads, broken or torn stitching, discoloration, abrasions, burn or chemical damage, ultraviolet deterioration and missing markings and/or labels.

b. Hardware: Check all components for signs of wear, cracks, corrosion and deformation.

21.H.03 Personal fall protection equipment shall be used, maintained and stored in accordance with manufacturer's

EM 385-1-1
15 Sep 08

instructions and recommendations or as prescribed by the Competent Person for fall protection.

21.H.04 Selection of personal fall protection equipment shall be based on the type of work; the work environment; the weight, size, and shape of the worker; the type and position/location of anchorage; and the length of the lanyard.

21.H.05 Personal Fall Arrest System (PFAS): Consists of body support (full body harness), connecting means, and an anchorage system. **> NOTE: All PFAS shall meet the requirements contained in ANSI/ASSE Z359.1- 2007.**

    a. PFAS are generally only certified for users within the capacity range of 130 to 310 lbs (59 to 140.6 kg) including the weight of the worker, equipment and tools. Workers shall not be permitted to exceed the 310 lbs (140.6 kg) limit unless permitted in writing by the manufacturer. For workers with body weight less than 130 lbs (59 kg), a specially designed harness and also a specially designed energy absorbing lanyard shall be utilized which will properly deploy if this person were to fall.

    b. When stopping a fall, PFAS shall:

    (1) Limit maximum arresting force on the body of the employee to 1,800 lbs (8.0 kN) when used with a full body harness;

    (2) Be rigged such that a worker can neither free fall more than 6 ft (1.8 m) nor contact any lower level or other physical hazard in the path of the fall;

    (3) Stop the fall with a maximum deceleration distance of not more than 3.5 ft (1.1 m).

    c. When designing new fall arrest systems, the Qualified Person for fall protection shall attempt to minimize fall distances (including free fall distances) and arrest forces. If it is necessary to increase free fall distances and arrest forces in order to accommodate existing and new structures or provide mobility to end users:

(1) Only the Qualified Person for fall protection shall make this determination; and,

(2) The maximum arrest force shall be kept below 1,800 lbs (8.0 kN).

d. PFAS Components.

(1) Full Body Harness. **> *Only full body harnesses meeting the requirements of ANSI/ASSE Z359.1 are acceptable. Full body harnesses labeled to meet the requirements of the ANSI A10.14 shall not be used.***

(a) PFAS require the use of a full-body harness. The use of body belts is not acceptable.

(b) The fall arrest attachment point on the full body harness shall be integrally attached and located at the wearer's upper back between the shoulder blades (dorsal D-ring).

> *A frontal D-ring attachment point integrally attached to wearer's front full body harness and located at the sternum, can be used for fall arrest, provided the free fall distance does not exceed 2 ft (0.6 m) and the maximum arresting force does not exceed 900 lbs (4 kN).*

(2) Lineman's equipment (electrically rated harnesses). The full body harness used around high voltage equipment or structures shall be an industry designed "linemen's FP harness" that will resist arc flashing and shall have either straps or plastic coated D-Rings and positioning side D-Rings in lieu of exposed metal D-Rings and exposed metal positioning side D-Rings. All other exposed metal parts of the linemen's harnesses shall also be plastic coated (i.e. buckles and adjusters).

(3) Hardware (connecting components).

EM 385-1-1
15 Sep 08

(a) Snaphooks and carabiners shall be self-closing and self-locking capable of being opened only by at least two consecutive deliberate actions. Snaphooks and carabiners having a gate strength of 3,600 lbs (16 kN), per ANSI Z359.1-2007, shall be used.

> *Existing snaphooks and carabiners meeting ANSI Z359.1-1992 (R1999) may continue to be used but shall be replaced with ANSI Z359.1 – 2007 compliant equipment within 2 years of effective date of this manual.*

(b) Snaphooks and carabiners shall have a minimum tensile strength of 5,000 lbs (22.2 kN); D-rings, O-rings, snaphooks and carabiners shall be proof-load tested by the manufacturer to a minimum tensile load of 3,600 lbs (16 kN) without cracking, breaking, or taking permanent deformation.

(c) Connectors and adjusters shall be drop forged, pressed or formed steel, or made of equivalent materials; shall have corrosion resistant finish; and all surfaces and edges shall be smooth to prevent damage to interfacing parts of the system.

(d) All connecting components used in PFAS shall be compatible and shall be used properly.

(4) Connecting Subsystem. Connecting subsystems may include energy absorbing lanyards (shock absorbing lanyards) with snaphooks or carabiners at each end, self-retracting lanyards (SRL), and/or fall arrestors (rope grabs).

(a) Lanyards. Lanyards shall be made of ropes, straps or webbing made from synthetic materials. Energy absorbing lanyards, (including rip stitch/tearing and deforming lanyards) shall be capable of sustaining a minimum tensile load of 5,000 lbs (22.2 kN). When the energy absorbers are dynamically tested by the manufacturers, the maximum arrest force shall not exceed 900 lbs (4kN).

> *Lanyards shall not be looped back over or through an object and then attached back to themselves unless permitted by the manufacturer.*

(b) When using lanyard with two integrally connected legs for 100% tie-off, attach only the snaphook at the center of the lanyard to the fall arrest attachment element of the harness (D-ring). The two legs of the lanyard and the joint between the legs shall withstand a force of 5,000 lbs (22.2 kN). When one leg of the lanyard is attached to the anchorage, the unused leg of the lanyard shall not be attached to any part of the harness except to attachment points specifically designated by the manufacturer for this purpose. Do not rig the lanyard to create a more than 6 ft (1.8 m) free fall and do not allow the legs of the lanyard to pass underarms, between legs and around the neck.

(c) Self-retracting lanyards (SRL) that automatically limit free fall distance to 2 ft (60 cm) or less shall be capable of sustaining a minimum tensile load of 3,000 lbs (13.3 kN).

> *SRL may only be used in vertical applications, unless otherwise permitted by the manufacturer.*

(d) Fall arrestors (rope grabs) designed to be used with a vertical lifeline and ladder climbing devices (rope, cable or sleeve) shall be approved by the manufacturer for such use. Fall arresters shall have a minimum ultimate strength of 3,600 lbs (16 kN).

> *For vertical lifelines or ladder climbing devices, use fall arrestors that move in one direction only.*

(5) Anchorage System. The anchorage system consists of anchorage (the rigid part of the building, facility, structure or equipment) and anchorage connector.

(a) Anchorages used for attaching the PFAS shall be independent of any anchorage used to support or suspend platforms. They shall be capable of supporting at least 5,000

EM 385-1-1
15 Sep 08

lbs (22.2 kN) per worker attached or designed by a Qualified Person for fall protection for twice the maximum arrest force on the body.

(b) Anchorage connectors are used to tie the PFAS to the anchorage and shall be capable of withstanding without breaking 5000 lbs (22.2 kN) load per worker attached.

(c) If cables are used as guardrails and also used as an anchorage for tying off a worker as part of a PFAS, they shall be designed to meet the Horizontal Life Line criteria, per 21.E.01.d (4)(c).

> *Do not use hoists, electric conduits, utility pipes, ductwork or unstable points as anchorages for PFAS.*

(6) Lifelines.

(a) Vertical lifeline (VLL). A VLL is a vertically suspended flexible line with a connector at the upper end for tying it to a 5000 lbs (22.2 kN) overhead anchorage along which a fall arrestor (rope grab) travels. VLL shall have a minimum tensile strength of 5000 lbs (22.2 kN). Each worker shall be attached to a separate lifeline system.

(b) Horizontal lifeline (HLL). A HLL is a fall arrest system consisting of flexible wire, rope or synthetic cable, spanned horizontally between two end anchorages. It may include in-line energy absorber, lifeline tensioner, turnbuckles or intermediate anchorages. Locally manufactured HLLs are not acceptable. Off-the-shelf commercial HLLs shall be installed, and used, under the supervision of a Qualified Person for fall protection only, as part of a complete fall arrest system that maintains a factor of safety of at least two. The design shall include drawings, required clearance, instructions on proper installation, and use procedures and inspection requirements.

EM 385-1-1
15 Sep 08

21.H.06 Positioning System. Positioning system consists of fall protection equipment including the use of a full body harness configured to allow a worker to be supported on an elevated vertical or inclined surface, and perform work with both hands free from body support (e.g., working on rebar assembly, towers, poles or ladders).

   a. A positioning system shall not be used as a primary fall arrest system. Positioning systems use some of the same equipment as a fall protection system (such as a harness), however a positioning system used alone does not constitute fall protection. While positioning (working with both hands free), a person is exposed to a fall hazard and is required under this section to use a separate system that provides backup protection from a fall.

   b. System requirements: Positioning System shall:

   (1) Be rigged such that a worker cannot free fall more than 2 ft (0.6 m);

   (2) Be secured to an anchorage capable of supporting at least twice the potential impact load of a worker's fall or 3,000 lbs (13.3 kN), whichever is greater;

   (3) When necessary, full-body harnesses used in a positioning system shall have two lanyards to ensure that a person is tied-off with at least one lanyard at all times to achieve continuous 100% tie-off; and,

   (4) The attachment point on thefull body harness used in positioning system shall be located on the sides or on the front of the harness.

21.H.07 Restraint Systems.

   a. Fall restraint systems shall prevent the user from reaching an area where a free fall could occur by restricting the length of the lanyard or by other means.

EM 385-1-1
15 Sep 08

b. The anchorage strength requirement for restraint systems shall be 3,000 lbs (13.3 kN) or designed by a Qualified Person for fall protection for two times the foreseeable force.

c. Restraint systems can be used only on sloped surfaces equal to or less than 18.4° (4:12 slope).

21.I LADDER-CLIMBING DEVICES (LCDS). A LCD is a sleeve or cable/rope attached to a fixed ladder over 20 ft (6 m) in length.

21.I.01 Anchorage strength for LCDs shall be a minimum of 3,000 lbs (13.3 kN).

21.I.02 The connector between the front D-ring of the harness and the ladder cable, rope or sleeve shall be 9 in (20 cm) long.

21.I.03 The free fall distance when using a LCD shall not exceed 2 ft (0.6 m).

21.I.04 There shall be 100% transition at the top of the LCD for safe access to above work surface or roof.

> *Do not install LCDs on ladders that have -in (1.9 cm) rungs (off- the-shelf-ladders) unless the ladders are designed to withstand the fall forces.*

21.J SCAFFOLDS, AERIAL LIFT EQUIPMENT, MOVABLE WORK PLATFORMS.

21.J.01 Scaffolds shall be equipped with a standard guardrail per 21.E.01 or other fall protection systems.

21.J.02 For workers erecting and dismantling scaffolds, an evaluation shall be conducted by a Competent Person for fall protection to determine the feasibility and safety of providing fall protection if fall protection is not feasible. An AHA detailing rationale for infeasbility of use of fall protection shall be submitted and accepted by the GDA.

EM 385-1-1
15 Sep 08

21.J.03 Suspended scaffolds.

a. Single point or two point suspended scaffold: In addition to railings, workers shall also be tied off to an independent vertical lifeline using a full body harness.

b. Other suspended scaffolds (e.g., catenary, float, needle-beam, Boatswain chairs): PFAS is required and workers shall be tied off to an independent vertical lifeline using a full body harness.

21.J.04 Elevating Work Platforms/Scissors Lifts: Scissors lifts shall be equipped with standard guardrails. In addition to the guardrail provided, if the scissor lift is equipped with a manufactured anchorage, a restraint system shall be used in addition to guardrails. Lanyards used with the restraint system shall be sufficiently short to prohibit workers from climbing out of, or being ejected from, the platform.

21.J.05 Aerial Lift Equipment: Workers shall be anchored to the basket or bucket in accordance with manufacturer's specifications and instructions (anchoring to the boom may only be used when allowed by the manufacturer and permitted by the Competent Person for fall protection). Lanyards used shall be sufficiently short to prohibit worker from climbing out of basket. Tying off to an adjacent pole or structure is not permitted unless a safe device for 100% tie-off is used for the transfer.

21.K WARNING LINE SYSTEM (WLS). A WLS is a barrier erected on a floor, roof, or edge of excavation area to warn workers that they are approaching an unprotected side or edge. A WLS may ONLY be used on floors or flat or low-sloped roofs (between 0-$18.4°$ or 4:12 slope) and shall be erected around all sides of the work area.

21.K.01 A WLS shall consist of wires, rope or chains 34-39 in (0.9-1.0 m) high with supporting stanchions. WLS shall be flagged at not more than 6 ft (1.8 m) intervals with a high visibility material.

EM 385-1-1
15 Sep 08

21.K.02 The wire, rope or chains shall have a minimum tensile strength of 500 lbs (2.2 kN) and after being attached to the stanchions shall be capable of supporting without braking, the loads applied to the stanchions.

21.K.03 Stanchions shall be capable of resisting without tipping a force of 16 lbs (71 N) applied horizontally against the stanchions 30 in (76.2 cm) above the walking/working surface, perpendicular to the warning line and in the direction of the roof floor or platform edge. The line consisting of wire rope or chains shall be attached at each stanchion in such a way that the pulling on one section of the line will not result in a slack being taken up in adjacent sections before the stanchion tips over.

21.K.04 Working within the WLS does not require fall protection. No worker shall be allowed in the area between the roof or floor edge and the WLS without fall protection. Fall protection is required when working outside the line.

21.K.05 For roofing work the WLS shall be erected not less than 6 ft (1.8 m) from the roof edge. For other work (i.e. use of mechanical equipment) the WLS shall be erected not less than 15 ft (4.5 m) from the edge of the roof.

21.K.06 Mechanical equipment on roofs shall be used or stored only in areas where workers are protected by a WLS, guardrail or PFAS.

21.L SAFETY MONITORING SYSTEM (SMS). The use of a SMS by itself as a fall protection method is prohibited. SMS may only be used in conjunction with other fall protection systems.

21.M RESCUE PLAN AND PROCEDURES. The employer is required to provide prompt rescue to all fallen workers.

21.M.01 A rescue plan (see ANSI Z359.2, Written Rescue Procedures) shall be prepared and maintained when workers are working at heights and using fall protection equipment.

EM 385-1-1
15 Sep 08

21.M.02 The plan shall contain provisions for self-rescue and assisted rescue of any worker who falls including rescue equipment. If other methods of rescue are planned (i.e. by a jurisdictional public or Government emergency rescue agencies), it shall be indicated in the rescue plan including how to contact and summon the agency to the mishap site.

21.M.03 Personnel conducting rescue shall be trained accordingly.

21.M.04 If required, anchorages for self-rescue and assisted – rescue shall be identified, selected, and documented in Site-Specific Fall Protection and Prevention Plan. Anchorages selected for rescue shall be capable of withstanding static loads of 3,000 lbs (13.3 kN) or five times the applied loads as designed by Qualified Person for fall protection.

21.M.05 Workers using fall protection equipment shall have an assigned safety person (spotter) also known as the "buddy system", who will be within visual/verbal range to initiate rescue of the fallen worker if required.

21.N WORKING OVER OR NEAR WATER (piers, wharves, quay walls, barges, aerial lifts, crane-supported work platforms, etc). PFDs are required for all work over or near water unless detailed below.

> ***All USACE and contractor workers, to include divers, shall comply with the requirements below.***

21.N.01 When continuous fall protection is used without exception to prevent workers from falling into the water, the employer has effectively removed the drowning hazard and PFDs are not required. > ***When using safety nets as fall protection, USCG-approved PFDs are usually required, unless rationale is provided in AHA.***

21.N.02 When working over or near water and the distance from walking/working surface to the water's surface is 25 ft (7.6 m) or

EM 385-1-1
15 Sep 08

more, workers shall be protected from falling by the use of a fall protection system and PFDs are not required.

21.N.03 When working over or near water where the distance from the walking/working surface to the water's surface is less than 25 ft (7.6 m) **and** the water depth is less than 10 ft (3.05 m), or hazards from currents, intakes, machinery or barges, etc., are present, fall protection shall be required and PFDs are not required.

21.N.04 When working over water, PFD, lifesaving equipment and safety skiffs meeting the requirements of this EM shall be used.

BLANK

EM 385-1-1
15 Sep 08

SECTION 22

WORK PLATFORMS AND SCAFFOLDING

22.A GENERAL

22.A.01 Manufactured work platforms shall be erected, used, inspected, tested, maintained, and repaired in accordance with ANSI A10.8 and the manufacturer's recommendations as outlined in the operating manual or in accordance with guidance from the Scaffolding, Shoring, and Forming Institute. A copy of the manufacturer's recommendations (operating manual) or guidance from the Scaffolding, Shoring, and Forming Institute shall be available at the work site.

22.A.02 Work platforms shall comply with fall protection and appropriate access requirements of Sections 21 and 24.

   a. All requirements of this section shall be applied to work platforms and means of access.

   b. Standard railing and handrails for work platforms shall be in compliance with the requirements of Section 24.C and E; personal fall protection devices shall be in compliance with Section 21.H; and safety (fall protection) nets shall be in compliance with the requirements of 21.G.

   c. Ladders used as work platforms shall be in compliance with the requirements of Section 24.

22.A.03 Prior to commencing any activity that requires work in elevated areas, all provisions for access and fall protection shall be delineated in the Site-Specific Fall Protection and Prevention Plan and AHA, per 21.C and accepted by the GDA for the activity. For specific guidance related to erecting and disassembling scaffolds, see paragraph 21.J.02.

EM 385-1-1
15 Sep 08

22.A.04 The following hierarchy and prohibitions shall be followed in selecting appropriate work platform.

    a. Scaffolds, platforms, or temporary floors shall be provided for all work except that can be performed safely from the ground or similar footing.

    b. Ladders may be used as work platforms only when use of small hand tools or handling of light material is involved.

    c. Ladder jacks, lean-to, and prop-scaffolds are prohibited.

    d. Emergency descent devices shall not be used as working platforms.

22.A.05 Erection, moving, dismantling, or altering of work platforms shall be under the supervision of a Competent Person.

22.A.06 Contractors shall use a scaffold tagging system in which all scaffolds are tagged by the Competent Person. Tags shall be color-coded: green indicates the scaffold has been inspected and is safe to use; red indicates the scaffold is unsafe to use. Tags shall be readily visible, made of materials that will withstand the environment in which they are used, be legible and shall include:

    a. The Competent Person's name and signature;

    b. Dates of initial and last inspections.

22.A.07 Work platforms shall not be erected or used in the immediate vicinity of power lines or electrical conductors until such are insulated, de-energized, or otherwise rendered safe against accidental contact. **> See 11.F.**

22.A.08 Where persons are required to work or pass under a working platform, a screen (consisting of No. 18 gauge US Standard wire -in (1.2 cm) mesh or the equivalent) shall be provided between the toe board and the guardrail and extending over the entire opening.

EM 385-1-1
15 Sep 08

22.A.09 Anyone involved in erecting, disassembling, moving, operating, using, repairing, maintaining or inspecting a scaffold shall be trained by a Competent Person to recognize any hazards associated with the work in question. Proof of training shall be available upon request.

22.B SCAFFOLDS - GENERAL

22.B.01 Capacities.

a. Scaffolds and their components shall meet the requirements contained in ANSI A10.8 and be capable of supporting without failure at least 4 times the maximum anticipated load.

b. Direct connections to roofs and floors, and counterweights used to balance adjustable suspension scaffolds, shall be capable of resisting at least 4 times the tipping moment imposed by the scaffold operating at the rated load of the hoist, or 1.5 (minimum) times the tipping moment imposed by the scaffold operating at the stall load of the hoist, whichever is greater.

22.B.02 Design.

a. The dimensions of the members and materials used in the construction of various working platforms or scaffolds shall conform to the sizes shown in the ANSI A10.8 tables.

b. Factory-fabricated scaffolds and components shall be designed and fabricated in accordance with the applicable ANSI standard. When there is a conflict between the ANSI standard and this manual concerning the design or fabrication of factory-fabricated scaffolds, the ANSI standard shall prevail.

c. Load-carrying timber members shall be a minimum of 1,500 lb-ft/in^2 (10,342.1 kPa) (stress grade) construction grade lumber.

(1) All dimensions are nominal sizes (except where rough sizes are noted) as provided by Voluntary Product Standard DOC PS 20, published by NIST of the US Department of Commerce.

EM 385-1-1
15 Sep 08

Where rough sizes are noted, only rough or undressed lumber of the size specified will satisfy minimum requirements.

(2) Lumber shall be reasonably straight-grained and free of shakes, checks, splits, cross grains, unsound knots or knots in groups, decay and growth characteristics, or any other condition that will decrease the strength of the material.

22.B.03 Supporting members and foundations shall be of sufficient size and strength to safely distribute loading.

a. Supporting members shall be placed on a firm, smooth foundation that will prevent lateral displacement.

b. Unstable objects such as barrels, boxes, loose bricks, or concrete blocks shall not be used as supports.

c. Vertical members (i.e., poles, legs, or uprights) shall be plumb and securely braced to prevent swaying or displacement.

22.B.04 The design and construction or selection of planking and platform for means of access shall be based upon either the number of persons for which they are rated or the uniform load distribution to which they will be subjected, whichever is the more restrictive, in accordance with Tables 22-1 and 22-2.

EM 385-1-1
15 Sep 08

TABLE 22-1

SELECTION CRITERIA FOR PLANKING AND PLATFORMS

Rated Load Capacity	Designed and Constructed To Carry	Load Placed
1 person	250 lb (115 kg)	At center of span
2 persons	250 lb (115 kg)	18 in (45.7 cm) to left of center of span and
	250 lb (115 kg)	18 in (45.7 cm) to right of center of span
3 persons	250 lb (115 kg)	At center of span and
	250 lb (115 kg)	18 in (45.7 cm) to left of center of span and
	250 lb (115 kg)	18 in (45.7 cm) to right of center of span

TABLE 22-2

MAXIMUM INTENDED LOAD

Rated Load Capacity	Maximum Intended Load
light duty	25 lb/ft^2 (120 kg/m^2) applied uniformly over entire span area
medium duty	50 lb/ft^2 (240 kg/m^2) applied uniformly over entire span area
heavy duty	75 lb/ft^2 (360 kg/m^2) applied uniformly over entire span area

EM 385-1-1
15 Sep 08

22.B.05 Scaffolds shall be plumb and level.

22.B.06 Scaffolds (other than suspended scaffolds) shall bear on base plates upon mudsills or other adequate foundation.

22.B.07 Working levels of work platforms shall be fully planked or decked.

22.B.08 Planking.

a. All wood planking shall be selected for scaffold plank use as recognized by grading rules established by a recognized independent inspection agency for the species of wood used.

(1) The maximum permissible spans for 2-in x 10-in (5-cm x 25.4-cm) (nominal) or 2-in x 9-in (5-cm x 22.8-cm) (rough) solid sawn wood planks shall be as shown in Table 22-3:

(2) The maximum permissible span for 1 in x 9 in (3.1 cm x 22.8 cm) or wider wood plank of full thickness with a maximum intended load of 50 lb/ft^2 shall be 4 ft (1.2 m).

b. Fabricated planks and platforms may be used in lieu of solid sawn wood planks. Maximum spans for such units shall be as recommended by the manufacturer based on the maximum intended load being calculated as specified in Table 22-3.

c. Planking shall be secured to prevent loosening, tipping, or displacement and supported or braced to prevent excessive spring or deflection. Intermediate beams shall be provided to prevent dislodgement of planks due to deflection. **> See 24.A.04.**

d. Planking shall be laid with edges close together across the entire access surface. There will be no spaces through which personnel, equipment, or material could fall.

EM 385-1-1
15 Sep 08

e. When planking is lapped, each plank shall lap its supports at least 12 in (30.4 cm). Scaffold planks shall extend over their end supports not less than 6 in (15.2 cm) (unless the planking is manufactured with restraining hooks or equivalent means of preventing movement) nor more than 12 in (30.4 cm).

f. Where the ends of planks abut each other to form a flush floor, the butt joint shall be at the centerline of a pole and abutted ends shall rest on separate bearers.

g. For outrigger scaffolds, the platform will be nailed or bolted to the outriggers and shall extend to within 3 in (7.6 cm) of the building wall.

h. Planking shall be supported or braced to prevent excessive spring or deflection and secured and supported to prevent loosening, tipping, or displacement.

i. When a scaffold materially changes its direction, the platform planks shall be laid to prevent tipping.

(1) The planks that meet the corner bearer at an angle shall be laid first, and extend over the diagonally placed bearer far enough to have a good safe bearing but not far enough to involve any danger from tipping, and

(2) The planking running in the opposite direction at an angle shall be laid so as to extend over and rest on the first layer of planking.

j. Planks shall be maintained in good condition. When cracks exceed 1.5 times the width of the board the plank will not be used. Planks with notches deeper than 1/3 the width of the plank will not be used. Planks with saw kerfs shall not be used.

22.B.09 Work platforms shall be securely fastened to the scaffold.

EM 385-1-1
15 Sep 08

TABLE 22-3

WOOD PLANK SELECTION

Maximum Intended Load lb/ft² (kg/m²)	Maximum Permissible Span - Full Thickness Undressed Lumber ft (m)	Maximum Permissible Span - Nominal Thickness Undressed Lumber ft (m)
25 (122)	10 (3.0)	8 (2.4)
50 (244)	8 (2.4)	6 (1.8)
75 (366)	6 (1.8)	n/a

22.B.10 When moving platforms to the next level, the old platform shall be left undisturbed until the new bearers have been set to receive the platform planks.

22.B.11 Access.

a. An access ladder or equivalent safe access shall be provided.

b. Where a built-in ladder is part of a scaffold system, it shall conform to the requirements for ladders.

c. Climbing of braces shall be prohibited.

d. Where end frames are designed to be used as a ladder or where bolted-on ladders are used, the maximum height will be limited to 20 ft (12 m) unless fall protection is used. The distance between rungs shall not exceed 12 in (30.5 cm) and shall be uniform throughout the length of the ladder. The minimum clear length of the rungs shall be 16 in (40.7 cm).

22.B.12 When the scaffold height exceeds four times the minimum scaffold base dimension (and including the width added by

EM 385-1-1
15 Sep 08

outriggers, if used), the scaffold shall be secured to the wall or structure.

    a. The first vertical and horizontal tie shall be placed at this point.

    b. Vertical ties shall be repeated at intervals not greater than 26 ft (7.9 m) with the top tie placed no lower than four times the base dimension from the top of the scaffold.

    c. Horizontal ties shall be placed at each end and at intervals not greater than 30 ft (9.1 m).

22.B.13 The use of brackets on scaffolds shall be prohibited unless the tipping effect is controlled.

22.B.14 Use of the following types of scaffolding are permitted if they are designed and constructed in accordance with ANSI A10.8:

    a. Outrigger scaffolds;

    b. Needle beam scaffolds;

    c. Interior hung scaffolds;

    d. Bricklayer's square scaffolds;

    e. Float/ship scaffolds;

    f. Boatswain's scaffolds;

    g. Window jack scaffolds, and

    h. Carpenter's bracket scaffolds.

22.B.15 Other types of scaffolding not included in ANSI A10.8 may be approved by the GDA provided the design is approved by a

EM 385-1-1
15 Sep 08

<u>Registered Professional Engineer (RPE) or they meet a nationally recognized design standard.</u>

22.C METAL SCAFFOLDS AND TOWERS

22.C.01 Scaffold components made of dissimilar metals shall not be used together unless a Competent Person has determined that galvanic action will not reduce the strength of any component to a level below that required by 22.B.01.

22.C.02 The sections of metal scaffolds shall be securely connected and all braces shall be securely fastened.

22.C.03 A ladder or stairway shall be provided for access and shall be affixed or built into all metal scaffolds and so located that, when in use, it will not have a tendency to tip the scaffold.

22.C.04 Tube and coupler scaffolds.

    a. Tube and coupler scaffolds shall have posts, runners, and bracing of nominal 2 in (5-cm) (outside diameter) steel tubing or pipe: other structural metals, when used, must be designed to carry an equivalent load. The size of bearers (outside diameter) and the spacing of posts shall meet the requirements contained in ANSI A10.8.

    b. Tube and coupler scaffolds shall be limited in heights and working levels to those permitted in ANSI A10.8. Drawings and specifications for tube and coupler scaffolds that exceed the limitations in ANSI A10.8 shall be designed by a <u>RPE.</u>

    c. All tube and coupler scaffolds shall be constructed to support four times the maximum intended loads, as set forth by ANSI A10.8 or as specified by a <u>RPE (with knowledge in structural design).</u>

    d. Runners shall be erected along the length of the scaffold and shall be located on both the inside and the outside posts at even heights.

EM 385-1-1
15 Sep 08

(1) When tube and coupler guardrails and midrails are used on outside posts, they may be used in lieu of outside runners. If guardrail systems are removed to other levels, extra runners shall be installed to compensate.

(2) Runners shall be interlocked to form continuous lengths and coupled to each post.

(3) The bottom runners shall be located as close to the base as possible.

(4) Runners shall be placed not more than 6 ft - 6 in (1.9 m) on center.

e. Bearers.

(1) Bearers shall be installed transversely between posts.

(2) When coupled to the post, the inboard coupler shall bear directly on the runner coupler. When coupled to the runners, the couplers shall be kept as close to the post as possible.

(3) Bearers shall extend beyond the posts and runners and shall provide full contact with the coupler.

f. Bracing across the width of the scaffold shall be installed at the ends of the scaffold at least every fourth level vertically and repeated every third set of posts horizontally.

(1) Such bracing shall extend diagonally from the outer post or runner at this level upward to the inner post or runner at the next level.

(2) Building ties shall be installed adjacent to bracing.

g. Longitudinal diagonal bracing across the inner and outer rows of poles shall be installed at approximately a 45° angle in

EM 385-1-1
15 Sep 08

both directions from the base of the end post upward to the extreme top of the scaffold.

(1) Where the longitudinal length of the scaffold permits, such bracing shall be repeated beginning at every fifth post.

(2) On scaffolds where the length is shorter than the height the longitudinal bracing shall extend diagonally from the base of the end posts upward to the opposite end posts and then in alternating directions until reaching the top of the scaffold.

(3) Where conditions preclude the attachment of bracing to the posts, it may be attached to the runners.

22.C.05 Metal frame scaffolds.

a. Spacing of tubular welded panels or frames shall be consistent with the loads imposed.

b. Scaffolds shall be properly braced by cross, horizontal, or diagonal braces (or combination of these) to secure vertical members together laterally, and the cross braces shall be of such length as will automatically square and align vertical members so that the erected scaffold is always plumb, square, and rigid. All brace connections shall be made secure.

c. Scaffold legs shall be set on adjustable bases or plain bases placed on mudsills or other foundations adequate to support the maximum rated loads.

d. Frames shall be placed one on top the other with coupling or stacking pins to provide vertical alignment of the legs.

e. Where uplift may occur, panels shall be locked together vertically by pins or other equivalent suitable means.

EM 385-1-1
15 Sep 08

f. Drawings and specifications for all frame scaffolds over 125 ft (38.1 m) in height above the base plates shall be designed by a RPE.

22.C.06 Manually propelled mobile scaffolds.

a. All wheels and casters on rolling scaffolds shall have a positive locking device, securely fastened to the scaffold, to prevent accidental movement.

b. All casters or wheels shall be locked when a scaffold is occupied.

c. The force necessary to move the mobile scaffold shall be applied as close to the base as practical and provision shall be made to stabilize the tower during movement from one location to another.

d. Rolling scaffolds shall be used only on firm, level, clean surfaces.

e. Free-standing mobile scaffold working platform heights shall not exceed three times the smallest base dimension.

f. No person shall be allowed to ride on manually propelled scaffolds unless all of the following conditions exist:

(1) The ground surface is within 3° of level and free from pits, holes, or obstructions;

(2) The minimum dimension of the scaffold base (when ready for rolling) is at least one-half of the height and outriggers, if used, are installed on both sides of staging;

(3) The wheels are equipped with rubber or similar resilient tires; and

4) All tools and materials are secured or removed from the platform before the scaffold is moved.

22.D WOOD POLE SCAFFOLDS

22.D.01 All wood scaffolds 60 ft (18.2 m) or less in height shall be constructed in accordance with Table 22-4 or Table 22-5: wood scaffolds over 60 ft (18.2 m) high shall be designed by a RPE and constructed in accordance with such design.

EM 385-1-1
15 Sep 08

TABLE 22-4

SINGLE WOOD POLE SCAFFOLDS
Minimum nominal size and maximum spacing of members of single pole scaffolds

Description	Light duty Up to 20 feet high	Light-duty Up to 60 feet high	Medium duty Up to 60 feet high	Heavy Duty Up to 60 feet high
Max. Intended Load(lbs./sq.ft.)	25	25	50	75
Poles or Uprights	2 x 4 in. (5 x 10.1 cm)	4 x 4 in. (10.1 x 10.1 cm)	4 x 4 in. (10.1 x 10.1 cm)	4 x 6 in. (10.1 x 15.2 cm)
Max. pole spacing (longitudinal)	6 ft. (1.8 m)	10 ft. (3 m)	8 ft. (2.4 m)	6 ft. (1.8 m)
Max. Pole spacing (transverse)	5 (1.5 m)	5 (1.5 m)	5 (1.5 m)	5 (1.5 m)
Runners	1 x 4 in (2.5 x 10.2 cm)	1 x9 in. (3.1 x 22.8 cm)	2 x 10 in. (5.1 x 25.4 cm)	2 x 10 in. (5.1 x 25.4 cm)
Maximum spacing of bearers				
3 feet	2 x 4 in (5.1 x 10.1 cm)	2 x 4 in (5.1 x 10.1 cm)	2 x 10 in (5.1 x 25.4 cm) or 3 x 4 in. (7.6 x 10.1 cm)	2 x 10 in (5.1 x 25.4 cm) or 3 x 5 in. (7.6 cm x 12.7 cm)
5 feet	2 x 6 in (5.1 x 15.2 cm) or 3 in. x 4 in. (7.6 x 10.1 cm)	2 x 6 in (5.1 x 15.2 cm) or 3 in. x 4 in (7.6 x 10.1 cm) (rough)	2 x 10 in (5.1 x 25.4 cm) or 3 x 4 in. (7.6 x 10.1 cm)	2 x 10 in (5.1 x 25.4 cm) or 3 x 5 in. (7.6 x 12.7 cm).

EM 385-1-1
15 Sep 08

TABLE 22-4 (Continued)

SINGLE WOOD POLE SCAFFOLDS

Description	Light duty Up to 20 feet high	Light-duty Up to 60 feet high	Medium duty Up to 60 feet high	Heavy Duty Up to 60 feet high
6 feet			2 x 10 in (5.1 x 25.4 cm) or 3 x 4 in. (7.6 x 10.1 cm)	2 x 10 in (5.1 x 25.4 cm) or 3 x 4 in. (7.6 x 10.1 cm)
8 feet			2 x 10 in (5.1 x 25.4 cm) or 3 x 4 in. (7.6 x 10.1 cm)	
Planking	1 in. x 9in. (3.1 x 22.8 cm)	2 x 10 in. (5.1 x 25.4 cm)	2 x 10 in. (5.1 x 25.4 cm)	2 x 10 in. (5.1 x 25.4 cm)
Max. vertical spacing of horiz. members	7 ft (2.1 m)	9 ft (2.1 m)	7 ft (2.7 m)	6 ft 6 in (2 m)
Bracing, horizontal	1 in x 4 in (2.5 cm x 10.2 cm)	1 in x 4 in (2.5 cm x 10.2 cm)	1 in x 6 in (2.5 cm x 15.2 cm) or 1 in x 4 in (3.2 cm x 10.2 cm)	2 in x 4 in (5 cm x 10.2 cm)
Bracing, diagonal	1 in x 4 in (2.5 cm x 10.1 cm)	1 in x 4 in (2.5 cm x 10.1 cm)	1 in x 6 in or 1 in. x 4 in. (3.2 cm x 10.2 cm)	2 in x 4 in (5 cm x 10.2 cm)
Tie-ins	1 in x 4 in (2.5 cm x 10.2 cm)	1 in x 4 in (2.5 cm x 10.2 cm)	1 in x 4 in (2.5 cm x 10.2 cm)	1 in x 4 in (2.5 cm x 10.2 cm)

Note: All members are used on edge. All wood bearers shall be reinforced with 3/16 x 2 inch steel strip, or the equivalent, secured to the lower edges for the entire length of the bearer

EM 385-1-1
15 Sep 08

TABLE 22-5

INDEPENDENT WOOD POLE SCAFFOLDS

	6 feet	10 feet	8 feet	8 feet
Runners	1 x 4 in (3.2 cm x 10.2 cm)	1 x 9 in (3.2 cm x 22.8 cm)	2 x 10 in. (5.1 x 25.4 cm)	2 x 10 in. (5.1 x 25.4 cm)
Bearers				
3 feet	2 x 4 (5.4 x 10.2 cm)	2 x 4 (5.4 x 10.2 cm)	2 x 10 in. (5.1 x 25.4 cm)	2 x 10 in. (rough) (5.1 x 25.4 cm)
6 feet	2 x 6 in (5.4 x 15.2 cm) Or 3 x 4 in (7.6 x 10.2 cm)	2 x 10 in (rough) (5.4 x 25.4 cm) Or 2 x 4 in (5.1 x 10.2 cm)	2 x 10 in. (5.1 x 25.4 cm)	2 x 10 in. (rough) (5.1 x 25.4 cm)
8 feet	2 x 6 in (5.4 x 15.2 cm) Or 3 x 4 in (7.6 x 10.2 cm)	2 x 10 in (rough) (5.4 x 25.4 cm) Or 2 x 8 in (5.1 x 20.3 cm)	2 x 10 in. (5.1 x 25.4 cm)	
10 feet	2 x 6 in (5.4 x 15.2 cm) Or 3 x 4 in (7.6 x 10.2 cm)	2 x 10 in (rough) (5.4 x 25.4 cm) Or 3 x 3 in (7.6 x 7.6 cm)	2 x 10 in. (5.1 x 25.4 cm)	
Planking	1 x 9 in (3.2 cm x 22.8 cm)	2 x 10 in. (5.1 x 25.4 cm)	2 x 10 in. (5.1 x 25.4 cm)	2 x 10 in. (5.1 x 25.4 cm)
Max. vertical spacing of horizontal members	7 feet (2.1 x 2.1 cm)	7 feet (2.1 x 2.1 cm)	6 feet (1.8 x 1.8 cm)	6 feet (1.8 x 1.8 cm)
Bracing horizontal	1 x 4 in (2.54 x 10.2 cm)	1 x 4 in (2.54 x 10.2 cm)	1 x 4 in (2.54 x 10.2 cm)	2 in x 4 in (5 cm x 10.2 cm)
Bracing vertical	1 x 4 in (2.54 x 10.2 cm)	1 x 4 in (2.54 x 10.2 cm)	1 x 4 in (2.54 x 10.2 cm)	2 in x 4 in (5 cm x 10.2 cm)
Tie-ins	1 x 4 in (2.54 x 10.2 cm)	1 x 4 in (2.54 x 10.2 cm)	1 x 4 in (2.54 x 10.2 cm)	1 x 4 in (2.54 x 10.2 cm)

Note: All members are used on edge. All wood bearers shall be reinforced with 3/16 x 2 inch steel strip, or the equivalent, secured to the lower edges for the entire length of the bearer.

22.D.02 Bracing.

a. Diagonal bracing shall be provided to prevent the poles from moving in a direction parallel with the wall of the building or from buckling.

b. Full diagonal bracing shall be erected across the entire face of pole scaffolds in both directions. Braces shall be spliced at the poles. The inner row of poles on medium and heavy-duty scaffolds shall be braced in a similar manner.

c. Cross bracing shall be provided between inner and outer sets of poles in independent pole scaffolds.

d. The free ends of pole scaffolds shall be cross-braced.

22.D.03 Splices.

a. Where wood poles are spliced, the ends shall be squared and the upper section shall rest squarely on the lower section.

b. Splice plates shall be provided on two adjacent sides and shall be not less than 4 ft (1.2 m) in length, overlapping the abutted ends equally, and have the same width and not less than the cross sectional area of the pole. The splice shall be capable of developing strength in any direction equal to the spliced members.

22.D.04 Ledgers and bearers.

a. Ledgers and bearers shall be installed on edge.

b. Ledgers and bearers shall not be spliced between poles.

c. Ledgers shall be long enough to extend over a minimum of two poles and shall be reinforced by bearing blocks nailed to the side of the pole to form a support for the ledger.

EM 385-1-1
15 Sep 08

d. Bearers shall be long enough to project at least 3 in (7.6 cm) over the ledgers of the inner and outer rows of poles for support.

e. Every wooden bearer on single pole scaffolds shall be reinforced with a 3/16-in x 2-in (.47-cm x 5-cm) steel strip, or equivalent, secured to its lower edge throughout the length.

22.D.05 Independent pole scaffolds shall be set as near to the wall of the building as practical.

22.D.06 All pole scaffolds shall be securely guyed or tied to the structure. Where the height or length exceeds 25 ft (7.6 m), the scaffold shall be secured at intervals not greater than 25 ft (7.6 m) vertically and horizontally.

22.E SUSPENDED SCAFFOLDS

22.E.01 Suspended scaffolds are scaffolds/work platforms that are suspended from anchorage points/hoists that allow the scaffold to move up and down as needed for work to be performed. Suspended scaffolds shall be designed, constructed, operated, inspected, tested, and maintained as specified in the operating manual for the device.

22.E.02 Inspections.

a. Suspended scaffold systems shall be inspected prior to being placed in service to determine that the system conforms to this manual and the manufacturer's specifications.

b. Every suspended scaffold shall be tested with twice the maximum anticipated load before being put into operation.
> *See 22.B.*

c. Each hoist shall be inspected before, and trial operated after, every installation and re-rigging in accordance with the manufacturer's specifications.

EM 385-1-1
15 Sep 08

    d. Connection and anchorage systems of suspended scaffold shall be inspected at the beginning of each shift.

    e. All wire ropes, fiber and synthetic ropes, slings, hangers, hoists, rigging, fall protection equipment, platforms, anchorage points and their connections, and other supporting parts shall be inspected before every installation, daily thereafter, and periodic while the scaffold is in use.

    f. Governors and secondary brakes for powered hoists shall be inspected and tested per the manufacturer's recommendations: at the minimum, inspections shall be made annually.

    (1) Inspections and tests shall include a verification that the initiating device for the secondary braking operates as intended.

    (2) A copy of the latest inspection and test report shall be maintained on the job site.

    g. Records of inspections conducted while the unit is at the work site shall be maintained at the work site.

22.E.03 Only personnel trained in the use of the suspended work platform shall be authorized to operate it. Training shall include:

    a. Reading and understanding the manufacturer's operating manual and any associated rules and instructions, or training by a Qualified Person on the contents on these documents, and

    b. Reading and understanding all decals, warnings, and instructions on the device.

22.E.04 All parts of all suspended scaffolds shall have a minimum safety factor of 4. A minimum safety factor of 6 is required for support ropes.

EM 385-1-1
15 Sep 08

22.E.05 Support ropes.

a. Support ropes shall be attached at the vertical centerline of the outrigger and the attachment shall be directly over the hoist machine.

b. Support ropes shall be vertical for their entire length. The scaffold shall not be swayed nor the support ropes fixed to any intermediate points to change the original path of travel.

c. Support ropes shall have the fixed end equipped with a proper size thimble and secured by eye splicing or equivalent means. Free ends shall be brazed or secured to prevent fraying.

d. The wire rope for traction hoists shall be of such length that the operator may descend to the lowest point of travel without the end of the wire rope entering the hoist. Where the wire rope is inadequate for the lowest descent, provision shall be made to prevent the hoist from running off the wire rope.

e. On winding drum type hoists, running ends of suspension ropes shall be attached by positive means to the hoisting drum and at least four wraps of the rope shall remain on the drum at all times.

f. Support ropes shall be capable of resisting chemicals or conditions to which they are exposed.

g. No welding, burning, riveting, or open flame work shall be performed on any platform suspended by fiber or synthetic rope.

h. Defective or damaged rope shall not be used as lifelines or suspension lines. The repairing of wire rope is prohibited.

22.E.06 All suspension scaffold support devices such as outrigger beams, cornice hooks, parapet clamps, or similar devices shall:

EM 385-1-1
15 Sep 08

    a. Be made of mild steel, wrought iron, or equivalent materials;

    b. Be supported by bearing blocks;

    c. Rest on surfaces capable of supporting the reaction forces imposed by the scaffold hoist operating at its maximum rated load; and

    d. Be secured against movement by tiebacks installed at right angles to the face of the building whenever possible and secured to a structurally sound portion of the building. Tiebacks shall be equivalent in strength to the hoisting rope.

22.E.07 Outrigger beams.

    a. Outrigger beams shall be made of structural metal and shall be restrained to prevent movement.

    b. The inboard ends of outrigger beams shall be stabilized by bolts or other direct connections to the floor or roof deck, or they shall have their inboard ends stabilized by counterweights, except mason's multiple point adjustable suspension scaffold outrigger beams shall not be stabilized by counterweights.

    c. Before use, direct connections shall be evaluated by a Competent Person who shall affirm that the supporting surfaces are capable of supporting the loads to be imposed. Mason's multiple point adjustable suspension scaffold connections shall be designed by a licensed engineer experienced in scaffold design.

    d. Counterweights shall be made of non-flowable solid material, shall be secured to the outrigger beams by mechanical means, and shall not be removed until the scaffold is disassembled.

    e. Outrigger beams shall be secured by tiebacks equivalent in strength to the suspension ropes. Tiebacks shall be secured to a structurally sound portion of the building or structure and shall be installed parallel to the centerline of the beam.

f. Outrigger beams shall be provided with stop bolts or shackles at both ends.

g. When channel iron beams are used in place of I-beams, the channels shall be securely fastened together with the flanges turned outward.

h. Outrigger beams shall be installed with all bearing supports perpendicular to the beam centerline.

i. Outrigger beams shall be set and maintained with the web in a vertical position.

j. Where a single outrigger beam is used, the steel shackle or clevises with which the wire ropes are attached to the beam shall be placed directly over the hoisting machines.

22.E.08 Hoisting machines

a. Hoisting machines shall be of a type tested and listed by a nationally recognized testing laboratory.

b. Each hoist shall contain a name plate(s) containing:

(1) Manufacturer's name;

(2) Maximum load rating;

(3) Identification number; and

(4) Wire rope specifications.

c. Powered hoists shall be electric-, air-, hydraulic-, or propane-powered. Gasoline-powered hoists are prohibited.

d. All powered hoists shall be equipped with speed reducers and shall be provided with a primary brake and a secondary brake.

(1) The primary brake shall automatically engage whenever power is interrupted or whenever the operator ceases to apply effort;

(2) The secondary brake shall stop and hold the hoist under over speed or abnormal conditions. Every secondary brake shall be periodically tested under simulated conditions in accordance with the manufacturer's recommendations.

e. Each powered hoist shall have its own separate control.

(1) If the control is of the push-button type, it shall be constant pressure;

(2) If the control is of the fixed-position type, it shall have provision for automatic locking when in the off position, or shall be guarded against accidental actuation; and

(3) If the control is of the lever type, it may be of the constant pressure type or of the fixed-position type.

f. Manual operation of powered hoists may be provided if the hoist is designed so that not more than one person per hoist is required to perform this operation.

(1) During manual operation, a means shall be provided to make the prime mover inoperative.

(2) Instruction shall be provided advising personnel to disconnect the power source before using a manual crank.

g. Manually-operated hoists.

(1) Manual operation shall provide a means to prevent rapid handle movement or fast un-spooling. Mechanisms used to allow fast un-spooling during the erection process shall not be in place on the scaffold.

(2) In the event a controlled descent device is used, it shall not bypass the secondary brake.

(3) All winding drum hoists shall be provided with a driving pawl and a locking pawl that automatically engages when the driving pawl is released.

(4) Gripping-type hoists shall be designed so that the hoist is engaged on the suspension rope at all times, including all travel actuations of the operating lever.

(5) Each winding drum hoist shall be provided with a positive means of attachment of the suspension hoist. The drum attachment shall develop a minimum of four times the rated capacity of the hoist.

(6) Each hoist shall require a positive crank force to descend.

22.E.09 Platforms.

a. Light metal platforms, when used, shall be of a type tested and listed by a nationally recognized testing laboratory.

b. Ladder-type platforms.

(1) Ladder-type platforms shall be constructed in accordance with Table 22-6.

(2) The side stringer for ladder-type platforms shall be of clear straight-grained spruce or materials of equivalent strength and durability.

(3) The rungs shall be of straight-grained oak, ash, or hickory, at least 1-1/8 in (2.8 cm) in diameter, with 7/8-in (2.2-cm) tenons mortised into the side stringers at least 7/8 in (2.2 cm).

TABLE 22-6

LADDER-TYPE PLATFORMS

Component	Length of platform (feet, m)				
	12 (3.7)	14 & 16 (4.3 & 4.9)	18 & 20 (5.5 & 6.1)	22 & 24 (6.7 & 7.3)	28 & 30 (8.5 & 9.1)
Side stringers, minimum cross sections (finished sizes, inches,):					
at ends	1-3/4 x 2-3/4 (4.4 x 6.9)	1-3/4 x 2-3/4 (4.4 x 6.9)	1-3/4 x 3 (4.4 x 7.6)	1-3/4 x 3 (4.4 x 7.6)	1-3/4 x 3-1/2 (4.4 x 8.9)
at middle	1-3/4 x 3-3/4 (4.4 x 9.5)	1-3/4 x 3-3/4 (4.4 x 9.5)	1-3/4 x 4 (4.4 x 10.1)	1-3/4 x 4-1/4 (4.4 x 10.8)	1-3/4 x 5 (4.4 x 12.7)
Reinforcing strips	(1)	(1)	(1)	(1)	(1)
Rungs	(2)	(2)	(2)	(2)	(2)
Tie rods: number (minimum) diameter (minimum) (in/cm)	3 1/4 (0.6)	4 1/4 (0.6)	4 1/4 (0.6)	5 1/4 (0.6)	6 1/4 (0.6)
Flooring, minimum finished sizes (in/cm)	1/2 x 2-3/4 (1.2 x 6.9)	1/2 x 2-3/4 (1.2 x 6.9)	1/2 x 2-3/4 (1.2 x 6.9)	1/2 x 2-3/4 (1.2 x 6.9)	1/2 x 2-3/4 (1.2 x 6.9)

NOTE:
(1) A 1/8 x 7/8 in (0.3 x 2.2 cm) steel reinforcing strip or its equivalent shall be attached to the side or underside, full length.
(2) Rungs shall be 1-1/8 in (2.8 cm) diameter tenons and the maximum spacing shall be 12 in (30.4 cm) center to center.
(4) The stringers shall be tied with tie rods not less than 1/4 in (0.6 cm) diameter passing through the stringers and riveted up tight against washers on both ends.
(5) The flooring strips shall be spaced not more than 5/8 in (1.5 cm) apart except at the side rails where the space may be 1 in (2.5 cm).

EM 385-1-1
15 Sep 08

c. Plank platforms.

(1) Plank platforms shall be composed of not less than nominal 2-in x 10-in (5-cm x 25.4-cm) unspliced planks, cleated together on the underside, starting 6 in (15.2 cm) from each end at intervals not to exceed 4 ft (1.2 m).

(2) The plank platform shall not extend beyond the hangers more than 12 in (30.4 cm). A bar or other effective means shall be securely fastened to the platform at each end to prevent its slipping off the hanger.

(3) The span between hangers for plank platforms shall not exceed 8 ft (2.4 m).

d. Beam platforms.

(1) Beam platforms shall have side stringers of lumber not less than 2 in x 6 in (5 cm x 15.2 cm), set on edge.

(2) The span between hangers shall not exceed 12 ft (3.6 m) when beam platforms are used.

(3) The flooring shall be of 1-in x 6-in (2.5-cm x 15.2-cm) material properly nailed. Floor boards shall not be spaced more than 1/2 in (1.2 cm) apart.

(4) The flooring shall be supported on 2-in x 6-in (5-cm x 15.2-cm) cross beams, laid flat and set into the upper edge of the stringers with a snug fit, at intervals of not more than 4 ft (1.2 m), nailed securely in place.

22.E.10 Suspended scaffolds shall be guyed, braced, guided, or equipped with tag line to prevent swaying.

22.E.11 Two-point suspension scaffolds.

a. Two-point suspension scaffold platforms shall not be less than 20 in (50.8 cm) or more than 36 in (91.4 cm) wide. The platform shall be securely fastened to the hangers by U-bolts or by other equivalent means.

b. The hangers of two-point suspension scaffolds shall be made of mild steel, or equivalent materials, having a cross sectional area capable of sustaining four times the maximum rated load and shall be designed with a support for a standard railing.

c. Two-point suspension scaffolds shall be securely lashed to the structure. Window cleaner's anchors shall not be used.

d. The platform on every two-point suspension scaffolds shall be of the light metal-, ladder-, plank-, or beam-type.

e. Two-point suspension scaffolds shall not be joined by bridging.

f. Two-point suspension scaffold platforms, when in use, shall be level within 1 in (2.5 cm) for every 1 ft (0.3 m) of platform length.

22.E.12 Mason's multiple-point adjustable suspension scaffolds.

a. When employees on the scaffold are exposed to overhead hazards, overhead protection equivalent in strength to 2-in (5-cm) planking shall be provided on the scaffold not more than 9 ft (2.7 m) above the platform, laid tight and extending the entire width of the scaffold.

b. The scaffold shall be capable of sustaining a load of 50 psf (2394 Pa) and shall not be overloaded.

c. The platform shall be suspended by wire ropes from overhead outrigger beams.

EM 385-1-1
15 Sep 08

22.E.13 Stonesetters' multiple-point adjustable suspension scaffolds.

a. Stonesetters' multiple-point adjustable suspension scaffolds shall be capable of sustaining a load of 25 psf (1197 Pa) and shall not be overloaded.

b. Stonesetters' multiple-point adjustable suspension scaffolds shall not be used for storage of stone or other heavy materials.

c. The scaffold platform shall be securely fastened to the hangers by U-bolts or other equivalent means.

d. Stonesetters' multiple-point adjustable suspension scaffolds shall be suspended from metal outriggers, iron brackets, wire rope slings, or iron hooks.

e. When two or more stonesetters' multiple-point adjustable suspension scaffolds are used on a structure, they shall not be bridged one to the other, but shall be maintained at even height with platforms abutting closely.

22.E.14 Working capacities.

a. On suspension scaffolds designed for a working load of 500 lb (226.8 kg), no more than two employees shall be permitted to work at one time.

b. On suspension scaffolds with a working load of 750 lb (340.2 kg), no more than three people shall be permitted to work at one time.

22.E.15 Fall protection.

a. Each person supported by a <u>single-point or two-point adjustable</u> suspended scaffold shall be protected from falling by the use of a fall arrest system. <u>A risk assessment shall be performed when persons are supported on a multi-point adjustable suspended scaffold to evaluate the effectiveness</u>

and feasibility of the use of personal fall protection systems. Results shall be documented in the AHA for the activity being performed. > *See 21.H.05.*

b. Full-body harnesses shall be attached by lanyard to a lifeline, trolley line, or structural member independent of the scaffold. However, when overhead obstructions or additional platform levels are part of a single-point or two-point adjustable suspension scaffold, then lifelines shall not be used.

(1) Lifelines, when used, shall be fastened to a fixed safe point of anchorage, shall be independent of the scaffold, and shall be protected from sharp edges and abrasion;

(2) Trolley lines, when used, shall be secured to two or more structural members of the scaffold and shall not be attached to the suspension ropes;

(3) When lanyards are connected to trolley lines or structural members on a single-point or two-point adjustable suspension scaffold, the scaffold shall be equipped with additional independent support lines and automatic locking devices capable of stopping the fall of the scaffold in the event one or both of the suspension ropes fail. The independent support lines shall be equal in number and strength to the suspension ropes; and

(4) Lifelines, independent support lines, and suspension ropes shall not be attached to one another and shall not be attached to or use the same point of anchorage.

c. To keep the lifeline continuously attached, with a minimum of slack, to a fixed structure, the attachment point of the lifeline shall be changed as the work progresses.

22.F HANGING SCAFFOLDS

22.F.01 A hanging scaffold is a scaffold/work platform that is hung from a location (such as a lock gate) for work to be performed and that remains stationary until it is them repositioned with a crane/hoisting device. Hanging scaffolds shall be designed by a Registered Professional Engineer (RPE) competent in structural design. Scaffold performance and components shall meet or exceed those for general scaffolds and platforms found in ANSI A10.8-2001. *> See Figure 22-1.*

22.F.02 Hanging scaffolds shall meet the following requirements:

a. The scaffold shall be securely fastened to a vertical structure (i.e. wall, lock gate, etc.) by hooks over a secured structural supporting member, bolt-on brackets, or other secure attachment. The maximum span between secure attachments is 8 ft (2.4 m). Fasteners shall be of adequate size to achieve design strength of scaffold.

b. The scaffold must be secured against an uplift force equal to two times the weight of the scaffold and its rated load by means of hooks, brackets, or other secure attachments designed and placed to counteract uplift.

c. The scaffold shall have a secondary attachment method to secure it against falling if the primary attachment fails. This should be a flexible attachment, such as wire rope or chain, designed to withstand a minimum of five (5) times the weight of the scaffold and its rated load. The secondary attachment shall be connected to an anchor point of the same load rating or greater.

d. The scaffold shall have only one working level. Working platform decks shall be slip resistant and securely attached to the scaffold frame. The maximum width, front to back, of decks is 42 in (106.6 cm). Grating used for deck surfaces shall have a maximum width opening between bars small enough to prevent the rigging components used (slings, chains) from entering.

e. Standard guardrail systems meeting the requirements of 21.E.01 shall be installed on all open sides and ends of the platform.

EM 385-1-1
15 Sep 08

f. The scaffold shall be conspicuously posted with a plate or other permanent marking that indicates:

(1) the weight of the scaffold;

(2) the number of personnel it was designed for;

(3) the rated weight capacity;

(4) the specific structure(s) it was designed to be attached to – this may be a code or other form of identification when designed for a number of different structures with similar structural attachment points;

(5) the name of the RPE who designed the scaffold;

(6) the date of manufacture;

g. Hanging scaffolds designed to also function as crane-supported work platforms shall meet the requirements of Section 16.T. This includes scaffolds that require a person to stand/ ride on the platform while the initial attachment to the structure is made.

h. The space between the platform deck edge and the face of the vertical structure shall not be more than 14 in. Prior to use on each jobsite application, the Competent Person shall determine if this space constitutes a hazard by being large enough to allow tools/ objects to fall on workers below, or if crane rigging may enter and entangle in the space. In these situations, the space shall be closed or blocked to remove the hazard.

22.F.03 Testing

a. Prior to initial use and after any modification of the structural members or secure attachment points, the platform shall be proof tested to 125% of its rated capacity. The test shall take place on a structure the scaffold was designed for or a test structure with similar support member characteristics.

b. Prior to use on each jobsite or placement location, hanging scaffolds shall be performance tested to 100% of the maximum intended load for the expected work. This test shall be performed with the scaffold attached to the structure in the work location.

22.F.04 Operations

a. Scaffolds and their attachments shall be inspected by a Competent Person prior to initial use on a worksite, before use on each work shift, and regularly during use until they are removed.

b. Workers shall use properly selected and anchored personal fall protection when accessing and working on hanging scaffolds. Personal fall protection system components shall meet the requirements of 21.H.05. No part of a hanging scaffold shall be used as an anchor point for personal fall protection.

c. The number of workers on the platform shall not exceed the number listed on the scaffold.

d. Ladders may not be used on hanging scaffolds, except as a means of access from above the deck. Ladders used for access must meet the requirements of 24.B.

e. Hanging scaffolds shall be coated or painted to minimize corrosion of the components. Storage between uses shall be designed to minimize damage to the scaffold.

FIGURE 22-1

Hanging Scaffold

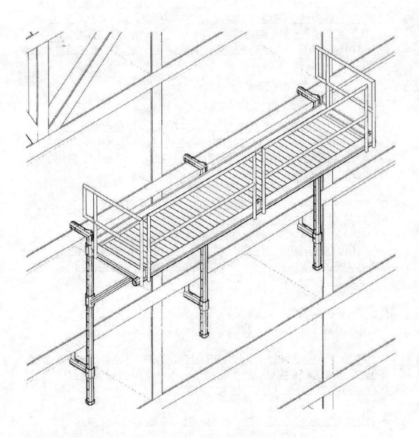

EM 385-1-1
15 Sep 08

22.G FORM AND CARPENTER'S BRACKET SCAFFOLDS

22.G.01 At the minimum, form scaffolds shall be designed in accordance with Table 22-7.

22.G.02 Each bracket, except for wooden-bracket form scaffolds, shall be attached to the supporting formwork or structure by means of one or more of the following:

    a. Nails;

    b. A metal stud attachment device;

    c. Welding;

    d. Hooking over a secured structural supporting member, provided the form walers are bolted to the form or secured by snap ties or tie-bolts extending through the form and securely anchored; or

    e. For carpenter's bracket scaffolds only, by a bolt extending through to the opposite side of the structure's wall.

22.G.03 Wooden form scaffolds shall be an integral part of the form panel.

22.G.04 Folding-type metal brackets, when extended for use, shall be either bolted or secured with a locking-type pin.

22.G.05 Brackets shall consist of a triangular shaped frame made of wood with a cross-section not less than 2-in x 3-in (5-cm x 7.6-cm) or of 1-1/4-in x 1-1/4-in x 1/8-in (3.1-cm x 3.1-cm x 0.3-cm) structural angle iron.

EM 385-1-1
15 Sep 08

TABLE 22-7

FORM SCAFFOLDS

Minimum design criteria for light-duty wooden bracket form scaffolds

Members	Dimensions
Bracket uprights	2 x 4 in or 2 x 6 in (5 x 10.1 cm or 5 x 15.2 cm)
Bracket support ledgers	2 x 6 in (5 x 15.2 cm)
Maximum bracket width	3 ft 6 in (1 m)
Bracket braces	1 x 6 in (2.5 x 15.2 cm)
Guardrail post	2 x 4 in (5 x 10.1 cm)
Guardrail height	36 to 42 in (91.4 to 106.6 cm)
Midrail	1 x 6 in (2.5 x 15.2 cm)
Toeboards	1 x 6 in (2.5 x 15.2 cm)
Bracket upright spacing	8 ft (2.4 m) (on centers)

TABLE 22-7 (CONTINUED)

FORM SCAFFOLDS

Minimum design criteria for light-duty figure-four form scaffolds

Members	Dimensions
Bracket uprights	2 x 4 in or 2 x 6 in (5 x 10.1 cm or 5 x 15.2 cm)
Bracket outrigger ledgers (2)	1 x 6 in (2.5 x 15.2 cm)
Bracket braces (2)	1 x 6 in (2.5 x 15.2 cm)
Maximum length of ledgers	3 ft 6 in (1 m) (unsupported)
Bracket upright spacing	8 ft (2.4 m) (on centers)

TABLE 22-7 (CONTINUED)

FORM SCAFFOLDS

Minimum design criteria for light-duty metal bracket form scaffolds

Members	Dimensions
Guardrail post	2 x 4 in (5 x 10.1 cm)
Guardrail	2 x 4 in (5 x 10.1 cm)
Guardrail height	36 to 45 in (91.4 to 114.3 cm)
Midrail	1 x 6 in (2.5 x 15.2 cm)
Toeboards	1 x 6 in (2.5 x 15.2 cm)
Metal bracket spacing (metal bracket or scaffold jack dimensions in accordance with manufacturer's design)	8 ft (2.4 m)

22.G.06 Bolts used to attach brackets to structures shall not be less than 5/8 in (1.5 cm) in diameter.

22.G.07 Maximum bracket spacing shall be 8 ft (2.4 m) on centers.

22.G.08 Figure-four form scaffolds shall have bearers consisting of two pieces of 1-in x 6-in (2.5-cm x 15.2-cm) lumber nailed on opposite sides of the vertical support; bearers shall project not more than 3.5 ft (1 m) from the outside of the form support and shall be braced and secured to prevent tipping or turning.

22.G.09 The knee or angle brace for figure four form scaffolds shall intersect the bearer at least 3 ft (0.9 m) from the form at an angle of 45° and the lower end shall be nailed to a vertical support.

EM 385-1-1
15 Sep 08

22.H HORSE SCAFFOLDS

22.H.01 Horse scaffolds shall not be constructed or arranged more than two tiers or 10 ft (3 m) in height: scaffolds shall be 5° feet or less in height and 5 ft (1.5 m) or more in width.

22.H.02 The members of horse scaffolds shall not be less than those specified in Table 22-8.

TABLE 22-8

MINIMUM DIMENSIONS FOR HORSE SCAFFOLD MEMBERS

Members	Dimensions
Horizontal members of bearers	3 x 3.9 in (7.6 x 10 cm)
Legs	2 x 3.9 in (5 x 10 cm)
Longitudinal brace between legs	1 x 5.9 in (2.5 x 15 cm)
Gusset brace at top of legs	1 x 7.9 in (2.5 x 20 cm)
Half diagonal braces	2 x 3.9 in (5 x 10 cm)

22.H.03 Horse scaffolds shall be spaced not more than 5 ft (1.5 m) for medium duty and not more than 8 ft (2.4 m) for light duty.

22.H.04 When arranged in tiers, each horse scaffold shall be placed directly over the horse scaffold in the tier below. The legs shall be nailed or otherwise secured to the planks to prevent displacement or thrust and each tier shall be cross braced.

22.I PUMP JACK SCAFFOLDS

22.I.01 Pump jack scaffolds shall not carry a working load exceeding 500 lb (226.8 kg). The components shall not be loaded in excess of the manufacturer's recommended limits.

EM 385-1-1
15 Sep 08

22.I.02 Pump jack brackets, braces, and accessories shall be fabricated from metal plates and angles and installed in accordance with the manufacturer's recommendations. Installation and operational manuals shall be available upon request of the GDA.

22.I.03 Poles.

   a. Pole lumber shall be two 2-in x 4-in (5-cm x 10.1-cm) stock, of Douglas fir, or equivalent, straight-grained, clear, free of cross-grain, shakes, large loose or dead knots, and other defects that might impair strength.

   b. Poles shall not exceed 30 ft (9.1 m) in height.

   c. When poles are constructed of two continuous lengths they shall be of 2-in x 4-in (5-cm x 10.1-cm) stock, spiked together with the seam parallel to the bracket, and with 10d nails, no more than 12 in (30.4 cm) center-to-center, staggered uniformly from opposite outside edges.

   d. If 2-in x 4-in (5-cm x 10.1-cm) stock is spliced to make up the pole, the splices shall be so constructed as to develop the full strength of the member.

   e. Poles shall be secured to the wall by triangular bracing, or equivalent, at the bottom, top, and other points to provide a maximum vertical spacing of not more than 10 ft (3 m) between braces. Each brace shall be capable of supporting a minimum of 225-lb (102-kg) tension or compression.

   f. When wood scaffold planks are used as platforms, poles used for pump jacks shall not be spaced more than 10 ft (3 m) on center. When fabricated platforms are used that comply with all other provisions of this Section, pole spacing may exceed 10 ft on center if permitted by the manufacturer.

22.I.04 Brackets.

a. Each pump jack bracket shall have two positive gripping mechanisms to prevent any failure or slippage.

b. Platform brackets shall be fully decked and the planking secured.

c. For the pump jack bracket to pass bracing already installed, an extra brace shall be used approximately 4 ft (1.2 m) above the one to be passed until the original brace is reinstalled.

22.I.05 Not more than two persons shall be permitted at one time upon a pump jack scaffold between any two supports.

22.I.06 When a work bench is used at an approximate height of 42 in (106.6 cm), the top guardrail may be eliminated if the work bench is fully decked, the planking secured, and is capable of withstanding 200 lb (90.7 kg) pressure in any direction. Employees shall not be permitted to use a workbench as a scaffold platform.

22.I.07 A ladder shall provide access to the platform during use.

22.J ADJUSTABLE SCAFFOLDS

22.J.01 Adjustable scaffolds shall be designed and constructed in accordance with ANSI/SIA A10.8.

22.J.02 A copy of the user's manual shall be kept of site at all times.

22.J.03 Adjustable scaffolds will be secured to the structure in accordance with the manufacturer's user manual.

22.J.04 Safe access will be provided in accordance with Section 24.

22.J.05 The leveling of adjustable scaffold will be accomplished by using leveling jacks.

22.J.06 Bridges will not be permitted on a single tower and used as a "mini-mast climbing scaffold".

22.K CRANE SUPPORTED WORK (PERSONNEL) PLATFORMS. See Section 16.T

22.L ELEVATING WORK PLATFORMS

22.L.01 Elevating work platforms shall be designed and constructed in accordance with ANSI/Scaffold Industry Association (SIA) A92.3, ANSI/SIA A92.5, and ANSI/SIA A92.6, as appropriate.

22.L.02 Elevating work platforms shall be operated, inspected, and maintained as specified in the operating manual for the equipment.

   a. Elevating work platforms shall also comply with requirements of this Section and 18.G.

   b. Records of inspections conducted while the unit is at the work site shall be maintained at the work site.

EM 385-1-1
15 Sep 08

    c. Height to base width ratio of the scaffold during movement is 2:1 or less, or per manufacturer's instructions.

22.L.03 All boom-supported elevating work platforms shall be equipped with an alarm, or other suitable warning device, at the platform. The alarm shall be in operable condition and shall automatically activate when the machine base is more than 5° out of level in any direction.

22.L.04 Only personnel trained in the use of the elevating work platform shall be authorized to operate it. Training shall consist of:

    a. Reading and understanding the manufacturer's operating manual and any associated rules and instructions, or training by a Qualified Person on the contents on these documents, and

    b. Reading and understanding all decals, warnings, and instructions on the elevating work platform.

22.L.05 Before operating the work platform the operator shall:

    a. Survey the work area for loose or soft ground, ditches, drop-offs or holes, bumps and floor obstructions, debris, overhead obstructions, ground and elevated energy sources, and other possible hazards;

    b. Ensure the elevating work platform is on a firm, level surface;

    c. Ensure the work platform is loaded in accordance with the manufacturer's specifications;

    d. Ensure that outriggers and/or stabilizers are used if required by the manufacturer;

    e. Ensure that, if the vehicle is on wheels, the wheels are locked or chocked; and

    f. Ensure that fall protection systems are in place.

EM 385-1-1
15 Sep 08

22.L.06 Elevating work platforms shall not be used by persons working on energized electrical wiring and/or equipment.

22.L.07 The use of personal fall protection devices shall be as specified in the manufacturer's operating manual. Personal fall protection devices, if used, may only be secured to manufacturer-approved hard points. **> See Section 21.J.**

22.M VEHICLE-MOUNTED ELEVATING AND ROTATING WORK PLATFORMS (Aerial Devices/Lifts).

22.M.01 Vehicle-mounted elevating and rotating work platforms (aerial lifts, to include articulating boom platforms/lifts (knuckle boom lifts), trailer-mounted boom lifts) shall be designed and constructed per ANSI/SIA A92.2.

22.M.02 Vehicle-mounted elevating and rotating work platforms shall be operated, inspected, tested, and maintained as specified in the operating manual for that piece of equipment.

   a. Vehicle-mounted elevating and rotating work platforms shall also comply with requirements of this Section and 18.G.

   b. Records of inspections conducted while the unit is at the work site shall be maintained at the work site.

   c. All aerial devices shall have manufacturer's operating manual readily available in or on the vehicle.

   d. If the unit is considered rated, and used as an insulating device, copies of the electrical insulating components and system tests conducted while the unit is at the work site shall be maintained at the work site.

   e. All required safety decals, labels and signs shall be in place and readable.

22.M.03 Only personnel trained in the use of the vehicle-mounted elevating and rotating work platform shall be authorized to operate it. Training shall consist of:

   a. Reading and understanding the manufacturer's operating manual and any associated rules and instructions, or training by a Qualified Person on the contents on these documents; and

   b. Reading and understanding all decals, warnings, and instructions on the vehicle-mounted elevating and rotating work platform.

22.M.04 Transporting.

   a. An aerial lift truck, to include cherry pickers, shall not be moved when the boom is elevated in a working position with personnel in the basket except for equipment that is specifically designed for this type of operation.

   b. Before moving an aerial lift, the boom(s) shall be inspected to see that it is properly cradled and outriggers are in stowed positions, except as provided in a, above.

   c. Aerial ladders shall be secured in the lower traveling position by the locking device on top of the truck cab and the manually operated device at the base of the ladder before the truck is moved for highway travel.

22.M.05 Operating practices.

   a. Brakes shall be set and outriggers, when used, shall be positioned on pads or a solid surface.

   b. Wheel chocks shall be installed before using an aerial lift on an incline.

   c. Lift controls shall be tested each day prior to use to ensure safe working condition.

EM 385-1-1
15 Sep 08

d. Boom and basket load limits specified by manufacturer shall not be exceeded.

e. Articulating boom and extensible boom platforms, primarily designed as personnel carriers, shall have both platform (upper) and lower controls.

(1) Upper controls shall be in or beside the platform within easy reach of the operator.

(2) Lower controls shall provide for overriding the upper controls.

(3) Controls shall be plainly marked as to their function.

(4) Lower level controls shall not be operated unless permission has been obtained from the employee in the lift except in case of emergency.

f. Climbers shall not be worn while performing work from an aerial lift.

g. The insulated portion of an aerial lift shall not be altered in any manner that might reduce its insulating value.

22.M.06 Fall protection.

a. Tying off to an adjacent pole, structure or equipment while working from an aerial lift shall not be permitted.

b. Employees shall always stand firmly on the floor of the basket and shall not sit or climb on the edge of the basket or use planks, ladders, or other devices for a work position.

c. A harness and lanyard, or deceleration device of length or design with a suitable height anchorage such that any fall over the platform edge shall not cause impact with the ground, shall be worn by a worker when working from the basket of a vehicle mounted aerial lift. > *See Section 21.*

22.N MAST CLIMBING WORK PLATFORMS

22.N.01 Mast Climbing work platforms shall be erected, used, inspected, tested, maintained, and repaired in accordance with ANSI A 92.9 and the manufacturer's recommendations as outlined in the operating manual.

22.N.02 An inspection will be performed prior to erecting the work platform.

   a. An overhead inspection will be done to ensure that the work platform will not come in contact with any obstructions while moving up or down the mast. Special attention will be given to high voltage conductors.

   b. An inspection of the ground will be done to ensure that there are no obstacles around the work platform and in the path of travel such as holes, drop-offs, debris, ditches, or soft fill.

   c. Daily maintenance and inspections will be performed and documented. Copies will be maintained on the job site.

22.N.03 Only a designated operator will use the platform.

22.N.04 The platform will not be raised on uneven or sloped surfaces unless outriggers are used to level the platform and the ground is suitable to support the load.

22.N.05 Platforms will not be raised without outriggers extended and locked in proper operating position. The unit will be leveled before raising the platform. **NOTE: Not all Mast Climbing Work Platforms are designed with freestanding capability. Check the machine and manual to see if the machine being operated has a freestanding height.**

22.N.06 The platform must be lowered when moved, and must be set up and leveled each time before it is elevated.

EM 385-1-1
15 Sep 08

22.N.07 A mast climbing work platform, with platform elevated or personnel on the platform, will not be driven. The manufacturer's instructions will be referred to when moving a mast climbing work platform to determine the safe mast height for ground conditions, ground slope, and overhead obstructions.

22.N.08 Mast climbing work platforms will be properly tied to the building (or structure) within the manufacturer's recommended guidelines unless it is designed to be freestanding.

22.N.09 Mast climbing work platforms will not be moved unless everyone on the platform is aware of the direction the platform is being moved.

22.N.10 No ladders or structures of any kind will be used to increase the size or working height of platform.

22.N.11 Climbing of braces and guardrails is prohibited. <u>When access ladders, including masts designed as ladders, exceed 20 ft (6 m) in height, positive fall protection shall be used.</u>

22.N.12 The work platform will not be raised in windy or gusty conditions. The operation manual will be followed to determine maximum in-service wind speed conditions. A copy of the operation manual will be available on the job site.

22.N.13 Platforms will not be altered or modified in any way. Changing the configuration may change load capacity, freestanding height, and tie frequency. Mechanical, hydraulic, or electrical changes may adversely affect operation of this machine.

22.N.14 A Competent Person will perform daily maintenance and inspections.

22.N.15 Training. Personnel will be trained before using and/or operating mast climbing work platforms. Each user and operator will:

a. Read and understand all cautions and danger warnings on the machine and in the operator's manual.

b. Have a solid working understanding of the controls.

c. Understand the hazards associated with the use of mast climbing work platforms.

d. Ensure that only authorized personnel use the platform.

22.N.16 A damaged or malfunctioning machine will not be used. Operation of damaged equipment shall be discontinued until the unit is repaired.

22.O ROOFING BRACKETS

22.O.01 Roofing brackets shall be secured by nailing in addition to the pointed metal projections. Nails will be driven into a rafter or beam; not just into the decking. Fasteners will be selected in accordance with the manufacturer's recommendations.

22.O.02 When it is impractical to nail brackets, rope supports shall be used. When rope supports are used, they shall consist of first-grade manila rope, 3/4 in (1.9 cm) diameter or equivalent.

22.O.03 Positive fall protection will be used when working at heights over six feet.

22.P STILTS

22.P.01 Stilts shall not be used on scaffolds.

22.P.02 Surfaces on which stilts are used shall be flat and free of pits, holes, obstructions, debris and other tripping or slipping hazards.

22.P.03 Stilts shall be properly maintained. Any alteration of the equipment shall be approved by the manufacturer.

22.P.04 Stilts shall not be used on stairs. When used adjacent to stairs or ramps where a fall to a different level could occur, guardrails or other fall protection shall be provided (increased in height by an amount equal to the height of the stilts).

22.P.05 Employees shall be trained in the proper use of stilts.

22.P.06 When using stilts exposes workers to a fall of 6 ft (1.8 m) or more in areas protected by guardrails, the height of the guardrail must be raised accordingly to maintain a protective height of 42 in (107cm) above the stilt. See 21.E.06.

BLANK

SECTION 23

DEMOLITION

23.A GENERAL

23.A.01 Demolition activities shall be performed in accordance with ANSI Standard A10.6, Safety Requirements for Demolition. Surveys and planning shall meet the following:

    a. Prior to initiating demolition activities the following survey and plan shall be accomplished: **> See lead and asbestos requirements in Section 6.B.05.**

    (1) An engineering survey by a Registered Professional Engineer (RPE) of the structure to determine the structure layout, the condition of the framing, floors, walls, the possibility of unplanned collapse of any portion of the structure (any adjacent structure where employees or property may be exposed shall be similarly checked), and the existence of other potential or real demolition hazards.

    (2) A demolition plan - by a RPE and based on the engineering and lead and asbestos surveys - for the safe dismantling and removal of all building components and debris.

    b. The GDA and the Contractor's designated authority shall be provided written evidence that the required surveys have been performed and shall be provided a copy of the demolition plan.

    c. All employees engaged in demolition activities shall be instructed in the demolition plan so that they may conduct their work activities in a safe manner.

23.A.02 All electric, gas, water, steam, sewer, and other service lines shall be shut off, capped, or otherwise controlled outside the building line before demolition is started.

EM 385-1-1
15 Sep 08

a. In each case, any utility company that is involved shall be notified in advance.

b. The Contractor shall provide the GDA and the Contractor's designated authority with an engineering drawing (e.g., site plans, utility plans) that indicates the location of all service lines and the means for their control.

c. If it is necessary to maintain any power, water, or other utilities during demolition, such lines shall be temporarily relocated and protected.

d. If the project includes the abandonment or demolition of existing gas lines, ensure that the existing lines are accurately located and that procedures and installations are accomplished in accordance with applicable sections of 29 CFR 1926.850.

23.A.03 It shall be determined if any hazardous building materials, hazardous chemicals, gases, explosives, flammable materials, or dangerous substances have been used in any building construction, pipes, tanks, or other equipment on the property.

a. When such hazards are identified, testing shall be conducted to determine the type and concentration of the hazardous substance and test results shall be provided to the GDA and the Contractor's designated authority.

b. Such hazards shall be controlled or eliminated before demolition is started.

23.A.04 When employees work within a structure to be demolished that has been damaged by fire, flood, explosion, or other cause, the walls or floor shall be shored or braced.

23.A.05 Work progression.

a. Except for cutting holes in floors for chutes, holes through which to drop materials, preparation of storage space, and similar preparatory work, the demolition of floors and exterior

EM 385-1-1
15 Sep 08

walls shall begin at the top of the structure and proceed downward.

b. Each story of exterior wall and floor construction shall be removed and dropped into the storage space before commencing the removal of exterior walls and floors in the next story below.

23.A.06 Hazards to anyone from the fragmentation of glass shall be controlled.

23.A.07 Mechanical equipment shall not be used on floors on working surfaces unless such floors or surfaces are of sufficient strength to support the imposed load.

23.A.08 Employee entrances to multistory structures being demolished shall be protected by sidewalk sheds, canopies, or both.

a. Protection shall be provided from the face of the building for a minimum of 8 ft (2.4 m).

b. All such canopies shall be at least 2 ft (0.6 m) wider than the building entrances or openings (1 ft (0.3 m) wider on each side), and shall be capable of sustaining a load of 150 psi (1,034.2 kPa).

23.A.09 Only those stairways, passageways, and ladders designated as means of access to the structure shall be used.

a. The designated means of access shall be indicated on the demolition plan. Other access ways shall be indicated as not safe for access and closed at all times.

b. The stairwell shall be covered at a point no less than two floors below the floor on which work is being performed.

EM 385-1-1
15 Sep 08

c. Access to a floor where work is in progress shall be through a separate lighted, protected passageway.

23.A.10 During demolition, continuing inspections by a competent person shall detect hazards resulting from weakened or deteriorated floors, walls, or loosened material. No employee shall be permitted to work where such hazards exist until they are corrected by shoring, bracing, or other means.

23.B DEBRIS REMOVAL

23.B.01 Any chute opening into which debris is dumped shall be protected by a guardrail 42 in (1.1 m) above the floor or other surface on which personnel stand to dump the material. Any space between the chute and the edge of openings in the floors through which it passes shall be covered.

23.B.02 When debris is dropped through openings in the floors without chutes, the openings and the area onto which the material is dropped shall be enclosed with barricades not less than 42 in (1.1 m) high and not less than 6 ft (1.8 m) back from the projected edge of the opening above.

a. Signs warning of the hazard of falling materials shall be posted at each side of the debris opening at each floor.

b. Debris removal shall not be permitted in lower areas until debris handling ceases on the floors above.

23.B.03 All material chutes, or sections thereof, at an angle of more than 45° from the horizontal shall be enclosed, except for openings equipped with closures at or about floor level for the insertion of materials.

a. The openings shall not exceed 48 in (1.2 m) in height measured along the wall of the chute.

b. Such openings, when not in use, shall be kept closed at all floors below the top floor.

23.B.04 A substantial gate shall be installed in each chute at or near the discharge end. A competent employee shall be assigned to control operation of the gate and the backing and loading of trucks.

23.B.05 When operations are not in progress, the area surrounding the discharge end of a chute shall be closed.

23.B.06 Where material is dumped from mechanical equipment or wheelbarrows, a toe board or bumper, not less than 4 in (10 cm) thick and 6 in (15 cm) high, shall be attached at each chute opening.

23.B.07 Chutes shall be designed and constructed of such strength as to eliminate failure due to impact of materials or debris loaded therein.

23.B.08 The storage of waste and debris on any floor shall not exceed the allowable floor loads.

23.B.09 In buildings having wood floor construction, the floor joists may be removed from not more than one floor above grade to provide storage space for debris provided falling material is not permitted to endanger the stability of the structure.

a. When wood floor beams serve to brace interior walls or free-standing exterior walls, such beams shall be left in place until other support can be installed to replace them.

b. Floor arches, to an elevation of not more than 25 ft (7.6 m) above grade, may be removed to provide storage area for debris provided such removal does not endanger the stability of the structure.

c. Storage space into which material is dumped shall be blocked off, except for openings for the removal of materials.

EM 385-1-1
15 Sep 08

Such openings shall be kept closed when material is not being removed.

d. Floor openings shall have curbs or stop-logs to prevent equipment from running over the edge.

e. Any opening cut in a floor for the disposal of materials shall be not longer in size than 25% of the aggregate of the total floor area, unless the lateral supports of the removed flooring remain in place. Floors weakened or otherwise made unsafe by demolition shall be shored to carry safely the intended imposed load for demolition.

23.C WALL REMOVAL

23.C.01 Masonry walls, or sections of masonry, shall not be permitted to fall upon the floors of the building in such masses as to exceed the safe carrying capacities of the floors.

23.C.02 No wall section that is more than 6 ft (1.8 m) in height shall be permitted to stand without lateral bracing, unless such wall was designed and constructed to stand without such lateral support and is in a condition safe enough to be self-supporting. No wall section shall be left standing without lateral bracing any longer than necessary for removal of adjacent debris interfering with demolition of the wall. Exception to this requirement will be allowed for such wall sections that are designed and constructed to stand without lateral support.

23.C.03 Employees shall not be permitted to work on the top of a wall when weather constitutes a hazard.

23.C.04 Structural or load-supporting members on any floor shall not be cut or removed until all stories above such a floor have been demolished and removed. This shall not prohibit the cutting of floor beams for the disposal of materials or for the installation of equipment, providing the requirements of 23.B.09 and 23.D. are met.

EM 385-1-1
15 Sep 08

23.C.05 Floor openings within 10 ft (3 m) of any wall being demolished shall be planked solid, except when employees are kept out of the area below.

23.C.06 In buildings of skeleton-steel construction, the steel framing may be left in place during the demolition of masonry. Where this is done, all steel beams, girders, and structural supports shall be cleared of all loose material as the masonry demolition progresses downward.

23.C.07 Walls that serve as retaining walls to support earth or adjoining structures shall not be demolished until such earth has been braced or adjoining structures have been underpinned.
> *See 23.A.05.*

23.C.08 Walls shall not be used to retain debris unless capable of safely supporting the imposed load.

23.D FLOOR REMOVAL

23.D.01 Openings cut in a floor shall extend the full span of the arch between supports.

23.D.02 Before demolishing any floor arch, debris and other material shall be removed from such arch and other adjacent floor area.

   a. Planks not less than 2-in x 10-in (5-cm x 25.4-cm) in cross section, full sized undressed, shall be provided for and shall be used by employees to stand on while breaking down floor arches between beams.

   b. Such planks shall be so located as to provide a safe support for personnel should the arch between the beams collapse.

   c. Straddle space between planks shall not exceed 16 in (40.6 cm).

EM 385-1-1
15 Sep 08

23.D.03 Safe walkways, not less than 18 in (45.7 cm) wide, formed of wood planks not less than 2 in (5 cm) thick or of equivalent strength, shall be provided and used by personnel when necessary to enable them to reach any point without walking upon exposed beams.

23.D.04 Stringers of ample strength shall support the flooring planks. The ends of such stringers shall be supported by floor beams or girders and not by floor arches alone.

23.D.05 Planks shall be laid together over solid bearings with the ends overlapping at least 1 ft (0.3 m).

23.D.06 When floor arches are being removed, employees shall not be allowed in the area directly underneath. The area shall be barricaded to prevent access and signed to warn of the hazard.

23.E STEEL REMOVAL

23.E.01 When floor arches have been removed, planking shall be provided for the workers razing the steel framing.

23.E.02 Steel construction shall be dismantled column-by-column and tier-by-tier (columns may be in two-story lengths).

23.E.03 Any structural member being dismembered shall not be overstressed.

23.F MECHANICAL DEMOLITION

23.F.01 No person shall be permitted in any area that can be affected by demolition when balling or clamming is being performed. Only those persons necessary for the operations shall be permitted in this area at any other time.

23.F.02 The weight of the demolition ball shall not exceed 50% of the crane's rated load, based on the length of the boom and the maximum angle of operation at which the demolition ball will be

EM 385-1-1
15 Sep 08

used, or it shall not exceed 25% of the nominal breaking strength of the line by which it is suspended, whichever is less.

23.F.03 The crane boom and load line shall be as short as possible.

23.F.04 The ball shall be attached to the load line with a swivel connection to prevent twisting of the load line and shall be attached by positive means so that the weight cannot accidentally disconnect.

23.F.05 When pulling over walls or portions of walls, all steel members affected shall have been cut free.

23.F.06 All roof cornices or other ornamental stonework shall be removed prior to pulling walls over.

BLANK

EM 385-1-1
15 Sep 08

SECTION 24

SAFE ACCESS, LADDERS, FLOOR & WALL OPENINGS, STAIRS AND RAILING SYSTEMS

24.A SAFE ACCESS - GENERAL

24.A.01 Safe access shall be provided to work areas and where danger exists of workers falling through floor, roof, or wall openings, or from platforms, runways, ramps, or fixed stairs.

   a. A stairway, ladder, ramp, or personnel hoist shall be provided where there is a break of 19 in (48.2 cm) or more in a route of access.

   b. Means of access constructed of metal shall not be used for electrical work or where the potential exists to contact electrical conductors.

   c. Means of access between levels shall be kept clear to allow free passage of workers. If work is performed in an area that restricts free passage, a second means of access shall be provided.

   d. For all USACE-owned/operated facilities, every open-sided floor or platform 4 ft (1.2 m) or more above adjacent floor or ground level shall be guarded by a railing system (or equivalent) along all open sides (except where there is an entrance to a ramp, stairway or fixed ladder. The railing system shall be provided with a toeboard when necessary. **> See 21.E.01.**

24.A.02 An AHA, accepted by the GDA for the activity in which means of access are to be used shall delineate the following:

   a. The design, construction, and maintenance of the means of access, and

EM 385-1-1
15 Sep 08

b. Erection and dismantling procedures of scaffolds, including provisions for providing fall protection during the erection or dismantling when the erection or dismantling involves work at heights. See Sections 21.J.02, Fall Protection; and 22.A.03, Work Platforms.

24.A.03 Job-made means of access shall be designed to support, without failure, at least four times the maximum intended load and shall be constructed according to Section 22 of this manual.

24.A.04 Means of access shall not be loaded beyond the maximum intended load for which they were designed or beyond their manufacture rated capacity. When loaded, planking and decking shall not deflect more than 1/60 the span length.

24.A.05 The width of access ways shall be determined by the purpose for which they are built, shall be sufficient to provide safe passage for materials and movement of personnel and (except for ladders) shall not be less than 18 in (45.7 cm).

24.A.06 Access ways shall have overhead protection equal to 2 in (5 cm) solid planking whenever work is performed over them or if personnel are exposed to hazards from falling objects.

24.A.07. Access ways shall be inspected daily.

a. The walkway must be free of tripping hazards, obstructions and cannot impede or restrict the travel of personnel. In addition, access ways shall be kept free of ice, snow, grease and mud or any other environmental hazards.

b. Where access ways are slippery, abrasive material shall be used to assure safe footing.

c. All obstructions or projections into an access way shall be removed or conspicuously marked. Obstructions or projections that are sharp, pointed or that may cause lacerations, contusions, or abrasions shall be covered with protective material.

EM 385-1-1
15 Sep 08

d. Access ways, including their accessories that become damaged or weakened shall not be used. These defective items shall be repaired or replaced.

24.A.08 When moving platforms to the next level, the old platform shall be left undisturbed until the new bearers have been set to receive the platform planks.

24.A.09 Safe Roof Access.

a. Level, guarded platforms shall be provided at the landing area on the roof.

b. Crawling boards.

(1) Crawling boards shall be not less than 10 in (25 cm) wide and 1 in (2.5 cm) thick, having cleats 1 in x 1.5 in (2.5 cm x 3.75 cm).

(2) Cleats shall be equal in length to the width of the board and spaced at equal intervals not to exceed 24 in (60 cm).

(3) Nails shall be driven through and clinched on the underside. Screws may be used in lieu of nails.

(4) Crawling boards shall be secured and extend from the ridge pole to the eaves when used with roof construction, repairs, or maintenance.

(5) A firmly fastened lifeline of at least 0.75 in (2 cm) diameter rope, or equivalent, shall be strung beside each crawling board for a handhold.

c. Access paths shall be erected as follows:

(1) Points of access, materials handling areas and storage areas shall be connected to the work area by a clear access path formed by two warning lines.

EM 385-1-1
15 Sep 08

(2) When the path to a point of access is not being used, one of the following shall be used:

(a) A rope, wire, or chain, equal in strength and height to the warning line, shall be placed across the path at the point where the path intersects the warning line erected around the work area, or

(b) The path shall be offset such that a person cannot walk directly into the work area.

24.B LADDERS

24.B.01 The construction, installation, and use of ladders shall conform to ANSI A14.1, ANSI A14.2, ANSI A14.3, and ANSI A14.4, as applicable.

24.B.02 Length of ladders.

a. All portable ladders shall be of sufficient length and shall be placed so that workers will not stretch or assume a hazardous position.

b. Portable ladders, used as temporary access, shall extend at least 3 ft (0.9 m) above the upper landing surface.

(1) When a 3 ft (0.9-m) extension is not possible, a grasping device (such as a grab rail) shall be provided to assist workers in mounting and dismounting the ladder.

(2) In no case shall the length of the ladder be such that ladder deflection under a load would, by itself, cause the ladder to slip from its support.

c. The length of portable stepladders shall not exceed 20 ft (6 m).

EM 385-1-1
15 Sep 08

    d. When splicing of side rails is required to obtain the required length, the resulting side rail must be at least equal in strength to a one-piece side rail made of the same material.

24.B.03 Width of ladders.

    a. The minimum clear distance between the sides of individual-rung/step ladders shall be 16 in (40.6 cm).

    b. The minimum clear distance between side rails for all portable ladders shall be 12 in (30.4 cm).

24.B.04 Spacing of rungs, cleats, and steps on ladders.

    a. On portable ladders, spacing of rungs shall be 8 in (20.3 cm) - 14 in (35.5 cm) on center and uniform.

    b. On step stools, spacing shall be not less than 8 in (20.3 cm) or more than 12 in (30.4 cm) apart, as measured from their centerlines.

    c. On extension trestle ladders, spacing on the base section shall be not less than 8 in (20.3 cm) or more than 18 in (45.7 cm) apart, as measured from their centerlines. On the extension section, spacing shall not be less than 6 in (15.2 cm) or more than 12 in (30.4 cm) apart, as measured from their centerlines.

24.B.05 Ladders shall be surfaced so as to prevent injury to an worker from punctures or lacerations and to prevent snagging of clothing.

24.B.06 Wooden ladders shall not be coated with any opaque covering, except for identification or warning labels that may be placed on only one face of a side rail.

EM 385-1-1
15 Sep 08

24.B.07 A metal spreader bar or locking device shall be provided on each stepladder to hold the front and back sections in an open position.

24.B.08 Set-up of ladders.

   a. Ladders shall not be placed in passageways, doorways, drives, or any locations where they may be displaced by any other work unless protected by barricades or guards.

   b. Portable ladders shall be used at such a pitch that the horizontal distance from the top support to the foot of the ladder will not be greater than   the vertical distance between these points.

   c. Wooden job-made ladders, with spliced rails, shall be used at an angle such that the horizontal distance is 1/8 the length of the ladder.

   d. Ladders shall be secured by top, bottom, and intermediate fastenings, as necessary to hold them rigidly in place and to support the loads that will be imposed upon them.

   e. The steps or rungs of all ladders shall be set to provide at least 7 in (17.7 cm) toe space from the inside edge of the rung to the nearest interference.

   f. The top of a non-self supporting ladder shall be placed with the two rails supported equally, unless the ladder is equipped with a single support attachment.

   g. Step-across distance. The step-across distance from the nearest edge of ladder to the nearest edge of equipment or structure shall be not more than 12 in (30.5 cm) or less than 2-1/2 in (6.4 cm).

EM 385-1-1
15 Sep 08

24.B.09 Use of ladders.

a. Ladders shall be restricted to their intended use.

b. Ladders shall be inspected for visible defects on a daily basis and after any occurrence that could affect their safe use. Broken or damaged ladders shall be immediately tagged "**DO NOT USE**," or with similar wording, and withdrawn from service until restored to a condition meeting their original design.

c. Ladders shall not be moved, shifted, or extended while occupied.

d. Ladders shall not be climbed by more than one person at a time, unless it is designed to be climbed by more than one person.

e. Portable ladders used as means of access to ascend and descend to a work location do not require fall protection, however only light work for short periods of time shall be performed on portable ladders. No work requiring lifting of heavy materials or substantial exertion shall be done from ladders.

f. When ladders are the only means of access to or from a working area for 25 or more workers, or when a ladder is to serve simultaneous two-way traffic, double-cleated ladders shall be used.

g. Portable ladders shall have slip-resistant feet.

h. The top or top step of a stepladder, shall not be used, as a step unless it has been designed to be so used by the manufacturer.

i. Ensure latches are in place before climbing an extension ladder.

j. Keep loose tools off the steps and top platform.

24.B.10 Job made ladders will be made in accordance with ANSI A14.4.

24.B.11 Single-rail ladders shall not be used. Three-legged ladders may be used for specific tasks, if accepted by the GDA.

24.B.12 The use of ladder climbing devices shall be in accordance with 21.I.

24.B.13 Articulated ladders are allowed if they meet ANSI A14.2 standard.

24.B.14 Any ladder accessory, including but not limited to, ladder levelers, ladder stabilizers or stand-off devices, ladder jacks or ladder straps or hooks, that may be installed or used in conjunction with ladders must be installed and used per manufacturer's instructions.

24.C HANDRAILS

24.C.01 A standard handrail shall be of construction similar to a standard guardrail (reference Section 21.E.01) except that it is mounted on a wall or partition and does not include a midair.

24.C.02 Handrails shall have smooth surfaces along the top and both sides.

24.C.03 Handrails shall have an adequate handhold for anyone grasping it to avoid falling.

24.C.04 Ends of handrails shall be turned into the supporting wall or partition or otherwise arranged so as to not constitute a projection hazard.

24.C.05 The height of handrails shall be not more than 38 in (86.3 cm) nor less than 34 in (76.2 cm) from upper surface of handrail to

EM 385-1-1
15 Sep 08

surface of tread, in line with face of riser or to surface of ramp. Existing installations need not be modified if they meet the building code that was in effect at the time the facility was built.

24.C.06 All handrails and railings shall be provided with a clearance of approximately 3 in (7.6 cm) between the handrail or railing and any other object.

24.D FLOOR, WALL AND ROOF HOLES AND OPENINGS.

24.D.01 Floor and roof holes/openings are any that measure over 2 in (51 mm) in any direction of a walking/working surface which persons may trip or fall into or where objects may fall to the level below. See 21.F for covering and labeling requirements.

< *Skylights located in floors or roofs are considered floor or roof hole/openings.*

24.D.02 All floor, roof openings or hole into which a person can accidentally walk or fall through shall be guarded either by a railing system with toeboards along all exposed sides or a load-bearing cover. When the cover is not in place, the opening or hole shall be protected by a removable guardrail system or shall be attended when the guarding system has been removed, or other fall protection system. See Sections 21.E and 21.F.

24.D.03 All floor and roof holes through which equipment, materials, or debris can fall shall be covered.

24.D.04 Conduits, trenches, and manhole covers and their supports, when exposed to vehicles or equipment, shall be designed to carry a truck rear axle load of 2 times the maximum anticipated load.

24.D.05 Every hatchway and chute floor opening shall be guarded by a hinged floor-opening cover. The opening shall be barricaded with railings so as to leave only one exposed side. The exposed side shall be provided either with a swinging gate or offset so that a person cannot walk into the opening. When operating conditions

EM 385-1-1
15 Sep 08

require the feeding of material into a hatchway or chute opening, protection shall be provided to prevent a person from falling through the opening.

24.D.06 Wall openings from which a fall could occur shall be protected with a standard guardrail or equivalent. A toe board shall be provided where the bottom of the wall opening, regardless of width, is less than 4 in (10.1 cm) above the working surface. See Section 21.E.01.

24.D.07 An extension platform outside a wall opening onto which materials can be hoisted for handling shall have a standard railing that meets criteria in Section 21.E.01 of this manual. However, one side of an extension platform may have removable railings to facilitate handling materials, if appropriate fall protection is used.

24.D.08 Roof openings and holes shall be provided with covers, guardrail systems or warning lines systems on all exposed sides.

    a. Roofing material, such as roofing membrane, insulation or felts, covering or partly covering openings or holes, shall be immediately cut out. No hole or opening shall be left unattended unless covered according to Section 21.F.

    b. All covers for openings shall be identified in accordance with Section 21.F.

    c. Non-load-bearing skylights shall be guarded by a load-bearing skylight screen, cover, or railing system along all exposed sides.

    d. Workers are prohibited from standing/walking on skylights.

EM 385-1-1
15 Sep 08

24.E STAIRWAYS

24.E.01 On all structures 20 ft (6 m) or more in height, stairways shall be provided during construction.

>   a. Where permanent stairways are not installed concurrently with the construction of each floor, a temporary stairway shall be provided to the work level.
>
>   b. Alternatives to the use of stairways shall be addressed in the AHA and shall be acceptable to the GDA.

24.E.02 Design of stairways.

>   a. Temporary stairways shall have landings not less than 30 in (76.2 cm) in the direction of travel and extend at least 22 in (55.8 cm) in width at every 12 ft (3.6 m) or less of vertical rise.
>
>   b. Stairs shall be installed between 30° and 50° from horizontal.
>
>   c. Risers shall be of uniform height and treads of uniform width.

24.E.03 Metal pan landings and metal pan treads, when used, shall be secured in place and filled with concrete, wood, or other material at least to the top of each pan.

24.E.04 Wooden treads shall be nailed in place.

24.E.05 Every flight of stairs with four or more risers or rising more than 30 in (76.2 cm) shall have standard stair railings (defined below) or standard handrails unless omitted by design.

>   a. On stairways less than 44 in (111.7 cm) wide having both sides enclosed, at least one standard handrail shall be installed, preferably on the right descending side.

b. On stairways less than 44 in (111.7 cm) wide having one side open, at least one standard stair railing shall be installed on the open side.

c. On stairways less than 44 in (111.7 cm) wide having both sides open, one standard stair railing shall be installed on each side.

d. On stairways more than 44 in (111.7 cm) wide, but less than 88 in (223.5 cm) wide, one standard handrail shall be installed on each enclosed side, and one standard stair railing installed on each open side.

e. On stairways more than 88 in (223.5 cm) wide, one standard handrail shall be installed on each enclosed side, one standard stair railing on each exposed side, and a standard handrail in the middle of the stairway.

24.E.06 Standard stair railing shall be installed around all stairwells.

a. The height of stair rails shall be 42+/- 3 in (cm) from the upper surface of the top rail to surface of tread in line with face of riser at forward edge of tread. Existing installations need not be modified. Existing installations need not be modified.

b. Midrails, screens, mesh, intermediate vertical members, or equivalent intermediate structural members shall be provided between the toprail and the stairway steps.

(1) Midrails shall be located at a height midway between the top edge of the stairway system and the stairway steps.

(2) Screens or mesh, when used, shall extend from the toprail to the stairway steps and along the entire opening between rail supports.

(3) Intermediate vertical members, when used, shall be not more than 19 in (48.2 cm) apart.

(4) Other structural members, when used, shall be installed in such a manner that there are no openings in the stair rail system that are more than 19 in (48.2 cm) wide.

24.E.07 Doors or gates opening onto a stairway shall have a platform; and swinging of the door shall not reduce the width of the platform to less than 20 in (50.8 cm).

24.E.08 Spiral stairways shall not be permitted, except for special limited usage and secondary access where it is not practical to provide a conventional stairway.

24.E.09 Three points of contact shall be maintained at all times when ascending or descending spiral stairs, ship stairs, or alternating tread stairs. Three point contact means that either both hands and one foot, or both feet and one hand are in contact with the climbing device at all times.

24.F RAMPS, RUNWAYS, AND TRESTLES

24.F.01 Ramps, runways, and platforms shall be as flat as conditions will permit. Where the slope exceeds 1ft:5 ft (0.3 m:1.5m), traverse cleats shall be applied to the working surface.

24.F.02 Vehicle ramps, trestles, and bridges on which foot traffic is permitted shall be provided with a walkway and guardrail outside the roadway. The roadway structures shall be provided with wheel guards, fender logs, or curbs not less than 8 in (20.3 cm) high placed parallel and secured to the sides of the runway.

24.F.03 All locomotive and gantry crane trestles that extend into or pass over a work area, except where a crane is hoisting between rails, shall be decked solid with not less than 2-in (5-cm) planking, or the equivalent, for the full length of the extension into the working area.

24.F.04 When used in lieu of steps, ramps shall be provided with cleats to ensure safe access.

EM 385-1-1
15 Sep 08

24.G PERSONNEL HOISTS AND ELEVATORS

24.G.01 Design, construction, installation or erection, operation, inspection, testing, and maintenance of personnel hoists and elevators shall be in accordance with the manufacturer's recommendations and the applicable ANSI standard.

   a. Track-guided personnel hoist systems and structures that are temporarily installed inside or outside buildings during construction, alteration, or demolition shall be in compliance with ANSI A10.4;

   b. Rope-guided personnel hoist systems that are temporarily erected during construction, alteration, or demolition shall be in compliance with ANSI A10.22;

   c. Non-guided personnel hoist systems that are temporarily erected during construction, alteration, or demolition shall be in compliance with ANSI A10.8 and ANSI A10.22. (An air-tugger hoist, or the equivalent meeting the criteria in section 4.2 of ANSI A10.22, may by substituted for a base-mounted hoist.)

   d. Elevators operating in permanent hoistways on the permanent guide rails for handling personnel during construction shall be in compliance with ANSI/ASME A17.1

   e. A copy of the manufacturer's manual covering construction, installation or erection, operation, inspection, testing, and maintenance and a copy of the applicable ANSI standard shall be available on site.

   f. Personnel hoists and elevators shall comply with applicable requirements from Section 16 of this manual.

24.G.02 Personnel hoists used in bridge tower construction shall be approved by a registered engineer and erected under the supervision of a registered engineer competent in this field.

EM 385-1-1
15 Sep 08

SECTION 25

EXCAVATION AND TRENCHING

25.A GENERAL

25.A.01 Excavation/Trenching Plan. An Excavation/Trenching Plan will be submitted and accepted by the GDA prior to beginning operations. At a minimum, the plan shall include:

a. Conditions: For excavations/trenches less than 5 ft (1.5 m) in depth, an AHA is required; plan is optional. For excavations or trenches greater than 5 ft (1.5 m) in depth an AHA and plan are required;

b. Identification and credentials of Competent Person;

c. Diagram or sketch of the area where the work is to be done, with adjacent and nearby structures shown;

d. Projected depth of the excavation;

e. Projected soil type and method of testing to determine soil type;

f. Planned method of shoring, sloping and/or benching;

g. Planned method for confined space entry, trench access and egress and atmospheric monitoring processes;

h. Location of utility shut offs (if required);

i. Proposed methods for preventing damage to overhead utility lines, trees designated to remain, and other man-made facilities or natural features designated to remain within or adjacent to the construction rights-of-way;

j. Plan for management of excavated soil/asphalt/concrete;

EM 385-1-1
15 Sep 08

k. Plan for traffic control;

l. Digging permits (Excavation permits). All underground lines/utilities (communication lines, water, fuel, electric lines) shall be located and protected from damage or displacement. Utility companies and other responsible authorities shall be contacted to locate and mark the locations and, if they so desire, direct or assist with protecting the underground installations. The Contractor shall obtain a "Digging Permit" (excavation permit) from Base Civil Engineers or other authority having jurisdiction prior the initiation of any excavation work. Requests for the permits will be processed through the GDA.

m. Certification of UXO clearance. Where excavations are to be performed in areas known or suspected to contain explosives, unexploded munitions, or military ordnance, surface and subsurface clearance by qualified explosive ordnance disposal (EOD) personnel shall be accomplished prior to excavation work.

n. For Cofferdams: Controlled flooding plan, Fall protection, Access/egress; Evacuation procedures.

25.A.02 Excavation inspection and testing.

a. When persons will be in or around an excavation, a Competent Person shall inspect the excavation, the adjacent areas, and protective systems daily: before each work shift; throughout the work shifts as dictated by the work being done; after every rainstorm; after other events that could increase hazards, e.g., snowstorm, windstorm, thaw, earthquake, etc.; when fissures, tension cracks, sloughing, undercutting, water seepage, bulging at the bottom or other similar conditions occur; when there is a change in size, location or placement of the spoil pile; and where there is any indication or change in adjacent structures.

EM 385-1-1
15 Sep 08

b. The Competent Person shall be able to demonstrate the following:

(1) Training, experience, and knowledge of:

(a) Soil analysis;

(b) Use of protective systems; and

(c) Requirements of this section, EM 385-1-1 and 29 CFR 1926 Subpart P.

(2) Ability to detect:

(a) Conditions that could result in cave-ins;

(b) Failures in protective systems;

(c) Hazardous atmospheres; and

(d) Other hazards including those associated with confined spaces.

(3) And have the Authority to take prompt corrective measures to eliminate existing and predictable hazards and stop work when required.

c. Testing for soil classification shall be of an approved method; pocket pentrometer, plasticity/ wet threadtest or visual test and shall be conducted at least daily or if conditions warrant as described in paragraph 25.A.02.a. above.

d. If evidence of a situation that could result in possible cave-ins, slides, failure of protective systems, hazardous atmospheres, or other hazardous condition is identified, exposed workers shall be removed from the hazard and all work in the excavation stopped until all necessary safety precautions have been implemented.

EM 385-1-1
15 Sep 08

    e. In locations where oxygen deficiency or gaseous conditions are known or suspected, or in excavations 4 ft (1.2 m) or greater in depth, air in the excavation shall be tested prior to the start of each shift or more often if directed by the GDA. A log of all test results shall be maintained at the work site. **> See Sections 5 and 6.**

25.A.03 Protective systems.

    a. The sides of all excavations in which employees are exposed to danger from moving ground shall be guarded by a support system, sloping or benching of the ground, or other equivalent means.

    b. Excavations less than 5 ft (1.5 m) in depth and which a Competent Person examines and determines there to be no potential for cave-in do not require protective systems, however, a fixed means of egress shall be provided.

    c. Sloping or benching of the ground shall be in accordance with 25.C.

    d. Support systems shall be in accordance with 25.D.

    e. Protective systems shall have the capacity to resist without failure all loads that are intended or could reasonably be expected to be applied to the system.

    f. Shoring shall be used for unstable soil or depths greater than 5 ft (>1.5 m) unless benching, sloping, or other acceptable plan is implemented by the Contractor and accepted by the GDA.

25.A.04 Stability of adjacent structures.

    a. Except in stable rock, excavations below the level of the base of footing of any foundation or retaining wall shall not be permitted unless:

EM 385-1-1
15 Sep 08

(1) A support system, such as underpinning, is provided to ensure the stability of the structure and to protect employees involved in the excavation work or in the vicinity thereof; or

(2) A Registered Professional Engineer (RPE) has approved the determination that the structure is sufficiently removed from the excavation so as to be unaffected by the excavation and that the excavation will not pose a hazard to employees.

b. If the stability of adjoining buildings or walls is endangered by excavations, shoring, bracing, or underpinning designed by a qualified person shall be provided to ensure the stability of the structure and to protect employees.

c. Sidewalks, pavements, and related structures shall not be undermined unless a support system is provided to protect employees and the sidewalk, pavement, or related structure.

25.A.05 Where it is necessary to undercut the side of an excavation, overhanging material shall be safely supported.

25.A.06 Protection from water.

a. Diversion ditches, dikes, or other means shall be used to prevent surface water entering an excavation and to provide good drainage of the area adjacent to the excavation.

b. Employees shall not work in excavations in which there is accumulated water or in which water is accumulating unless the water hazards posed by accumulation is controlled.

(1) Freezing, pumping, drainage, and similar control measures shall be planned and directed by a registered engineer. Consideration shall be given to the existing moisture balances in surrounding soils and the effects on foundations and structures if it is disturbed.

(2) When continuous operation of ground water control equipment is necessary, an emergency power source shall be

EM 385-1-1
15 Sep 08

provided. Water control equipment and operations shall be monitored by a Competent Person to ensure proper operation.

25.A.07 Protection from falling material.

a. Employees shall be protected (by scaling, ice removal, benching, barricading, rock bolting, wire mesh, or other means) from loose rock or soil that could create a hazard by falling from the excavation wall: special attention shall be given to slopes that may be adversely affected by weather, moisture content, or vibration.

b. Materials, such as boulders or stumps, that may slide or roll into the excavation shall be removed or made safe.

c. Excavated material shall be placed at least 2 ft (0.6 m) from the edge of an excavation or shall be retained by devices that are sufficient to prevent the materials from falling into the excavation. In any case, material shall be placed at a distance to prevent excessive loading on the face of the excavation.

25.A.08 Mobile equipment and motor vehicle precautions.

a. When vehicles or mobile equipment are used or allowed adjacent to an excavation, substantial stop logs or barricades shall be installed. The use of a ground guide is recommended.

b. Workers shall stand away from vehicles being loaded or unloaded to avoid being struck by spillage or falling materials.

c. Excavating or hoisting equipment shall not be allowed to raise, lower, or swing loads over <u>or adjacent to</u> personnel in the excavation without substantial overhead protection. <u>Personnel shall maintain a safe distance from hoisting operation until the load has been placed.</u>

d. <u>Employees exposed to public vehicular traffic shall be provided with, and shall wear, high visibility apparel as per Section 05.F.</u>

EM 385-1-1
15 Sep 08

25.A.09 Employees shall not be permitted to work on the faces of sloped or benched excavations at levels above other employees except when employees at lower levels are adequately protected from the hazard of falling material or equipment.

25.A.10 When operations approach the location of underground utilities, excavation shall progress with caution until the exact location of the utility is determined. Workers shall be protected from the utility and the utility shall be protected from damage or displacement.

25.A.11 <u>Employees entering excavations classified as confined spaces or that otherwise present the potential for emergency rescue such as bell-bottom pier holes or similar deep and confined footing, shall wear rescue equipment and maintain communication with the (confined space) attendant.</u> **> See Section 34.**

25.B SAFE ACCESS

25.B.01 Protection shall be provided to prevent personnel, vehicles, and equipment from falling into excavations. Protection shall be provided according to the following hierarchy **> See Appendix Q for definitions of Perimeter protection: Class I, Class II, and Class III.**

   a. If the excavation is exposed to members of the public or vehicles or equipment, then Class I perimeter protection is required;

   b. If the excavation does not meet the requirements for Class I perimeter protection but is (1) routinely exposed to employees, and (2) either is deeper than 6 ft (1.8 m) or (3) contains hazards (e.g., impalement hazards, hazardous substances), then Class II perimeter protection is the minimum protection required. When workers are in the zone between the warning barricades/flagging and the excavation, they shall be provided with fall protection as specified in Section 21;

EM 385-1-1
15 Sep 08

    c. If the excavation does not meet the requirements for either Class I or Class II perimeter protection, then Class III perimeter protection is the minimum protection required.

25.B.02 All wells, calyx holes, pits, shafts, etc., shall be barricaded or covered.

25.B.03 Excavations shall be backfilled as soon as possible. Upon completion of exploration and similar operations, test pits, temporary wells, calyx holes, etc., shall be backfilled immediately.

25.B.04 Walkways or bridges shall be provided <u>with standard guardrails</u> where people or equipment are required or permitted to cross over excavations.

25.B.05 Where personnel are required to enter excavations/trenches over 4 ft (1.2 m) in depth, sufficient stairs, ramps, or ladders shall be provided to require no more than 25 ft (7.6 m) of lateral travel.

    a. At least two means of exit shall be provided for personnel working in excavations. Where the width of the excavation exceeds 100 ft (30.4 m), two or more means of exit shall be provided on each side of the excavation.

    b. When access to excavations in excess of 20 ft (6 m) in depth is required, ramps, stairs, or mechanical personnel hoists shall be provided.

25.B.06 Ramps *<See 24.B. and 24.F.*

    a. Ramps used solely for personnel access shall be a minimum width of 4 ft (1.2 m) and provided with standard guardrails.

    b. Ramps used for equipment access shall be a minimum width of 12 ft (3.6 m). Curbs not less than 8-in x 8-in (20.3-cm x 20.3-cm) timbers, or equivalent protection, shall be provided. Equipment ramps shall be designed and constructed in accordance with accepted engineering practice.

25.B.07 Ladders used as access ways shall extend from the bottom of the excavation to not less than 3 ft (0.9 m) above the surface.

25.C SLOPING AND BENCHING.

25.C.01 Sloping or benching of the ground shall be in accordance with one of the systems outlined in a through d below as per OSHA (*29 CFR 1926, Subpart P, Appendix B*): **> See Figure 25-1.**

a. For excavations less than 20 ft (6 m) in depth, the maximum slope shall be 34° measured from the horizontal (1-1/2 horizontal to 1 vertical).

b. All excavations less than 20 ft (6m) in depth which have vertically lowered portions shall be shielded or supported to a height at least 18 in (.5 m) above the top of the vertical side with a maximum allowable slope of 1-1/2:1.

c. The design shall be selected from and be in accordance with written tabulated data, such as charts and tables approved by a RPE. At least one copy of the tabulated data shall be maintained at the job site during excavation. The tabulated data shall include:

(1) Identification of the parameters that affect the selection of a sloping or benching system drawn from the data;

(2) Identification of the limits of use of the data, to include the magnitude and configuration of slopes determined to be safe;

(3) Explanatory information as may be necessary to aid the user in correctly selecting a protective system from the data; and

(4) The identity of the RPE who approved the data.

EM 385-1-1
15 Sep 08

d. The sloping or benching system shall be designed by a RPE. At least one copy of the design shall be maintained at the job site during excavation. Designs shall be in writing and include:

(1) The magnitudes and configurations of the slopes that were determined to be safe for the particular excavation, and

(2) The identity of the RPE who approved the design.

25.D SUPPORT SYSTEMS

25.D.01 Support systems shall be in accordance with one of the systems outlined in a through c below:

a. Designs drawn from manufacturer's tabulated data shall be in accordance with all specifications, limitations, and recommendations issued or made by the manufacturer.

(1) Deviation from the specifications, recommendations, and limitations are only allowed after the manufacturer issues specific written approval.

(2) A copy of the manufacturer's specifications, recommendations, and limitations (and the manufacturer's approval to deviate from these, if required) shall be in written form and maintained at the job site during excavation.

b. Designs shall be selected from and be in accordance with tabulated data (such as tables and charts). At least one copy of the tabulated data shall be maintained at the job site during excavation. The tabulated data shall include:

(1) Identification of the parameters that affect the selection of the protective system drawn from such data,

(2) Identification of the limits of use of the data, and

EM 385-1-1
15 Sep 08

(3) Explanatory information as may be necessary to aid the user in correctly selecting a protective system from the data, and

(4) The identity of the RPE who approved the data.

c. Designed by a RPE. At least one copy of the design shall be maintained at the job site during excavation. Designs shall be in writing and include:

(1) A plan indicating the sizes, types, and configurations of the materials to be used in the protective system, and

(2) The identity of the RPE who approved the design.

25.D.02 Materials and equipment used for protective systems.

a. Materials and equipment shall be free from damage or defects that might impair their proper function.

b. Manufactured materials and equipment shall be used and maintained in a manner consistent with the recommendations of the manufacturer and in a manner that will prevent employee exposure to hazards.

c. When material or equipment is damaged, a Competent Person shall examine the material or equipment and evaluate its suitability for continued use.

25.D.03 Installation and removal of support systems **> See Examples of Support Systems at Figures 25-1 through 25-3.**

a. Members of support systems shall be securely connected together to prevent sliding, falling, kickouts, or other predictable failure.

EM 385-1-1
15 Sep 08

b. Support systems shall be installed and removed in manners that protect employees from cave-ins, structural collapses, or from being struck by members of the support system.

c. Individual members of a support system shall not be subjected to loads exceeding those <u>for</u> which they were designed to withstand.

d. Before temporary removal of individual members, additional precautions shall be taken to ensure the safety of employees, such as installing other structural members to carry the loads imposed on the support system.

e. Removal shall begin at and progress from the bottom of the excavation. Members shall be released slowly as to note any indication of possible failure of the remaining members or possible cave-in of the sides of the excavation.

f. Backfilling shall progress together with the removal of support systems from excavations.

g. <u>For trench excavations: excavation material shall be permitted to a level not greater than 2 ft (.6 m) below the bottom of the members of a support system, only if the system is designed to resist the forces calculated for the full depth of the trench, and there is no indication while the trench is open of a possible loss of soil from behind or below the bottom of the support system.</u>

25.D.04 Shield systems.

a. <u>Shield systems shall not be subjected to loads exceeding those that the system was designed to withstand.</u>

b. Shields shall be installed in a manner to restrict lateral or other hazardous movement of the shield in the event of the application of sudden lateral loads.

c. Employees shall be protected from the hazard of cave-ins when entering or exiting the area protected by shields.

d. Employees shall not be allowed in shields when shields are being installed, removed, or moved vertically.

e. For shield systems used in trench excavations: excavations of earth material to a level not greater than 2 ft (.6 m) below the bottom of the shield shall be permitted, only if the shield is designed to resist the forces calculated for the full depth of the trench, and there is no indications while the trench is open of a possible loss of soil from behind or below the bottom of the shield.

25.D.05 Additional requirements for trenching.

a. Installation of support systems shall be closely coordinated with excavations of trenches.

b. Bracing or shoring of trenches shall be carried along with the excavation.

c. Backfilling and removal of trench supports should progress together from the bottom of the trench. Jacks or braces shall be released slowly and, in unstable soil, ropes shall be used to pull out the jacks or braces from above after personnel have cleared the trench. > *See Examples of Jacks at Figure 25-3.*

d. Excavation of material to a level no greater than 2 ft (0.6 m) below the bottom of the members of a trench support system (including a shield) shall be permitted, only if the system is designed to resist the forces calculated for the full depth of the trench and there are no indications while the trench is open of a possible loss of soil from behind or below the bottom of the support system.

EM 385-1-1
15 Sep 08

25.E COFFERDAMS

25.E.01 If overtopping of the cofferdams by high water is possible, design shall include provisions for controlled flooding of the work area.

25.E.02 If personnel or equipment are required or permitted on cofferdams, standard railings, or equivalent protection, shall be provided.

<u>25.E.03 Walkways, bridges, or ramps with at least two means of rapid exit, with standard guardrails, shall be provided for personnel and equipment working on cofferdams</u>.

25.E.04 A plan (including warning signals) for evacuation of personnel and equipment in case of emergency and for controlled flooding shall be developed and posted.

25.E.05 Cofferdams located close to navigable shipping channels shall be protected from vessels in transit.

TABLE 25-1

SOIL CLASSIFICATION*

Soil Type	Criteria	Other Considerations
Stable Rock	Natural solid mineral that can be excavated with vertical sides and remain intact while exposed.	
Type A	Cohesive soil with an unconfined compressive strength of 1.5 tons per square foot (tsf) (144 kPa) or greater.	Can **not** be Type A if soil is: 1) fissured; 2) subject to vibration from heavy traffic, pile driving, etc.; 3) previously disturbed; 4) part of sloped, layered system where layers dip into excavation on a slope of 4H:1V or greater; or 5) subject to other factors requiring it to be classified as less stable material.

TABLE 25-1 (Continued)

SOIL CLASSIFICATION*

Soil Type	Criteria	Other Considerations
Type B	Cohesive soil with an unconfined compressive strength greater than 0.5 tsf (48 kPa) but less than 1.5 tsf (144 kPa).	Type B soil can also be: 1) granular cohesionless soils such as angular gravel, silt, silt loam, sandy loam, and in some cases, silty clay loam and sandy clay loam; 2) previously disturbed soils except those which would otherwise be classed as Type C soil; 3) soil that meets the requirements of Type A, but is fissured or subject to vibration; 4) dry rock that is not stable; or 5) part of sloped, layered system where layers dip into excavation on a slope of 4H:1V, but only if the soil would otherwise be classed as Type A.
Type C	Cohesive soil with an unconfined compressive strength of 0.5 tsf (48 kPa) or less.	Type C soil can also be: 1) granular soils including gravel, sand, and loamy sand; 2) submerged soil or soil from which water is freely seeping; 3) submerged rock that is not stable; or 4) part of sloped, layered system where layers dip into excavation on a slope of 4H:1V or steeper.

* Soil classification must be determined by a Competent Person as defined in 25.A.02

EM 385-1-1
15 Sep 08

FIGURE 25-1

SLOPING AND BENCHING

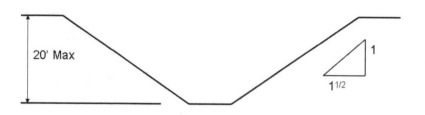

SINGLE SLOPE - TYPE C SOIL

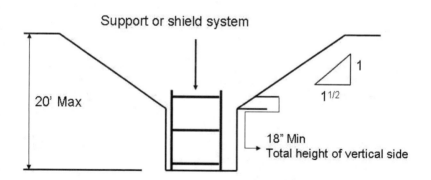

SUPPORTED OR SHIELDED VERTICALLY-SIDED
LOWER PORTION - TYPE C SOIL

EM 385-1-1
15 Sep 08

FIGURE 25-1 (CONTINUED)

SLOPING AND BENCHING

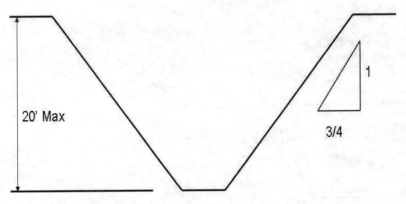

SINGLE SLOPE – GENERAL - TYPE A SOIL*

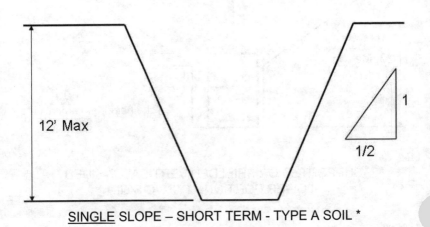

SINGLE SLOPE – SHORT TERM - TYPE A SOIL *

EM 385-1-1
15 Sep 08

FIGURE 25-1 (CONTINUED)

SLOPING AND BENCHING

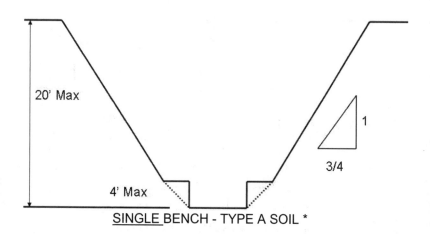

SINGLE BENCH - TYPE A SOIL *

FIGURE 25-1 (CONTINUED)

SLOPING AND BENCHING

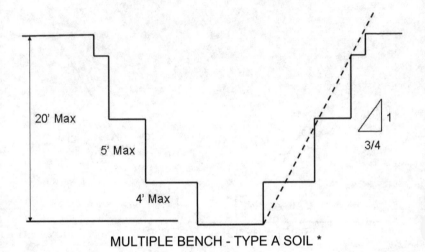

MULTIPLE BENCH - TYPE A SOIL *

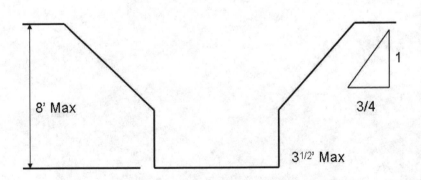

UNSUPPORTED VERTICALLY SIDED LOWER PORTION - MAXIMUM 8 FEET IN DEPTH - TYPE A SOIL *

EM 385-1-1
15 Sep 08

FIGURE 25-1 (CONTINUED)

SLOPING AND BENCHING

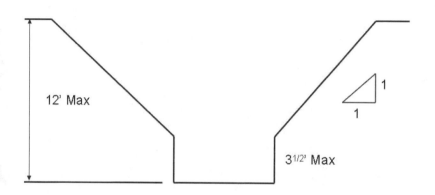

UNSUPPORTED VERTICALLY SIDED LOWER PORTION –
(MAXIMUM 12 FEET IN DEPTH) - TYPE A SOIL *

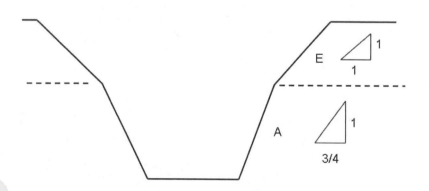

EXCAVATIONS MADE IN LAYERED SOILS - B OVER A *

FIGURE 25-1 (CONTINUED)

SLOPING AND BENCHING

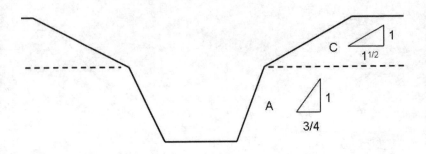

EXCAVATIONS MADE IN LAYERED SOILS - C OVER A *

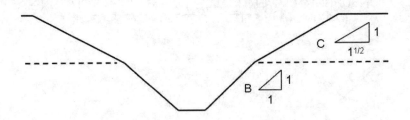

EXCAVATIONS MADE IN LAYERED SOILS - C OVER B *

* Requires the approval and identity of a Registered Professional Engineer.

EM 385-1-1
15 Sep 08

FIGURE 25-2

TRENCH SHIELDS

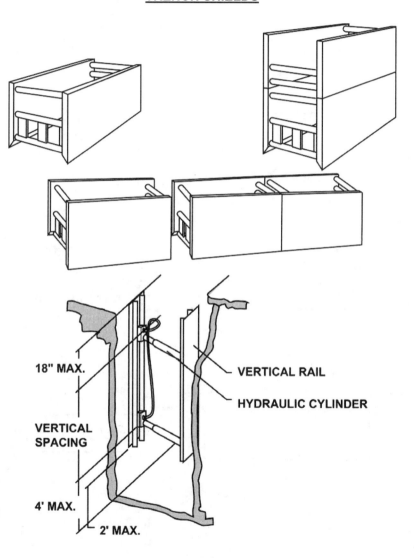

Aluminum Hydraulic Shoring

FIGURE 25-3

TRENCH JACKS

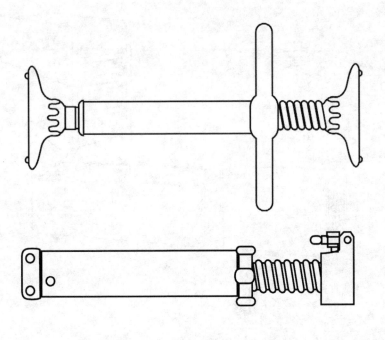

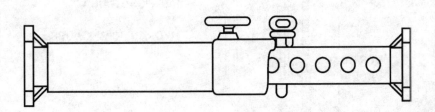

Pneumatic/hydraulic Shoring

EM 385-1-1
15 Sep 08

SECTION 26

UNDERGROUND CONSTRUCTION (TUNNELS), SHAFTS, AND CAISSONS

26. GENERAL

26.A.01 Access.

a. Access to all underground openings shall be controlled to prevent unauthorized entry.

b. Unused access ways or other openings shall be tightly covered or fenced off and shall be posted with warning signs indicating "**KEEP OUT**" or similar language.

c. Completed or unused sections of underground structures shall be barricaded.

d. See Section 34 of this manual for confined space requirements.

26.A.02 Every location of underground construction shall have a check-in/check-out system that will ensure that above-ground personnel can determine the identification of all underground personnel.

26.A.03 Oncoming shifts shall be informed of any hazardous occurrences or conditions that have affected or might affect employee safety, including liberation of gas, equipment failures, earth or rock slides, cave-ins, flooding, fires, or explosions.

26.A.04 Communications.

a. In situations where unassisted voice communication is inadequate, power-assisted means shall be used to provide communication among workers and support personnel.

b. At least two effective means of communication (at least one of which shall be voice communication) shall be provided in all shafts that are being developed or used either for personnel access or for hoisting.

c. Powered communication systems shall operate on an independent power supply and shall be installed so that the use of or disruption of any one phone or signal location will not disrupt the operation of the system from any other location.

d. Communication systems shall be tested upon initial entry of each shift to the underground and as often as necessary thereafter to ensure proper operation.

e. Any employee working alone underground, who is both out of range of natural unassisted voice communication and not under observation by other persons, shall be provided with effective means to communicate the need for and to obtain emergency assistance. Employees working alone shall be required to check in with their supervisor at least once an hour.

26.A.05 Emergency rescue plans and equipment.

a. Plans for rescuing personnel who might become injured or incapacitated while underground or in a shaft or caisson shall be developed.

(1) Plans shall be incorporated in either the APP or the AHA and posted at the job site.

(2) Plans shall be periodically reviewed with all affected personnel so that they maintain a working knowledge of emergency responsibilities and procedures.

(3) Emergency plans shall be drilled on a periodic basis to ensure their efficacy.

b. Emergency equipment specified in the emergency plan shall be provided within 15 minutes of each portal or shaft entry.

Inspections and workability tests of the equipment shall be made and documented monthly.

c. When a shaft is used as a means of egress, arrangements shall be made for power-assisted hoisting capability to be readily available in an emergency, unless the regular hoisting means can continue to function during a power failure.

d. Hoisting devices used for emergencies shall be designed so that the load hoist drum is powered in both directions of rotation and so that the brake is automatically applied upon power release or failure.

e. Self-rescuing/emergency respirators shall be immediately available to all employees at workstations in underground areas where they may be trapped by smoke or gas. > *See 5.G.*

f. At least one designated person shall be on duty above ground whenever personnel are underground.

(1) The designated person shall be responsible for keeping an accurate count of employees' underground and securing immediate aid in case of emergency.

(2) The designated person shall not be given other responsibilities that could affect his emergency response duties.

g. Each worker underground shall have an acceptable portable hand lamp or cap lamp in his work area for emergency use, unless natural light or an emergency lighting system provides adequate illumination for escape.

26.A.06 Rescue teams.

a. On job sites where less than 25 persons are underground at one time, provisions shall be made for at least one five-person rescue team to be either on the job site or within 30-minutes travel time from the underground entry point. This rescue team may be provided by local emergency response services.

b. On job sites where 25 or more persons are underground at one time, provisions shall be made for at least two five-person rescue teams. One <u>rescue team shall be</u> on the job site or <u>be</u> within 30-minutes travel time from the underground entry point, and the other <u>rescue team shall be</u> within 2-hours travel time. These rescue teams may be provided by local emergency response services.

c. Rescue team members shall be qualified in rescue procedures, the use and limitations of breathing apparatus, and the use of firefighting equipment.

d. On job sites where flammable or noxious gases are encountered or anticipated in hazardous quantities, rescue team members shall practice donning and using SCBA monthly.

e. Rescue teams shall be kept informed of conditions at the job site with may impact their response.

26.A.07 In addition to the requirements of Section 5, personnel in wet underground areas shall wear rubber boots (and rain gear, as necessary).

26.A.08 First-aid facilities.

a. A fully equipped first-aid station and emergency transportation shall be provided at each underground construction project regardless of the number of persons employed.

b. If an underground construction project has multiple portals a first-aid station(s) shall be provided at each portal or entry shaft or shall be so located between them that the distance from the station to each portal/entry shaft is less than 5 mi (8 km) and travel time less than 15 minutes.

26.A.09 Electrical and lighting.

a. All electrical systems used in hazardous locations must be approved for that location > *See 11.H.*

b. Lighting circuits shall be installed on one side of the tunnel near the spring line and shall be mounted on insulators at each point of suspension.

c. Light fixtures shall be nonmetallic and weatherproof and mounted in a manner that provides safe clearance for personnel and equipment.

d. Only portable lighting equipment that is approved for the hazardous location shall be used within:

(1) Storage areas, or

(2) 50 ft (15.2 m) of any underground heading during explosives handling.

26.A.10 Inspections and testing.

a. A program for testing all rock bolts for tightness shall be established. The frequency of testing shall be determined by rock conditions and the distance from vibration sources.

b. The employer shall examine and test the roof, face, and walls of the work area at the start of each shift and frequently thereafter.

c. Ground conditions along underground haulways and access ways shall be inspected as frequently as necessary to maintain safe passage.

d. All drilling and associated equipment to be used during a shift shall be inspected before each shift by a competent person.

EM 385-1-1
15 Sep 08

e. Drilling areas shall be inspected for hazards before drilling operations are started.

f. A competent person shall inspect haulage equipment before each shift.

g. Whenever defects affecting safety or health are identified, the defects shall be corrected before activities are initiated or continued.

26.A.11 Protection from falling material.

a. Portal openings and access areas shall be guarded by shoring, fencing, head walls, shotcreting, or other equivalent means to ensure safe access of employees and equipment. Adjacent areas shall be scaled or otherwise secured to prevent loose soil or rock from endangering the portal and access areas.

b. Ground stability in hazardous subsidence areas shall be ensured by shoring or filling in, or by erecting barricades and posting warning signs to prevent entry.

c. Loose ground in underground areas that might be hazardous to employees shall be taken down, scaled, or supported.

d. Rock masses separated from the main mass by faults, joints, or fractures shall be secured by rock bolting or other suitable means or shall be removed. The means of securing shall be designed by a foundation engineer, an engineering geologist, or other qualified person.

e. Anchored chain-link fabric or other method approved by the GDA shall be provided on rock faces subject to spalling.

f. Where tunnels are excavated through earth or shale, any excavation above or adjacent to portal areas shall be sloped to the angle of repose or held in place by ground supports. When undercutting occurs on these slopes (whether due to erosion or other causes) the overhanging material shall be promptly removed.

g. Where the need is indicated, a protective shelter shall be provided at each underground portal to protect persons and equipment from the hazards of falling rock or other material. The protective shelter shall project at least 15 ft (4.5 m) out from the portal.

h. Ice or snow buildup on rock faces or earth slopes that create a hazard shall be promptly removed.

26.A.12 Tunneling in soil.

a. Where tunnels are excavated by conventional methods, the excavation shall not be extended more than 24 in (60.9 cm) ahead of ground supports; where continuous mining machines are used for tunnel excavation, the excavation shall not be extended more than 48 in (121.9 cm) ahead of ground supports.

b. Under no circumstances shall persons be permitted to work in unsupported sections of the tunnels.

c. All voids in back of ground supports shall be filled, blocked, braced, or treated to prevent further cave-ins.

d. Where liner plate is not used for tunnel support, 2in (5cm) wire mesh or chain-link fabric shall be installed over the crown section, extending down to the spring line on each side of the tunnel and secured in place.

26.A.13 Ground support systems.

a. Torque meters and/or torque wrenches shall be used where rock bolts are used for ground support.

EM 385-1-1
15 Sep 08

b. Frequent tests shall be made to determine if bolts meet the required torque. The test frequency shall be determined by rock conditions and distance from vibration sources.

c. Rock bolt support systems shall be designed by a foundation engineer, a geologist, or other qualified person. Suitable protection shall be provided for employees exposed to the hazard of loose ground while installing ground support systems.

d. Support sets shall be installed so that the bottoms have sufficient anchorage to prevent ground pressures from dislodging the support base of the sets. Lateral bracing shall be provided between immediately adjacent sets to provide added stability.

e. Damaged or dislodged ground supports shall be repaired or replaced. Whenever possible, new supports shall be installed before removing the damaged supports.

f. A shield or other type of support shall be used to maintain a safe travel way for personnel working in dead-end areas ahead of any support replacement operation.

26.A.14 Material handling equipment.

a. Powered mobile haulage equipment shall have audible warning devices to inform personnel to stay clear. The operator shall sound the warning device before moving the equipment and whenever necessary during travel.

b. All vehicles and mobile equipment required to move in and out of underground construction areas shall have a revolving, flashing amber light, mounted so as to be visible in all directions. The flashing light shall be on whenever a vehicle or mobile equipment is in operation.

c. Haulage equipment shall be equipped with two headlights at both ends, a backup light, and an automatic backup alarm.

EM 385-1-1
15 Sep 08

d. Conveyors used to transport muck from tunnels shall be installed, guarded, and maintained as required by Section 17. Fire extinguishers or equivalent protection shall be provided at the head and tail pulleys of underground belt conveyors and at 300 ft (91.4 m) intervals along the belt line.

e. No person shall ride haulage equipment unless it is equipped with seating for each passenger and passengers are protected from being struck, crushed, or caught between other equipment or surfaces.

f. When dumping cars by hand, the car dumps shall be provided with tie-down chains or bumper blocks to prevent cars from overturning.

g. Where narrow-gage railroads are used for haulage, the tracks shall be secured to prevent shifting. No "humping" of mine dump cars shall be permitted.

h. Whenever rails serve as a return for a trolley circuit, both rails shall be bonded at every joint and cross-bonded every 200 ft (60.9 m).

i. Mine dump cars shall be equipped with automatic safety couplings, and cradle cars shall be equipped with a positive locking device to prevent accidental dumping.

j. Berms, bumper blocks, safety hooks, or equivalent means shall be provided to prevent overtravel and overturning of haulage equipment at dumping locations.

k. Bumper blocks or equivalent shall be provided at all track dead ends.

26.A.15 Vehicles not directly involved in work shall be kept away from portals and separated from construction activities.

EM 385-1-1
15 Sep 08

26.A.16 A caution sign reading "**BURIED LINE**" (or similar wording) shall be posted where air lines are buried or otherwise hidden by water or debris.

26.A.17 Where underground openings are located adjacent to sources of water with potential for causing flooding in the underground work area, measures shall be taken to ensure that the underground area cannot be flooded.

26.B HAZARDOUS CLASSIFICATIONS

26.B.01 Underground construction operations shall be classified in accordance with the following.

   a. Underground construction operations shall be classified as potentially gassy operations if either:

   (1) Air monitoring discloses 10% or more of the lower explosive limit for methane or other flammable gases measured at 12 in +/- 0.25 in (30.4 cm +/- 0.6 cm) from the roof, face, floor, or walls for a period of more than 24 hours; or

   (2) The history of the geological area or geological formation indicates that 10% or more of the lower explosive limit for methane or other flammable gas is likely to be encountered.

   b. Underground operations shall be classified as gassy operations if:

   (1) Air monitoring discloses 10% or more of the lower explosive limit for methane or other flammable gases measured at 12 in +/- 0.25 in (30.4 cm +/- 0.6 cm) from the roof, face, floor, or walls for three consecutive days; or

   (2) There has been an ignition of methane or other flammable gases emanating from the strata that indicates the presence of such gases; or

(3) The underground construction operation is both connected to an underground work area that is currently classified as gassy and is also subject to a continuous course of air containing the flammable gas concentration.

26.B.02 Underground construction gassy operations may be downgraded to potentially gassy operations when air monitoring results remain under 10% of the lower explosive limit for methane or other flammable gases for 3 consecutive days.

26.B.03 Requirements for gassy operations.

a. Only equipment approved for the hazardous location and maintained in suitable condition shall be used in gassy operations.

b. Mobile diesel-powered equipment used in gassy operations shall be approved in accordance with the requirements of 30 CFR 36 by MSHA and State regulations and shall be operated in accordance with these requirements and the manufacturer's instructions.

c. Each entrance to a gassy operation shall be prominently posted with signs notifying all entrants of the gassy classification.

d. Smoking shall be prohibited in all gassy operations and the employer shall be responsible for collecting all personal sources of ignition, such as matches and lighters, from all persons entering a gassy operation.

e. A fire watch shall be maintained when hot work is performed.

f. Once an operation has been classified as gassy, all activities in the affected area (except those in (1) through (3), below) shall be discontinued until the operation either is in compliance with all gassy operation requirements or has been downgraded to potentially gassy:

(1) Activities related to the control of the gas concentration;

(2) Installation of new equipment, or conversion of existing equipment, to comply with subparagraph (1), above; and

(3) Installation of above-ground controls for reversing the air flow.

26.C AIR MONITORING, AIR QUALITY STANDARDS, AND VENTILATION

26.C.01 Air monitoring requirements.

a. Air monitoring devices shall be inspected, calibrated, maintained, and used in accordance with the manufacturer's instructions. Back-up monitoring devices shall be maintained in calibrated and working condition at the worksite. **> See Section 6.**

b. When air monitoring is required "as often as necessary," the competent person shall determine which substances to monitor and how frequently to monitor. Such determination shall be based on:

(1) The location of the job site and proximity to fuel tanks, sewers, gas lines, old landfills, coal deposits, and swamps;

(2) The geology of the job site, particularly the soil types and their permeability;

(3) Any history of air contaminants in nearby job sites or any changes in air quality monitored during a previous shift; and

(4) Work practices and job site conditions (use of diesel engines, explosives, or fuel gas, ventilation characteristics, visible atmospheric conditions, decompression of the atmosphere, welding, cutting, or hot work, etc.).

EM 385-1-1
15 Sep 08

c. A record (including location, date, time, substance, monitoring results, and name of person conducting the test) of all air quality tests shall be maintained at the job site.

d. The atmosphere in all underground work areas shall be tested as often as necessary to assure that the atmosphere at normal atmospheric pressure contains at least 19.5% oxygen and no more than 22% oxygen.

e. The atmosphere in all underground work areas shall be tested quantitatively for CO, nitrogen dioxide, hydrogen sulfide, and other toxic gases, dusts, vapors, mists, and fumes as often as necessary to ensure that the PEL are not exceeded.

f. The atmosphere in all underground work areas shall be tested quantitatively for methane and other flammable gases as often as necessary to determine whether action is to be taken under 26.C.02.f-h and to determine whether an operation is to be classified gassy or potentially gassy under 26.B.01.

g. The atmosphere in all underground work areas shall be tested as often as necessary to ensure that the ventilation requirements of 26.C.03-05 are met.

h. If diesel-engine or gasoline-engine driven ventilating fans or compressors are used, an initial test shall be made of the inlet air of the fan or compressor, with the engine operating, to ensure that the air supply is not contaminated by engine exhaust.

i. When rapid excavation machines are used, a continuous flammable gas monitor shall be operated at the face with the sensor(s) placed as high and close to the front of the machine's cutter head as possible.

j. Operations that meet the criteria for potentially gassy or gassy operations shall be subjected to the following monitoring:

(1) Tests for oxygen content shall be conducted in all affected work areas and work areas immediately adjacent to such areas at least at the beginning and midpoint of each shift;

(2) When using rapid excavation machines, continuous automatic flammable gas monitoring equipment shall be used to monitor the air at the heading, on the rib, and in the return air duct. The continuous monitor shall signal the heading and shut down electric power in the affected underground work area, except for acceptable pumping and ventilation equipment, when 20% or more of the lower explosive limit for methane or other flammable gases is encountered.

(3) A manual flammable gas monitor shall be used as needed, but at least at the beginning and midpoint of each shift, to ensure that the limits prescribed in 26.B 01 and 26.C.01.d and f are not exceeded. In addition, a manual electrical shut down control shall be provided near the heading.

(4) Local gas tests shall be made prior to and continuously during any welding, cutting, or other hot work.

(5) In underground operations driven by drill-and-blast methods, the air in the affected area shall be tested for flammable gas prior to re-entry after blasting and continuously when employees are working underground.

26.C.02 Air quality standards.

a. Whenever air monitoring indicates the presence of 5 ppm or more of hydrogen sulfide, a test shall be conducted in the affected underground work areas, at least at the beginning and midpoint of each shift, until the concentration of hydrogen sulfide has been less than 5 ppm for 3 consecutive days.

b. Whenever hydrogen sulfide is detected in an amount exceeding 10 ppm, a continuous sampling and indicating hydrogen sulfide monitor shall be used to monitor the affected work areas.

EM 385-1-1
15 Sep 08

c. Employees shall be informed when a concentration of 10 ppm hydrogen sulfide is exceeded.

d. The continuous sampling and indicating hydrogen sulfide monitor shall be designed, installed, and maintained to provide a visual and aural alarm when the hydrogen sulfide concentration reaches 10 ppm to signal that additional measures might be necessary to maintain hydrogen sulfide exposure below the PEL.

e. When the competent person determines, on the basis of air monitoring results or other information, that air contaminants may be present in sufficient quantities to be dangerous to life, the employer shall:

(1) Prominently post a notice at all entrances to the underground area to inform all entrants of the hazardous condition, and

(2) Ensure that the necessary precautions are taken.

f. Whenever 5% or more of the lower explosive limit for methane or other flammable gases is detected in any underground work area or in the air return, steps shall be taken to increase ventilation air volume or otherwise control the gas concentration, unless operations are conducted in accordance with the potentially gassy or gassy operation requirements: such additional ventilation controls may be discontinued when gas concentrations are reduced below 5% of the lower explosive limit.

g. Whenever 10% or more of the lower explosive limit for methane or other flammable gases is detected in the vicinity of welding, cutting, or other hot work, such work shall be suspended until the concentration of such flammable gas is reduced to less than 10% of the lower explosive limit.

EM 385-1-1
15 Sep 08

h. Whenever 20% or more of the lower explosive limit for methane or other flammable gases is detected in any underground work area or in the return:

(1) All employees, except those necessary to eliminate the hazard, shall be immediately withdrawn to a safe location above ground; and

(2) Electrical power, except for acceptable pumping and ventilation equipment, shall be cut off to the area endangered by the flammable gas until the concentration of such gas is reduced to less than 20% of the lower explosive limit.

i. When ventilation has been reduced to the extent that hazardous levels of methane or other flammable gas may have accumulated, all affected areas shall be tested after ventilation has been restored and before any power, other than for acceptable equipment, is restored or work is resumed and shall determine whether the atmosphere is within flammable limits.

j. Whenever the ventilation system has been shut down with all employees out of the underground area, only competent persons authorized to test for air contaminants shall be allowed underground until the ventilation has been restored and all affected areas have been tested for air contaminants and declared safe.

26.C.03 Ventilation.

a. Fresh air shall be supplied to all underground work areas in sufficient quantities to prevent dangerous accumulation of dusts, fumes, mists, gases, or vapors.

b. Mechanical ventilation shall be provided in all underground work areas except where it is demonstrated that natural ventilation provides the necessary air quality through sufficient air volume and airflow.

(1) Ventilation and exhaust systems for tunnel excavation shall be of sufficient capacity to maintain an adequate supply of uncontaminated air at all points in the tunnel.

(2) The supply of fresh air shall not be less than 200 cfm (94.4 liters per second (L/s)) for each employee underground plus that necessary to operate the equipment.

(3) The linear velocity of air flow in all underground work areas shall be at least 30 ft/min (0.15 m/s) where blasting or rock drilling is conducted or where there are other conditions likely to produce dusts, fumes, vapors, or gases in harmful quantities.

(4) The direction of mechanical airflow shall be reversible.

(5) Ventilation doors shall be designed and installed so that they remain closed when in use, regardless of the direction of airflow.

c. Following blasting, ventilation systems shall exhaust smoke and fumes to the outside atmosphere before work is resumed in affected areas.

d. Potentially gassy or gassy operations shall have ventilation systems installed which are constructed of fire-resistant materials and have acceptable electrical systems, including fan motors.

e. Gassy operations shall be conducted with controls for reversing the airflow of ventilation systems located above ground.

f. In potentially gassy or gassy operations, wherever mine-type ventilation systems using an offset main fan installed on the surface are used, they shall be equipped with explosion-doors or a weak-wall having an area at least equivalent to the cross sectional area of the airway.

g. Air that has passed through underground oil or fuel-storage areas shall not be used to ventilate work areas.

26.C.04 When drilling rock or concrete, appropriate dust control measures shall be taken to maintain dust levels within safe limits.

26.C.05 Internal combustion engines, except diesel-powered engines on mobile equipment, are prohibited underground. Mobile diesel-powered equipment used underground in atmospheres other than gassy operations shall be either approved by MSHA (30 CFR 36), or shall be demonstrated to be fully equivalent to such MSHA-approved equipment, and shall be operated in accordance 30 CFR 36.

26.D FIRE PREVENTION AND PROTECTION

26.D.01 Fire prevention and protection plans.

a. For every underground construction project, a fire prevention and protection plan shall be developed and implemented. The plan shall detail:

(1) The specific work practices to be implemented for preventing fires;

(2) Response measures to be taken in case of fire to control and extinguish the fire;

(3) Equipment required for fire prevention and protection;

(4) Personnel requirements and responsibilities for fire prevention and protection; and

(5) Requirements for daily and weekly fire prevention and protection inspections.

b. Fire prevention and protection plans shall be incorporated in either the APP or the AHA and posted at the job site.

EM 385-1-1
15 Sep 08

c. Fire prevention and protection plans shall be reviewed with all affected personnel as often as is necessary for them to maintain a working knowledge of emergency responsibilities and procedures.

d. Plans shall be drilled as often as is necessary to ensure their efficacy.

26.D.02 Fire extinguishers.

a. Fire extinguishers shall be provided and maintained in accordance with the requirements of Section 9.

b. Fire extinguishers (or equivalent protection) shall be provided and maintained at each portal and shaft entry, within 100 ft (30.4 m) of the advancing face of each tunnel, and at locations containing combustible materials.

c. A fire extinguisher of at least 4A:40B:C rating or other equivalent extinguishing means shall be provided at the head pulley and tail pulley of underground belt conveyors.

26.D.03 Open flames/fires and smoking.

a. Open flames and fires are prohibited in all underground construction operations except as permitted for welding, cutting, and other hot work operations.

b. Smoking may be allowed only in areas free of fire and explosion hazards.

c. Readily visible signs prohibiting smoking and open flames shall be posted in areas having fire or explosion hazards.

26.D.04 Heating devices used in tunnels shall be approved for such locations by a nationally-recognized testing laboratory.

26.D.05 Gasoline shall not be taken, stored, or used underground.

26.D.06 Acetylene, LP-Gas, and methylacetylene propadiene stabilized gas may be used underground only for welding, cutting, and other hot work. No more than the amount necessary for work during the next 24-hour period shall be permitted underground.

26.D.07 Only fire-resistant hydraulic fluids approved by a nationally-recognized authority or agency shall be used in hydraulically actuated underground machinery and equipment unless the machinery or equipment is protected by a fire suppression system or a multi-purpose fire extinguisher rated for sufficient capacity for the type and size of hydraulic equipment involved (but at least 4A:40B:C).

26.D.08 Storage of flammable and combustible materials.

   a. Not more than a 1-day supply of diesel fuel may be stored underground.

   b. Oil, grease, and diesel fuel stored underground shall be kept in tightly sealed containers in fire-resistant areas at least 300 ft (91.4 m) from underground explosive magazines and at least 100 ft (30.4 m) from shaft stations and steeply inclined passageways.

   c. Flammable or combustible materials shall not be stored above ground within 100 ft (30.4 m) of any access opening to any underground operation unless they are located as far as practical from the opening and either a fire-resistant barrier of not less than a 1-hour rating is placed between the stored material and the opening.

   d. Electrical installations in underground areas where oil, grease, or diesel fuel are stored shall be used only for lighting fixtures.

   e. Lighting fixtures in storage areas or within 25 ft (7.6 m) of underground areas where oil, grease, or diesel fuel are stored shall be approved for Class I, Division 2 locations > See 11.H.

EM 385-1-1
15 Sep 08

26.D.09 The piping of diesel fuel from the surface to an underground location is permitted only if:

a. Diesel fuel is contained at the surface in a tank whose maximum capacity is no more than the amount required to supply the equipment serviced by the underground fueling station for a 24-hour period;

b. The surface tank is connected to the underground fueling station by an acceptable pipe or hose system controlled at the surface by a valve, and at the shaft bottom by a hose nozzle (nozzle shall not be of the latch-open type);

c. The pipe is empty at all times except when transferring diesel fuel from the surface tank to a piece of equipment in use underground; and

d. Hoisting operations in the shaft are suspended during refueling operations if the supply piping in the shaft is not protected from damage.

26.D.10 Any structure located underground or within 100 ft (30.4 m) of an opening to the underground shall be constructed of material having a fire-resistance rating of at least 1 hour.

26.D.11 Oil-filled transformers shall not be used underground unless they are located in a fire-resistant enclosure and surrounded by a dike to contain the contents of the transformers in event of a rupture.

26.D.12 Noncombustible barriers shall be installed below welding or burning operations in or over shaft or raise.

EM 385-1-1
15 Sep 08

26.E DRILLING

26.E.01 Drilling machines.

a. Employees shall not be allowed on a drill mast while the drill bit is in operation or the drill machine is being moved.

b. When drill machines are being moved from one drilling area to another, drill steel, tools, and other equipment shall be secured and the mast placed in a safe position.

c. Drills on columns shall be anchored firmly before drilling is started and shall be retightened frequently.

d. Jumbos.

(1) Safe access shall be provided to all working levels of drill jumbos.

(2) Jumbo decks and stair treads shall be designed to be slip-resistant and secured to prevent accidental displacement.

(3) Only employees assisting the operator shall be allowed to ride on jumbos, unless the jumbo meets the requirements for adequate seating arrangements that protect passengers from being struck, crushed, or caught between equipment or surfaces and has safe access.

(4) Employees working under jumbo decks shall be warned whenever drilling is about to begin.

(5) On jumbo decks over 10 ft (3 m) in height, guardrails, which are removable, or equal protection shall be provided on all open sides, excluding access openings of platforms, unless an adjacent surface provides equivalent fall protection.

(6) Stair access to jumbo decks wide enough to accommodate two persons if the deck is over 10 ft (3 m) in height.

(7) Receptacles or racks shall be provided for drill steel stored on jumbos.

(8) The employer shall provide mechanical means for lifting drills, roof bolts, mine straps, and other material to the top decks of jumbos over 10 ft (3 m) in height.

26.E.02 Scaling bars shall be available at scaling operations and shall be maintained in good conditions at all times. Blunted or severely worn bars shall not be used.

26.E.03 Blasting holes shall not be drilled through blasted rock (muck) or water.

26.E.04 Before commencing the drill cycle after a blast, the face and any remaining blasting holes shall be examined for misfires that, if found, shall be removed.

26.E.05 Employees in a shaft shall be protected either by location or by suitable barriers if powered mechanical loading equipment is used to remove muck containing unfired explosives.

26.F SHAFTS

26.F.01 All wells or shafts over 5 ft (1.5 m) in depth that employees must enter shall be supported by lagging, piling, or casing of sufficient strength to withstand shifting of the surrounding earth.

a. The full depth of the shaft shall be supported by casing or bracing except where the shaft penetrates into solid rock having characteristics that will not change because of exposure.

(1) Where the shaft passes through earth into solid rock or through solid rock into earth and where there is potential for

EM 385-1-1
15 Sep 08

shear, the casing or bracing shall extend at least 5 ft (1.5 m) into the solid rock.

(2) When the shaft terminates in solid rock, the casing of bracing shall extend to the end of the shaft or 5 ft (1.5 m) into the solid rock, whichever is less.

b. The casing or bracing shall extend 42 in +/- 3 in (106.6 cm +/- 7.6 cm) above ground level, except that the minimum casing height may be reduced to 12 in (30.4 cm) provided that a standard railing is installed, that the ground adjacent to the top of the shaft is sloping away from the shaft collar to prevent entry of liquids, and that effective barriers are used to prevent mobile equipment operating near the shaft from jumping over the 12 in (30.4 cm) barrier.

26.F.02 After blasting operations in shafts, a competent person shall inspect the walls, ladders, timbers, blocking, and wedges to determined if they have loosened. Where found unsafe, corrections shall be made before shift operations are started.

26.F.03 No employee shall be permitted to enter an unsupported auger-type excavation in unstable material for any purpose. In such cases, necessary clean-out shall be accomplished without entry.

26.F.04 There shall be two safe means of access in shafts at all times: this may include the ladder and hoist.

26.G HOISTING

26.G.01 A warning light suitably located to warn employees at the shaft bottom and subsurface shaft entrances shall flash whenever a load is being moved in the shaft, except in fully enclosed hoistways.

26.G.02 Whenever a hoistway is not fully enclosed and employees are at the shaft bottom, conveyances or equipment shall be stopped at least 15 ft (4.5 m) above the bottom of the shaft and held there until the signalman at the bottom of the shaft directs the

EM 385-1-1
15 Sep 08

operator to continue lowering the load; except that the load may be lowered without stopping if the load or conveyance is within full view of a bottom signalman who is in constant voice communication with the operator.

26.G.03 Before maintenance, repairs, or other work is commenced in a shaft served by a cage, skip, or bucket, the operator and other employees shall be informed and given suitable safety precautions. A sign warning that work is being performed in the shaft shall be installed at the shaft collar, at the operator's station, and at each underground landing.

26.G.04 Any connection between the hoisting rope and the cage or skip shall be compatible with the type of wire rope used for hoisting.

26.G.05 Spin-type connections, where used, shall be maintained in a clean condition and protected from foreign matter that could affect their operation.

26.G.06 Cage, skip, and load connections to the hoist rope shall be made so that the force of the hoist pull, vibration, misalignment, release of lift force, or impact will not disengage the connection. Moused or latched open-throat hooks do not meet this requirement.

26.G.07 When using wire rope wedge sockets, means shall be provided to prevent wedge escapement and to ensure that the wedge is properly seated.

26.H CAISSONS

26.H.01 In caisson work in which compressed air is used and the working chamber is less than 11 ft (3.3 m) in length, whenever such caissons are at any time suspended or hung while work is in progress so that the bottom of the excavation is more than 9 ft (2.7 m) below the deck of the working chamber, a shield shall be erected for the protection of the workers.

26.H.02 Shafts shall be subjected to a hydrostatic test, at which pressure they shall be tight. The shaft shall be stamped on the

EM 385-1-1
15 Sep 08

outside shell about 12 in (30.4 cm) from each flange to show the safe working pressure.

25.H.03 Whenever a shaft is used, it shall be provided, where space permits, with a safe, proper, and suitable staircase for its entire length, including landing platforms (not more than 20 ft (6 m) apart). Where this is impractical, ladders not more than 20 ft (6 m) high shall be installed with each section offset from adjacent sections and a guarded landing provided at each offset.

26.H.04 All caissons having a diameter or side greater than 10 ft (3 m) shall be provided with a man lock and shaft for the exclusive use of employees.

26.H.05 In addition to gauges in the locks, an accurate gauge shall be maintained on the outer and inner side of each bulkhead. These gauges shall be accessible at all times and kept in accurate working order.

26.H.06 In caisson operations where employees are exposed to compressed air working environments, the requirements of 26.I shall be complied with.

26.I COMPRESSED AIR WORK

26.I.01 All safety requirements for compressed air work will be carefully detailed in a compressed air work plan that shall be included as a part of the accident prevention plan or AHA.

26.I.02 The compressed air work plan shall include the following considerations:

    a. Requirements for a medical lock and its operation,

    b. An identification system for compressed air workers,

    c. Communications system requirements,

d. Requirements for signs and recordkeeping,

e. Special compression and decompression requirements,

f. Man lock and decompression chamber requirements,

g. Requirements for compressor systems and air supply,

h. Ventilation requirements,

i. Electrical power requirements,

j. Sanitation considerations,

k. Fire prevention and fire protection considerations, and

l. Requirements for bulkheads and safety screens.

26.I.03 Work in compressed air environments shall be performed in compliance with the requirements of 29 CFR 1926.803.

26.J UNDERGROUND BLASTING > *See Section 29.*

26.J.01 Explosives.

a. Dynamite used in tunnel blasting should be Fume Class 1. Fume Class 2 and Fume Class 3 explosives may be used if adequate ventilation is provided.

b. Storage of explosives, blasting agents, and detonators in tunnels or underground work areas shall be prohibited.

c. Trucks used for the transportation of explosives underground shall have the electrical system checked weekly to detect any failures that may constitute an electrical hazard. A written record of such inspections shall be kept on file and available for review. The installation of auxiliary lights on truck beds that are powered by the truck's electrical system shall be prohibited.

d. Explosives or blasting agents, not in original containers, shall be placed in a suitable container when transported manually. Detonators, primers, and other explosives shall be carried in separate containers when transported manually.

26.J.02 Blasting circuits.

a. All underground blasts fired by external power shall be by a power blasting switch system shown in Figure 29-1.

b. Blasting power circuits shall be separate and distinct from, and kept clear of, other power and lighting circuits and pipes, rails, and other conductive material (excluding earth) to prevent explosives initiation or employee exposure to electric current.

c. Sectioning switches or equivalent shall be installed in the firing line at 500-ft (150.4-m) intervals.

26.J.03 Loading.

a. Prior to loading, all power, water, and air lines shall be disconnected from the loading jumbo and power lines, including lighting circuits, shall be moved back a minimum of 50 ft (15.2 m).

b. The loading area shall be illuminated (minimum 10 foot-candles (107.6 lx)) by floodlights located 50 ft (15.2 m) from the face. If additional illumination is needed, the loading crew shall be provided with head lamps approved by the United States Bureau of Mines.

c. Equipment used for pneumatic placement of non-cap-sensitive blasting agents shall be designed for that purpose and shall be grounded while in use.

EM 385-1-1
15 Sep 08

26.J.04 Blasting.

a. The person in charge of blasting shall be the last to leave the blast area, shall see that no one remains in the blast area, and shall operate the sectioning switches in the firing line while proceeding out of the blast area.

b. No persons shall enter the tunnel blast area until the ventilation system has cleared the heading of harmful gases, smoke, and dust.

c. After each blast, the underground supports in the blast area shall be inspected and secured as necessary work is resumed. Rock surfaces shall be inspected, scaled, and if required, provided with shoring, bracing, rock bolts, shotcrete, or chain-link fabric, before mucking is started. Rock bolts within 100 ft (30.4 m) of a blast shall be tested after each blast before drilling for the next round begins.

d. The muck pile shall be wet down prior to mucking and kept wet during mucking operations.

26.J.05 Blasting in excavation work under compressed air.

a. When detonators or explosives are brought into an air lock, no employee (except the blaster, lock tender, and employees necessary for transport) shall be permitted to enter the air lock; no other material, supplies, or equipment shall be locked through with the explosive materials.

b. Detonators and explosives shall be taken separately into pressure working chambers.

c. All metal pipes, rails, air locks, and steel tunnel lining shall be electrically bonded and grounded at or near the portal or shaft. Such pipes and rails shall be cross-bonded at not less than 1000-ft (304.8-m) intervals throughout the length of the tunnel. In addition, each low air supply pipe shall be grounded at its delivery end.

EM 385-1-1
15 Sep 08

d. The explosive suitable for use in wet holes shall be water resistant and shall be Fume Class 1.

e. When tunnel excavation in rock face is approaching mixed face, and when tunnel excavation is in mixed face, blasting shall be performed with light charges and with light burden on each hole. Advance drilling shall be performed as tunnel excavation in rock face approaches mixed face to determine the nature and extent of rock cover and the remaining distance ahead to soft ground.

26.J.06 See Section 29 for blasting requirements.

EM 385-1-1
15 Sep 08

SECTION 27

CONCRETE, MASONRY, STEEL ERECTION AND RESIDENTIAL CONSTRUCTION

27.A GENERAL. The fall protection threshold height requirement is 6 ft (1.8 m) for ALL WORK covered by this manual, unless specified differently below, whether performed by Government or Contractor work forces, to include steel erection activities, systems-engineered activities (prefabricated) metal buildings, residential (wood) construction and scaffolding work. *> See Section 21*.

27.A.01 Construction loads shall not be placed on a structure or portion of a structure unless the employer determines, based on information from a person who is qualified in structural design, that the structure or portion of the structure is capable of supporting the loads.

27.A.02 Employees shall not be permitted to work above or in positions exposed to protruding reinforcing steel, fasteners, or other impalement hazards unless provisions have been made to control the hazard.

27.A.03 Working under loads.

    a. No employee shall be permitted to work under concrete buckets, bundled material loads, or other suspended loads (riggers securing lower loads to multi-lift rigging and workers setting suspended structural components such as beams, trusses, and precast members are excluded from this requirement. In these cases, work controls should be used to minimize the time spent directly under loads).

    b. Elevated concrete buckets and loads shall be routed, to the extent practical, to minimize the exposure of workers to hazards associated with falling loads or materials from the loads.

EM 385-1-1
15 Sep 08

<u>Vibrator crews shall be kept out from under concrete buckets suspended from cranes of cableways.</u>

<u>c. Riding on concrete buckets or other suspended loads shall be prohibited.</u>

27.B CONCRETE AND MASONRY CONSTRUCTION

27.B.01 Post-tensioning operations.

a. No employee (except those essential to the post-tensioning operations) shall be permitted to be behind jacks or end anchorages during post-tensioning operations.

b. Signs and barriers shall be erected to limit employee access to the post-tensioning area during tensioning operations.

27.B.02 Equipment.

a. Bulk storage bins, containers, or silos shall have conical or tapered bottoms with mechanical or pneumatic means of starting the flow of material.

b. Concrete mixers equipped with 1yard^3 (0.8 m^3) or larger loading skip shall be equipped with a mechanical device to clear the skip of material and shall have guardrails installed on each side of the skip.

c. Handles on bull floats used where they may contact energized electrical conductors shall be constructed of nonconductive material or insulated with a nonconductive sheath whose electrical and mechanical characteristics provide equivalent protection.

d. Powered and rotating concrete troweling machines that are manually guided shall be equipped with a control switch that will automatically shut off the power whenever the operator removes his/her hands from the equipment handles.

EM 385-1-1
15 Sep 08

e. Concrete pumping systems using discharge pipes shall be provided with pipe supports designed for 100% overload.

f. Handles of concrete buggies shall not extend beyond the wheels on either side of the buggy.

g. Concrete buckets equipped with hydraulic or pneumatically operated gates shall have positive safety latches or similar safety devices installed to prevent premature or accidental dumping. The buckets shall be designed to prevent material from accumulating on the top and sides of the bucket.

h. Sections of tremies and similar concrete conveyances shall be secured with wire rope (or equivalent material) in addition to the regular couplings or connections.

27.B.03 Structural and reinforcing steel for walls, piers, columns, and similar vertical structures shall be supported and/or guyed to prevent overturning or collapse. Support systems for reinforcing steel that are independent of other form or shoring support systems shall be designed by a Registered Professional Engineer.

a. Connections of equipment used in plumbing-up shall be secured.

b. The turnbuckles shall be secured to prevent unwinding while under stress.

c. Plumbing-up guys and related equipment shall be placed so that employees can get at the connection points.

d. Plumbing-up guys shall be removed only under the supervision of a Competent Person.

e. Measures shall be taken to prevent unrolled wire mesh from recoiling.

EM 385-1-1
15 Sep 08

27.C FORMWORK AND SHORING

27.C.01 Formwork, shoring, and bracing shall be designed, fabricated, erected, supported, braced, and maintained so that it will safely support all vertical and lateral loads that might be applied until such loads can be supported by the structure.

27.C.02 Planning and design.

> a. The planning and design of formwork and shoring shall be in accordance with provisions of American Concrete Institute (ACI) Publication 347.
>
> b. The design and the erection and removal plans for formwork and shoring shall be submitted for review to the GDA.
>
> c. The manufacturer's specifications for fabricated shoring systems shall be available at the job site during job planning and execution.

27.C.03 Base support.

> a. Supporting ground or completed construction upon which formwork and shoring is to be placed shall be of adequate strength to carry the vertical and lateral loads to be imposed.
>
> b. Sills for shoring shall be sound, rigid, and capable of carrying the maximum intended load.
>
> c. <u>Base plates</u>, shore heads, extension devices, or adjustment screws shall be in firm contact with the footing sill and form material and <u>when necessary, shall be secured to them</u>.

27.C.04 Splices shall be designed and constructed to prevent buckling and bending.

EM 385-1-1
15 Sep 08

27.C.05 Diagonal bracing shall be provided in vertical and horizontal planes to provide stiffness and to prevent buckling of individual members.

27.C.06 Inspection.

>   a. Shoring equipment shall be inspected prior to erection to determine that it is as specified in the shoring design. Any equipment found to be damaged shall not be used.

>   b. Erected shoring equipment shall be inspected immediately prior to, during, and immediately after the placement of concrete. Any shoring equipment that is found to be damaged, displaced, or weakened shall be immediately reinforced or re-shored.

27.C.07 Re-shoring shall be provided to safely support slabs and beams after stripping or where such members are subjected to superimposed loads due to construction.

27.C.08 Fabricated shoring shall not be loaded beyond the safe working load recommended by the manufacturer.

27.C.09 Single post shores.

>   a. Wherever single post shores are used in more than one tier, the layout shall be designed and inspected by an <u>RPE qualified in structural design.</u>

>   b. Single post shores shall be vertically aligned and spliced to prevent misalignment.

>   c. When shoring is at an angle, sloping, or when the surface shored is sloping, the shoring shall be designed for such loading.

>   d. Adjustment of single post shores to raise formwork shall not be made after concrete is in place.

EM 385-1-1
15 Sep 08

e. Fabricated single post shores and adjusting devices shall not be used if heavily rusted, bent, dented, rewelded, or have broken weldments or other defects; if they contain timber, they shall not be used if timber is split, cut, has sections removed, is rotted, or otherwise structurally damaged.

f. All timber and adjusting devices to be used for adjustable timber single post shores shall be inspected before erection.

g. All nails used to secure bracing or adjustable timber single post shores shall be driven home and the point of the nail bent over if possible.

h. For stability, single post shores shall be horizontally braced in both the longitudinal and transverse directions.

(1) Single-post shores shall be adequately braced in two mutually perpendicular directions at the splice level.

(2) Each tier shall also be diagonally braced in the same two directions.

(3) Bracing shall be installed as the shores are erected.

27.C.10 Tube and coupler shoring.

a. The material used for the couplers shall be of a structural type such as drop-forged steel, malleable iron, or structural grade aluminum. Gray cast iron shall not be used. No dissimilar metals shall be used together.

b. Couplers shall not be used if they are deformed, broken, or have defective or missing threads on bolts, or other defects.

c. When checking the erected shoring towers with the shoring design, the spacing between posts shall not exceed that shown on the layout and all interlocking of tubular members and tightness of couplings shall be checked.

EM 385-1-1
15 Sep 08

27.C.11 Tubular welded-frame shoring.

a. All locking devices on frames and braces shall be in good working order, coupling pins shall align the frame or panel legs, pivoted cross braces shall have their center pivot in place, and all components shall be in a condition similar to that of original manufacture.

b. When checking the erected shoring frames with the shoring design, the spacing between towers and cross brace spacing shall not exceed that shown in the design and all locking devices shall be closed.

c. Devices for attaching external lateral stability bracing shall be fastened to the legs of the shoring frames.

27.C.12 Vertical slip forms.

a. The steel rods or pipe on which the jacks climb or by which the forms are lifted shall be designed specifically for that purpose. Such rods shall be braced where not encased in concrete.

b. Jacks and vertical supports shall be positioned in such a manner that the vertical loads are distributed equally and do not exceed the capacity of the jacks.

c. The jacks or other lifting devices shall be provided with mechanical dogs or other automatic holding devices to provide protection in case of failure of the power supply or the lifting mechanism.

d. Lifting shall proceed steadily and uniformly and shall not exceed the predetermined safe rate of lift.

e. Lateral and diagonal bracing of the forms shall be provided to prevent excessive distortion of the structure during the jacking operation.

EM 385-1-1
15 Sep 08

f. During jacking operations, the form structure shall be maintained in line and plumb.

g. All vertical lift forms shall be provided with scaffolding or work platforms completely encircling the area of placement.

27.C.13 Removal of formwork.

a. Forms and shores (except those on slab or grade and slip forms) shall not be removed until the individual responsible for forming and/or shoring determines that the concrete has gained sufficient strength to support its weight and all superimposed loads. Such determination shall be based on one of the following:

(1) Satisfaction of conditions stipulated in the plans and specifications for removal of forms and shores, or

(2) Concrete testing (in accordance with ASTM standard test methods) indicates that the concrete has achieved sufficient strength to support its weight and superimposed loads.

b. Re-shoring shall not be removed until the concrete being supported has attained adequate strength to support its weight and all loads placed on it.

27.C.14 Fall Protection. Each employee engaged in masonry or concrete activities who is on a walking/working surface with an unprotected side or edge more than 6 ft (1.8 m) above a lower level shall be protected from fall hazards by guardrail systems, safety net systems, engineered fall protection systems, personal fall arrest systems, positioning, or restraint systems in accordance with Section 21.

27.D PRECAST CONCRETE OPERATIONS

27.D.01 Precast Concrete operations shall be planned and designed by a Registered Professional Engineer (RPE). Such plans and designs shall include detailed instructions and sketches indicating the prescribed method of erection and shall be submitted to the GDA for review.

27.D.02 Precast concrete members shall be adequately supported to prevent overturning or collapse until permanent connections are complete.

27.D.03 Lifting inserts and hardware.

   a. Lifting inserts which are embedded or otherwise attached to tilt-up precast concrete members shall be capable of supporting at least two times the maximum intended load applied or transmitted to them.

   b. Lifting inserts which are embedded or otherwise attached to precast concrete members, other than tilt-up members, shall be capable of supporting at least four times the maximum intended load applied or transmitted to them.

   c. Lifting hardware shall be capable of supporting at least five times the maximum intended load applied or transmitted to the lifting device.

27.D.04 No employee shall be permitted under precast concrete members being lifted or tilted into position except employees required for the erection of those members.

27.E LIFT-SLAB OPERATIONS

27.E.01 Lift-slab operations shall be planned and designed by a RPE. Such plans and designs shall include detailed instructions and sketches indicating the prescribed method of erection and shall be submitted to the GDA for review.

27.E.02 Jacking equipment.

   a. The manufacturer's rated capacity shall be legibly marked on all jacks and shall not be exceeded.

EM 385-1-1
15 Sep 08

b. Threaded rods and other members that transmit loads to the jacks shall have a minimum safety factor of 2.5.

c. Jacks shall be designed and installed so that they will not continue to lift when overloaded.

d. All jacks shall have a positive stop to prevent overtravel.

e. Hydraulic jacks used in lift slab construction shall have a safety device that will cause the jacks to support the load in any position if the jack malfunctions.

27.E.03 Jacking operations.

a. When it is necessary to provide a firm foundation, the base of the jack shall be blocked or cribbed. Where there is a possibility of slippage of the metal cap of the jack, a wood block shall be placed between the cap and the load.

b. The maximum number of manually-controlled jacks on one slab shall be limited to 14, and in no event shall the number be too great to permit the operator to maintain the slab level within specific tolerances.

c. Jacking operations shall be synchronized to ensure even and uniform lifting of the slab.

d. During lifting, all points of the slab support shall be kept within   in (1.2 cm) of that needed to maintain the slab in a level position.

(1) If leveling is automatically controlled, a device shall be installed which will stop the operation when the   in (1.2 cm) leveling tolerance is exceeded.

(2) If leveling is manually controlled, such controls shall be located in a central location and attended by a trained operator while lifting is in progress.

EM 385-1-1
15 Sep 08

e. No one shall be permitted under the slab during jacking operations.

27.F STRUCTURAL STEEL ASSEMBLY

27.F.01. Prior to beginning the erection of any structural steel, a Steel Erection Plan shall be submitted to the GDA for review and acceptance. The plan will include the identification of the site and project; and will be signed and dated by the Qualified Person(s) responsible for its preparation and modification. This plan shall include the following information, as applicable to the particular project.

a. The sequence of erection activity, developed in coordination with the Controlling contractor, that includes the following:

(1) Material deliveries;

(2) Material staging and storage; and

(3) Coordination with other trades and construction activities.

b. A description of the crane and derrick selection and placement procedures, including the following:

(1) Site preparation;

(2) Path for overhead loads; and

(3) Identification of any lifts classified as Critical lifts, requiring separate plans.

c. A description of steel erection activities and procedures, including the following:

(1) Stability considerations requiring temporary bracing and guying;

(2) Erection bridging terminus point;

(3) Anchor rod (anchor bolt) notifications regarding repair, replacement and modifications;

(4) Columns and beams (including joists and purlins);

(5) Connections;

(6) Decking; and

(7) Ornamental and miscellaneous iron.

d. A description of the fall protection procedures that will be used;

e. A description of the procedures that will be used to comply with this section;

f. Activity hazard analysis in accordance with Section 1 of this manual;

g. A certification for each employee who has received training for performing steel erection operations as required by 29 CFR 1926.761;

h. A list of the Qualified and Competent Persons; and

i. A description of the procedures that will be utilized in the event of rescue or emergency response.

27.F.02. Steel erection activities include:

a. Hoisting, laying out, placing, connecting, welding, burning, guying, bracing, bolting, plumbing, and rigging structural steel, steel joists and metal buildings;

EM 385-1-1
15 Sep 08

b. Installing metal decking, curtain walls, window walls, siding systems, miscellaneous metals, ornamental iron, and similar materials; and

c. Moving point-to-point while performing these activities.

27.F.03 The following activities are covered by this Section when they occur during and are a part of steel erection activities: rigging, hoisting, laying out, placing, connecting, guying, bracing, dismantling, burning, welding, bolting, grinding, sealing, caulking, and all related activities for construction, alteration and/or repair of materials and assemblies such as structural steel; ferrous metals and alloys; non-ferrous metals and alloys; glass; plastics and synthetic composite materials; structural metal framing and related bracing and assemblies; anchoring devices; structural cabling; cable stays; permanent and temporary bents and towers; false work for temporary supports of permanent steel members; stone and other non-precast concrete architectural materials mounted on steel frames; safety systems for steel erection; steel and metal joists; metal decking and raceway systems and accessories; metal roofing and accessories; metal siding; bridge flooring; cold formed steel framing; elevator beams; grillage; shelf racks; multi-purpose supports; crane rails and accessories; miscellaneous, architectural and ornamental metals and metal work; ladders; railings; handrails; fences and gates; gratings; trench covers; floor plates; castings; sheet metal fabrications; metal panels and panel wall systems; louvers; column covers; enclosures and pockets; stairs; perforated metals; ornamental iron work, expansion control including bridge expansion joint assemblies; slide bearings; hydraulic structures; fascias; soffit panels; penthouse enclosures; skylights; joint fillers; gaskets; sealants and seals; doors; windows; hardware; detention/security equipment and doors, windows and hardware; conveying systems; building specialties; building equipment; machinery and plant equipment, furnishings and special construction.

27.F.04 Written notifications. Before authorizing the commencement of steel erection, the Controlling contractor shall

EM 385-1-1
15 Sep 08

ensure that the steel erector is provided with the following written notifications:

a. The concrete in the footings, piers, and walls has attained, on the basis of an appropriate ASTM standard test method of field-cured samples, either 75% of the intended minimum compressive design strength or sufficient strength to support the loads imposed during steel erection.

b. Any repairs, replacements, and modifications to the anchor bolts were conducted in accordance with contract specifications and/or <u>project structural engineer of record.</u>

c. A steel erection Contractor shall not erect steel unless it has received written notification that the concrete in the footings, piers and walls has attained, on the basis of an appropriate ASTM standard test method of field-cured samples, either 75% of the intended minimum compressive design strength or sufficient strength to support the loads imposed during steel erection.

d. Both Contractors will keep a copy of this written notification on-site.

27.<u>F</u>.05 Site layout. The Controlling contractor shall ensure that the following is provided and maintained:

a. Adequate access roads into and through the site for the safe delivery and movement of derricks, cranes, trucks, other necessary equipment, and the material to be erected; and means and methods for pedestrian and vehicular control. **Exception: This requirement does not apply to roads outside of the construction site.**

b. A firm, properly graded, drained area readily accessible to the work with adequate space for the safe storage of materials and the safe operation of the erector's equipment.

EM 385-1-1
15 Sep 08

c. Pre-planning of overhead hoisting operations. All hoisting operations in steel erection shall be pre-planned.

27.F.06 Hoisting and rigging. All the applicable requirements of Sections 15 and 16 apply to this Section.

27.F.07 Inspection of cranes. A Competent Person shall visually inspect cranes being used in steel erection activities prior to each shift as per Section 16.D.

27.F.08 Deficiencies. If any deficiency is identified, an immediate determination shall be made by the Competent Person as to whether the deficiency constitutes a hazard.

a. If the deficiency is determined to constitute a hazard, the hoisting equipment shall be removed from service until the deficiency has been corrected.

b. The operator shall be responsible for those operations under the operator's direct control. Whenever there is any doubt as to safety, the operator shall have the authority to stop and refuse to handle loads until safety has been assured.

27.F.09 A Qualified Rigger shall inspect the rigging prior to each shift.

27.F.10 The headache ball, hook, or load shall not be used to transport personnel.

27.F.11 Cranes or derricks may be used to hoist employees on a personnel platform when all applicable provisions of 16.T have been met.

27.F.12 Safety latches on hooks shall not be deactivated or made inoperable. **EXCEPTION:** When a Qualified Rigger has determined that the hoisting and placing of purlins and single joists can be performed more safely by doing so and precautions related to this practice are included in the accepted steel erection plan.

EM 385-1-1
15 Sep 08

27.F.13 Structural <u>steel assembly</u>.

a. Structural stability shall be maintained at all times during the erection process.

b. The following additional requirements shall apply for multi-story structures:

(1) The permanent floors shall be installed as the erection of structural members progresses, and there shall be not more than eight stories between the erection floor and the upper-most permanent floor, except where the structural integrity is maintained as a result of the design.

(2) At no time shall there be more than four floors or 48 ft (14.6 m), whichever is less, of unfinished bolting or welding above the foundation or uppermost permanently secured floor, except where the structural integrity is maintained as a result of the design.

27.F.14 Walking/working surfaces.

a. Shear connectors and other similar devices.

(1) Tripping hazards. Shear connectors (such as headed steel studs, steel bars, or steel lugs), reinforcing bars, deformed anchors or threaded studs shall not be attached to the top flanges of beams, joists, or beam attachments so that they project vertically from or horizontally across the top flange of the member until after the metal decking, or other walking/working surface, has been installed.

(2) Installation of shear connectors on composite floors, roofs, and bridge decks. When shear connectors are used in construction of composite floors, roofs, and bridge decks, employees shall lay out and install the shear connectors after the metal decking has been installed, using the metal decking as a working platform.

EM 385-1-1
15 Sep 08

b. Plumbing-up.

(1) When deemed necessary by a Competent Person, plumbing-up equipment shall be installed in conjunction with the steel erection process to ensure the stability of the structure.

(2) When used, plumbing-up equipment shall be in place and properly installed before the structure is loaded with construction material such as loads of joists, bundles of decking, or bundles of bridging.

(3) Plumbing-up equipment shall be removed only with the approval of a Competent Person.

c. Metal decking - Hoisting, landing, and placing of metal decking bundles.

(1) Bundle packaging and strapping shall not be used for hoisting unless specifically designed for that purpose.

(2) If loose items such as dunnage, flashing, or other materials are placed on the top of metal decking bundles to be hoisted, such items shall be secured to the bundles.

(3) Bundles of metal decking on joists shall be landed in accordance with 27.F.27.

(4) Metal decking bundles shall be landed on framing members so that enough support is provided to allow the bundles to be unbanded without dislodging the bundles from the supports.

(5) At the end of the shift or when environmental or jobsite conditions require, metal decking shall be secured against displacement.

(6) Roof and floor holes and openings. Metal decking at roof and floor holes and openings shall be installed as follows:

(a) Framed metal deck openings shall have structural members turned down to allow continuous deck installation except where not allowed by structural design constraints or constructability.

(b) Roof and floor holes and openings shall be decked over <u>or protected in accordance with Section 24</u>.

(c) Metal decking holes and openings shall not be cut until immediately prior to being permanently filled with the equipment or structure needed or intended to fulfill its specific use and that meets the strength requirements of Section 24, or shall be immediately covered.

27.F.15 Installation of metal decking.

a. Metal decking shall be laid tightly and secured upon placement to prevent accidental movement or displacement. <u>A maximum of 3,000 ft^2 may be laid before securing.</u>

b. During initial placement metal-decking panels shall be placed to ensure full support by structural members.

27.F.16 Derrick floors.

a. A derrick floor shall be fully decked and/or planked and the steel member connections completed to support the intended floor loading.

b. Temporary loads placed on a derrick floor shall be distributed over the underlying support members so as to prevent local overloading of the deck material.

27.F.17 Column anchorage.

a. General requirements for erection stability.

(1) All columns shall be anchored by a minimum of four anchor rods <u>or</u> anchor bolts.

EM 385-1-1
15 Sep 08

(2) Each column anchor rod <u>or</u> anchor bolt assembly, including the column-to-base plate weld and the column foundation, shall be designed to resist a minimum eccentric gravity load of 300 lbs (136.2 kg) located 18 in (45.7 cm) from the extreme outer face of the column in each direction at the top of the column shaft.

(3) Columns shall be set on level finished floors, pre-grouted leveling plates, leveling nuts, or shim packs that are adequate to transfer the construction loads.

(4) All columns shall be evaluated by a Competent Person to determine whether guying or bracing is needed; if guying or bracing is needed, it shall be installed.

b. Repair, replacement or field modification of anchor rods or anchor bolts.

(1) Anchor rods <u>or</u> anchor bolts shall not be repaired, replaced, or field-modified without the approval of the project structural engineer of record.

(2) Prior to the erection of a column, the Controlling Contractor shall provide written notification to the steel erector if there has been any repair, replacement, or modification of the anchor rods or anchor bolts of that column.

27.<u>F.18</u> Beams and columns.

a. During the final placing of solid web structural members, the load shall not be released from the hoisting line until the members are secured with at least two bolts per connection (of the same size and strength as shown in the erection drawings) drawn up wrench-tight or the equivalent as specified by the project structural engineer of record, except as specified in 27.F.19.

EM 385-1-1
15 Sep 08

   b. A Competent Person shall determine if more than two bolts are necessary to ensure the stability of cantilevered members; if additional bolts are needed, they shall be installed.

27.F.19 Diagonal bracing. Solid web structural members used as diagonal bracing shall be secured by at least one bolt per connection drawn up wrench-tight or the equivalent as specified by the project structural engineer of record.

27.F.20 Double connections

   a. Double connections at columns and/or at beam webs over a column. When two structural members on opposite sides of a column web, or a beam web over a column, are connected sharing common connection holes, at least one bolt with its wrench-tight nut shall remain connected to the first member unless a shop-attached or field-attached seat or equivalent connection device is supplied with the member to secure the first member and prevent the column from being displaced.

   b. If a seat or equivalent device is used, the seat (or device) shall be designed to support the load during the double connection process. It shall be adequately bolted or welded to both a supporting member and the first member before the nuts on the shared bolts are removed to make the double connection.

27.F.21 Column splices. Each column splice shall be designed to resist a minimum eccentric gravity load of 300 lbs (136.2 kg) located 18 in (45.7 cm) from the extreme outer face of the column in each direction at the top of the column shaft.

27.F.22 Perimeter columns. Perimeter columns shall not be erected unless:

   a. The perimeter columns extend a minimum of 48 in (121.9 cm) above the finished floor to permit installation of perimeter safety cables prior to erection of the next tier, except where constructability does not allow.

b. The perimeter columns have holes or other devices in or attached to perimeter columns at 42-45 in (106.6-114.3 cm) above the finished floor and the midpoint between the finished floor and the top cable to permit installation of perimeter safety cables except where constructability does not allow.

27.F.23 Open web steel joists.

a. Except as provided in paragraph (b)(2) below, where steel joists are used and columns are not framed in at least two directions with solid web structural steel members, a steel joist shall be field-bolted at the column to provide lateral stability to the column during erection. For the installation of this joist:

(1) A vertical stabilizer plate shall be provided on each column for steel joists. The plate shall be a minimum of 6-in x 6-in (15.2-cm x 15.2-cm) and shall extend at least 3 in (7.6 cm) below the bottom chord of the joist with a 13/16-in (2.1-cm) hole to provide an attachment point for guying or plumbing cables.

(2) The bottom chords of steel joists at columns shall be stabilized to prevent rotation during erection.

(3) Hoisting cables shall not be released until the seat at each end of the steel joist is field-bolted, and each end of the bottom chord is restrained by the column stabilizer plate.

b. Where constructability does not allow a steel joist to be installed at the column:

(1) An alternate means of stabilizing joists shall be installed on both sides near the column and shall:

(a) Provide stability equivalent to paragraph 27.F.23.a (1) above,

(b) Be designed by a Qualified Person,

EM 385-1-1
15 Sep 08

(c) Be shop installed, and

(d) Be included in the erection drawings.

(2) Hoisting cables shall not be released until the seat at each end of the steel joist is field-bolted and the joist is stabilized.

c. Where steel joists at or near columns span 60 ft (18.3 m) or less, the joist shall be designed with sufficient strength to allow one employee to release the hoisting cable without the need for erection bridging.

d. Where steel joists at or near columns span more than 60 ft (18.3 m), the joists shall be set in tandem with all bridging installed unless an alternative method of erection, which provides equivalent stability to the steel joist, is designed by a Qualified Person and is included in the site-specific erection plan.

e. A steel joist or steel joist girder shall not be placed on any support structure unless such structure is stabilized.

f. When steel joist(s) are landed on a structure, they shall be secured to prevent unintentional displacement prior to installation.

g. No modification that affects the strength of a steel joist or steel joist girder shall be made without the approval of the project structural engineer of record.

h. Field-bolted joists.

(1) Except for steel joists that have been pre-assembled into panels, connections of individual steel joists to steel structures in bays of 40 ft (12.1 m) or more shall be fabricated to allow for field bolting during erection.

(2) These connections shall be field-bolted unless constructability does not allow.

EM 385-1-1
15 Sep 08

i. Steel joists and steel joist girders shall not be used as anchorage points for a fall arrest system unless written approval to do so is obtained from a Qualified Person.

j. A bridging terminus point shall be established before bridging is installed.

27.F.24 Attachment of steel joists and steel joist girders.

a. Each end of "K" series steel joists shall be attached to the support structure with a minimum of two 1/8-in (0.3-cm) fillet welds 1 in (2.5 cm) long or with two 1/2-in (1.2-cm) bolts, or the equivalent.

b. Each end of "LH" and "DLH" series steel joists and steel joist girders shall be attached to the support structure with a minimum of two 1/4-inch (0.6-cm) fillet welds 2 in (5 cm) long, or with two 3/4-in (1.9-cm) bolts, or the equivalent.

c. Except as provided in paragraph d below, each steel joist shall be attached to the support structure, at least at one end on both sides of the seat, immediately upon placement in the final erection position and before additional joists are placed.

d. Panels that have been pre-assembled from steel joists with bridging shall be attached to the structure at each corner before the hoisting cables are released.

27.F.25 Erection of steel joists.

a. Both sides of the seat of one end of each steel joist that requires bridging under Tables 27-1 and 27-2 shall be attached to the support structure before hoisting cables are released.

b. For joists over 60 ft (18.2 m), both ends of the joist shall be attached as specified in 27.F.24 and the provisions of 27.F.26 are met before the hoisting cables are released.

EM 385-1-1
15 Sep 08

c. On steel joists that do not require erection bridging under Tables 27-1 and 27-2, only one employee shall be allowed on the joist until all bridging is installed and anchored.

d. Employees shall not be allowed on steel joists where the span of the steel joist is equal to or greater than the span shown in Tables 27-1 and 27-2 in accordance with 27.F.26.

e. When permanent bridging terminus points cannot be used during erection, additional temporary bridging terminus points are required to provide stability.

EM 385-1-1
15 Sep 08

TABLE 27-1

ERECTION BRIDGING FOR SHORT SPAN JOISTS

JOIST	SPAN	JOIST	SPAN
8L1	NM	22K6	36-0
10K1	NM	22K7	40-0
12K1	23-0	22K9	40-0
12K3	NM	22K10	40-0
12K5	NM	22K11	40-0
14K1	27-0	24K4	36-0
14K3	NM	24K5	38-0
14K4	NM	24K6	39-0
14K6	NM	24K7	43-0
16K2	29-0	24K8	43-0
16K3	30-0	24K9	44-0
16K4	32-0	24K10	NM
16K5	32-0	24K12	NM
16K6	NM	26K5	38-0
16K7	NM	26K6	39-0
16K9	NM	26K7	43-0
18K3	31-0	26K8	44-0
18K4	32-0	26K9	45-0
18K5	33-0	26K10	49-0
18K6	35-0	26K12	NM
18K7	NM	28K6	40-0
18K9	NM	28K7	43-0
18K10	NM	28K8	44-0
20K3	32-0	28K9	45-0
20K4	34-0	28K10	49-0
20K5	34-0	28K12	53-0
20K6	36-0	30K7	44-0
20K7	39-0	30K8	45-0
20K9	39-0	30K9	45-0
20K10	NM	30K10	50-0
22K4	34-0	30K11	52-0

EM 385-1-1
15 Sep 08

TABLE 27-1 (CONTINUED)

ERECTION BRIDGING FOR SHORT SPAN JOISTS

JOIST	SPAN	JOIST	SPAN
22K5	35-0	30K12	54-0
10KCS1	NM	20KCS2	36-0
10KCS2	NM	20KCS3	39-0
12KCS1	NM	20KCS4	NM
12KCS2	NM	24KCS5	NM
12KCS3	NM	26KCS2	39-0
14KCS1	NM	26KCS3	44-0
14KCS2	NM	26KCS4	NM
14KCS3	NM	26KCS5	NM
16KCS2	NM	28KCS2	40-0
16KCS3	NM	28KCS3	45-0
16KCS4	NM	28KCS4	53-0
16KCS5	NM	28KCS5	53-0
18KCS2	35-0	30KC53	45-0
18KCS3	NM	30KCS4	54-0
18KCS4	NM	30KCS5	54-0
18KCS5	NM		

NM=diagonal bolted bridging not mandatory for joists under 40 ft (12.1 m).

EM 385-1-1
15 Sep 08

TABLE 27-2

ERECTION BRIDGING FOR LONG SPAN JOISTS

JOIST	SPAN	JOIST	SPAN
18LH02	33-0	28LH06	42-0
18LH03	NM	28LH07	NM
18LH04	NM	28LH08	NM
18LH05	NM	28LH09	NM
18LH06	NM	28LH10	NM
18LH07	NM	28LH11	NM
18LH08	NM	28LH12	NM
18LH09	NM	28LH13	NM
20LH02	33-0	32LH06	47-0 through 60-0
20LH03	38-0	32LH07	47-0 through 60-0
20LH04	NM	32LH08	55-0 through 60-0
20LH05	NM	32LH09	NM through 60-0
20LH06	NM	32LH10	NM through 60-0
20LH07	NM	32LH11	NM through 60-0
20LH08	NM	32LH12	NM through 60-0
20LH09	NM	32LH13	NM through 60-0
20LH10	NM	32LH14	NM through 60-0
24LH03	35-0	32LH15	NM through 60-0
24LH04	39-0	36LH07	47-0 through 60-0
24LH05	40-0	36LH08	47-0 through 60-0
24LH06	45-0	36LH09	57-0 through 60-0
24LH07	NM	36LH10	NM through 60-0
24LH08	NM	36LH11	NM through 60-0
24LH09	NM	36LH12	NM through 60-0
24LH10	NM	36LH13	NM through 60-0
24LH11	NM	36LH14	NM through 60-0
28LH05	42-0	36LH15	NM through 60-0

NM = diagonal bolted bridging not mandatory for joists under 40 feet (12.1 m).

27.F.26 Erection bridging.

a. Where the span of the steel joist is equal to or greater than the span shown in Tables 27-1 and 27-2, the following shall apply:

(1) A row of bolted diagonal erection bridging shall be installed near the mid-span of the steel joist,

(2) Hoisting cables shall not be released until this bolted diagonal erection bridging is installed and anchored, and

(3) No more than one employee shall be allowed on these spans until all other bridging is installed and anchored.

b. Where the span of the steel joist is over 60 ft (18.2 m) through 100 ft (30.4 m), the following shall apply:

(1) All rows of bridging shall be bolted diagonal bridging,

(2) Two rows of bolted diagonal erection bridging shall be installed near the third points of the steel joist,

(3) Hoisting cables shall not be released until this bolted diagonal erection bridging is installed and anchored, and

(4) No more than two employees shall be allowed on these spans until all other bridging is installed and anchored.

c. Where the span of the steel joist is over 100 ft (30.4 m) through 144 ft (43.9 m), the following shall apply:

(1) All rows of bridging shall be bolted diagonal bridging,

(2) Hoisting cables shall not be released until all bridging is installed and anchored, and

(3) No more than two employees shall be allowed on these spans until all bridging is installed and anchored.

EM 385-1-1
15 Sep 08

d. For steel members spanning over 144 ft (43.9 m), the erection methods used shall be in accordance with 27.F.18 through 27.F.22.

e. Where any steel joist specified in paragraphs b above and 27.F.27.a-c is a bottom chord-bearing joist, a row of bolted diagonal bridging shall be provided near the support(s). This bridging shall be installed and anchored before the hoisting cable(s) is released.

f. When bolted diagonal erection bridging is required by this section, the following shall apply:

(1) The bridging shall be indicated on the erection drawing;

(2) The erection drawing shall be the exclusive indicator of the proper placement of this bridging;

(3) Shop-installed bridging clips, or functional equivalents, shall be used where the bridging bolts to the steel joists;

(4) When two pieces of bridging are attached to the steel joist by a common bolt, the nut that secures the first piece of bridging shall not be removed from the bolt for the attachment of the second; and

(5) Bridging attachments shall not protrude above the top chord of the steel joist.

27.F.27 Landing and placing loads.

a. During the construction period, the employer placing a load on steel joists shall ensure that the load is distributed so as not to exceed the carrying capacity of any steel joist.

b. Except for paragraph d below, no construction loads are allowed on the steel joists until all bridging is installed and anchored and all joist-bearing ends are attached.

c. The weight of a bundle of joist bridging shall not exceed a total of 1,000 lbs (454 kg). A bundle of joist bridging shall be placed on a minimum of three steel joists that are secured at one end. The edge of the bridging bundle shall be positioned within 1 ft (0.3 m) of the secured end.

d. No bundle of decking may be placed on steel joists until all bridging has been installed and anchored and all joist bearing ends attached, unless all of the following conditions are met:

(1) The employer has first determined from a Qualified Person and documented in a site-specific erection plan that the structure or portion of the structure is capable of supporting the load,

(2) The bundle of decking is placed on a minimum of three steel joists,

(3) The joists supporting the bundle of decking are attached at both ends,

(4) At least one row of bridging is installed and anchored,

(5) The total weight of the bundle of decking does not exceed 4,000 lbs (1816 kg), and

(6) Placement of the bundle of decking shall follow paragraph e below.

e. The edge of the construction load shall be placed within 1 ft (0.3 m) of the bearing surface of the joist end.

27.G SYSTEMS-ENGINEERED METAL BUILDINGS

27.G.01 All of the requirements of the previous section apply to the erection of systems-engineered metal buildings except 27.F.17 (column anchorage) and 27.F.23 (open web steel joists).

EM 385-1-1
15 Sep 08

a. Each structural column shall be anchored by a minimum of four anchor rods or anchor bolts.

b. Rigid frames shall have 50% of their bolts or the number of bolts specified by the manufacturer (whichever is greater) installed and tightened on both sides of the web adjacent to each flange before the hoisting equipment is released.

c. Construction loads shall not be placed on any structural steel framework unless such framework is safely bolted, welded, or otherwise adequately secured.

d. In girt and eave strut-to-frame connections, when girts or eave struts share common connection holes, at least one bolt with its wrench-tight nut shall remain connected to the first member unless a manufacturer-supplied, field-attached seat or similar connection device is present to secure the first member so that the girt or eave strut is always secured against displacement.

e. Purlins and girts shall not be used as an anchorage point for a fall arrest system unless written approval is obtained from a Qualified Person.

f. Purlins may only be used as a walking/working surface when installing safety systems, after all permanent bridging has been installed and fall protection is provided.

g. Construction loads may be placed only within a zone that is within 8 ft (2.4 m) of the centerline of the primary support member.

h. Both ends of all steel joists or cold-formed joists shall be fully bolted and/or welded to the support structure before:

(1) Releasing the hoisting cables,

(2) Allowing an employee on the joists, or

(3) Allowing any construction loads on the joists.

27.G.02 Falling object protection.

a. Securing loose items aloft. All materials, equipment, and tools, which are not in use while aloft, shall be secured against accidental displacement.

b. Protection from falling objects other than materials being hoisted shall be provided. The Controlling contractor shall bar other construction processes below steel erection unless overhead protection for the employees below is provided.

27.G.03 Fall protection.

a. Each employee engaged in a steel erection activity who is on a walking/working surface with an unprotected side or edge more than 6 ft (1.8 m) above a lower level shall be protected from fall hazards by guardrail systems, safety net systems, engineered fall protection systems, personal fall arrest systems, positioning, or restraint systems in accordance with Section 21.

b. Perimeter safety cables. On multi-story structures, perimeter safety cables shall be installed at the final interior and exterior perimeters of the floors as soon as the metal decking has been installed.

27.G.04 Each connector shall:

a. Be protected, in accordance with 27.G.03, from fall hazards of more than 6 feet (1.8 m) above a lower level.

b. Be provided special training in the following areas: the nature of the hazards associated with connecting; and the establishment, access, and proper connecting techniques; and

c. Have completed fall protection training in accordance with 27.G.10.

27.G.05 Controlled Decking Zones (CDZ) are not permitted.

27.G.06 Guardrail systems, safety net systems, engineered fall protection systems, personal fall arrest systems, positioning device systems, and their components shall conform to Section 21.

27.G.07 Perimeter safety cables shall meet the criteria for guardrail systems.

27.G.08 Custody of fall protection. Fall protection provided by the steel erector shall remain in the area where steel erection activity has been completed, to be used by other trades, only if the Controlling Contractor or his authorized representative:

> a. Has directed the steel erector to leave the fall protection in place, and
>
> b. Has inspected and accepted control and responsibility of the fall protection prior to authorizing persons other than steel erectors to work in the area.

27.G.09 Training personnel. Training required by this Section shall be provided by a Qualified Person(s).

27.G.10 Fall hazard training. The employer shall provide a training program for all employees exposed to fall hazards. The program shall include training and instruction in the following areas:

> a. The recognition and identification of fall hazards in the work area;
>
> b.. The use and operation of guardrail systems, including perimeter safety cable systems, engineered fall protection systems, personal fall arrest systems, positioning device systems, fall restraint systems, safety net systems, and other protection to be used;

c. The correct procedures for erecting, maintaining, disassembling, and inspecting the fall protection systems to be used;

　　d. The procedures to be followed to prevent falls to lower levels and through or into holes and openings in walking/working surfaces and walls to meet requirements of Section 21, 27.E and Section 24.

27.H MASONRY CONSTRUCTION

27.H.01 A limited access zone shall be established whenever a masonry wall is being constructed. The limited access zone shall:

　　a. Be established prior to the start of construction on the wall.

　　b. Be equal to the height of the wall to be constructed plus 4 ft (1.2 m), and shall run the entire length of the wall.

　　c. Be established on the side of the wall that will be unscaffolded.

　　d. Be restricted to entry by employees actively engaged in constructing the wall; no other employees shall be permitted to enter the zone.

　　e. Remain in place until the wall is adequately supported to prevent overturning and to prevent collapse unless the height of the wall is over 8 ft (2.4 m), in which case the limited access zone shall remain in place until the requirements of 27.H.02 have been met.

27.H.02 All masonry walls over 8 ft (2.4 m) in height shall be adequately braced to prevent overturning and to prevent collapse unless the wall is adequately supported so that it will not overturn or collapse. The bracing shall remain in place until permanent supporting elements of the structure are in place.

EM 385-1-1
15 Sep 08

27.H.03 Scaffolds for masonry construction workers shall not be used to provide temporary lateral support of masonry walls.

27.H.04 Cleanouts shall be on the side of the masonry wall opposite to the scaffolding.

27.H.05 Fall protection shall be provided to masonry workers exposed to falls of 6 ft (1.8 m) or more. **> See Section 21.**

27.I ROOFING

27.I.01 Before work begins, a Competent Person shall complete a daily inspection of each job site. This individual, designated by management, shall be capable of identifying existing predictable hazards and has the authority to take prompt corrective action to eliminate them. Hazards shall be eliminated by engineering methods and if this cannot be accomplished, guarding to isolate the hazard from the exposed employees shall be implemented. In no case shall warnings or instructions be used as a substitute for elimination of hazards by engineering means or guarding.

27.I.02 Prior to the start of work, a structural analysis of the roof shall be conducted by a Qualified Person to assure that the load capacity of the rood deck will not be exceeded.

27.I.03 Where the work presents a potential hazard to the public, the Contractor shall set up and maintain barricades with proper postings to alert public to the hazards. They shall be set up in accordance with ANSI D6.1. Applicable statutes and local regulations shall be examined and the more restrictive requirements shall be followed.

27.I.04 Work on the roof shall be halted during severe weather such as strong winds, electrical storms, icing conditions, heavy rain, or snow as soon as practical.

27.I.05 The employer shall establish emergency plans and fire prevention plans. All employees shall be trained in accordance with these plans.

27.I.06 Roof openings and holes shall be protected in accordance with Section 24.

27.I.07 In the construction, maintenance, repair, and demolition, of roofs, fall protection systems shall be provided which will prevent personnel from slipping and falling from the roof and prevent personnel on lower levels from being struck by falling objects in accordance with Section 21.

27.I.08 On all roofs greater than 16 ft (4.8 m) in height, a hoisting device, stairways, or progressive platforms shall be furnished for supplying materials and equipment.

27.I.09 Roofing materials and accessories that could be moved by the wind, including metal roofing panels, which are on the roof and unattached, shall be secured when wind speeds are greater than, or are anticipated to exceed, 10 mph (16.1 km/h).

27.I.10 Access to roofs and sections of roofs shall comply with Sections 22 and 24.

27.I.11 Materials may not be stored within 6 ft (1.8 m) of the roof edge unless guardrails are erected at the roof edge. Materials that are to be piled, stacked, or grouped shall be stable and self-supporting.

27.J RESIDENTIAL CONSTRUCTION

27.J.01 All wood used for residential construction shall meet applicable building codes and design criteria. Wood used for temporary work platforms and/ or fall protection must be inspected for compliance with Sections 21 and 22, as structural lumber from the site may not meet the requirements for protective systems.

27.J.02 Hand and power tools shall be equipped and used in accordance with the requirements of Section 13.

EM 385-1-1
15 Sep 08

27.J.03 Raising Walls.

a. Before manually raising framed walls that are 10 ft (3 m) or more in height, temporary restraints such as cleats on the foundation/floor system or straps on the wall bottom plate shall be installed to prevent inadvertent horizontal sliding or uplift of the framed wall bottom plate.

b. Anchor bolts alone shall not be used for blocking or bracing when raising framed walls 10 ft (3 m) or more in height.

27.J.04 Employees shall not work from or walk on top plates, joists, rafters, trusses, beams or other structural members until they are securely braced and supported.

27.J.05 Truss Support Plate. Where a truss support plate is used during the installation of trusses, it shall be constructed of a 2-in x 6-in (5 cm x 15.2 cm) plank laid flat, secured linearly to a 2-in x 6-in plank laid on edge, supported with 2-in x 4-in (5.4 x 10.2 cm) wood members (legs) spaced no more than 6 ft (1.8 m) on center and attached to diagonal bracing adequately secured to support its intended load. All material dimensions are minimum and nominal.

27.J.06 Trusses installed without a ridge beam or other horizontal structural connection shall be connected temporarily to each other and to a secured end gable by a minimum of one 1-in x 4-in (2.5 cm x 10.2 cm) plank face-nailed to every rafter on each slope of the truss. The number of planks shall be sufficient to protect against wind-related collapse of the truss rows.

27.J.07 During construction, proper work platforms such as scaffolds and decks, in accordance with Section 22 shall be used. Walking on plates, beams, joists, and other members more than 6 ft (1.8m) above the ground or floor is prohibited unless workers meet the fall protection practices outlined in Section 21.

BLANK

EM 385-1-1
15 Sep 08

SECTION 28

HAZARDOUS WASTE OPERATIONS AND EMERGENCY RESPONSE (HAZWOPER)

28.A. GENERAL.

28.A.01 This Section applies to:

a. Hazardous waste site cleanup operations performed under the Comprehensive Environmental Response, Compensation, Liability Act (CERCLA) or RCRA as specified by OSHA in 29 CFR 1910.120 and 29 CFR 1926.65 (a) (1) (i), (ii) and (iii) (e.g., site investigations, remedial action construction, treatment process operation, and maintenance at: Formerly Used Defense Sites (FUDS) projects, Installation Restoration Program (IRP) projects, Base Realignment and Closure (BRAC) projects, Formerly Used Sites Remedial Action Program (FUSRAP) projects, U.S. Environmental Protection Agency (EPA) Superfund projects, and hazardous waste site cleanup operations performed under the civil works program).

b. Facilities or construction projects holding RCRA Treatment Storage and Disposal (TSD) permits as specified by OSHA in 29 CFR 1910.120 and 29 CFR 1926.65 (a) (1) (iv).

c. Facilities or construction projects where emergency response as specified by OSHA in 29 CFR 1910.120 and 29 CFR 1926.65 (a) (1) (v) may be required.

28.B SITE SAFETY AND HEALTH PLAN (SSHP)

28.B.01 Hazardous waste site cleanup operations require development and implementation of a SSHP that shall be attached to the APP as an appendix.

a. The APP/SSHP shall address all occupational safety and health hazards associated with site cleanup operations.

EM 385-1-1
15 Sep 08

b. Contracted work on the cleanup projects shall be performed in compliance with the APP/SSHP.

c. Cleanup operations performed by in-house (Government) personnel do not require development of an APP, but shall be performed in compliance with local district safety and health policies for in-house activities and shall comply with the SSHP.

d. Changes and modifications to the SSHP are permitted and shall be made in writing with the knowledge and concurrence of the safety and health manager (SHM) and accepted by the GDA.

28.B.02 The SSHP shall cover the following in project-specific detail. General information adequately covered in the APP (introduction, site background, SOH organization and lines of authority, general site control and layout and general site safety procedures, logs, reports and inspections) need not be duplicated.

a. Site description and contamination characterization - a description of the contamination with the exposure potential to adversely affect safety and occupational health and likely to be encountered by the on-site work activities;

b. Hazard/Risk analysis. An AHA shall be developed for each task/operation to be performed per 01.A.13. The AHA shall account for all hazards (classic safety, chemical, physical, biological, ionizing radiation) likely to be encountered while performing the work;

c. Staff organization, qualifications, and responsibilities per 28.C;

d. Training, general and project-specific per 28.D;

e. PPE. PPE used to protect workers from site-related hazards (construction safety and health and contaminant-related) shall comply with requirements specified in Section 5;

EM 385-1-1
15 Sep 08

f. Medical surveillance per 28.E. Certification of medical surveillance program participation shall be appended to the SSHP. The certification shall include: employee name, date of last examination, and name of examining physician(s). The required written physician's opinion shall be made available upon request to the GDA;

g. Exposure monitoring/Air sampling program. Exposure monitoring and air sampling shall be performed to evaluate effectiveness of prescribed PPE and to evaluate worker exposure to site-related contaminants and hazardous substances used in the cleanup process. Project-specific exposure monitoring/air sampling requirements shall comply with requirements specified Section 6;

h. Heat and cold stress. The procedures and practices for protecting workers from heat and cold stress shall comply with the requirements 06.I;

i Standard operating safety procedures, engineering controls, and work practices. Safety and occupational health procedures, engineering controls and work practices shall be addressed for the following as appropriate:

(1) Site rules/prohibitions (buddy system, eating/drinking/ smoking restrictions, etc.);

(2) Work permit requirements (radioactive work, excavation, hot work, confined space, etc.);

(3) Material handling procedures (soil, liquid, radioactive materials, spill contingency);

(4) Drum/container/tank handling (opening, sampling, overpacking, draining, pumping, purging, inerting, cleaning, excavation and removal, disassembly and disposal, spill contingency;

(5) Comprehensive AHA of treatment technologies employed at the site;

j. Site control measures. Work zones shall be established so that on-site activities do not spread contamination. The site shall be set up so that there is a clearly defined exclusion zone (EZ) and a clearly defined support zone (SZ) with a contamination reduction zone (CRZ) as a transition between the EZ and SZ;

k. Personal hygiene and decontamination. A personal hygiene and decontamination station shall be set up in the CRZ for personnel to remove contaminated PPE and to wash when exiting the EZ;

l. Equipment decontamination. An equipment decontamination station shall be set up in the CRZ for equipment to be decontaminated when exiting the EZ;

m. Emergency equipment and first aid. The equipment and personnel required for first aid and CPR shall comply with the requirements in Section 3. Emergency equipment required to be on-site shall have the capacity to respond to project-specific emergencies. Site emergencies may require (but should not be limited to) PPE and equipment to control fires, leaks and spills, or chemical (contaminant or treatment process) exposure;

n. Emergency response and contingency procedures (ERP). An ERP shall be developed that addresses the following emergency response and contingency procedures:

(1) Pre-emergency planning. An agreement shall be established between the Contractor (or the GDA for in-house work), local emergency responders, and the servicing emergency medical facility that specifies the responsibilities of on-site personnel, emergency response personnel, and the emergency medical facility in the event of an on-site emergency;

(2) Personnel and lines of authority for emergency situations;

EM 385-1-1
15 Sep 08

(3) Criteria and procedures for emergency recognition and site evacuation (e.g., emergency alarm systems, evacuation routes and reporting locations, site security);

(4) Decontamination and medical treatment of injured personnel;

(5) A route map to emergency medical facilities and phone numbers for emergency responders;

(6) Criteria for alerting the local community responders.

28.C RESPONSIBILITIES

28.C.01 Safety and Health Manager (SHM) is required at cleanup operations. The SHM, dependent upon the contaminant-related hazards on the project, shall be a Certified Industrial Hygienist (CIH), Certified Safety Professional (CSP) or Certified Health Physicist (CHP).

a. The SHM shall have 3 years of experience managing safety and occupational health at hazardous waste site cleanup operations.

b. The SHM shall enlist the support of safety and occupational health professionals with appropriate education and experience when working on sites with multiple (chemical, safety, ionizing radiation) hazards.

c. The SHM shall be responsible for the following actions:

(1) Developing, maintaining, and overseeing implementation of the SSHP;

(2) Visiting the project as needed to audit the effectiveness of the SSHP;

(3) Remaining available for project emergencies;

EM 385-1-1
15 Sep 08

(4) Developing modifications to the SSHP as needed;

(5) Evaluating occupational exposure monitoring/air sampling data and adjusting SSHP requirements as necessary;

(6) Serving as a QC staff member;

(7) Approving the SSHP by signature.

28.C.02 Site Safety and Health Officer (SSHO). The SSHO is required at cleanup operations.

a. The SSHO shall have a minimum 1 year experience implementing safety and occupational health procedures at cleanup operations.

b. The SSHO shall have training and experience to conduct exposure monitoring/air sampling and select/adjust protective equipment use.

c. The SSHO shall have the authority and is responsible for the following actions:

(1) Being present anytime cleanup operations are being performed to implement the SSHP;

(2) Inspecting site activities to identify safety and occupational health deficiencies and correct them;

(3) Coordinating changes/modifications to the SSHP with the SHM, site superintendent, and contracting officer; and

(4) Conducting project specific training.

28.D TRAINING. Personnel shall comply with the following general and project-specific training requirements:

EM 385-1-1
15 Sep 08

28.D.01 General training. General training requirements apply to project personnel exposed to contaminant-related health and safety hazards. General training must comply with the following requirements:

a. 40-hour off-site hazardous waste site instruction. Off-site instruction shall comply with the 40-hour training requirements in OSHA standards 29 CFR 1910.120 and 29 CFR 1926.65.

(1) Instructor qualifications: Personnel responsible for planning and teaching/facilitating the 40-hour training course shall be thoroughly knowledgeable of the 40-hour training topics specified by OSHA in 29 CFR 1910.120 and 29 CFR 1926.65 and shall possess the knowledge and experience to instruct on each of the topics. Instructors shall retain qualifications for teaching on organizationally relevant 40-hour training safety and occupational health topics by regularly attending and participating in formal industrial hygiene or safety related courses, seminars and conferences. Five (5) days of training over a five (5)-year period is required.

(2) 40-hour training course outline for cleanup operations. 40-hour training courses shall cover the following topics in a manner that is relevant to organizational operations:

(a) Names of personnel and alternates responsible for site safety and health;

(b) Safety, health and other hazards;

(c) Use of personal protective equipment;

(d) Work practices by which employees can minimize risks from hazards;

(e) Safe use of engineering controls and equipment to minimize exposure to hazards;

(f) Medical surveillance implemented for the protection of employees;

(g) Decontamination procedures for personnel and equipment;

(h) Emergency response plan development and implementation for site work;

(i) Confined space hazards and awareness;

(j) Spill containment.

(3) Computer-based interactive 40-hour training. Computer-based interactive training is acceptable as long as the following criteria are met:

(a) The course shall cover each of the topics required by OSHA for cleanup operations 40-hour training. See paragraph 28.D.01.a(2);

(b) Students shall be able to ask questions and receive answers in a timely manner from a qualified instructor with hazardous waste site cleanup safety and health experience;

(c) Students shall participate in 16-hours of hands-on exercises to demonstrate equipment use and procedural proficiency.

b. 3-Days On-the-Job-Training (OJT). In addition to the classroom training, the training shall include 3 days of OJT (in field) experience under the direct supervision of a trained, experienced supervisor.

c. 8-hour annual refresher training. Refresher training shall comply with the requirements in OSHA standards 29 CFR 1910.120 and 29 CFR 1926.65. USACE employees shall comply with local district hazardous waste refresher training policies.

EM 385-1-1
15 Sep 08

(1) The following is the minimum for the 8-hour refresher training course outline for cleanup operations. Refresher training courses shall cover the following topics in a manner that is relevant to organizational operations:

(a) Names of personnel and alternates responsible for site safety and health;

(b) Safety, health and other hazards;

(c) Use of personal protective equipment;

(d) Work practices by which employees can minimize risks from hazards;

(e) Safe use of engineering controls and equipment to minimize exposure to hazards;

(f) Medical surveillance implemented for the protection of employees;

(g) Decontamination procedures for personnel and equipment;

(h) Emergency response plan development and implementation for site work;

(i) Confined space hazards and awareness;

(j) Spill containment.

(2) Computer-based interactive 8-hour refresher training. Computer based interactive training is acceptable as long as the following criteria are met:

(a) The course shall cover each of the topics required by OSHA for cleanup operations refresher training. See paragraph 4 a (ii);

(b) Students shall be able to ask questions of and receive answers in a timely manner from a qualified instructor with hazardous waste site cleanup health and safety experience;

(c) Students shall have access to hands on exercises when necessary for thorough learning.

d. Supervisory training. On-site supervisors shall comply with the 8-hour supervisory training requirements in OSHA standards 29 CFR 1910.120 and 29 CFR 1926.65.

28.D.02 Project-specific training. Training specific to other sections of this manual or OSHA standards applicable to site work and operations shall be provided to workers before on-site work begins.

28.D.03 DOT and DOD training is required for all persons who prepare DOT shipping papers (including hazardous waste manifests), label, package and/or mark containers for purposes of transportation. Training shall be documented and employees should be issued an appointment letter by their command.
> See EP 415-1-266 and DOD 4500.9-R/

28.E. MEDICAL SURVEILLANCE. All personnel performing on-site work that will result in exposure to contaminant-related health and safety hazards shall be enrolled in a medical surveillance program that complies with OSHA standards 29 CFR 1910.120 (f) and 29 CFR 1926.65 (f).

28.E.01 Certification of medical surveillance program participation shall be appended to the SSHP. The certification shall include: employee name, date of last examination, and name of examining physician(s).

28.E.02 The required written physician's opinion shall be made available upon request to the GDA.

28.E.03 All medical records shall be maintained in accordance with 29 CFR 1910.1020.

EM 385-1-1
15 Sep 08

28.E.04 USACE employees must comply with USACE medical surveillance policies.

28.E.05 Should any unforeseen hazard become evident during the performance of work, the SSHO shall bring such hazard information to the attention of the SHM and the GDA (both verbally and in writing) for resolution as soon as possible. In the interim, necessary action shall be taken to reestablish and maintain safe working conditions.

28.F RCRA TSD FACILITIES. Requirements specified in 29 CFR 1910.120 and 29 CFR 1926.65(p), and the terms of the facility RCRA permit shall be complied with for operations at TSD facilities.

28.G FACILITY OR CONSTRUCTION PROJECT EMERGENCY RESPONSE. Projects using, storing, or handling hazardous substances and whose employees will be engaged in emergency response operations shall comply with 29 CFR 1910.120 (q) and 29 CFR 1926.65 (q) (a) (1) (v) when a hazardous substance release may result in exposure causing adverse affects to the health or safety of employees.

EXCEPTION: Projects that will evacuate their employees from the danger area when an emergency occurs, and do not permit any of their employees to assist in handling the emergency, (if they provide an emergency response plan (ERP) in accordance with 29 CFR 1910.38(a) and 29 CFR 1926.35).

28.G.01 If applicable, the site manager shall develop and implement an ERP that addresses the following items:

a. Operations. Identify operations requiring use of hazardous substances;

b. Pre-emergency planning with local emergency responders. Describe emergency response agreements, including roles and responsibilities, made with local emergency responders for hazardous material response, fire, rescue, emergency medical care, and security and law enforcement;

c. Personnel roles, lines of authority, training, and communication. Describe key personnel roles, command structure/lines of authority and communications requirements for responding to site-specific hazardous substance releases;

d. Emergency recognition and prevention. Identify the likely emergency scenarios for the project and how employees can expect to identify and recognize emergency scenarios;

e. Safe distances and places of refuge. Select safe places of refuge to be used in emergency situations, identify these locations in the ERP, and require employees to report to selected places of refuge during emergencies;

f. Site security and control. Describe how the facility will be secured and describe access to the site controlled during emergencies;

g. Evacuation routes and procedures. Describe and map out evacuation routes to safe places of refuge and any special safety and health procedures employees must follow while evacuating the facility;

h. Decontamination. Develop and describe plans and procedures for decontaminating personnel if/when they come in contact with leaking hazardous substances;

i. Emergency medical treatment and first aid. Explain how emergency medical treatment and first aid will be provided in the event of a hazardous substance spill;

j. Emergency alerting and response procedures. Describe how personnel will be alerted in the event of a hazardous substance spill, and how facility personnel must respond after emergency alerting procedures are initiated;

k. Critique of response and follow-up. Describe how lessons learned from emergency response will be documented and used to improve future emergency response actions;

l. PPE and emergency equipment. Describe the PPE and emergency response equipment that will be available for use by response personnel at the facility;

m. ERT. Designate a facility-specific ERT. Describe the team's emergency responsibilities for interacting with local emergency response providers (i.e., where the facility team's responsibilities end and the local response providers begin);

28.G.02 Personnel training requirements. At a minimum, ERT personnel at the project shall be trained to the "First Responder Operations Levels" specified in 29 CFR 1910.120 (q)(6)(ii). Response above and beyond defensive requires additional training and highly qualified supervision under 29 CFR 1910.120(q) and 29 CFR 1926.65(q) and must be specified on a project specific basis.

28.G.03 ERT responsibilities. The ERT shall, at a minimum, respond in a defensive manner to hazardous substance releases at the facility or construction project using the equipment and procedures specified in the ERP for defensive response. The ERT shall only provide response services beyond defensive if qualified and only according the procedures specified in the facility or construction project-specific ERP.

BLANK

EM 385-1-1
15 Sep 08

SECTION 29

BLASTING

29.A GENERAL

29.A.01 Prerequisites.

    a. Permission in writing shall be obtained from the GDA before explosive materials are brought onto the job site. Periodic replenishment of approved supplies does not require written approval.

    b. Prior to bringing explosives on site, the contractor shall develop a blasting safety plan. As a minimum, this plan shall be accepted by the GDA and include the following:

(1) List the names, qualifications, and responsibilities of personnel involved with explosives;

(2) The Contractor's requirements for handling, transportation, and storage of explosives; employee training programs <u>and certifications</u>; <u>types of explosives; schedule of activities and</u> loading procedures; <u>detailed blasting schedule;</u> <u>explosives transportation route;</u> safety signals <u>methods and locations;</u> danger area clearance; methods for securing the site; <u>seismograph,</u> vibration and damage control; <u>test shots,</u> post-blast inspection and misfire procedures; provisions for disposal of explosives, blasting agents, <u>unused and</u> associated material; and post-blast ventilation requirements;

<u>(3) Public relations requirements before and after blasting (e.g.; community communication, protection of structures and personnel).</u>

    <u>c. If work is performed with military explosives, the blasting plan is required to be submitted (throughout the chain of command,</u>

ref. EM 385-1-97, Chapter IV.C) to DDESB upon request. (DoD 6055.09-STD, paragraph C1.3.1 and EM 385-1-97).

29.A.02 The transporting, handling, storage, and use of explosives, blasting agents, and blasting equipment shall be directed and supervised by a person of proven experience and ability in blasting operations in accordance with ANSI A10.7; 29 CFR 1910.109; 29 CFR 1926, Subpart U; 27 CFR 555; the manufacturers, the Institute of Makers of Explosives (IME), and, where applicable, DoD 6055.9-STD. > *See 26.J.*

29.A.03 All persons working with explosives shall be in good physical condition and be able to understand and give written and verbal orders.

29.A.04 Warning signs shall be provided at points of access to blasting area.

29.A.05 Operations involving the handling or use of explosive materials shall be discontinued and personnel moved to a safe area during the approach or progress of a thunderstorm or dust storm; controls will be established to prevent accidental discharge of electric blasting caps from extraneous electricity.

29.A.06 Blasting operations near overhead power lines, communications lines, utility services, or other structures shall not be carried on until the operators and/or owners have been notified and measures for safe control have been taken.

29.A.07 All loading and firing shall be directed and supervised by one designated person.

29.A.08 A positive system to detect and measure the probability of lightning or massive static electrical discharges shall be used.

29.A.09 Before adopting any system of electrical firing, a thorough survey shall be made for extraneous currents and all dangerous currents shall be eliminated before any holes are loaded.

EM 385-1-1
15 Sep 08

29.A.10 Blasts using electric detonators shall be fired with an electric blasting machine or a properly designed power source.

   a. Blasts using non-electric detonators shall be fired by a blasting machine or starting device prescribed by the manufacturer.

   b. When blasting near radar or radio transmission facilities or near electrical energy sources where testing has shown that RF energy or stray electrical current may present a hazard to electrical blasting, an approved non-electrical initiation system shall be employed.

   c. When electric detonators are used, leg wires shall be short circuited (shunted) until connected into the circuit for firing.

29.A.11 Detonating cord shall be initiated by non-electric detonator (cap and fuse), electric detonator, shock tube detonator or gas initiated detonator in accordance with the manufacturer's recommendation.

29.A.12 Delay electric detonators, non-electric delay detonators, detonating cord connectors, or sequential blasting machines shall be used for all delayed blasts; the practice shall conform to the manufacturer's recommendations.

29.A.13 Blasting machines.

   a. Blasting machines shall be operated, maintained, tested, and inspected as prescribed by the manufacturer.

   b. Blasting machines shall be tested prior to use and periodically thereafter as prescribed by the manufacturer.

   c. Blasting machines shall be secured and accessible only to the blaster; only the blaster shall connect the leading wire to the machine.

EM 385-1-1
15 Sep 08

29.A.14 When energy for blasting is taken from power circuits, the voltage shall not exceed 550 volts. The wiring controlling arrangements shall conform to the following (see Figures 29-1 and 29-2):

FIGURE 29-1

POWER FIRING SYSTEMS FOR SERIES AND PARALLEL SERIES FIRING (NO ARCONTROLLER)

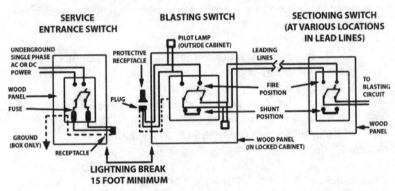

FIGURE 29-2

RECOMMENDED INSTALLATION OF SHOOTING STATION AND ACCESSORY ARRANGEMENT FOR USING ARCONTROLLER

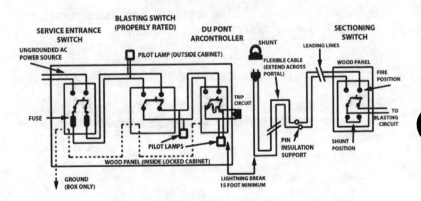

EM 385-1-1
15 Sep 08

a. The blasting switch shall be an ungrounded UL (or other nationally-recognized testing laboratory) listed, enclosed, externally operated double-pole double-throw switch that, when locked in the open position, will shunt the firing lines.

b. A grounded switch shall be installed between the blasting switch and the power circuit at a distance not less than 15 ft (4.5 m) from the blasting switch.

c. A lightning gap of at least 15 ft (4.5 m) shall be provided between the two switches; the gap connection shall be made by cable, plug, and receptacle.

29.A.15 The cable between switches shall be disconnected and both switches shall be locked in the open position immediately after firing the shot.

29.A.16 Keys to the switches shall remain in the possession of the blaster at all times.

29.A.17 Insulated solid core wires of an appropriate gage in good condition shall be used for all lines.

29.A.18 Sufficient firing line shall be provided to permit the blaster to be located at a safe distance from the blast.

29.A.19 Mechanized equipment (including drills) shall not be operated within 50 ft (15.2 m) of a loaded hole. **EXCEPTION:** Mechanized equipment may be permitted to operate within 50 ft (15.2 m) of a loaded hole when placing blasting mats or back covering.

29.A.20 The use of black powder shall be prohibited.

29.A.21 All refuse from explosive loading such as empty boxes, paper, and fiber packing shall not be used again for any purpose, but shall be destroyed by burning at an approved location.

29.A.22 Storage of explosives.

EM 385-1-1
15 Sep 08

a. The storage of explosives shall be in accordance with requirements of the Bureau of Alcohol, Tobacco, and Firearms (as outlined in 27 CFR 555, Subpart K) or the State in which they are stored.

b. An accurate running inventory of all explosives and blasting agents stored at the project shall be maintained: two copies shall be maintained - one at the magazine and one in a facility which is at least 50 ft (15.2 m) from the magazine.

29.A.23 Security of Explosives.

a. Area shall be guarded to control access to the explosives and ensure no tapping with explosives during non-working times.

b. Explosive materials shall not be abandoned.

29.B TRANSPORTATION OF EXPLOSIVE MATERIALS

29.B.01 Transportation of explosives by the following modes shall be in accordance with the prescribed federal regulations and the applicable state requirements.

a. Transportation of explosive materials over public highways shall be in accordance with DOT requirements.

b. Marine transportation of explosive materials shall be in accordance with USCG requirements.

c. Transportation of explosive materials by aircraft shall be in accordance with FAA requirements.

29.B.02 Vehicles used for transportation of explosive materials shall not be loaded beyond their rated capacity and the explosive materials shall be secured to prevent shifting of load or dislodgment from the vehicle; when explosive materials are transported by a vehicle with an open body, a magazine or closed container shall be securely mounted on the bed to contain the cargo.

29.B.03 Vehicles transporting explosive materials shall display all placards, lettering, and/or numbering required by DOT.

29.B.04 Explosive materials and blasting supplies shall not be transported with other materials or cargoes. Blasting caps (including electric) shall not be transported in the vehicle or conveyance with other explosives unless the conditions of 49 CFR 177.835(g) are met.

29.B.05 Personnel.

    a. Vehicles for transportation of explosive materials shall be in the charge of and operated by a person who is physically fit, careful, reliable, able to read and understand safety instructions, and not under the influence of intoxicants or narcotics.

    b. Only the authorized driver and a properly trained helper shall be permitted to ride on any conveyance transporting explosive materials or detonators.

29.B.06 Vehicles used in the transportation of explosives shall be substantially constructed, in good repair, and shall have tight beds to prevent explosives from falling from the vehicle. The ends and sides of vehicles shall be high enough to prevent containers from falling off.

29.B.07 Explosives shall not be exposed to sparking metal during transportation. When steel or part steel bodies are used, non-sparking cushioning materials shall separate the containers of explosives from the metal.

29.B.08 No spark-producing tools, carbides, oils, matches, firearms, electric storage batteries, flammable substances, acids, or oxidizing or corrosive compounds shall be carried in the bed or body of any vehicle transporting explosive materials.

EM 385-1-1
15 Sep 08

29.B.09 Vehicles transporting explosive materials shall be equipped with one or more fire extinguishers having a rating of 10-B:C and placed at strategic points.

   a. The extinguishers shall be of a type listed by a nationally-recognized testing laboratory and shall be ready for use.

   b. The driver will be trained in the use of the extinguisher.

29.B.10 A vehicle containing explosive materials shall not be taken into a garage or repair shop, parked in congested areas, or stored at any time in a public garage or similar building.

29.B.11 Vehicles transporting explosive materials shall be operated with extreme care. Full stops shall be made at approaches to all railroad crossings and main highways, and the vehicles shall not proceed until it is known that the way is clear.

29.B.12 No vehicle shall be refueled while explosive materials are on the motor vehicle except in an emergency.

29.B.13 Persons employed in the transportation, handling, or other use of explosive materials shall not smoke or carry on their persons or in the vehicle, matches, firearms, ammunition, or flame-producing devices.

29.B.14 Provision shall be made for safe transfer of explosive materials to magazine vessels including substantial ramps or walkways free of tripping hazards.

29.B.15 Vehicles transporting explosive materials shall not be left unattended.

29.B.16 The hoist operator shall be notified before explosive materials are transported in a shaft conveyance.

EM 385-1-1
15 Sep 08

29.B.17 Explosive materials shall be hoisted, lowered, or conveyed in a powder car. No other materials, supplies or equipment shall be transported in the same conveyance at the same time.

29.B.18 No person shall ride in any shaft conveyance transporting explosive materials. Loading and unloading shall be accomplished only when the conveyance is stationary.

29.B.19 No explosive materials shall be transported on any locomotive. At least two car lengths shall separate the locomotive from the powder car.

29.B.20 No explosive materials shall be transported on a man haul trip.

29.B.21 The car or conveyance containing explosive materials shall be pulled, not pushed, whenever possible.

29.B.22 The powder car or conveyance built for transporting explosive materials shall bear a reflectorized sign with a sharply contrasting background on each side with the word **"EXPLOSIVES"** in letters not less than 4 in (10.1 cm) in height.

29.C HANDLING OF EXPLOSIVE MATERIALS

29.C.01 There shall be no smoking, open lights, or fire of any kind within 50 ft (15.2 m) of any area where explosives are being handled. No source of ignition, except necessary means to light fuses or fire electric detonators, shall be permitted in an area containing loaded holes.

29.C.02 Containers of explosive materials shall be opened only with non-sparking tools or instruments. Metal cutters may be used for opening fiberboard boxes, paper bags or plastic tubes.

29.C.03 Explosive materials shall be removed from containers only as they are needed for immediate use.

EM 385-1-1
15 Sep 08

29.C.04 Explosive materials and detonators or primers shall be separated and taken to the blasting area in original containers, Type 3 Magazines, or containers prescribed by 49 CFR 177.835.

29.C.05 Primers shall not be made up in excess of immediate need for holes to be loaded.

29.C.06 Primers shall not be made up in or near magazines or excessive quantities of explosive materials.

29.C.07 After loading of a blast is completed, all excess explosive materials and detonators shall be removed to a safe location or returned at once to the storage magazines, observing the same rules as when being conveyed to the blasting area.

29.C.08 The quantity of explosive materials taken to an underground loading area shall not exceed the amount estimated to be necessary for the blast.

29.C.09 Detonators and explosive materials shall be taken separately into pressure working chambers.

29.D ELECTROMAGNETIC RADIATION

29.D.01 Blasting operations or storage of electrical detonators shall be prohibited in vicinity of operating RF transmitters or other RF producing devices except where the clearances in ANSI C95.4 can be maintained.

29.D.02 When necessary to perform blasting operations at a distance less than those shown in ANSI C95.4 tables, an approved non-electric initiation system shall be used.

29.D.03 Mobile radio transmitters, which are less than 100 ft (30.4 m) away from electric blasting caps in other than original containers, shall be de-energized and effectively locked, except in blasting areas where a non-electric initiation system as described in 29.A.11 is used.

EM 385-1-1
15 Sep 08

29.E VIBRATION AND DAMAGE CONTROL

29.E.01 Blasting operations in or adjacent to cofferdams, piers, underwater structures, buildings, structures, or other facilities shall be carefully planned with full consideration for all forces and conditions involved.

29.E.02 Prior to initiation of vibration controlled blasting operations, a written plan for monitoring the operations shall be established.

29.E.03 When appropriate, owners, occupants, and the public shall be notified of the nature of blasting operations to be undertaken and controls to be established.

29.E.04 Where vibration damage may occur, energy ratios and peak particle velocities shall be limited in accordance with state requirements or the requirements in Table 29-1, whichever is more stringent. When any recording indicates either the energy ratio or peak particle velocity limits have been exceeded, blasting shall be suspended and the designated authority (Government and Contractor) shall be immediately notified; blasting shall not be resumed until the probable cause has been determined and corrective measures taken.

EM 385-1-1
15 Sep 08

TABLE 29-1

ENERGY RATIO AND PEAK PARTICLE VELOCITY FORMULA

The maximum total energy ratio (ER) shall be limited to 1.0, calculated as follows: $$ER = (3.29FA)^2$$ where: F = frequency in cycles per second   A = amplitude in inches   The total energy ratio is equal to the arithmetic sum of the energy ratios in the 3 mutually perpendicular planes of motion in the vertical and horizontal directions at any one instant of time.
The maximum total peak particle velocity (PV) shall be limited to 1.92, calculated as follows: $$PV = A/t$$ where: A = amplitude in inches   t = time in seconds   The total peak particle velocity is equal to the vector sum of the particle velocities in the 3 mutually perpendicular planes of motion in the vertical and horizontal directions at any one instant of time.

29.E.05 Where required by State regulations, scaled distances shall be determined before each shot and included in the records. Scaled distances shall not exceed limitations set by the State.

29.E.06 Air blast pressure exerted on structures resulting from blasting shall not exceed 133 dB (0.013 psi).

EM 385-1-1
15 Sep 08

29.E.07 The monitoring, recording, and interpreting of vibrations shall be by qualified personnel. Records and interpretations shall be furnished to the GDA.

29.F DRILLING AND LOADING

29.F.01 All drill holes shall be sufficiently large enough to freely allow for the insertion of the explosives.

29.F.02 Drilling shall not be done in an area already blasted until remaining "bootlegs" are examined for unexploded charges and the total area has been examined to make sure that there are no unexploded charges remaining.

   a. Never insert a drill, pick, or bar into bootlegs even if examination fails to disclose explosives.

   b. When misfires have occurred and drilling must be done in an area where undetonated holes may exist, holes shall not be drilled where there is danger of intersecting a misfired hole.

   c. All drilling necessary to neutralize misfires must be done under the supervision of a competent person who has a working knowledge of the explosive materials involved and is familiar with the conditions under which the misfired holes were drilled, loaded, primed, and initiated, and is familiar with the drilling equipment capabilities that will be used during the neutralization.

29.F.03 Drilling and loading operations shall not be carried on in the same area. Drilling shall be separated from loaded holes by at least the depth of the loaded hole but in no case less than 50 ft (15.2 m).

29.F.04 No person shall be allowed to deepen drill holes that have contained explosives or blasting agents.

29.F.05 Holes shall not be drilled so that they disturb or intersect a loaded hole.

EM 385-1-1
15 Sep 08

29.F.06 See Section 18.H for earth drilling requirements.

29.F.07 The loading or loaded area shall be kept free of any equipment, operations, or persons not essential to loading; no vehicle traffic shall be permitted over loaded holes; the blast site shall be guarded or barricaded and posted with danger signs to restrict unauthorized entry.

29.F.08 No holes shall be loaded except those to be fired in the next round of blasting; after loading, all remaining explosive materials and detonators shall be immediately returned to an authorized magazine; no explosive materials or loaded holes shall be left unattended at the blast site at any time.

29.F.09 Loading of sprung or jet-pierced holes shall be prohibited until it is established that the hole has cooled sufficiently to allow loading.

29.F.10 No explosive shall be loaded or used underground in the presence of combustible gases or combustible dusts unless the conditions of use have been thoroughly identified and accepted, in writing, as safe by a competent person qualified by a thorough knowledge of the factors to be evaluated or by the written permission of the authority having jurisdiction where an authority exercises jurisdiction.

29.F.11 Cartridges shall be primed only in the number required for a single round of blasting.

29.F.12 No detonator shall be inserted in explosive materials which do not have a cap well without first making a hole in the cartridge with a non-sparking punch of proper size, or the appropriate pointed handle of a cap crimper.

29.F.13 Cartridges shall be seated by even steady pressure only.

29.F.14 Tamping shall be done with wood rods without exposed metal parts. Non-sparking metal connectors may be used for joint poles. An approved plastic tamping pole may also be used.

EM 385-1-1
15 Sep 08

29.F.15 Springing boreholes.

   a. A borehole shall never be sprung when it is adjacent to or near a hole that is loaded.

   b. Flashlight batteries shall never be used as a power source to replace a blasting machine when springing boreholes.

29.F.16 Use of detonating cord.

   a. Detonating cord shall be handled and used with the same respect and care given other explosives. Care shall be made to avoid damaging or severing cord during and after loading and hooking-up.

   b. When using a detonating cord down line, after the primer is loaded in the hole, the detonating cord shall be cut from the supply reel before loading the rest of the charge.

   c. Detonating cord connections shall be positive in accordance with recommended methods. Knot or other cord-to-cord connections shall be made only with detonating cord in which the explosive core is dry.

   d. All detonating cord trunk lines and branch lines shall be free of loops, sharp kinks, or angles that direct the cord back toward the oncoming line of detonation.

   e. When connecting a detonator to detonating cord, the detonators shall be taped or otherwise attached securely along the side or the end of the detonating cord, with the end of the detonator containing the explosive charge pointing in the direction in which the detonation is to proceed.

   f. Detonators for firing the trunk line shall not be brought to the loading area nor attached to the detonating cord until everything else is in ready for the blast.

EM 385-1-1
15 Sep 08

29.F.17 The blaster shall keep an accurate, up-to-date record of explosives, blasting agents, and blasting supplies used in a blast.

29.F.18 Loaded holes shall be stemmed to the collar with non-combustible material.

29.F.19 All loaded holes or charges shall be checked and located and all detonating cord connections shall be inspected before firing the blast.

29.F.20 All charges shall be covered with blasting mats or back covered before firing where blasting may cause injury or damage by flying rock or debris. Where mats are used, care shall be taken to protect electric blasting circuits.

29.G WIRING

29.G.01 In any blast using electric detonators, all blasting caps shall be from the same manufacturer.

29.G.02 Wiring.

    a. Bus wires shall be single solid wires of sufficient current carrying capacity.

    b. The insulation on all firing lines shall be adequate and in good condition.

29.G.03 The number of electric blasting caps in a circuit shall not exceed the capacity of blasting machine or power source.

29.G.04 A power circuit used for firing electric detonators shall not be grounded.

29.G.05 Whenever the possibility exists that a leading wire might be thrown onto a live power source by the force of the explosion, care shall be taken to see that the total length of wires is kept too short to contact the source or that the wires are securely anchored

EM 385-1-1
15 Sep 08

to the ground. Alternatively, de-energize the live power until it is certain during the post blast inspection that the lines have not crossed. If these requirements cannot be met, a non-electric system shall be used.

29.G.06 The manufacturer's shunt shall not be removed from the cap leg wires until the cap is connected to the lead line or to another cap in preparation for the assembly of two or more caps into a series circuit or when the cap is to be tested.

29.G.07 No lead wire shall be connected to the circuit until it has been grounded to dissipate any static charge.

29.G.08 The circuit, including all caps, shall be tested with an approved blasting instrument (blasting galvanometer, blasting ohmmeter, blaster's ohmmeter, or blaster's multimeter) before being connected to a firing line.

29.G.09 No firing line shall be connected to a blasting machine or other power source until the shot is to be fired. The firing line shall be checked with an approved blasting instrument before being connected to the blasting machine or other power source.

29.G.10 When a single series of caps is to be fired, or a number of series of caps is to be fired as a series-in-parallel circuit, the resistance of the circuit shall be checked with an approved blasting instrument.

29.G.11 For series-in-parallel circuits, each series shall have the same resistance.

29.G.12 Each series circuit shall be separately tested for two readings:

   a. To ensure that the series is complete; and

   b. To ensure that each series shows the same resistance and that this resistance is as close to the calculated resistance for such a series of caps as the testing instrument will read. If the

EM 385-1-1
15 Sep 08

first reading shows a series to be incomplete, the faulty cap or connection shall be located and corrected. If the second reading shows incorrect resistance, the cause shall be found and corrected.

29.H FIRING

29.H.01 Prior to the firing of a shot, all persons in the danger area shall be warned of the blast and ordered to a safe distance from the area. Blasts shall not be fired until it is certain that every person has retreated to a safe distance and no one remains in a dangerous location.

29.H.02 Prior to the firing of a shot, a competent flag person shall be posted at all access points to danger areas.

29.H.03 Prior to the firing of a shot, drill boats and other vessels shall be moved a safe distance from the danger area.

   a. Prior to and while the drill boat or vessel is being moved from the danger area, a series of short signals by horn or whistle similar to the usual navigation warning signals shall be given.

   b. No blast shall be fired while any vessel under way is closer than 1,500 ft (457.2 m) to the underwater blasting area. Those on board vessels or craft moored or anchored within 1,500 ft must be notified before a blast is fired.

   c. No blast shall be fired closer than 250 ft (76.2 m) to a boat or vessel containing an explosive magazine; personnel engaged in drilling operations on another drill boat within 500 ft (152.4 m) shall leave the drill frames for cover if any holes have been loaded.

   d. No blast shall be fired while any swimming or diving is in progress near the blasting area.

   e. Whenever a drill boat is moved from the drilling setting, all loaded under water holes shall be fired.

EM 385-1-1
15 Sep 08

29.H.04 Safety signals.

  a. All blasting operations shall use the following safety signals:

  (1) **WARNING SIGNAL** - a one-minute series of long audible signals 5 minutes prior to blast signal;

  (2) **BLAST SIGNAL** - a series of short audible signals 1 minute prior to the shot; and

  (3) **ALL CLEAR SIGNAL** - a prolonged audible signal following the inspection of blast area.

  b. The safety signals shall be given by use of a compressed air whistle, a horn, or equivalent means, and shall be clearly audible at the most distant point in the blast area. The boat whistle on a drill boat shall not be used as a blasting signal.

  c. The code for safety signals and warning signs and flags shall be posted at all access points.

  d. Employees shall be made familiar with the signals and instructed accordingly.

29.H.05 The person making leading wire connections shall fire the shot. All connections shall be made from the borehole back to the source of firing current and the leading wire shall remain shorted and not be connected to the blasting machine or other source of current until the charge is to be fired.

29.H.06 After firing an electric blast, the leading wires shall be immediately disconnected from the power source and shunted.

29.H.07 When firing a circuit of electric blasting caps, care shall be exercised to ensure that an adequate quantity of delivered current is available in accordance with the manufacturer's recommendations.

EM 385-1-1
15 Sep 08

29.I POST-BLAST PROCEDURES

29.I.01 Immediately after blast has been fired, the firing line shall be disconnected from the blasting machine or power source. Power switches shall be locked open. Atmospheres in confined areas shall be tested and/or ventilated after blast.

29.I.02 An inspection shall be made by the blaster to determine that all charges have been exploded. All wires shall be traced and search made for unexploded cartridges.

29.I.03 Other persons shall not be allowed to return to the area of the blast until an "all clear" signal is given.

29.I.04 Loose pieces of rock and other debris shall be scaled down from the sides of the face of excavation and the area made safe before proceeding with the work.

29.I.05 Misfires.

   a. Misfires shall be handled under the direction of the blaster. The blaster shall determine the safest method for handling the hazards of misfires (some misfires may require consultation with the supplier or manufacturer of the explosive material).

   b. When a misfire is <u>declared</u>, the blaster shall <u>wait 1-hour before inspecting the site and</u> provide proper safeguards for excluding all employees, except those necessary to do the work, from the danger zone.

   c. No other work shall be done except that necessary to remove the hazard of the misfire. Only those employees necessary to do the work shall remain in the danger zone.

   d. No drilling, digging, or picking shall be permitted until all <u>misfire</u> holes have been detonated or the blaster has approved that work can proceed.

EM 385-1-1
15 Sep 08

e. Based on contractor experience, a secondary/dual initiation system to prevent misfires should be considered.

29.J UNDERWATER BLASTING

29.J.01 A blaster shall conduct all blasting operations. No shot shall be fired without his approval.

29.J.02 Loading tubes and casings of dissimilar metals shall not be used because of possible electric transient currents from galvanic action of the metals and water.

29.J.03 Only water-resistant blasting caps and detonating cords shall be used for all marine blasting. Loading shall be done through a non-sparking metal loading tube when necessary.

29.J.04 Blasting flags shall be displayed.

29.J.05 The storage and handling of explosive materials aboard vessels used in underwater blasting operations shall be according to provisions in 29.A and 29.C.

29.J.06 When more than one hole is loaded to be fired underwater, a steel shot line shall be anchored and floated over the row of loaded holes.

   a. The detonation down line from each loaded hole shall be tied to the steel line and the loose end shall be tied to the detonation trunk line.

   b. After the trunk line fires, the steel shot line shall be inspected for misfires. Misfires shall be handled in accordance with the requirements of 29.I.05.

29.J.07 When drilling near or adjacent to a loaded hole, drilling shall be limited to vertical holes only. Drilling shall be separated from loaded holes by the depth of water plus the depth of the loaded hole.

EM 385-1-1
15 Sep 08

a. If a solid casing or drill mast - vertically plumbed with an inclinometer - is extended from the barge and firmly seated on bedrock, the distance between a loaded hole and one being drilled shall be 1/3 the depth of the hole, with a minimum of 8 ft (2.4 m) between the loaded hole and the one being drilled.

b. Drilling shall be halted to check alignment with an inclinometer every 4 ft (1.2 m) of hole depth.

EM 385-1-1
15 Sep 08

SECTION 30

DIVING OPERATIONS

30.A GENERAL

30.A.01 All USACE diving operations, both government and contractor shall be performed in accordance with this manual. Failure to meet these requirements will be cause for rejection or cessation of operations. Unless otherwise delegated in this section, requests for waivers or variance to the requirements of this section must be made in accordance with Appendix N of this manual through the local Designated Dive Coordinator (DDC) or the Alternate Dive Coordinator (ADC) acting on their behalf.

30.A.02 The USACE Command, at their discretion, may elect to implement and enforce more conservative diving requirements than stated herein, but under no circumstances will the operational requirements be less than specified in this Section.

30.A.03 Diving shall not be used as a work method if the work objective can be more safely and efficiently accomplished by another means (e.g., using remote controlled television systems in lieu of divers).

30.A.04 Surface-Supplied Air (SSA) shall be used whenever possible in accordance with the practical constraints of diving operations.

30.A.05 Live boating will not be used without prior specific acceptance by the DDC.

30.A.06 Training documentation shall be in compliance with the OSHA Diving Standards 29 CFR 1910.410 and shall show that the dive team members have successfully completed training to the appropriate level (e.g., SSA diver's certificate, surface supplied mixed-gas diver certificate). Such training shall be provided by:

a. A commercial diving school, military school, Federal school (e.g., USACE), or an Association of Commercial Diving Educators (ACDE) accredited school;

b. An in-house training program that meets the requirements contained in ANSI/ACDE-01, or in the Association of Diving Contractors International (ADCI) Consensus Standards;

c. Training for Scientific Divers using compressed air (SCUBA or SSA), shall be in compliance with 29 CFR 1910.410 and shall meet the above requirements or the training guidelines in the Standards for Scientific Diving published by the American Academy of Underwater Scientists (AAUS).

30.A.07 In substitution for a training certificate, an ADCI member company may show proof of a dive team member's qualification or experience by submitting a valid "ADCI Card" for the appropriate training level issued by the current employer.

30.A.08 Contractors shall provide evidence that each dive team member has training and experience consistent with the performance requirements of the scope of work. As a minimum, each team member shall have at least 1 year of commercial experience in the applicable position; divers shall have completed at least four (4) working dives with similar decompression techniques as in the contract, using the particular diving techniques and equipment to be used under the contract. Divers shall demonstrate that at least one (1) of the four (4) qualification dives was performed in the last 6 months prior to the contract award date. The DDC will ensure USACE divers meet the training and qualification requirements of ER 385-1-86.

30.A.09 Each dive team member shall have current certification in CPR, first aid, the use of emergency oxygen systems, and, if provided on the dive site, the use of Automated External Defibrillators (AEDs). Evidence of this will be a photocopy of the certificates.

EM 385-1-1
15 Sep 08

30.A.10 Divers will receive an annual diving physical. A statement that each diver has been medically examined within the previous 12 months and has been determined fit and approved to dive shall be signed by a licensed physician. The DDC will maintain a file of physician clearance certifications for all USACE divers. Contractors shall submit physician's certification to the DDC in accordance with 30.A.14. After any serious diving injury or illness, divers shall be re-examined by a physician and approved for diving.

30.A.11 Divers will wait at least 12 hours before flying after any dive: this interval should be extended to 24 hours following multiple days of repetitive dives.

30.A.12 When diving at altitudes of 1000 ft (304.8 m) or more of elevation above sea level, Dive Supervisors shall use appropriate high altitude decompression tables that compensate for the increased elevation.

30.A.13 Contract diving operations will be monitored and/or inspected by personnel qualified as USACE Dive Inspectors. Individual USACE Dive teams shall be inspected during operations at least once annually by the DDC, ADC and/ or Dive Safety Representative (DSR)

   a. Qualified Dive Inspectors shall hold current USACE training certification as Dive Inspector, Diver/ Dive Supervisor, Dive Safety Administrator, or Dive Coordinator; however, use of trained monitors/inspectors with other credentials will be considered on a case-by-case basis and may be approved in writing by the DDC. All USACE personnel used as dive inspectors must be approved by the DDC prior to performing inspector duties.

   b. Inspectors shall conduct on-site monitoring/ inspections of contractor dive sites during pre-dive conference, equipment inspection, and initial dives. Monitoring may be continuous for the duration of the contract dive activity or intermittent, as determined by the DDC based on an evaluation of the job complexity and degree of hazards.

EM 385-1-1
15 Sep 08

30.A.14 The following documents are required for all USACE and Contractor diving operations. All documents will be reviewed and found acceptable by two of the following: DDC/ ADC/ DSR, prior to start of diving operations. Contractors shall submit the documents through the Contracting Officer. Additional documentation may be required depending on the scope of the diving operation:

    a. Safe Practices Manual. **> See 30.A.16.**

    b. Dive Operations Plan(s). **> See 30.A.17.**

    c. AHA to cover all aspects of the job. **> See 30.A.18.**

    d. Emergency Management Plan. **> See 30.A.19.**

    e. Dive Personnel Qualifications. **> See 30.A.06 – 10.**

> Note: The above review requirement is that two qualified USACE personnel independently evaluate the documents prior to acceptance. The ADC may substitute for either the DDC or DSR in the review and/or acceptance process if these personnel are not available at the time of review.

30.A.15 A Dive Operations Plan, AHA, emergency management plan, and personnel list with qualifications will be developed for each separate diving operation. These documents will be submitted to the DDC for review and found acceptable prior to commencement of diving operations and will be at the diving location at all times. Each of these documents will become a part of the project file. Potential high-hazard conditions, such as penetration diving, contaminated environment diving, dives outside the no decompression limits, and in areas where differential pressure entrapment hazards exist, will be specifically addressed in each document when they are anticipated as part of the diving operation.

30.A.16 Safe Practices Manual. Contractors and USACE Districts/ Labs with in-house dive teams shall develop and maintain a safe practices manual that encompasses their entire diving program.

EM 385-1-1
15 Sep 08

The safe practices manual shall be available at all times to the Government representative and all dive team members at each diving location. The safe practices manual shall include, as a minimum, the following:

a. Dive safety procedures and checklists;

b. Assignments and responsibilities of dive team members;

c. Equipment certifications, procedures, and inspection checklists;

d. Emergency procedures for fire, equipment failure, adverse weather conditions, and medical illness or injury and <u>specific procedures for:</u>

(1) <u>Entrapped or fouled diver including fouled umbilical (suction and entanglement/debris);</u>

(2) <u>Actions upon loss of vital support equipment;</u>

(3) <u>Actions upon loss of gas supply;</u>

(4) <u>Action upon loss of communication;</u>

(5) <u>Lost diver plan;</u>

(6) <u>Injured diver plan;</u>

(7) <u>Actions upon discovery of fire;</u>

(8) <u>Diver blow up/over rapid ascent to surface;</u>

(9) <u>Diver loss of consciousness; and</u>

(10) <u>Injury/illness of member of surface crew with diver in the water.</u>

EM 385-1-1
15 Sep 08

    e. Procedures for internal safety inspections (frequency, checklists, etc.);

    f. A complete copy of OSHA, 29 CFR 1910, Subpart T, and a statement of the employer's policy for ensuring compliance with the standard;

    g. The appropriate U.S. Navy Table(s), including as a minimum;

    (1) U.S. Navy Table of No-Decompression Limits and Repetitive Group Designation for No-Decompression Air Dives;

    (2) U.S. Navy Residual Nitrogen Timetables for Repetitive Air Dives;

    (3) U.S. Navy Standard Air Decompression Table.

    h. A sample of the diving log sheets to be used;

    i. A sample of the repetitive dive worksheets or equivalent (dive profile method) to be used;

    j. An outline of the fitness for duty (including medical) requirements for dive team members, and

    k. An outline of administrative and recordkeeping procedures.

30.A.17 Dive Operations Plan. This plan is a general overview of all tasks to be performed, dive modes and equipment, site access, etc. Complex projects involving more than one work task, location, and/or dive team require task-specific dive plans as part of the overall Dive Operations Plan. As a minimum the Dive Operations Plan will contain the following:

    a. Date of dive plan submission;

    b. Name and contact information for diving supervisor preparing the dive plan;

c. Names and duties of on-site dive team members, including diving supervisor;

d. List of diving equipment to be used;

e. Type of diving platform to be used;

f. Detailed description of the mission; Identify how/ if work will be divided into separate tasks or phases of work;

g. Date(s), time(s), duration, and location of operation;

h. Diving mode used (SCUBA, SSA, and snorkeling) including a description of the backup air supply, as required;

i. Nature of work to be performed by the divers, including tools used and materials to be handled or installed;

j. Anticipated surface and underwater conditions, to include visibility, temperature, currents, etc. Thermal protection will be considered as appropriate;

k. Maximum single dive bottom time for the planned depth of dive for each diver. Altitude adjustments to dive tables will be calculated for dives made at altitudes of 1000 ft (304.8 m) or more above sea level;

l. <u>Identification of</u> topside assistance/support to the dive team (i.e., crane operator, lock operator, etc.);

m. Means of direct communication between the dive site and <u>the project office, the lockmaster/USACE project manager, and the contracting officer (if applicable);</u>

n. <u>Plans submitted for Contractor operations shall also include the name of Contractor (and diving subcontractor if applicable), Contract number, and names and contact information for key personnel.</u>

EM 385-1-1
15 Sep 08

> *< NOTE: The dive plan will include the following statement: "If for any reason the dive plan is altered in mission, depth, personnel, or equipment, the DDC will be contacted in order to review and accept the alteration prior to actual operation."*

30.A.18 <u>Activity Hazard Analysis.</u> An AHA represents the dive team's best effort to anticipate and mitigate or prevent the adverse effects of equipment failure, extreme weather/environmental conditions, or other hazardous/unexpected situations.

a. <u>AHA's shall address risk to personnel, property and to impacts to the overall USACE mission. When required, a new AHA shall be conducted to reflect changes in site conditions, operational changes, etc.</u>

b. <u>Each AHA will be job specific and address each phase of work, to include the hazards associated with flying after diving.</u>

c. <u>For USACE dive teams, a Risk Assessment Code should be applied to high hazard jobs, with residual risk being approved by the appropriate level of command.</u>

d. <u>Control of Hazardous Energy (Lockout/ Tagout) procedures in accordance with Section 12 of this manual</u> and procedures for dealing with differential pressures will be included if appropriate. If <u>Hazardous Energy Control</u> procedures are required for the diving operation, the diving supervisor will visually check all lockout/tagout and other control procedures/devices to assure they are in place and redundant where possible prior to the commencement of the diving operation. A copy of any clearances/permits to be issued to deal with identified hazards will be attached to the AHA.

e. <u>Some dives may be sufficiently complex to warrant several separate analyses.</u>

f. <u>The AHA will be covered in detail at the pre-dive conference.</u>

EM 385-1-1
15 Sep 08

30.A.19 Emergency management plan. An emergency management plan will be prepared for each dive operation. The minimum content of the plan will be as follows:

a. Location and phone number of nearest operational recompression chamber if not located at the dive site and the Divers Alert Network (DAN) phone number (919-684-8111);

b. Location, directions to and phone number(s) of nearest hospital(s) or available physicians capable of treating dive injuries;

c. Location and phone number of nearest USCG Rescue Coordination Center, where appropriate;

d. Description of an emergency victim transport plan including phone numbers of appropriate emergency transport services;

e. Procedures and phone numbers or other means of communications to activate emergency services at the facility where the work is being performed;

f. Diver rescue procedures conducted by the dive team, including responsibilities of team members, best location(s) where injured divers may be removed from the water, and best location(s) for performing first aid/ stabilization prior to emergency medical assistance arrival.

30.A.20 Prior to the initial work on each dive operation, a Pre-Dive Conference shall be held with key personnel designated by the DDC to discuss the Dive Operations plan, AHA, and Emergency Plan and any modifications needed. For contractor operations, the pre-dive conference will also be attended by the USACE dive inspector or DDC and a representative of the Contractor with sufficient authority to implement any changes required by the USACE diving inspector or coordinator.

30.A.21 Prior to each dive, the entire dive team will be briefed in detail on the following (as a minimum):

a. Description of mission and location, including drawings and/or photographs pertinent to the mission and equipment and materials that are to be installed as part of the mission;

b. Description of diving apparatus/equipment and craft to be used;

c. Maximum working depth with estimated bottom times and water temperatures;

d. Names and duties of personnel on the team (when possible, incorporate at least one person on the dive that has previously performed the same or similar mission);

e. Discussion of AHA; and

f. Emergency procedures.

30.A.22 Upon completion of each diving operation or at the conclusion of each day, a dive team debriefing shall be conducted by the dive supervisor. At the debriefing divers are advised of the location of the nearest recompression chamber (if not located on site), the phone number for DAN or local dive medical facility, and cautioned on the limitations of their post dive activities including repetitive dives and flying.

30.A.23 If for any reason the dive mission is altered, minor to moderate revisions to the accepted dive plan will be reviewed and accepted by the DDC or ADC prior to continuing the operation. These revisions may include differences in time, date, dive team members, work methods/ tools used, and other changes that do not affect overall risk. This review may be conducted electronically or verbally and confirmed in writing after completion of the dive operation. Major changes or those which modify high-risk activities, such as modifying pressure differential and hazardous energy controls, adding penetration diving, changing dive equipment modes (i.e. from SCUBA to SSA), discovery of unexpected contaminated diving conditions, etc. require a two-person review as outlined in 30.A.14. For contract operations, the

EM 385-1-1
15 Sep 08

project superintendent or the dive supervisor shall submit/ request the revised plan through the GDA for DDC acceptance.

30.A.24 All diving activities shall be conducted with full knowledge and close coordination with the GDA and on-site authorities such as the lockmaster/project manager, etc.

30.A.25 For each diver and dive, the following dive log information, as a minimum, shall be recorded and maintained at the dive location:

 a. Full name;

 b. Date, time and location of dive;

 c. Maximum depth and bottom time;

 d. Surface interval between dives;

 e. Breathing medium and type of equipment used;

 f. Group classification at the beginning and end of each interval and repetitive dive worksheet;

 g. Underwater and surface conditions;

 h. Depth(s) and duration(s) of any decompression stops;

 i. Date and time of last previous dive if it occurred in the last 48 hours;

 j. Name of Dive Supervisor(s) during dive;

 k. General description of work performed; AND

 l. For dives outside the no-decompression limits, deeper than 100 (30.5m) feet salt water (fsw), or using mixed-gas, include depth-time and breathing-gas profiles and decompression tables (including any modifications).

EM 385-1-1
15 Sep 08

30.A.26 For each dive in which decompression sickness and/or pulmonary barotraumas is suspected or symptoms are evident, the following information shall be recorded and maintained:

    a. Descriptions of signs and symptoms (including depth and time of onset);

    b. Description and results of treatment; and

    c. Name, address, and phone number of attending physician.

30.A.27 Prior to the dive, the <u>Dive Supervisor</u> shall assure, as a minimum, the following pre-dive checks are performed:

    a. Breathing air tanks contain <u>sufficient</u> air supply to perform the required work (i.e., standby air tanks are on site and full to the capacity);

    b. All diving equipment shall be checked for proper function prior to diver entry;

    c. All necessary safety equipment specified herein is on site and functioning properly;

    d. Lockout/tagout procedures are followed;

    e. When applicable, crane signals are reviewed and radio communication with the crane operator is functioning properly;

    f. When applicable, welding or cutting procedures are clearly reviewed, the proper welder polarity is set, and precautions have been taken to ensure that electrocution will not occur;

    g. When applicable, blasting procedures are clearly reviewed and precautions have been taken to ensure unplanned/unscheduled blasts will not occur;

EM 385-1-1
15 Sep 08

h. A pre-dive briefing shall be given that includes, but is not limited to, the accident management plan, AHA, equipment checklist, diving logs, diving conditions, and diving procedures;

i. When applicable, manbaskets used for diver access shall be inspected and load tested prior to use.

30.A.28 Copies of the dive logs shall be submitted to the DDC after completion of the dive operation. For USACE dive teams, these records shall be maintained on file for two years.

30.B DIVING OPERATIONS

30.B.01 Staging areas, where the fully suited and equipped diver enters the water, shall be selected and configured based on a hazard analysis that includes an examination of:

a. ease of diver access to the water;

b. hazards to diver (currents, equipment, etc.) in route from surface to work area;

c. ability of standby diver to access the water immediately and to reach the diver quickly;

d. if used as the topside dive team station, the ability to protect topside members and the standby diver from weather, operational, and other hazards;

e. whether topside equipment can be stowed safely and function properly;

f. if diver entry to water is remote from the staging area, the standby diver shall be placed at the water entry or immediately accessible to it.

30.B.02 All Dive teams shall be manned in accordance with the criteria established in Appendix O.

EM 385-1-1
15 Sep 08

30.B.03 A standby diver will be provided whenever a diver(s) is in the water to serve as immediate emergency assistance to the primary diver(s). Untethered SCUBA divers, working in "buddy" pairs, shall have one standby at the surface for each pair. A standby will deploy only after the dive supervisor assesses the situation and instructs him/ her to do so.

   a. The standby diver shall be fully equipped to dive and readily available the entire time the diver is in the water. The standby shall don all specific gear (suits, harnesses, and equipment) they will wear/use and test all for proper operation before the primary diver leaves the surface. All gear shall be maintained operational and ready for immediate use for the duration of the dive. If any of the tested gear is exchanged or replaced during the dive, it shall be donned and tested by the standby.

   b. The standby diver shall be dressed appropriately for the water and air temperature and remain fully suited up with helmet/ mask ready for immediate donning from the time the primary diver leaves the surface until reaching the work area/ working depth. At that point, the standby may remove the portions of his or her gear needed to prevent heat/cold stress and prevent fatigue. If the AHA identifies a need for the standby to remain fully dressed to deploy, it will address measures that will be taken to control these hazards (i.e., standby in water at surface). Any gear that has been removed must be maintained ready for immediate donning and use, accessible to the standby at the entry to the water.

   c. If configuration of the surface staging area prevents safe, immediate entry of the standby into the water, the standby diver will be placed in the water fully dressed prior to the primary diver leaving the surface, and remain at the surface ready for deployment if needed.

30.B.04 Dive operations that require surface decompression as an integral part of the dive operation shall have a trained competent person, whose sole purpose is to attend to the chamber operation. In dive operations where the chamber is required for emergency, first aid, or used for other unexpected recompression events, a team member with other team duties (tender, console operations, etc.) not diving during the current dive may serve as the chamber operator so long as he is specifically trained and competent in hyperbaric chamber operations. If used for the latter purpose, all diving shall be suspended during the chamber operations. Whenever a chamber is on site, the competent chamber operator shall be capable of communicating with a diving physician. Divers completing a recompression dive will remain within 30 minutes drive time from a fully operable and staffed recompression chamber for a minimum of 2 hours after completing the recompression dive.

30.B.05 Dive operations will be conducted in full coordination with external operations and processes that may impact the safety of the dive.

> a. When the operation of machinery or release of hazardous energy will affect the diver or dive team safety, the dive supervisor will develop a Hazardous Energy Control Plan (see Section 12). When diving at a facility with an existing Hazardous Energy Control Plan, the dive supervisor will review the facility's plan and establish positive control procedures with the facility leader.
>
> b. When water traffic, land-based traffic, industrial operations, heavy equipment operation, or other operations exist that present a hazard to the diver or dive team, the dive supervisor shall coordinate with the controlling authorities to minimize the hazards.

30.B.06 Crane operations conducted to support diving operations shall follow the requirements of Section 16 of this manual. All working dives requiring communications between the divers and topside to direct crane load movements, etc., shall be performed in Surface Supplied Air mode. The crane operator will take direction from the tender or supervisor directly in communication with the diver. Crane operations where the load is placed or removed underwater shall be considered Critical Lifts and the diver/ load

EM 385-1-1
15 Sep 08

director will participate in the Critical Lift Plan development as outlined in Section 16.H.

30.B.07 When dives will take place in an area or facility where potential or actual pressure differentials exist (locks, dams, spillways, powerhouses, etc.), the dive supervisor will develop specific plans and procedures, in coordination with the facility operator, to prevent diver exposure to pressure differentials. The plans and procedures shall be site-specific and include the following:

a. Identification of all potential exposure points (gate sills, valve openings, holes, etc.);

b. Means for identifying whether control structures/ mechanisms are fully in place (measurements of stop gates and openings, valve indicators, etc.);

c. Methods for checking pressure differential openings (observing current/ water flow, remote testing of opening area with objects (rope, sandbags, cinders, etc.);

d. Route diver will take from staging area to work area with specific designs to prevent diver and umbilical from uncontrolled pressure differential openings;

e. Procedures for immediate emergency pressure equalization or reduction, if possible, AND

f. Procedures for emergency diver extraction or rescue due to pressure differential exposure, including standby diver deployment precautions.

EM 385-1-1
15 Sep 08

30.C SCUBA OPERATIONS

30.C.01 SCUBA diving operations shall not be conducted:

a. At depths greater than 100 ft (30.5 m);

b. On dives outside the no-decompression limits unless a dual lock, multi-place, recompression chamber (capable of recompressing diver at the surface to a depth equivalent to 165 ft (50.3 m) of sea water) is available at the dive location and is immediately available for use, a trained competent operator is on site, and the chamber is of sufficient size to accommodate the diver as well as an inside tender;

c. Against currents exceeding one knot;

d. In enclosed or physically confining spaces;

e. Using closed circuit or semi-closed circuit SCUBA;

f. In visibility less than 3 ft (0.9 m) unless line tended with diver/surface two-way voice communications;

g. In areas where pressure differentials exist and it cannot be positively verified that all potential leaks have been eliminated;

h. When the diver does not have direct access to the surface.

30.C.02 Specific operational requirements for SCUBA operations are as follows:

a. Each SCUBA diver shall be equipped with a bailout bottle with a minimum of 30 ft^3 (0.85 m^3) of air and separate regulator. An octopus is not considered to be an alternate air source.

b. Each diver shall be equipped with a buoyancy compensation device (BCD) and/or an inflatable flotation device capable of maintaining the diver at the surface in a face-up position, having

EM 385-1-1
15 Sep 08

<u>a manually activated inflation source independent of the breathing supply, an oral inflation device, and an exhaust valve.</u>

c. Each SCUBA diver shall be equipped with a submersible cylinder pressure gauge capable of being monitored by the diver during the dive.

d. Each SCUBA diver shall be equipped with a weight belt or assembly capable of quick release.

e. Each SCUBA diver shall be equipped with a depth gauge and knife.

f. SCUBA air cylinders shall comply with the following requirements:

(1) Air cylinders of seamless steel or aluminum that meet DOT 3AA and DOT 3AL specifications are approved for used on USACE projects;

(2) Each cylinder used on USACE projects must have identification symbols stamped into the shoulder of the tank; and

(3) SCUBA tanks used on USACE projects must be visually inspected internally at least annually and hydrostatically tested at least once every 5 years in accordance with DOT and the CGA regulations; test dates will be stamped into the shoulder of each tank.

g. A timekeeping device shall be used for recording diving times for all SCUBA diving operations. When two-way voice communications are not used, each dive supervisor and diver shall have a timekeeping device. When two-way voice communications are used, the dive supervisor, at a minimum shall have a timekeeping device.

h. Each tethered SCUBA diver shall wear a safety harness with a positive buckling device, attachment point for the safety line, and a lifting point to distribute the pull force of the line over the

EM 385-1-1
15 Sep 08

diver's body while maintaining the body in a heads-up vertical position when unconscious or inert.

30.D SURFACE SUPPLIED AIR (SSA) OPERATIONS

30.D.01 SSA operations shall not be conducted at depths greater than 190 ft (57.9 m) except that dives with bottom times of 30 minutes or less may be conducted to depth of 220 ft (67 m). Exceptional exposure dives, as defined by the US Navy Diving Manual, shall not be conducted except in emergency lifesaving situations. <u>USACE in-house SSA operations shall not exceed a depth of 110 ft unless a waiver is requested by the DDC and approved by the HQUSACE Dive Safety Program Manager.</u>

30.D.02 SSA equipment components shall be a type specifically designed to be used in diving support systems.

30.D.03 Dual lock, multi-place, recompression chambers shall be available and ready for used at the dive location for any dive outside the no-decompression limits or deeper than 100 ft (30.4 m). <u>Sufficient</u> oxygen shall be available <u>to complete</u> chamber operations.

30.D.04 A bell shall be used for dives with an in-water decompression time greater than 120 minutes, unless heavy gear is worn or diving is conducted in physically confining spaces.

30.D.05 Minimum specific operational requirements for SSA diving operations are as follows:

   a. Each diver shall be continuously tendered while in the water, with one diver per tender, regardless of depth;

   b. An underwater tender/diver shall be stationed at the underwater point of entry when <u>any penetration</u> diving is conducted <u>or</u> in enclosed or physically confining spaces;

EM 385-1-1
15 Sep 08

c. Each diving operation shall have a primary breathing air supply sufficient to support divers for the duration of the planned dive, including decompression;

d. Each diver must have a reserve breathing supply available that can be turned on immediately by the diver in the event of loss of air. The reserve breathing air supply shall be of sufficient capacity to <u>recover the diver and complete emergency recompression (if required)</u> in the event of loss of primary air but no less than 30 ft^3 (0.85 m^3). <u>Heavy-gear diving is exempted from these provisions because the gear carries its own reserve</u>;

e. Each dive location shall have a reserve breathing air supply integral or in-line with the primary air source sufficient to safely terminate the dive and recover the diver(s) in the event of loss of the primary air supply;

f. For dives deeper than 100 ft (30.5 m) or outside the no decompression limits and using heavy gear, <u>a spare air supply</u> hose, <u>to replace the diver's air hose should it become damaged,</u> shall be available to the standby diver. An in-water support stage shall be provided to divers in water when using heavy gear, regardless of depth;

g. Electronic communication systems with an external speaker shall be incorporated in all SSA diving operations so the entire dive team can monitor communications. <u>Communications devices shall be tested prior to each dive, maintained in an operable condition, and protected from damage during use and storage IAW the manufacturer's recommendations.</u> All <u>dive operations will be terminated in a safe, orderly fashion using line-pull signals if voice communications are lost. Defective electronic communication equipment shall not prevent a standby diver from deploying in an emergency if the dive supervisor determines it is safe for the diver to deploy and line-pull signals are used.</u>

EM 385-1-1
15 Sep 08

30.E MIXED-GAS DIVING OPERATIONS

30.E.01 Dual lock, multi-place, recompression chambers with a trained, competent operator shall be available and ready for use at the dive location for any mixed-gas dive. Sufficient oxygen shall be available to complete chamber operations. At extreme depth, mixed gas diving can only be done if:

    a. A bell is used at depths greater than 220 ft (67 m) or when the dive involves in-water decompression time of greater than 120 minutes (except when heavy gear is worn or when diving in physically confining spaces), or

    b. A closed bell is used at depths greater than 300 ft (91.4 m), except when diving is conducted in physically confining spaces.

30.E.02 Each diving operation shall have a primary breathing gas supply sufficient to support divers for the duration of the planned dive, including decompression.

30.E.03 Each diving operation shall have a reserve breathing gas supply integral or in-line with the primary air source sufficient to safely recover the diver(s) in the event of failure of the primary breathing gas supply.

30.E.04 When heavy gear is worn:

    a. An extra breathing gas hose capable of supplying breathing gas to the diver in the water shall be available to the standby diver, and

    b. An in-water stage shall be provided to divers in the water.

30.E.05 An in-water stage shall be provided for divers without access to a bell for dives deeper than 100 ft (30.4 m) or outside the no-decompression limits.

30.E.06 When a closed bell is used, one dive team member in the bell shall be available and tend the diver in the water.

EM 385-1-1
15 Sep 08

30.E.07 Oxygen Enriched Air.

a. The use of "Oxygen Enriched Air" (OEA) such as Nitrox (EANx) breathing mixtures <u>by USACE in-house dive teams requires the specific initial approval of the HQUSACE Dive Safety Program Manager prior to the first use of such equipment. Requests for approval will be accompanied by a written program that identifies training, certification, and procedures for OEA use. Use of OEA by Contractors requires approval by the local DDC.</u>

b. <u>Navy or NOAA Nitrox Dive Tables or other decompression tables designed specifically for the OEA mixture being used shall be followed without exception.</u>

c. <u>The use of OEA/ Nitrox is considered mixed gas diving and requires a decompression chamber on site and ready for use.</u>

30.E.08 Contractors must provide evidence of training and experience with OEA breathing mixtures prior to actual diving operations.

30.E.09 OEA breathing mixture shall be analyzed/ tested by the diver to assure proper mix prior to each use. <u>No more than 40% OEA is allowed for normal diving operations. Higher OEA concentrations are allowable for in-water decompression at shallow safety stops.</u>

30.F EQUIPMENT REQUIREMENTS

30.F.01 Equipment modifications, repairs, tests, calibrations, or maintenance shall be recorded by means of a tagging or logging system, and include the date and nature of work performed and the name of the individual performing the work.

30.F.02 Air compressor systems used <u>on-site as a direct source</u> to supply air to SSA divers (Direct Source Compressors) shall be

EM 385-1-1
15 Sep 08

equipped with a volume tank with a check valve on the inlet side, a pressure gauge, a relief valve, and a drain valve.

30.F.03 Direct Source compressors shall be of sufficient capacity to overcome any line loss or other losses and deliver a minimum 4.5 cfm (2.1 L/s) (actual) to each diver at the maximum diving depth.

30.F.04 All air compressor intakes shall be located away from/ upwind of areas containing exhaust or other contaminants. Compressors used in areas where there is known or suspected chemical air contamination (sandblasting operations, painting, etc.) shall be equipped with appropriate in-line air purifying absorbent beds and filters inserted into the supply line to assure breathing air quality. Oil -lubricated compressors containing a petroleum or potential CO-producing lubricant for the air pressurization pistons will not be used. Direct Source compressors shall be equipped specifically for their intended use and shall have a suitable approved means to regulate the pressure and a low air pressure alarm in the system. All monitor alarm systems shall be so designed and placed so that the dive supervisor will be made aware of the hazardous conditions. Direct Source compressors will have a Carbon Monoxide (CO) monitor with alarm in the following situations:

   a. The compressor is powered by an internal combustion engine, and

   b. Compressors used in close proximity to internal combustion engines that may/ will be running during dive operations (boat motors, generators, cranes, etc.). Air intake pipes shall be placed away from/ upwind of the exhaust source.

30.F.05 Air compressor systems will be tested by means of sampling at the connection to the distribution system.

   a. All air compressors with a working pressure greater than 500 psi will be tested every six months by an accredited testing laboratory. Compressors with a working pressure less than 500 psi may be tested in-house with documentation every six months and must be tested by an accredited testing laboratory every two years. Lab accreditation shall be from NIST/NVLAP, American Association of Laboratory Accreditation (A2LA – for environmental or calibration) or similar recognized accreditation. Purchased air must be certified by the supplier that it has been tested and meets the standards below.

b. A copy of the certificate of analysis showing the breathing air meets the minimum acceptable criteria shall be provided to the GDA.

c. Air purity standards are as follows:

(1) Air shall not contain a level of carbon monoxide greater than 10 ppm;

(2) Air shall not contain a level of carbon dioxide greater than 1,000 ppm;

(3) Air shall not contain a level of oil mist greater than 5 milligrams per cubic meter (mg/m3);

(4) Air shall not contain a level of hydrocarbons other than methane greater than 25 ppm; and

(5) Air shall not contain a noxious or pronounced odor.

30.F.06 Breathing supply hoses.

a. Breathing air supply hoses shall be suitable for breathing gas service or shall be specifically manufactured for SSA use. Hoses shall have a maximum allowable working pressure equal to or greater than the maximum depth of dive relative to supply source plus 150 psi, and have a rated bursting pressure at least four times the working pressure.

b. Breathing air supply hoses shall have connectors made of corrosion resistant materials and have a working pressure at

EM 385-1-1
15 Sep 08

least equal to the working pressure of the hose to which they are attached: connectors must not be able to become accidentally disengaged.

c. Umbilicals shall be marked, beginning at the divers end, in 10 ft (3 m) increments to 100 ft (30.5 m) and in 50 ft (15.2 m) increments thereafter. USACE in-house dive teams shall use the following umbilical marking system found in the ADCI Consensus Standard 006 in order to assure consistency and interoperability:

Table 30-1
Umbilical Markings

Distance (from diver's end)	Marking
10 ft [3 m]	one white band
20 ft [6.1 m]	two white bands
30 ft [9.2 m]	three white bands
40 ft [12.2 m]	four white bands
50 ft [15.2 m]	one yellow band
60 ft [18.3 m]	1 yellow/1 white
70 ft [21.3 m]	1 yellow/2 white
80 ft [24.4 m]	1 yellow/3 white
90 ft [27.4 m]	1 yellow/4 white
100 ft [30.5 m]	1 red band
150 ft [45.7 m]	1 red/1 yellow
200 ft [61 m]	2 red bands
250 ft [76.2 m]	2 red/1 yellow
300 ft [91.5 m]	3 red bands

For each 50 ft (15.2 m) thereafter the sequence continues by increasing the number of red bands at each even increment of 100 ft (30.5 m). In cases where the umbilical color matches an

EM 385-1-1
15 Sep 08

<u>above band color, a reasonable substitute may be used (contrasting outline on same-color tape, contrasting diagonal pattern, replacement with color not used above).</u>

d. Umbilicals shall have a nominal breaking strength of <u>1000 lb (453.6kg)</u> and shall be made of kink resistant materials.

e. Hoses must be tested <u>prior to being placed into initial service and after any repair, modification, or alteration, and at least every 12 months</u> to 1.5 times the working pressure. <u>Umbilical assemblies shall be tensile tested at the same time intervals by subjecting each hose-to-fitting connection to a 200 pound axial load.</u>

f. When hoses are not in use, their open ends must be closed by taping or other means.

<u>g. The umbilical assembly used for the standby diver must be of sufficient length to reach the primary diver at the furthest distance he can proceed from the dive station or beyond.</u>

<u>h. Umbilicals shall be carefully tended to maintain them and the diver clear of hazards such as propellers (including those of ROV's) or intakes present in the diving zone so that the diver or umbilical cannot be drawn into them.</u>

30.F.07 SSA and mixed-gas helmets and masks shall have a non-return valve at the attachment between the helmet or mask and hose which will close readily and also have an exhaust valve; helmets and masks shall have a minimum ventilation rate capacity of 4.5 cfm (2.1 L/s) (actual) at the depth at which they are operated. The use of Jack Brown masks is prohibited on <u>SSA operations</u> unless it incorporates electronic communication and a means of incorporating a diver carried bailout system.

30.F.08 SSA and mixed-gas helmets and masks must be capable of supporting a reserve breathing supply which can be immediately turned on by the diver in event of loss of air.

EM 385-1-1
15 Sep 08

30.F.09 SSA and mixed-gas helmets and masks must be capable of supporting a two-way or four way diver-surface communication system.

30.F.10 Weights and harnesses. Unless heavy gear is worn, each <u>tethered</u> diver shall wear a safety harness with a positive buckling device, attachment point for the safety line, and a lifting point to distribute the pull force of the line over the diver's body while maintaining the body in a heads-up vertical position when unconscious or inert.

30.F.11 The following emergency and first-aid equipment shall be located at all dive sites:

   a. A first-aid kit meeting the requirements of Section 3;

   b. An oxygen resuscitation system capable of delivering oxygen for a minimum of 30 minutes <u>or until emergency medical assistance can be administered</u>; and

   c. A stokes litter or backboard, <u>with flotation capability</u>.

30.F.12 <u>When diving from vessels</u>, International alpha code and recreational dive flags with a minimum dimension of 23 in (58.4 cm) will be displayed a minimum of 3 ft (0.9 m) above the working surface at the dive location during diving operations. <u>When diving from surfaces other than vessels in areas capable of supporting marine traffic, a rigid replica of the international code flag "A" at least one meter in height shall be displayed at the dive location in a manner which allows all-round visibility, and shall be illuminated during night diving operations.</u>

30.F.13 Hand-held power tools shall be tested and certified to be safe for underwater use; these tools shall be de-energized <u>at the surface</u> before being placed into or retrieved from the water and shall not be supplied with power until requested by the diver.

EM 385-1-1
15 Sep 08

30.F.14 The use of one-atmosphere suits (e.g., Newt Suits) requires the specific approval of the MSC DDC and FOA DDC prior to the use of such equipment.

30.G SCIENTIFIC SNORKELING

30.G.01 Scientific snorkeling will be conducted only with prior acceptance of the DDC.

30.G.02 Scientific snorkeling will be allowed only for environmental assessments such as fish surveys, stream surveys, and the like. It will not be used for structural inspections or other work.

30.G.03 An on-site snorkeling team shall be made up of no less than two persons: snorkeler, and observer/assistant. Additional site personnel may be required by the DDC or Safety Office Diving Safety Representative based on site hazards and conditions. Snorkeling team plans and procedures shall be developed and enacted by a team supervisor who is qualified and experienced in scientific snorkeling.

30.G.04 Quality assurance for contractor snorkeling operations will be provided by USACE certified Diving Inspectors or qualified USACE scientific snorkelers.

30.G.05 Scientific snorkeling will only be done on the surface of the water. No diving of any kind is permitted. Untethered scientific snorkeling will NOT be allowed in waters deeper than 5 ft (1.5 m), in bodies of water that a snorkeler cannot wade across, or anywhere a pressure differential may exist. Scientific snorkeling in open waters greater than 5 feet deep may be allowed by the local DDC based on an acceptable AHA and compliance with all of the following:

   a. The snorkeler shall be tethered with a harness and a maximum of 40 ft (12.2 m) of floating line;

   b. The tether must be constantly tended from the shore or boat;

EM 385-1-1
15 Sep 08

c. The snorkeler must wear a device providing a minimum of 15.5 pounds (7 kg) of positive buoyancy (Type III PFD, fully inflated snorkeling vest, etc.), and

d. There are no potential tether entanglement hazards in the snorkeling area (overhanging branches, surface stumps, rocks, etc.).

30.G.06 All snorkelers and observers/assistants will be certified as skin divers (snorkelers) or open water divers by a nationally-recognized organization (e.g., Professional Association of Diving Instructors (PADI), National Association of Underwater Instructors (NAUI), etc.) or the U.S. Forest Service Snorkel Safety Program.

30.G.07 An observer/assistant will accompany each untethered snorkeler either along the shore or in a boat and be within 50 ft (15.2 m) of the snorkeler at all times. Two untethered snorkelers in the same body of water may act as observer/ assistant for each other if they remain within 50 ft (15.2 m) of each other. Non-snorkeling observer/assistants shall wear a PFD and be equipped with a throw bag and/or ring buoy with at least 70 ft (21.3) of line, and must be capable of performing a rescue on the specific snorkeler(s) in an emergency.

30.G.08 Areas of extreme water velocity and turbulence will be avoided especially those immediately upstream from debris jams or bedrock outcrops.

30.G.09 Snorkelers will be provided with appropriate thermal protection.

30.G.10 Employees will be determined medically fit by a licensed physician prior to snorkeling. This certification shall be signed by the physician and state that each snorkeler is physically and medically fit to perform snorkeling activities. The Contractor shall submit such certification to the GDA for acceptance.

30.G.11 All snorkeling team members shall be certified in CPR and first aid.

30.G.12 A first-aid kit meeting the requirements of Section 03 will be available at each location where snorkeling is being performed. A means of securely transporting an unconscious person, such as a litter or stretcher, shall be provided when snorkeling is conducted in areas inaccessible to vehicles or boats.

30.G.13 A means of communication capable of contacting emergency services must be available at locations where snorkeling is performed.

30.G.14 Each snorkeler will be equipped with a professional grade diving mask and snorkel.

30.G.15 A snorkeling protocol will be developed and included in the project file. It will contain as a minimum, the following:

a. An AHA for each specific snorkeling mission. Particular detail will be given to currents and other environmental considerations;

b. Records for snorkeling activities will be maintained. These records will include as a minimum: snorkeler's annual physician certifications, AHAs, and a snorkeling plan. The latter will be based on the requirements of 30.A16.a-e. Contractors shall submit these to the GDA for acceptance by the DDC/SOH Dive Safety Officer a minimum of 10 days prior to start of work.

30.G.16 Snorkelers will wear apparel which provides appropriate environmental protection. The apparel must include fins or other appropriate foot protection.

SECTION 31

TREE MAINTENANCE AND REMOVAL

31.A GENERAL

31.A.01 References.

a. ANSI Z133.1 - Tree Care Safety Standard;

b. 29 CFR 1910.266 - Logging Operations;

c. 29 CFR 1910.269 - Electrical Power Generation, Transmission, and Distribution;

d. International Society of Arborist Safety Standards.

31.A.02 Tree maintenance or removal shall be performed under the direction of a qualified tree worker and in accordance with references above. The services of a certified arborist may also be necessary to properly access the required maintenance to be performed.

31.A.03 Working near electrical equipment and systems. *> See Section 11 and 29 CFR 1910.269.*

a. Employees working in the proximity of electrical equipment or conductors shall consider them to be energized.

b. A qualified tree worker shall make a visual inspection to determine whether an electrical hazard exists before climbing or before performing any work in or on a tree. If electrical lines or equipment cannot be safely avoided, arrangements shall be made with the power company to de-energize the power.

c. Only a qualified line-clearance tree trimmer or line-clearance trainee under the direct supervision of a qualified person shall be assigned to work in close proximity to electrical hazards.

d. There shall be a second qualified line-clearance tree trimmer or line-clearance tree trimmer trainee within normal voice communication during the clearing operations aloft under the following conditions:

(1) When the line-clearance tree trimmer or line-clearance tree trimmer trainee must approach any closer than 10 ft (3 m) to any conductor or electrical apparatus energized in excess of 750 volts;

(2) When branches or limbs being removed cannot first be cut (with a pole pruner/pole saw) sufficiently clear of the equipment or conductors so as to avoid contact; or

(3) When roping is required to remove branches or limbs from such equipment or conductors.

e. Line-clearance tree trimmers and trainees shall maintain the distances from energized conductors as specified in Table 11-3. All other tree workers shall maintain a safe distance of 10 ft (3 m) or greater according to Table 11-1.

f. Bucket Trucks and Aerial Lifts that are electrically rated above the electrical voltages of adjacent power lines are exempt from the 10 ft (3 m) rule, and can follow Table 11-3 if workers have been electrically qualified. Ladders on aerial lift devices may not be brought closer to an energized part than the distance listed in Table 11-3.

g. Electrically rated buckets shall be tested yearly with approved test equipment.

31.A.04 Equipment.

a. Equipment shall be inspected, maintained, repaired, and used in accordance with the manufacturer's instructions.

EM 385-1-1
15 Sep 08

b. Employees shall be instructed in the safe and proper use of all equipment provided to them.

c. See Appendix P for Climbing Equipment Requirements.

31.A.05 Climbing ropes shall not be used to lower limbs or other parts of trees or to raise or lower equipment.

31.A.06 Tool handles shall be used when raising and lowering tools.

31.A.07 Tools used for cabling, bark tracing, cavity work, etc., shall be carried in a bag, belt, or sheath designed to hold tools and not put in the pockets or stuck in the top of a boot.

31.A.08 Aerial Platforms and Buckets.

a. Tree Workers in a bucket or work platform shall use fall protection in accordance with manufacturer's recommendations. Workers shall be positively secured to the work platform at all times but especially during transit between the tree and platform. The employee shall be safely secured to the tree prior to removing the lanyard attached to the basket.

b. If a lanyard longer than 1 ft (.3 m) is used, and the fall potential is greater than 2 ft (.6 m) , then a full body harness will be used. If a short lanyard is used for restraint only and the fall potential is less than 2 ft (.6 m), then a climber's belt may be used with attachment points on the sides or front. Lanyards longer than 1 ft (.3 m) used for fall arrest rather than restraint shall be of the shock absorbing type that reduces the arresting force to 900 lbs (4 kN). The shock absorbing side of the lanyard shall be attached to the back of the harness. All snap hooks and carabineers shall be of the triple action type and rated for 5000 lbs (22.2 kN) meeting ANSI Z359.1 standard.

EM 385-1-1
15 Sep 08

31.B TREE CLIMBING

31.B.01 Tree Climbing Techniques.

a. All tree work operations above a height of 12 ft (3.6 m), whether there are electrical hazards or not, shall require a second worker in the area. If climbing is being performed, the 2nd worker shall also be a qualified climber, capable and knowledgeable of rescue techniques, including self rescue.

b. Use of Rope Access techniques should only be used where other means of access or undertaking the work such as mechanically operated work platforms or pole saws are not practical. **> See Appendix P for recommended rope climbing equipment, techniques, and safety practices.**

31.B.02 The climber shall inspect the tree and surrounding area for hazards and perform a risk assessment of the tree and work site. Some issues to be considered are: power lines, tree hangers or broken and dead branches, entanglement with adjacent or downed trees, shape and lean of the tree, tree damage from wind, lightening, disease, location of septic lines and tanks and other potential at-grade or below-grade utilities that could be impacted. Debris and other objects shall be removed from beneath the climber whenever possible. Weather conditions shall be assessed as well as location of adjacent structures. Adverse weather conditions may include lightening and thunderstorms in the area.

31.B.03 Tree crews, where climbing is required, shall have a secondary climber that could assist in a rescue if necessary or the crew shall be working in proximity to nearby crews with a climber who could assist in a rescue if needed.

31.B.04 A tree worker shall be tied in with an approved type of climbing rope and safety saddle when working above the ground This does not necessarily apply to a worker ascending into a tree. Work may be performed while standing on a self-supporting ladder only when the worker is tied off as required.

EM 385-1-1
15 Sep 08

31.B.05 The climbing rope (working line) shall be passed around the trunk of the tree as high above the ground as possible using branches with a wide crotch to prevent any binding of the safety rope (safety line). **Exception: Palms and other trees with similar growth characteristics that will not allow a climbing rope to move freely.** The crotch selected for tying should be directly above the work area, or as close to such a position as possible, but located in such a way that a slip or fall would swing the worker away from any electrical conductor. The rope shall be passed around the main leader or an upright branch, using the limb as a stop. Feet, hands, and ropes shall be kept out of tight V-shaped crotches.

31.B.06 A figure-eight knot shall be tied in the end of the rope, particularly when climbing high trees, to prevent pulling the rope accidentally through the taut-line hitch and possibly falling.

31.B.07 The tree worker shall be completely secured with the climbing line before starting the operation. The climbing line shall be crotched as soon as practicable after the employee is aloft, and a taut-line hitch tied and checked. The worker shall remain tied in until the work is completed and he/she has returned to the ground. If it is necessary to recrotch the rope in the tree, the worker shall re-tie in or use the safety strap before releasing the previous tie.

31.B.08 A 5/8 in (1.5 cm) metal shackle shall be secured to the end of a support line that meets minimum standards for a climbing line. The support line shall be tied to the pin of the shackle with the climbing line placed through the shackle. The support line shall be tied off at the base of the tree or any other acceptable anchor.

31.B.09 Tree workers shall not carry tools in their hands while climbing. Chain saws and Tools shall be raised and lowered one at a time by means of a line, except when working from an aerial-lift device or during topping or removing operations.

31.B.10 Climbers should use chain saws less than 15 lbs (6.8 kg) and they should be connected to the climber by means of a saw lanyard.

EM 385-1-1
15 Sep 08

31.B.11 Climbing of dead and dying trees shall only be performed where no other safe and feasible alternative exists for removal of the tree. Climbers shall not trust the capability of a dead branch to support his/her weight. If possible, dead branches should be broken off on the way up and hands and feet should be placed on separate limbs.

31.B.12 Climbing with tree spurs on live trees is generally not allowed. Tree spurs used for large bark trees shall have longer gaffs, such as 2   in (7 cm). Gaff lengths of 1   in (4.5 cm) are intended only for pole climbing. Gaff lengths shall be suitable for the tree being climbed.

31.B.13 The climber may apply a variety of climbing techniques, but they must be approved by the GDA.

   a. Climbing without the use of tree spurs may be required.

   b. The most commonly used arborist rope climbing technique is the Advancing the Rope and Body Thrusting technique/Alternate Lanyard Technique.

   c. If the climber can remain near the trunk of the tree, he may use both the Belt Lanyard/Flip line and the Rope Advance (lifeline) technique. Otherwise, a single line access is permitted. If a lifeline (Access Line) cannot be set in the tree, then the use of two flip lines may be used.

   d. The use of auto-locking belays devices or tree climber's hitches are both permitted.

   e. Tree climbers shall not climb above their tie off point. Tie in points shall be well above the climber to prevent an uncontrolled pendulum swing in the event of a slip.

   f. Once in the tree, climbers shall be tied off at two points while working or using the chain saw, (this includes the primary support of the access line, and the flip line/lanyard/or buck

EM 385-1-1
15 Sep 08

strap). Climbers may ascend or descend from the tree using only the access line by using approved single rope techniques. Once the worker is at the tie in point (TIP), a secure climbing system shall be installed and the climber should only disconnect from the access line when a new pitch and line have been established as required when moving higher into the tree.

g. Use of three point contact climbing is recommended if possible. Climbers may also use ground personnel to help pull them up the tree.

31.B.14 Climbers over the age of 40 years shall have obtained a medical clearance for heavy exertion work within the past 2 years.

31.C FELLING

31.C.01 Prior to felling operations, the employee shall consider:

a. The tree and the surrounding area for anything that may cause trouble when the tree falls;

b. The shape of the tree, the lean of the tree, and decayed or weak spots;

c. Wind force and direction;

d. The location of other people;

e. Electrical hazards; and

f. Other obstructions such as curb stops, meter pits, sewer clean outs, and gas lines.

31.C.02 Prior to felling operations, the work area shall be cleared to permit safe working conditions and an escape route shall be planned. Tree trimmers shall ensure that homes and structures are evacuated where trimming and felling operations are in close proximity.

EM 385-1-1
15 Sep 08

31.C.03 Felling paths shall be at least twice the distance as the height of the tree (due to limbs and debris being thrown after hitting the ground). Where this distance cannot be maintained, limbing may be required. Power lines may also need to be dropped or de-energized.

31.C.04 Each worker shall be instructed as to exactly what he is to do. All workers not directly involved in the operation shall be kept clear of the work area.

31.C.05 Before starting to cut, the operator shall be sure of his footing and must clear away brush, fallen trees, and other materials that might interfere with cutting operations.

31.C.06 A notch and backcut shall be used in felling trees over 5 in (12.7 cm) in diameter (measured at breast height). No tree shall be felled by "slicing" or "ripping" cuts.

   a. The depth or penetration of the notch shall be about one-third the diameter of the tree.

   b. The opening or height of the notch shall be about 2.5 in (6.3 cm) for each 1 ft (0.3 m) of the tree's diameter.

   c. The backcut shall be made higher (approximately 2 in (5 cm)) than the base of the notch to prevent kickback.

31.C.07 If sections of the tree are to be removed, sections shall be limited in length to 1/3 the distance to the nearest structure (e.g., If the tree is 30 ft (9 m) from the structure, sections shall be no more than 10 ft (3 m)).

>Note: the discretion of the tree trimmer must be used. In some instances it may be safer to fell a large trunk away from the structure rather than to remove it in small sections, especially where the tree has grown very close to the house or structure. If this is done, a rope should be used to help guide

the direction of the fall along with the use of proper notch and backcut.

31.C.08 The employee shall work from the uphill side whenever possible. Wind effect shall be considered when falling. The use of tag lines may be used to help in the direction of the fall provided the workers on the tagline are well clear of the fall path, such as twice the distance of the fall area.

31.C.09 Just before the tree or limb is ready to fall, an audible warning shall be given to all those in the area. All persons shall be safely out of range when the tree falls.

31.C.10 If there is danger that the trees being felled may fall in the wrong direction or damage property, wedges, block and tackle, rope, or wire cable (except when an electrical hazard exists) shall be used. All limbs shall be removed from trees to a height and width sufficient to allow the tree to fall clear of any wires and other objects in the vicinity. Manufacturer's recommendations will be strictly followed when using a loader, skid steer, or similar piece of equipment to push directly against the tree.

31.C.11 Special precautions shall be taken when roping rotten or split trees due to the potential for falling in an unexpected direction even though the cut is made on the proper side.

31.C.12 Persons shall be kept back from the butt of a tree that is starting to fall.

31.D BRUSH REMOVAL AND CHIPPING

31.D.01 Brush and logs shall not be allowed to create a hazard at the work site.

31.D.02 Employees working with a brush chipper shall be trained in its safe operation. The chipper shall be operated in accordance with the manufacturer's recommendations.

31.D.03 Brush chippers.

a. Rotary drum and disk-type tree or brush chippers not equipped with a mechanical in-feed system shall be equipped with an in-feed hopper not less than 85 in (2.2 m) (the sum of the horizontal distance from the chipper blade out along the center of the chute to the end of the chute and the vertical distance from the chute down to the ground) and shall have sufficient height on its side members to prevent personnel from contacting the blades or knives of the machine during normal operations.

b. Rotary drum and disk-type tree or brush chippers not equipped with a mechanical in-feed system shall have a flexible anti-kickback device installed in the in-feed hopper for the purpose of protecting the operator and other persons in the machine area from the hazards of flying chips and debris.

c. Disk-type tree or brush chippers equipped with a mechanical in-feed system shall have a quick stop and reversing device on the in-feed. The activating mechanism for the quick stop and reversing device shall be located across from the top, along each side of, and as close as possible to the feed end of the in-feed hopper and within easy reach of the operator.

d. The feed chute or feed table of a chipper shall have sufficient height on its side members to prevent operator contact with the blades or knives during normal operation.

e. A swinging baffle shall be mounted in front of the knives to prevent throwback of material.

f. Brush chippers shall be equipped with an exhaust chute of sufficient length or design to prevent contact with the blade.

g. Brush chippers shall be equipped with a locking device on the ignition system to prevent unauthorized starting of the equipment.

EM 385-1-1
15 Sep 08

h. Brush chipper cutting bars and blades shall be kept sharp, properly adjusted, and otherwise maintained in accordance with the manufacturer's recommendations.

31.D.04 Trailer brush chippers detached from trucks shall be chocked or otherwise secured.

31.D.05 All workers feeding brush into chippers shall wear eye protection. Loose clothing, gauntlet-type gloves, rings, and watches shall not be worn by workers feeding the chipper.

31.D.06 Employees shall never place hands, arms, feet, legs, or any other part of the body on the feed table when the chipper is in operation or the rotor is turning. Push sticks (of material that can be consumed by brush chipper) shall be used.

31.D.07 Brush chippers shall be fed from the side of the centerline, and the operator shall immediately turn away from the feed table when the brush is taken into the rotor. Chippers shall be fed from the curbside whenever possible.

31.D.08 Material such as stones, nails, sweepings, etc. shall not be fed into brush chippers.

31.D.09 The brush chipper chute shall not be raised while the rotor is turning.

31.E OTHER OPERATIONS AND EQUIPMENT

31.E.01 Pruning and trimming.

    a. Pole pruners, pole saws, and similar tools shall be equipped with wood or nonmetallic poles. Actuating cords shall be of a nonconducting material.

    b. Pole pruners and pole saws shall be hung securely in a vertical position with the sharp edges away from employees.

EM 385-1-1
15 Sep 08

They shall not be hung on utility wires or cables or left overnight in trees.

c. When necessary, warning shall be given by the worker in the tree before a limb is dropped.

d. A scabbard or sheath shall be hooked to the belt or safety saddle to carry a handsaw when not in use.

e. A separate line shall be attached to limbs that cannot be dropped safely or are too heavy to be controlled by hand. The line should be held by workers on the ground end of the rope. Use of the same crotch for both the safety rope and the work rope shall be avoided.

f. Cut branches shall not be left in trees overnight.

g. A service line shall be put up for operations lasting overnight or longer and shall be used to bring the climbing rope back into position at the start of the next day's work.

31.E.02 Limbing and bucking.

a. Whenever it is possible to do so, the tree worker shall work on the side on which the limb is being cut.

b. Branches bent under tension shall be considered hazardous.

c. When topping or lowering limbs, consideration shall be given to the use of taglines to control the limbs. A separate line shall be attached to limbs that cannot be dropped or are too heavy to be controlled by hand. The use of the same crotch for both safety rope and work rope shall be avoided.

d. In bucking, tree workers shall stand on the uphill side of the work whenever possible. The tree worker shall block the log to prevent rolling when necessary.

EM 385-1-1
15 Sep 08

    e. When bucking, wedges shall be used as necessary to prevent binding of the guide bar or chain.

31.E.03 Stump cutters shall be equipped with enclosures or guards that effectively protect the operator. When flush cutting stumps with a chain saw, all persons assisting the sawyer shall wear the same level of PPE that is required of the sawyer.

31.E.04 Cabling.

    a. Branches that are to be cabled shall be brought together to the proper distance by means of a block and tackle, a hand winch, a rope, or a rope with a come-along.

    b. No more than two persons shall be in a tree working at opposite ends during cabling installation.

    c. When the block and tackle are released, workers in trees shall be positioned off to one side in order to avoid injury in case the lag hooks pull out under the strain.

    d. Ground men shall not stand under the tree when cable is being installed.

31.E.05 Topping/Lowering Limbs.

    a. Workers performing topping operations shall ensure the trees can stand the strain of a topping procedures; if not, some other means of lowering the branches shall be used.

    b. If large limbs are lowered in sections, the worker in the tree shall be above the limb being lowered.

31.E.06 Trucks.

    a. A steel bulkhead or equivalent protection shall be provided to protect the occupants of vehicles from load shifts.

EM 385-1-1
15 Sep 08

b. Logs or brush shall be securely loaded onto trucks in such a manner as not to obscure taillights or brake lights and vision, or to overhang the side.

c. In order to avoid the hazard of spontaneous combustion or the production of undesirable products, wood chips shall not be left in trucks for extended periods.

31.E.07 Power saws.

a. Power saws weighting more than 15 lbs (6.8 kg) shall be supported by a separate line, except when used from an aerial lift device or on the ground.

b. Where there are no lateral branches on which to crotch a separate support line for power saws weighing more than 15 lb (6.8 kg), a false crotch shall be used.

c. Use of hydraulic power saws is permissible.

d. Climbers shall use a saw lanyard to carry the saw.

e. The engine shall be started and operated only when all co-workers are clear of the saw and then in accordance with the manufacturer's recommendations and instructions.

f. The operator will shut off the saw when carrying it over slippery surfaces, through heavy brush, and when adjacent to personnel. The saw may be carried running (idle speed with the brake set) for a short distances (less than 50 ft (15.2 m)) as long as it is carried to prevent contact with the chain or muffler.

g. All saws shall be equipped with a clutch, chain brake (gas only), throttle trigger latch, stop switch, rear hand guard, chain catcher, vibration damper, spark arrestor, and muffler.

h. Chain saws shall be kept sharp and operated per Section 13.F.

EM 385-1-1
15 Sep 08

i. Proper PPE for chain saw use includes, eye protection, chaps, safety boots, hearing protection, and head protection. Hearing protection may not be needed on hydraulic saws.

j. Saws shall be equipped with a control that will return the saw to idling speed when released.

k. A power saw may not be operating while a climber is climbing up in the tree.

31.E.08 Chopping tools.

a. Chopping tools that have loose or cracked heads or splintered handles shall not be used.

b. Chopping tools shall never be used while working aloft.

c. Chopping tools shall be swung away from the feet, legs, and body, using the minimum power practical for control.

d. Chopping tools shall not be driven as wedges or used to drive metal wedges.

e. All edged tools and blades shall be properly sheathed when not in use.

31.E.09 Cant hooks, cant dogs, tongs, and carrying bars.

a. Hooks shall be firmly set before applying pressure.

b. Workers shall be warned and shall be in the clear before logs are moved.

c. The points of hooks shall be at least 2 in (5 cm) long and shall be kept sharp.

d. Workers shall stand to the rear and uphill when rolling logs.

31.E.10 Wedges and chisels.

  a. Wedges and chisels shall be properly pointed and tempered.

  b. Only wood, plastic, or soft metal wedges shall be used with power saws.

  c. Wood-handled chisels should be protected with a ferrule on the striking end.

EM 385-1-1
15 Sep 08

SECTION 32

AIRFIELD <u>AND</u> <u>AIRCRAFT</u> OPERATIONS

32.A AIRFIELDS - GENERAL

32.A.01 The following safety requirements shall be in addition to the airfield's safety requirements. When an airfield has safety requirements that differ from those of this Section, the more stringent requirements shall prevail.

32.A.02 Prior to the performance of any work upon or around an airfield, the <u>Air Field Manager</u> shall be informed <u>14 days prior to performance with a written description of work activities</u>, work locations, work equipment and personnel requirements, and work schedules.

    a. The GDA shall also be informed <u>of proposed revisions to approved work activities</u> in writing, or any changes to this information.

    b. The GDA shall keep the airport operator informed so that Notice to Airmen can be issued to reflect hazardous conditions.

32.A.03 Unless a runway is closed by the airfield operator and properly marked, it shall not be used for purposes other than aircraft operation without permission of the GDA.

32.A.04 All paved surfaces, such as runways, taxiways, and hardstands, shall be kept clean at all times, particularly with regards to stones and other small objects that might damage aircraft propellers or jet aircraft. <u>Sweeping operations shall be performed by truck mounted vacuum sweeper capable of using water to minimize dust generation.</u>

32.A.05 When mobile equipment is not <u>actively being utilized</u> to perform work on an airfield, it shall be removed to a location(s) that is approved by the GDA <u>and at a</u> minimum distance required by the

EM 385-1-1
15 Sep 08

GDA (plus any additional distance necessary to ensure the safety of airfield operations) from the runway centerline.

32.A.06 Excavations.

    a. An excavation shall not be opened unless there is material on hand and ready to complete that work item.

    b. As soon as practicable after material has been placed and work approved, the excavation shall be backfilled and compacted IAW contract documents. Meanwhile, all hazardous conditions shall be identified as specified in this section.

32.A.07 Nothing shall be placed upon the landing areas without authorization of the GDA.

32.A.08 <u>All vehicle access shall be at an entry control point (ECP) and approved by the Airfield Manager</u>. Effective control of vehicles required to enter or cross aircraft movement areas shall be maintained <u>as directed by the Airfield Manager</u>.

32.A.09 Those landing areas hazardous to aircraft shall be <u>submitted to the Air Field manager for a FAA Notum on displaced threshold or other changes on non use or caution</u> (unless otherwise directed by the GDA).

    a. During daylight, areas shall be outlined with red flags spaced every 200 ft (60.9 m).

    b. During periods of darkness, areas shall be outlined with battery-operated low-intensity red flashing lights spaced every 200 ft (60.9 m).

    c. During dawn and dusk, and when weather conditions reduce visibility, areas shall be outlined with both red flags and battery-operated low-intensity red flashing lights spaced every 200 ft (60.9 m).

EM 385-1-1
15 Sep 08

32.A.10 When work is to be performed at an airfield where flying is controlled, permission to enter a landing area shall be obtained from the control tower operator every time entry is required, unless the landing area has been closed by the airfield operator and marked as hazardous in accordance with 32.A.09 a-c.

>   a. All vehicles which operate in landing areas shall be identified by means of a checkered flag on a staff attached to, and flying above, the vehicle: the flag shall be 3 ft (0.9 m) square and consist of a checkered pattern of international orange and white squares of 1 ft (0.3 m) on each side.

>   b. All other equipment and materials in the landing area shall be marked as specified in 32.A.09.a - c.

32.A.11 When working in landing areas, work shall be performed so as to leave that portion of the landing area that is available to aircraft free from hazards, including holes, piles, or material, and projecting shoulders that might damage an airplane tire. <u>Each vehicle, piece of equipment, or work crew shall be equipped with a two-way radio capable of maintaining communications with the air traffic control tower while performing work in landing areas.</u>

32.A.12 <u>No equipment, materials or contractor plant</u> shall be placed upon or within a safety precaution area without approval of the GDA.

32.A.13 All equipment and materials in a safety precaution area shall be marked as specified in 32.A.09.a-c. If an object in a safety precaution area projects above the approach-departure clearance surface or above the transitional surface, the object shall be marked with a red light.

32.B AIRCRAFT

<u>32.B.01</u> All non-military aircraft shall be registered, certified in the appropriate category and maintained in accordance with the airworthiness standards of the FAA. (If used OCONUS, and not prohibited by other regulation such as ER 95-1-1, registration, certification and maintenance in accordance with the standards of a comparable governing body of foreign or international authority may be substituted for those of the FAA.)

<u>32.B.02</u> All contract pilots or pilots of chartered aircraft shall hold at least a commercial pilot certificate with instrument rating. All pilots of non-military aircraft shall possess ratings to comply with the FAA Regulation governing the aircraft and operations involved.

<u>32.B.03</u> All non-military aircraft shall be equipped with a two-way radio.

<u>32.B.04</u> All non-military flight operations shall be in accordance with the FAA rules governing conduct for the specific operation (i.e., 14 CFR 133, 14 CFR 135 and 14 CFR 91).

<u>32.B.05</u> All military flight operations shall be conducted under appropriate DOT/DOD regulations.

<u>32.B.06 All USACE-owned aircraft will use approved Government Flight Representatives' (GFRs) approved procedures as outlined in AR 95-20 and AR 95-1. GFRs are appointed in accordance with AR 95-20.</u>

EM 385-1-1
15 Sep 08

SECTION 33

MUNITIONS AND EXPLOSIVES OF CONCERN ENCOUNTERED DURING USACE ACTIVITIES

33.A GENERAL

33.A.01 All Munitions and Explosives of Concern (MEC) or suspect MEC encountered on jobsites shall be treated as extremely dangerous. MEC can be Unexploded Ordnance (UXO), Discarded Military Munitions (DMM), or Munitions Constituents (MC). Follow the **3Rs: RECOGNIZE, RETREAT, REPORT** and take the following actions:

> a. **RECOGNIZE:** see examples in paragraph 33.B. Do not touch, disturb or move the item (munitions can become very unstable over time). They can detonate with movement or sometimes due to ground vibration. Munitions come in all shapes, sizes, and color but exposure to weather and time can alter or remove these markings.
>
> b. **RETREAT**: Mark the general location of the MEC hazard with tape, colored cloth, or colored ribbon. If available, attach the marker to a branch, structure or other existing object so that it is about 3 ft (.9 m) off the ground and visible from all approaches. Place the marker no closer than the point where you first recognized the MEC hazard and do not drive stakes into the ground or otherwise disturb the surface.
> c. Leave by the same route you entered the area if possible. Clear site of all workers and secure from unauthorized entry.
>
> d. Do not transmit on any radio frequencies. Do not talk on a cell phone near a suspected MEC. Signals transmitted from items such as cell phones, short-wave radios, single side-band radios or other communications and navigation devices may detonate the MEC.

EM 385-1-1
15 Sep 08

e. Note the location where the suspect munitions is found, the direction, any landmarks or other features that would aid others in locating the munitions.

f. **REPORT**: Once area has been evacuated, notification shall be made immediately. Provide as much information as possible, including location, approximate size, shape, color, and any other distinguishing features such as nomenclature or writing, fins, etc.,

(1) If not on DoD installation, anytime suspected MEC is encountered, immediately call the local emergency response authority (e.g., local police, sheriff, or 911) to report the finding. GDA and Corps PM shall be notified immediately as well. Before work can begin, the District Commander will determine the level of construction support required at the project site by assessing the probability of encountering MEC.

(2) If on DoD installation, immediately notify supervisor, GDA and Corps PM, installation POC (who shall contact and facilitate Explosive Ordnance Disposal (EOD) response). Before work can begin, the Installation Commander will determine the level of construction support required at the project site by assessing the probability of encountering MEC.

33.A.02 The site is now considered a potential munitions response site (MRS). Further work shall proceed in accordance with requirements found in EM 358-1-97, ER 385-1-95, and EPs 75-1-2, 75-1-3, 385-1-95a and 385-1-95b.

33.A.03 Military munitions (MM), regardless of age or condition, shall be handled by trained UXO-qualified personnel, Government Ordnance and Explosives (OE) Safety Specialists, or Military Explosives Ordnance Disposal (EOD) personnel.

33.B MEC Examples (may be encountered on a USACE project site).

EM 385-1-1
15 Sep 08

33.B.01 GRENADES. There are three types of grenades discussed here: hand grenades; rifle grenades; and projectile grenades.

a. Hand grenades are small explosives or chemical-type munitions that are designed to be thrown at a short distance. Various types of hand grenades may be encountered as UXO, including fragmentation, smoke, and illumination grenades. All hand grenades have three main parts: a body, a fuse and filler. *< See Figure 33-1.a.*

FIGURE 33-1

GRENADES

FIGURE 33-1.A

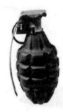

Mk-II Fragmentation Grenade

Hazards: Cocked Striker, High Explosives (HE) & Fragmentation (Frag)

Weight: 1.3 lbs
Length: 4.5 in

EM 385-1-1
15 Sep 08

b. Fragmentation grenades are the most common type of hand grenade used. They have metal or plastic bodies filled with an explosive material. Other types of hand grenades may be made of metal, plastic, cardboard, or rubber and may contain, white phosphorus (WP), chemical agents (CA), or illumination flares, depending on their intended use. Most use a burning (pyrotechnic) delay fuse that functions 3 to 5 seconds after the safety lever is released, but some are activated instantly when the lever is released. **< *See Figure 33.1.b below.***

FIGURE 33-1.B

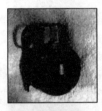

M33/67 Fragmentation Grenade

Hazards: Cocked Striker, HE & Frag

Weight: 0.875 lbs
Height: 3.530 in

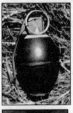

M-26 Fragmentation Grenade

Hazards: Cocked Striker, HE & Frag

Weight: 1.00 lb
Length: 3.33 in

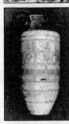

M34 - WP Grenade

Hazards: Cocked Striker, HE & Frag, WP, Smoke & Fire

Weight: 1.5 lbs
Length: 5.5 in

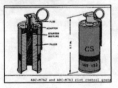

M7 Chemical Grenade (Riot Control) CS-Filled

Hazards: Cocked Striker, Chemical & Fire

Weight: 1.2 lbs
Length: 4.5 in

EM 385-1-1
15 Sep 08

c. Rifle grenades look like small mortars and range from 9 - 17 in (23 - 43 cm) in length. They may be filled with high explosives (HE), WP, CS, illumination flares, or chemicals that produce colored screening/signal smoke. Rifle grenades are fired from standard infantry rifles. They have an opening at the tail-end of a fin assembly that allows the rifle grenade to be placed on the barrel of a rifle. **< *See Figure 33.1.c.***

FIGURE 33-1.C

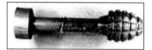

M17 Fragmentation Rifle Grenade

Hazards: Impact/Inertia, HE & Frag

Weight: 2.2 lbs
Length: 9.4 in

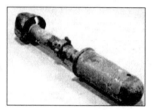

M19 Rifle Grenade, Smoke WP

Hazards: HE, Frag, Fire, WP, Smoke/Incendiary, & Impact/Inertia

Weight: 1.50 lbs
Length: 11.31 in

EM 385-1-1
15 Sep 08

d. The most commonly used projected grenade is the 40 mm grenade. This grenade is also among the most commonly found UXO item. The 40mm grenade is about the same size and shape as a chicken egg. It can contain a variety of fillers such as HE, CS, illumination flares, or various colored screening/signal smoke mixtures. Because of their relatively small size, they are easily concealed by vegetation. They are extremely dangerous because of their sensitive internal fusing systems and can be detonated by simple movement of if handled. **< See Figure 33.1.d.**

FIGURE 33-1.D

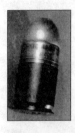

Projected Grenade M406 – 40MM HE (New Unfired)

Hazards: HE, Frag & Movement

Weight: 0.503 lbs
Length: 3.894 in

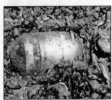

Projected Grenade M406 – 40MM HE (Fired)

Hazards: HE, Frag & Movement

Weight: 0.31 lbs
Length: 3.08 in

EM 385-1-1
15 Sep 08

33.B.02 PROJECTILES. Projectiles can range from approximately 1 in (2.54 cm) to 16 in (40.6 cm) in diameter and from 2 in (5 cm) to 4 ft (1.2 m) in length. Projectiles can be fused either in the nose or the base of the projectile. A wide variety of fuses and fillers can be found in the various types of projectiles. Some projectile fuses are extremely sensitive to movement and will detonate if jarred or accidentally moved. *< See Figure 33.2.*

FIGURE 33-2

PROJECTILES

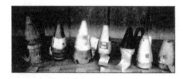

Miscellaneous Projectile Fuzes

Hazards: Electromagnetic Radiation (EMR), HE, Frag, Cocked Striker, Movement & Static

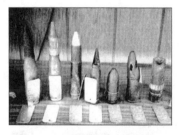

Projectiles Ranging from 20MM and Up

Hazards: EMR, HE, Frag, Movement & Missile

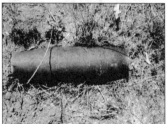

M1 105MM HE Projectile

Hazards: HE & Frag

Weight: 39.92 lbs
Length: 28.60 in

FIGURE 33-2 (CONTINUED)

PROJECTILES

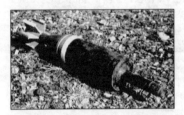

M456 105MM Heat Projectile

Hazards: EMR, HE, Frag, Jet (Shaped Charge), Lucky (Piezoelectric), Movement & Static

Weight: 20 lbs
Length: 26 in

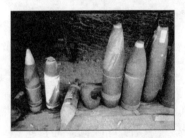

Miscellaneous Spin Stabilized Projectiles

Hazards: EMR, HE, Frag, Jet (Shaped Charge), Cocked-Striker, Movement & Static

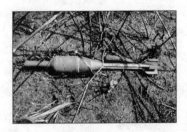

M371 90MM HEAT Recoilless Rifle Projectile

Hazards: EMR, HE, Frag, Jet (Shape Charge), Lucky (Piezoelectric), Movement & Static

Weight: 9.25 lbs
Length: 27.78 in

EM 385-1-1
15 Sep 08

33.B.03 MORTARS. Mortars range form approximately 2 in (5 cm) to 11 in (28 cm) in diameter and can by filled with explosives, WP, or illumination flares. Mortars generally have thinner metal casing than artillery projectiles. They normally use fin stabilization but, some types can be found that uses spin stabilization. *≤ See Figure 33.3.*

FIGURE 33-3

MORTARS

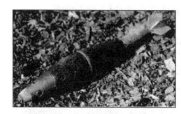

M374 81MM HE Mortar
Hazards: HE, Frag & Movement
Weight: 9.340 lbs
Length: 20.838 in

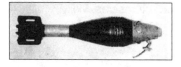

M49 60MM HE Mortar (New)
Hazards: HE, Frag & Movement
Weight: 3.07 lbs
Length: 9.61 in

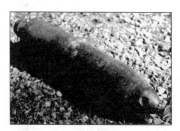

M3 4.2", 107MM HE Mortar
Hazards: HE, Frag & Movement
Weight: 26.20 lbs
Length: 23.05 in

EM 385-1-1
15 Sep 08

FIGURE 33-3 (CONTINUED)

MORTARS

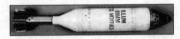

81 mm M301A3 Illumination Mortar Projectile

Hazards: Ejection & Fire

Weight: 0.10 lbs
Length: 24.73 in

33.B.04 ROCKETS. A rocket uses gas pressure from rapidly burning material (propellant) to propel a payload (warhead) to a desired location. Rockets can range from 1 (3.8 cm) to more than 15 in (38.1 cm) in diameter, and that can vary from 1 ft (.3 m) to over 9 ft (2.8 m) in length. All rockets consist of a warhead section and a motor section. Rockets are unguided after launch and are stabilized during flight by fins attached to the motor section or by canted nozzles built into the base of the motor section. The warhead section can be filled with either, explosives, WP, submunitions, or illumination flares. **< See Figure 33.4.**

FIGURE 33-4

ROCKETS

Warning: Fired rockets may still contain residual propellant that could ignite and burn violently!

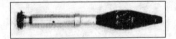

M7A2 2.36" Rocket Heat (Bazooka)
Hazards: EMR, HE, Fire, Frag, Jet (Shaped Charge), & Movement
Weight: 3.5 lbs
Length: 21.5 in

EM 385-1-1
15 Sep 08

FIGURE 33-4 (CONTINUED)

ROCKETS

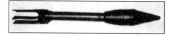

M72 Law 66MM Rocket

Hazards: Cocked Striker, HE, Frag, Jet (Shaped Charge), Lucky (Piezoelectric) & Missile

Weight: 2.300-lbs
Length: 19.987-inches

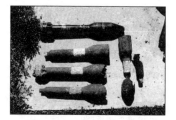

M28 3.5 in Heat Rocket

Hazards: EMR, HE, Frag, Jet (Shaped Charge), & Movement

Weight: 9 lbs
Length: 23.55 in

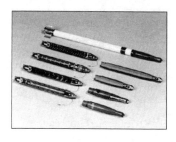

2.75 in Aerial Rocket System

Hazards: EMR, HE, Frag, Jet (Shaped Charge), Static, Movement, Missile, Cock Striker, Submunitions, White Phosphorus, & Fire

Weight: 18.1 lbs
Length: 70 in

EM 385-1-1
15 Sep 08

33.B.05 GUIDED MISSILES. Guided missiles are similar to rockets; however, they are guided to their target by various guidance systems. Some are wire-guided, and internal or external devices guide others. Fins controlled by internal electronics usually stabilize guided missiles. Guided missiles vary in size from man-portable, shoulder launched to very large intercontinental ballistic missiles. *< See Figure 33.5.*

FIGURE 33-5

GUIDED MISSILES

Warning: Some guidance systems contain toxic materials, do not touch or handle missile components!

Warning: Fired guided missiles may still contain residual propellant that could ignite and burn violently!

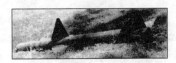

AIM-7 Sparrow Missile (Air to Air)

Hazards: EMR, HE, Frag, Fire, High Pressure (Accumulator), Mechanical, Electrical & Missile

Weight: 319 lbs
Length: 12 ft

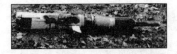

BGM-71 TOW (Surface to Surface)

Hazards: EMR, HE, Frag, Fire, High Pressure (Accumulator), Mechanical, Electrical & Missile

Weight: 39.60 lbs
Length: 45.67 in

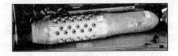

M47 Dragon Missile

Hazards: EMR, HE, Frag, Fire, High Pressure (Accumulator), Electrical, Missile, Static, & Unexpended Rocket Motors May Exist After Impact

Weight: 22.1 lbs
Length: 33.3 in

EM 385-1-1
15 Sep 08

33.B.06 BOMBS. Bombs are dropped from aircraft and vary in weight from 100 - 20,000 lbs ((45.4 kg - 9.07 MT), with lengths ranging from 6 in – 10 ft (15.2 cm - 3 m). Bombs consist of a bomb body and some form of stabilizing device (fin assembly) and may be fused in either the nose or the tail. There are two general types of bombs, "Old-Style" which date from the early 1920's to the 1950's and what are know as "Mk-80-Series" which date from the late 1950's to the present. **< *See Figure 33.6.***

FIGURE 33-6

BOMBS

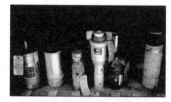

Bomb Fuzes

Hazards: EMR, HE, Frag, Electrical, & Movement

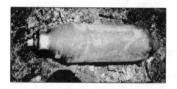

Old Style Series of Aerial Bomb

Hazards: HE, Frag, Movement, & Cock-Striker

Weight: From 100 to 2000-lbs
Length: Varied

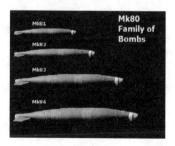

Mk-80 Series New Style Aerial Bombs

Hazards: HE, Frag, Movement, EMR, Static, Cock-Striker, & Influence (Magnetic/Acoustic)

Weight: 250 lb, 500 lb, 2000-lb, & 3000 lb
Length: Varied

EM 385-1-1
15 Sep 08

33.B.07 PRACTICE BOMBS. Practice bombs are used to simulate the explosive filled bomb and will duplicate the same weight and dimensions of those bombs. They can also be found with very distinctive shapes and sizes. All practice bombs contain a "Spotting Charge" consisting of in some cases up to 23 lbs (11.3 kg) of HE. Although most practice bombs contain pyrotechnic charges that consist of red/white phosphorus and a propellant such as smokeless or black powder. **≤ *See Figure 33.7.***

FIGURE 33-7

PRACTICE BOMBS

Warning: Practice bombs contain very dangerous pyrotechnic charges!

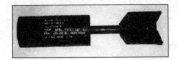

MK106 5 lbs Practice Bomb

Hazards: Ejection, HE, Movement, & Smoke/Incendiary

Weight: 2.68 lbs
Length: 8.25 inches

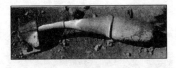

BDU-33 Practice Bomb

Hazards: Ejection, HE, & Smoke/Incendiary

Weight: 23.8 lbs
Length: 22.5 in

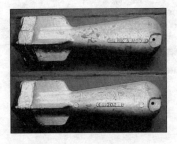

Mk 5 Mod 0 Practice Bomb

Hazards: Ejection, Smoke, & Incendiary

Weight: .5 lb
Length: 8 in

EM 385-1-1
15 Sep 08

33.B.08 DISPENSERS. Dispensers are used to carry and dispense submunitions payloads. They can be found either as aircraft dispensers or as artillery projectiles that eject (dispense) their submunition payloads. ≤ *See Figure 33.8.*

a. Aerial dispensers generally look like medium size aerial bombs, except the construction of dispenser body is normally out of lightweight aluminum.

b. Projectiles that are designed to eject their submunition payload generally appear like any other projectile except there are some design features that allow the projectile body to eject its payload.

FIGURE 33-8

DISPENSERS

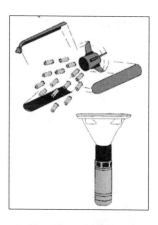

When the fuze in the dispenser functions above the target area, a length of explosive det-cord opens the dispenser container. When that occurs the individual submunitions within the container is spread-out over a large area.

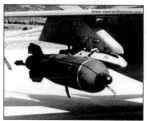

SUU-30H/H (Dispenser) loaded on the wing of an attack aircraft.

EM 385-1-1
15 Sep 08

33.B.09 SUBMUNITIONS. Submunitions are delivered in a container such as a projectile body or a dispenser that will dispense the submunitions in-flight over a target area. Submunitions come in a variety of sizes and shapes. Submunitions include bomblete, grenades, and mines that can be filled with explosives or chemical agent. They may be anti-personnel, anti-material, anti-tank, dual-purpose, incendiary, or chemical submunitions. Submunitions are activated in a variety of ways, depending on their intended use. Some are activated by pressure, impact, or movement/disturbance. Others are activated in flight or when they come near metallic objects. Some submunitions contain a self-destruct fuse as a backup. The self destruct time can vary from a couple of hours to several days. **≤ *See Figure 33.9.***

FIGURE 33-9

SUBMUNITIONS

Warning: Submunitions are extremely hazardous because even very slight movement can cause them to detonate.

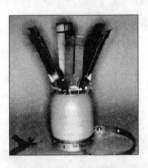

BLU-3 Aerial Dispersed Anti-Personnel Frag Bomb (New)

Hazards: HE, Frag, & Movement

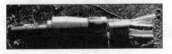

MK118 Aerial Dispersed Anti-Tank Shape Charge (Field)

Hazards: EMR, HE, Jet (Shaped Charge), Lucky (Piezoelectric), & Movement

EM 385-1-1
15 Sep 08

FIGURE 33-9 (CONTINUED)

SUBMUNITIONS

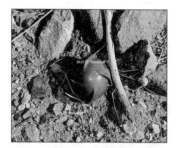

M42 Projectile Dispersed Dual-Purpose Submunitions.

Hazards: HE, Frag, Jet (Shape Charge), & Movement

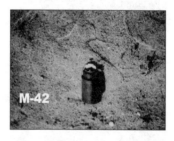

BLU-26 Aerial Dispersed Anti-Personnel Submunition.

Hazards: HE, Frag, & Movement

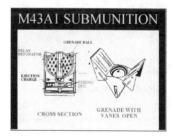

Projectile Dispersed M43 Anti-Personnel Submunition

Hazards: HE, Frag, Ejection, & Movement

EM 385-1-1
15 Sep 08

33.B.10 PYROTECHNICS. Pyrotechnics and pyrotechnic devices contain chemical compound that when ignited will burn at extreme temperatures. They are primarily designed to produce either illumination (light) and/or various colors of smoke for signaling or screening purposes. Pyrotechnic devices can be found in a wide variety of sizes and shapes ranging from small hand held signal flares to large aerial illumination flares. **< *See Figure 33.10.***

FIGURE 33-10

PYROTECHNICS

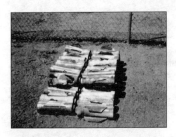

155MM Illumination Candles

Hazards: Ejection, EMR, HE, & Smoke/Incendiary

Weight: 4.3-5.8 lbs
Length: 23 in

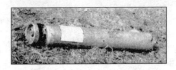

MK-45 Parachute Flare (Field)
Hazards: Ejection, EMR, HE, & Smoke/Incendiary
Weight: 28.6 lbs
Length: 3 ft

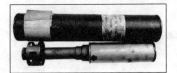

M18A1 White Star Cluster

Hazards: Ejection, & Incendiary

Weight: 17.49 oz
Length: 10.14 in

EM 385-1-1
15 Sep 08

33.B.11 Items That Might Contain Chemical Warfare Materiel ≤ *See Figures 33.11.a-e.*

FIGURE 33-11.A

Figure 33-11.a 4 in (10.16 cm) Stokes mortar, an example of a round that could have an unknown filler. The differences between the chemical mortar and the smoke-filled and the high explosive filled mortars are in the length.

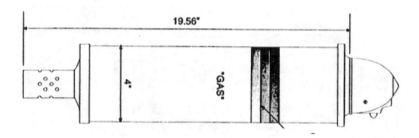

FIGURE 33-11.B

Figure 33-11.b 8 in (20.32 cm) Livens projectile, an example of a round that could have an unknown filler. There are virtually no external differences between the chemical projectile and the smoke-filled projectile

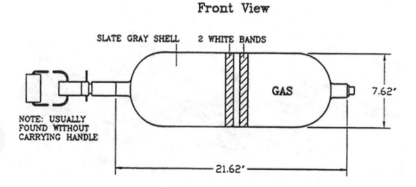

785

EM 385-1-1
15 Sep 08

FIGURE 33-11.C

Figure 33-11.c 4.2 in (10.67 cm) Gas Mortar. This is an example of an item that might have an unknown filler. This model of mortar can have CA, WP smoke, and tearing agent, to mention a few. There are virtually no external differences, except possible fusing combinations.

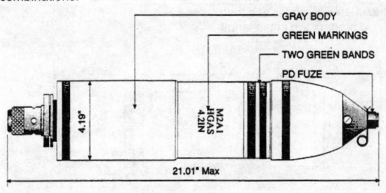

FIGURE 33-11.D

Figure 33-11.d. K941 Chemical Agent Identification Set (CAIS). This is an example of a suspect chemical item. It typically contains 24 bottles (2.5 liters (2500 ml) total weight) of distilled mustard (HD) or mustard (H and HS) agent.

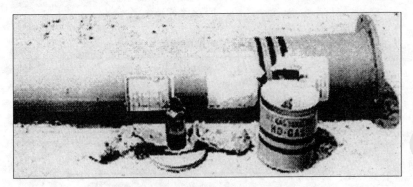

FIGURE 33-11.E

Figure 33-11-e. K951/K952 CAIS. This is an example of a suspect chemical item. Typically it could contain 48 pyrex, flame sealed ampules, 12 each containing 1.4 oz (2.66 ml) Zunce solution of mustard (H), a 5% solution in chloroform, Lewisite (L), a 5% solution in chloroform, Chloropicrin (PS), 50% solution in chloroform, and Phosgene (CG), 40 ml, full strength

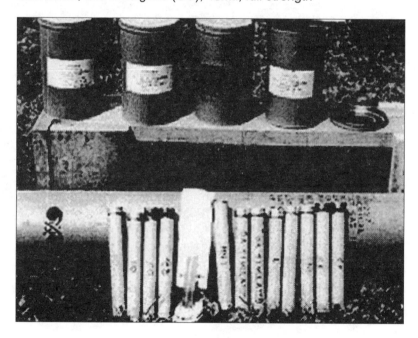

BLANK

EM 385-1-1
15 Sep 08

Section 34

CONFINED SPACE ENTRY

34.A CONFINED SPACES – NON-MARINE FACILITIES

34.A.01 General. Confined space work performed in permanent facilities and/or performed on Construction sites shall be performed in accordance with this Section, 29 CFR 1910.146 and ANSI Z117.1. In addition, employer shall consult the OSHA Regional authority to determine if the requirements of 29 CFR 1910.146 and those provided herein are sufficient to be considered compliant for the specific confined space work tasks to be performed.

34.A.02 For USACE-conducted confined space work activities associated with ship and vessel repair and maintenance operations covered by 29 CFR 1915, see Section 34.B. Confined space work covered by OSHA's Shipyard (29 CFR 1915) standard or USCG regulations shall be performed in accordance with those regulations.

34.A.03 The following definitions apply to all confined spaces except those in ships or vessels:

a. Confined Space – A space that is large enough and so configured that an employee can bodily enter and perform assigned work and, has limited or restricted means for entry or exit and, is not designed for continuous employee occupancy;

b. Non-Permit Required Confined Space (NPRCS) – a confined space that does not contain or have the potential to contain an atmospheric hazard capable of causing death or physical harm. The atmosphere should be proven by air monitoring to be free of hazard;

c. Permit Required Confined Space (PRCS) – Is a confined space that has one or more of the following characteristics:

(1) Contains or has a potential to contain a hazardous atmosphere;

(2) Contains a material that has the potential for engulfing an entrant;

(3) Has an internal configuration such that an entrant could be trapped or asphyxiated by inwardly converging walls or by a floor which slopes downward and tapers to a smaller cross section; AND

(4) Contains any other recognized serious safety or health hazard.

d. Confined Space Competent Person (CSCP) – A person with thorough knowledge of OSHA's Confined Space Standard, 29 CFR 1910.146, experience with PRCS space entry procedures and, the authority to supervise and influence how work is performed on job sites and in facilities.

34.A.04 Confined Space Identification. Facilities and job sites shall assign a Confined Space Competent Person (CSCP) to identify all confined spaces and determine entry rules. Permit Required Confined Space (PRCSs) may be entered under PRCS procedures only. Non-Permit Required Confined Spaces (NPRCSs) may be entered under NPRCS entry procedures.

a. PRCS Entry Procedures. Entry into PRCSs shall comply with 29 CFR 1910.146.

b. NPRCS Entry Procedures. Entry into NPRCS shall comply with paragraph (c) (5) of 29 CFR 1910.146.

34.A.05 CSCP Responsibilities:

a. Identification and Labeling. The CSCP shall identify and label all confined spaces at the facility/site. The label shall identify the space as a NPRCS or a PRCS;

EM 385-1-1
15 Sept 08

b. Program Development. The CSCP shall develop an activity/site-specific confined space program. The program shall contain the confined space program elements defined in this section;

c. PRCS Permit Development. The CSCP shall develop and enforce confined space permits for entry into all PRCSs at the facility/site;

d. Coordination with local emergency responders. The CSCP shall coordinate with local emergency responders to determine if they are capable of a rescue from the specific confined space. If the local emergency responders do not have the appropriate rescue capability, the rescue capability should be developed on-site.

34.A.06 Confined Space Program Elements. The confined space program shall address each of the following elements with facility/site- specific detail:

a. Identification and Labeling. Describe the process for regularly inspecting facilities/sites and the work tasks performed at them to identify confined spaces. Describe labeling and enforcement procedures that will assure personnel do not enter confined spaces in an unauthorized fashion;

b. Confined space hazard identification. Describe the air monitoring or ventilation monitoring conducted to identify the space as a PRCS or a NPRCS;

c. Safe confined space entry conditions. Describe the practices and procedures that will be followed to assure that confined spaces will be entered safely. Procedures and practices shall include but are not limited to the following:

(1) NPRCSs – Describe any monitoring and employee training that will assure non-permit conditions are maintained and that employees entering the NPRCS understand how to maintain a safe working environment while working in the NPRCS;

(2) PRCSs – At a minimum, describe how each of the elements below will be enforced at each PRCS:

(a) PRCS entry permit development and maintenance procedures for all PRCS;

(b) Acceptable entry conditions;

(c) Observation by the authorized entrant of monitoring or testing in PRCSs;

(d) Isolation of the PRCSs;

(e) Purging, inerting, flushing or ventilating the PRCS as necessary to eliminate or control atmospheric hazards;

(f) Installation of barriers to protect entrants from external hazards;

(g) Monitoring to verify acceptable entry conditions for the duration of the authorized entry;

d. Equipment (and equipment maintenance procedures) to be used for confined space entry at the facility/site. Equipment shall include the following at a minimum:

(1) Atmospheric testing and monitoring equipment to assure safe entry;

(2) Ventilation equipment to assure maintenance of safe entry conditions;

(3) Communication equipment for entry;

(4) Personal Protective Equipment (PPE) necessary in the event that engineering controls and work practices do not adequately protect entrants (does not apply to NPRCS);

EM 385-1-1
15 Sept 08

(5) Lighting equipment for entry;

(6) Barriers and shields to keep unauthorized entrants out of the confined spaces during entry;

(7) Ladders or other equipment necessary for entrant access and egress;

(8) Rescue and emergency equipment needed to remove entrants in the event of an emergency;

(9) Any other equipment necessary for safe entry into or rescue from confined spaces;

e. Procedures for evaluating PRCS conditions when entry is conducted. Address each of the following in facility/site-specific detail;

(1) Atmosphere conditions required to be maintained during entry to ensure safe entry;

(2) At a minimum, test the PRCS atmosphere for the following in the order specified:

(a) Oxygen;

(b) Combustible gases and vapors; and

(c) Toxic gases and vapors.

f. Policies and procedures to assure that at least one attendant is available outside the PRCS during entry to respond to emergencies;

g. Designate by name, personnel at the facility/site with active roles in confined space entry. Specify their responsibilities for PRCS entry. All permits shall be signed by each employee entering the confined space, the CSCP, attendant and a responsible entry supervisor;

h. Document procedures and agreements with local emergency responders for summoning rescue and emergency services for rescuing PRCS entrants;

i. Document a facility/site procedure for preparing, issuing, using and canceling PRCS entry permits;

j. Document procedures for coordinating with employees from outside organizations who will be participating in PRCS entry;

k. Document procedures for concluding an entry after entry operations have been completed;

l. Develop procedures for reviewing PRCS entries and documenting lessons learned from them; and

m. Establish a policy to review cancelled permits to modify the PRCS entry procedures.

34.A.07 Employee Training – Employees entering confined spaces shall be trained to understand the requirements of the facility/site-specific confined space program.

34.A.08 Rescue and Emergency Services – The CSCP shall develop or establish rescue and emergency services for PRCS entry.

EM 385-1-1
15 Sept 08

34.B WORK PERFORMED IN CONFINED AND ENCLOSED SPACES ON SHIPS AND VESSELS. The following applies only to ship and vessel repair and maintenance, not regular ship and vessel activities. > *See Section 19.*

34.B.01 Definitions

a. Adjacent spaces are spaces which border an area on a vessel or vessel section such as, cargo tanks or holds, pump or engine rooms, storage lockers, tanks containing flammable or combustible liquids, gases, or solids, and crawl spaces, in all directions, including all points of contact, corners, diagonals, decks, tank tops, and bulkheads.

b. A Competent Person for confined spaces in ships and vessels (CPCSSV) is a person who has knowledge of the designation of spaces where the work is done; ability to understand and follow through on the air sampling, PPE and instructions of a Marine Chemist, Coast Guard authorized persons, or Certified Industrial Hygienist.

c. A confined space on a ship or vessel is a compartment of small size and limited access such as a double bottom tank, cofferdam, or other space which by its small size and confined nature can readily create or aggravate a hazardous exposure.

d. An enclosed space means any space, other than a confined space, which is enclosed by bulkheads and overhead. It includes cargo holds, tanks, quarters, and machinery and boiler spaces.

e. "Enter with restrictions" refers to entry into a confined space when engineering controls, PPE and time limitations are imposed by the competent person.

f. "Safe for Workers" denotes a space that meets the following criteria:

(1) The oxygen content of the atmosphere is at least 19.5 percent and below 22 percent by volume;

(2) The concentration of flammable vapors is below 10 percent of the lower explosive limit (LEL);

(3) Any toxic materials in the atmosphere associated with cargo, fuel, tank coatings, or inerting media are within permissible concentrations at the time of the inspection.

34.B.02 All spaces on a vessel or ship or floating plant that could be considered a "potential confined space", shall be posted as a "Potential Confined Space". An inventory of these spaces shall be maintained in the pilot house and the land based office.

34.B.03 Before and during entry into the types of spaces listed below, the CPCSSV shall test for oxygen content, flammability, and toxicity. These tests and all entries shall be recorded on a entry form or in an entry log and reviewed by the GDA:

a. Unventilated confined spaces that have been closed up or freshly painted;

b. Confined spaces that have contained or do contain combustible or flammable liquids or gases;

c. Confined spaces that have contained or do contain toxic, corrosive, or irritant liquid, gases, or solids.

34.B.04 If the testing determines the oxygen is below 19% or above 22%, or the lower explosive limit (LEL) of 10% is exceeded, or other toxic substances are measured, then entry shall proceed under the direction of a CPCSSV.

EM 385-1-1
15 Sep 08

APPENDIX A

MINIMUM BASIC OUTLINE FOR ACCIDENT PREVENTION PLANS

An <u>Accident Prevention Plan (APP)</u> is a safety and health policy and program document. The following areas are typically addressed in an APP, but an APP shall be job-specific and shall also address any unusual or unique aspects of the project or activity for which it is written.

The APP shall interface with the employer's overall safety and health program, <u>and a copy shall be available on the work site</u>. Any portions of the overall safety and health program that are referenced in the APP shall be included as appropriate.
<u>ANSI/ASSE A10.38 should be referenced for Programmatic Issues.</u>

> For LIMITED-SCOPE SERVICE, SUPPLY AND R&D CONTRACTS, for example, mowing (only), park attendant, rest room cleaning, the Contracting Officer and SOHO may allow an ABBREVIATED APP (customized APP requirements and waive the more stringent elements of this section). **> See 01.A.11, and Appendix A, paragraph 11.**

1. SIGNATURE SHEET. Title, signature, and phone number of the following:

    a. Plan preparer (Qualified Person<u>, Competent Person</u>, such as corporate safety staff person, QC);

    b. Plan must be approved, by company/corporate officers authorized to obligate the company;

    c. Plan concurrence (e.g., Chief of Operations, Corporate Chief of Safety, Corporate Industrial Hygienist, project manager or superintendent, project safety professional, project QC). Provide concurrence of other applicable corporate and project personnel (Contractor).

EM 385-1-1
15 Sep 08

2. **BACKGROUND INFORMATION.** List the following:

   a. Contractor;

   b. Contract number;

   c. Project name;

   d. Brief project description, description of work to be performed, and location; phases of work anticipated (these will require an AHA).

3. **STATEMENT OF SAFETY AND HEALTH POLICY.** Provide a copy of current corporate/company Safety and Health Policy Statement, <u>detailing commitment to providing a safe and healthful workplace for all employees. The Contractor's written safety program goals, objectives, and accident experience goals for this contract should be provided</u>.

4. **RESPONSIBILITIES AND LINES OF AUTHORITIES.** <u>Provide the following:</u>

   a. A statement of the employer's ultimate responsibility for the implementation of his SOH program;

   b. Identification and accountability of personnel responsible for safety at both corporate and project level. Contracts specifically requiring safety or industrial hygiene personnel shall include a copy of their resumes. <u>Qualifications shall include the OSHA 30-hour course or equivalent course areas as listed here:</u>

   <u>(1) OSH Act/General Duty Clause;</u>

   <u>(2) 29 CFR 1904, Recordkeeping;</u>

   <u>(3) Subpart C: General Safety and Health Provisions, Competent Person;</u>

(4) Subpart D: Occupational Health and Environmental Controls, Citations and Safety Programs;

(5) Subpart E: PPE, types and requirements for use;

(6) Subpart F: understanding fire protection in the workplace;

(7) Subpart K: Electrical;

(8 Subpart M: Fall Protection;

(9) Rigging, welding and cutting, scaffolding, excavations, concrete and masonry, demolition; health hazards in construction, materials handling, storage and disposal, hand and power tools, motor vehicles, mechanized equipment, marine operations, steel erection, stairways and ladders, confined spaces or any others that are applicable to the work being performed.

c. The names of Competent and/or Qualified Person(s) and proof of competency/qualification to meet specific OSHA Competent/Qualified Person(s) requirements must be attached. The District SOHO will review the qualifications for acceptance;

d. Requirements that no work shall be performed unless a designated competent person is present on the job site;

e. Requirements for pre-task safety and health analysis;

f. Lines of authority;

g. Policies and procedures regarding noncompliance with safety requirements (to include disciplinary actions for violation of safety requirements) should be identified;

h. Provide written company procedures for holding managers and supervisors accountable for safety.

EM 385-1-1
15 Sep 08

5. SUBCONTRACTORS AND SUPPLIERS. If applicable, provide procedures for coordinating SOH activities with other employers on the job site:

   a. Identification of subcontractors and suppliers (if known);

   b. Safety responsibilities of subcontractors and suppliers.

6. TRAINING.

   a. Requirements for new hire SOH orientation training at the time of initial hire of each new employee.

   b. Requirements for mandatory training and certifications that are applicable to this project (e.g., explosive actuated tools, confined space entry, crane operator, diver, vehicle operator, HAZWOPER training and certification, PPE) and any requirements for periodic retraining/recertification.

   c. Procedures for periodic safety and health training for supervisors and employees.

   d. Requirements for emergency response training.
   > *See paragraph 9.b. below for a list of requirements that may require emergency response training.*

7. SAFETY AND HEALTH INSPECTIONS.

   a. Specific assignment of responsibilities for a minimum daily job site safety and health inspection during periods of work activity: Who will conduct (e.g., SSHO, PM, safety professional, QC, supervisors, employees – depends on level of technical proficiency needed to perform said inspections), proof of inspector's training/qualifications, when inspections will be conducted, procedures for documentation, deficiency tracking system, and follow-up procedures;

EM 385-1-1
15 Sep 08

b. Any external inspections/certifications that may be required (e.g., USCG).

8. ACCIDENT REPORTING. The Contractor shall identify person(s) responsible to provide the following:

a. Exposure data (man-hours worked);

b. Accident investigations, reports, and logs: Report all accidents as soon as possible but not more than 24 hours afterwards to the Contracting Officer/Representative (CO/COR). The contractor shall thoroughly investigate the accident and submit the findings of the investigation along with appropriate corrective actions to the CO/COR in the prescribed format as soon as possible but no later than five (5) working days following the accident. Implement corrective actions as soon as reasonably possible;

c. The following require immediate accident notification:

(1) A fatal injury;

(2) A permanent total disability;

(3) A permanent partial disability;

(4) The hospitalization of three or more people resulting from a single occurrence;

(5) Property damage of $200,000 or more.

9. PLANS (PROGRAMS, PROCEDURES) REQUIRED BY THE SAFETY MANUAL. Based on a risk assessment of contracted activities and on mandatory OSHA compliance programs, the Contractor shall address all applicable occupational risks and compliance plans. Using the EM 385-1-1 as a guide, plans may include but not be limited to:

EM 385-1-1
15 Sep 08

a. Layout plans (04.A.01);

b. Emergency response plans:

(1) Procedures and tests (01.E.01);

(2) Spill plans (01.E.01, 06.A.02);

(3) Firefighting plan (01.E.01, Section 19);

(4) Posting of emergency telephone numbers (01.E.05);

(5) Man overboard/abandon ship (Section19.A.04);

(6) Medical Support. Outline on-site medical support and off-site medical arrangements including rescue and medical duties for those employees who are to perform them, and the name(s) of on-site Contractor personnel trained in first aid and CPR. A minimum of two employees shall be certified in CPR and first-aid per shift/site (Section 03.A.02; 03.D);

c. Plan for prevention of alcohol and drug abuse (01.C.02);

d. Site sanitation plan (Section 02);

e. Access and haul road plan (4.B);

f. Respiratory protection plan (05.G);

g. Health hazard control program (06.A);

h. Hazard communication program (06.B.01);

i. Process Safety Management Plan (06.B.04);

j. Lead abatement plan (06.B.05 & specifications);

k. Asbestos abatement plan (06.B.05 & specifications);

EM 385-1-1
15 Sep 08

l. Radiation Safety Program (06.E.03.a);

m. Abrasive blasting (06.H.01);

n. Heat/Cold Stress Monitoring Plan (06.I.02)

o. Crystalline Silica Monitoring Plan (Assessment) (06.M) ;

p. Night operations lighting plan (07.A.08);

q. Fire Prevention Plan (09.A);

r. Wild Land Fire Management Plan (09.K);

s. Hazardous energy control plan (12.A.01);

t. Critical lift Plan (16.H);

u. Contingency plan for severe weather (19.A.03);

v. Float Plan (19.F.04);

w. Site-Specific Fall Protection & Prevention Plan (21.C);

x. Demolition plan (to include engineering survey) (23.A.01);

y. Excavation/trenching plan (25.A.01);

z. Emergency rescue (tunneling) (26.A.);

aa. Underground construction fire prevention and protection plan (26.D.01);

bb. Compressed air plan (26.I.01);

cc. Formwork and shoring erection and removal plans (27.C);

dd. PreCast Concrete Plan (27.D);

EM 385-1-1
15 Sep 08

    ee. Lift slab plans (27.E);

    ff. Steel erection plan (27.F.01);

    gg. Site Safety and Health Plan for HTRW work (28.B);

    hh. Blasting Safety Plan (29.A.01);

    ii. Diving plan (30.A.13);

    jj. Confined space Program (34.A).

10. RISK MANAGEMENT PROCESSES. Detailed project-specific hazards and controls shall be provided by an Activity Hazard Analysis (0I.A.13) for each major phase/activity of work.

11. ABBREVIATED APP for LIMITED-SCOPE SERVICE, SUPPLY AND R&D CONTRACTS. If service, supply and R&D contracts with limited scopes are awarded, the contractor may submit an abbreviated Accident Prevention Plan. This APP shall address the following areas **at a minimum**. If other areas of the EM 385-1-1 are pertinent to the contract, the contractor must assure these areas are addressed as well.

    a. Title, signature, and phone number of the plan preparer.

    b. Background Information to include: Contractor; Contract number; Project name; Brief project description, description of work to be performed, and location (map); The project description shall provide a means to evaluate the work being done (see AHA requirements in 01.A.13) and associated hazards involved. Contractor's APP shall address the identified hazards involved and the control measures to be taken.

    c. Statement of Safety and Health Policy detailing their commitment to providing a safe and healthful workplace for all employees.

EM 385-1-1
15 Sep 08

d. Responsibilities and Lines of Authorities – to include a statement of the employer's ultimate responsibility for the implementation of his SOH program; Identification and accountability of personnel responsible for safety at all levels to include designated site safety and health officer (SSHO) and associated qualifications. The District SOHO will review the qualifications for acceptance.

e. Training - new hire SOH orientation training at the time of initial hire of each new employee and any periodic retraining/recertification requirements.

f. Procedures for job site inspections - assignment of responsibilities and frequency.

g. Procedures for reporting man-hours worked and reporting and investigating any accidents as soon as possible but not more than 24 hours afterwards to the Contracting Officer/Representative (CO/COR). An accident that results in a fatal injury, permanent partial or permanent total disability shall be immediately reported to the Contracting Officer.

h. Emergency Planning. Employees working alone shall be provided an effective means of emergency communication. This may be cellular phone, two-way radio or other acceptable means. The selected means of communication must be readily available and must be in working condition.

i. Drinking Water provisions, toilet and washing facilities.

j. First Aid and CPR training (at least two employees on each shift shall be qualified/certified to administer first aid and CPR) and provision of first aid kit (types/size).

k. Personal Protective Equipment.

(1) WORK CLOTHING - Minimum Requirements. Employees shall wear clothing suitable for the weather however minimum requirements for work shall be short-sleeve shirt, long pants

(excessively long or baggy pants are prohibited) and leather work shoes. If analysis determines that safety-toed (or other protective) footwear is necessary (i.e., mowing, weedeating, chain saw use, etc), they shall be worn.

(2) Eye and Face Protection. Eye and face protection shall be worn as determined by an analysis of the operations being performed HOWEVER, all involved in chain saw use, chipping, stump grinding, pruning operations, grass mowing, weedeating and blowing operations shall be provided safety eyewear (Z87.1) as a minimum.

(3) Hearing Protection. Hearing protection must be worn by all those exposed to high noise activities (to include grass mowing and trimming, chainsaw operations, tree chipping, stump grinding and pruning).

(4) Head Protection. Hard hats shall comply with ANSI Z89.1 and shall be worn by all workers when a head hazard exists. At a minimum, hard hats shall be worn when performing activities identified in (2) above.

(5) High Visibility Apparel shall comply with ANSI/ISEA 107, Class 2 requirements at a minimum and shall be worn by all workers exposed to vehicular or equipment traffic.

(6) Protective Leg chaps shall be worn by all chainsaw operators.

(7) Gloves of the proper type shall be worn by persons involved in activities that expose the hands to cuts, abrasions, punctures, burns and chemical irritants.

(8) If work is being performed around water and drowning is a hazard, PFDs must be provided and worn as appropriate.

l. Machine Guards and safety devices. Lawn maintenance equipment must have appropriate guards and safety devices in place and operational.

EM 385-1-1
15 Sep 08

m. Hazardous Substances. When any hazardous substances are procured, used, stored or disposed, a hazard communication program must be in effect and MSDSs shall be available at the worksite. Employees shall have received training in hazardous substances being used. When the eyes or body of any person may be exposed to corrosives, irritants or toxic chemicals, suitable facilities for quick drenching or flushing of the eyes and body shall be provided within 10 seconds of the worksite.

n. Traffic control shall be accomplished in accordance with DOT's MUTCD.

o. Control of Hazardous Energy (Lockout/Tagout). Before an employee performs any servicing or maintenance on any equipment where the unexpected energizing or startup of the equipment could occur, procedures must be in place to ensure adequate control of this energy.

p. Driving, working on (i.e., working with equipment/mowers) while on slopes, working from/in boats/skiffs, etc shall also be considered and dealt with accordingly.

BLANK

EM 385-1-1
15 Sep 08

APPENDIX B

EMERGENCY OPERATIONS

1. SAFETY AND HEALTH REQUIREMENTS

a. During emergency operations, it is extremely important that safety and health requirements are implemented. Personnel often perform unusual, difficult, hazardous tasks while in a challenging environment, and these conditions may increase risk and the potential for accidents. Additionally, resources are in short supply, and the loss of any resource to an accident reduces the USACE ability to respond. The safety and occupational health of USACE employees, Contractors, and members of the public exposed to USACE activities will be a primary concern during all USACE emergency operations. Safety and Occupational Health Offices (SOHO) shall provide the necessary input to their Emergency Management counterparts to ensure that planning for safety and health concerns (including risk and hazard analysis) is addressed prior to and during emergency operations.

b. Contract Requirements. Safety and occupational health program requirements shall be included in all Government and contract operations. FAR Clause 52.236-13 shall be included in contracts and memoranda of agreement/understanding (MOAs/MOUs) for emergency operations and recovery assistance.

c. Accident Prevention Plan (APP) and Activity Hazard Analyses(AHAs). In addition to the APP already submitted by the Controlling Contractor, activity-specific AHA shall be developed and submitted to the on-site USACE safety and health professional for review and acceptance prior to beginning any operation (debris removal, tree removal, blue-roof activities, leaners and hangers, etc).

EM 385-1-1
15 Sep 08

d. Structural Demolition. For structural demolition activities, consideration shall be given to combine like-structures under a common engineering survey and demolition plan (see 23.A.01.a). For example, single-story residential structures that would pose no hazards to neighboring structures or personnel could be demolished using a common engineering survey and demolition plan, whereas multiple-story structures or others that would pose risks to personnel or other structures would have individual surveys and plans per 23.A.01.

2. INITIAL RESPONSE. A qualified safety and health professional shall be immediately alerted of the disaster and shall be included in the planning and execution of response and recovery efforts. This individual shall assess safety and health issues and shall assure precautions are taken prior to deployment of personnel. Issues to consider include: sanitation, drinking water, power supply, living quarters, driving conditions, environmental conditions, and health issues.

3. STAFFING. SOHO in the Geographic District experiencing the disaster will be temporarily staffed with additional safety, industrial hygiene, and medical personnel as necessary to ensure a comprehensive safety and occupational health program is administered for all emergency operations. If a Recovery Field Office (RFO) is established, SOH staffing is usually accomplished by use of safety and occupational health functional planning and response teams (PRT). If a RFO is not established, the Geographic District shall establish an emergency operations safety office (minimum staffing to include a safety manager and administrative support person) dedicated totally to emergency operations. Also, each Emergency Field Office established shall have a minimum of one SOH professional.

a. Medical personnel shall provide medical assistance, assessments, and advice to USACE management and employees.

b. SOH personnel shall: manage safety and health aspects of emergency operations; provide advice on safety and health

EM 385-1-1
15 Sep 08

issues; provide safety and health technical oversight for USACE employees, other Federal employees engaged in fulfilling the Corps' mission, and quality assurance for Contractor employees.

c. Prime Contractors for emergency operations are required to have as a minimum a full-time, qualified safety professional on-site. Qualifications of the safety professional shall be provided to the GDA for <u>review and acceptance</u>. Additional Contractor personnel may be required as determined by the GDA.

4. QUALIFICATIONS OF GOVERNMENT EMPLOYEES

a. All Government employees reporting for emergency recovery operations shall be medically fit to perform assigned duties for extended hours and endure the additional stress related to this type of work. Prior to assignment to deployment teams and prior to voluntary deployment assignments, the GDA shall ensure employees are medically screened and/or examined by a licensed physician.

(1) The medical screening and/or examination will provide the basis for a determination of fitness for deployment.

(2) Medical screening and/or examination procedures shall be developed by a licensed physician and shall be in accordance with 5 CFR 339.

(3) The medical screening and/or examination shall fully consider the employee's current medical status to include the use of prescription and non-prescription maintenance medications, use of medical appliances, deployment job duties and physical capacities required, use of PPE (such as respirators), extended work hours, potential adverse living and environmental factors, anticipated availability of medical resources at the deployment site in case of emergency, immunizations required, and other factors determined appropriate by the physician.

EM 385-1-1
15 Sep 08

b. Medical documentation shall be on applicable medical screening and/or medical history and medical examination forms and shall be maintained in accordance with 5 CFR 293 and Privacy Act requirements.

c. Physicians shall provide the GDA with recommendations regarding employee <u>deployability</u> status to include the length of medical certification (1 year, 2 years, etc.).

d. Employees with known pre-existing non-work-related medical conditions such as uncontrollable diabetes, cardiovascular or pulmonary problems, back conditions, or hypertension should not deploy to emergency operations sites unless specific medical clearance is provided by the USACE medical provider in conjunction with their personal physician(s) indicating their current medical condition will not jeopardize their health or their ability to fully perform their duty assignments at deployment sites.

<u>e.</u> Employees may be returned to their duty station if during the course of duty they experience health problems that may endanger their well-being.

<u>f.</u> Employees shall be notified that pharmacies and medical services may be limited at the emergency operations site.

5. MOBILIZATION OF USACE PERSONNEL. <u>USACE personnel will be provided the following (prior to departing their duty station for emergency operations when possible):</u>

a. PPE (e.g., head, eye, hearing, foot protection, and PFDs) appropriate for the hazards of the field activities that they will perform, and

b. Immunizations appropriate for their field exposure (follow-up immunizations will be the responsibility of each employee's home duty station). <u>Deploying USACE personnel shall update their immunization data in ENGLink before departing their home</u>

EM 385-1-1
15 Sep 08

station and carry with them their immunization record (USPHS Form 731).

6. **SAFETY ORIENTATION.** Safety and health in-briefings and orientation shall be conducted as personnel arrive at the emergency area and prior to beginning work activities.

7. **COMMUNICATIONS**

   a. Paging equipment, two-way radios, cellular phones, computers, facsimile machines shall be used as needed to establish and enhance communications. > ***See 18.C.01.***

   b. Safety and health programs, documents, signs, tags, instructions, etc., shall be communicated to employees and the public in a language they understand.

8. **DUTY SCHEDULE**

   a. During the first 2 weeks of an emergency response operation extended work hours are allowed. Supervisors shall monitor employees for signs of stress-related health problems and seek medical assistance as appropriate.

   b. For operations lasting longer than 2 weeks, USACE and contractor employees shall not work in excess of 84 hours per week. The duty hours an employee would be required to work during emergency operations are 12 hours per day, 7 days a week. Work and travel time must allow for 8 hours continuous rest between each work shift.

   c. Employees shall be provided the opportunity for 24 hours of rest after working 14 days and 48 hours of rest after working 21 days. Employees shall be required to take at least 24 hours off for rest after a continuous 29-day period of work and shall be required to take at least 24 hours every 2 weeks thereafter. Supervisors shall monitor employees for signs of stress-related health problems and seek medical assistance as appropriate.

EM 385-1-1
15 Sep 08

9. MACHINERY AND MECHANIZED EQUIPMENT > *See Sections 16 and 18.*

a. Inspection of equipment is critical as mobilization can be extremely short and equipment may not be up to USACE safety standards. Whenever feasible, contract specifications shall provide adequate mobilization time to allow equipment to be inspected and brought up to USACE standards. Equipment not meeting the requirements of this manual will not be used.

b. Trucks hauling debris on public highways shall have physical barriers (covers and either tail gates or chain link fencing) to preclude debris from falling from the truck.

(1) Back-up alarms shall be provided.

(2) The need for rollover warning devices shall be considered for long-bed end-dump trucks.

(3) Sideboards shall not be added to trucks to increase their capacity unless specific design specifications are provided to Contractors as part of the scope of work. Single or double boards added to trailers designed for normal operation with the additional boards are permitted.

c. Prior to operation, Contractors shall develop written safe operating procedures for each brush chipper, shredder, and/or grinder.

(1) SOPs shall incorporate the manufacturer's recommendations for safe operation of this equipment as well as the use of an exclusion zone (EZ) and fire prevention efforts.

(2) Operations and maintenance manuals for chippers, grinders, and shredders shall be kept on-site.

(3) A minimum 200 ft (61.0 m) EZ is required for authorized persons during operation of chippers, shredders, and grinders

EM 385-1-1
15 Sep 08

unless documentation or actual practice indicates otherwise. Signs shall be placed at 200 ft (61.0 m) identifying the EZ.

(4) The public shall be kept a minimum of 300 ft (91.4 m) from all chipper operations.

(5) Unauthorized personnel shall not enter the EZ while the chipper is in operation.

(6) Front-end loaders and knuckle booms working in debris reduction areas or feeding grinders, shredders or chippers shall have completely enclosed cabs to protect the operators from debris. Protection shall include heavy metal grating of sufficient strength to protect the operators from logs, limbs, and woods or other debris thrown from grinders.

(7) Whenever chipper operations are shut down for any significant length of time (e.g., overnight or when the chipper will be left unattended), equipment walls, crevice drums, cutter heads and hammers, and drive mechanisms shall be cleared of all combustible materials by blowing, washing, and wetting down.

(8) Any material contaminated by leakage of hydraulic fluids, oils, or fuel shall be immediately removed. Leakage shall be minimized through preventive maintenance.

(9) Because piles of chipped wood are susceptible to spontaneous combustion, fire controls such as segregation, separation, and adequate water supply shall be used.

d. The number of workers in proximity to loaders, trucks, and other equipment shall be the minimum necessary to accomplish the job.

(1) In restricted areas or areas with reduced access or visibility, special precautions will be taken to ensure the safety of workers on the ground.

EM 385-1-1
15 Sep 08

(2) Sequencing of work shall minimize equipment movement when personnel are in the work area.

(3) Workers in the area of operating machinery or vehicular traffic shall wear high-visibility apparel, in accordance with 05.F. These workers include, but are not limited to flag persons, signalpersons, spotters, survey crews and inspectors.

e. Loaders, trackhoes, and other construction equipment in debris reduction areas shall have functional lights in the front and back in order to work at night or during periods of reduced visibility.

f. Aerial Lifts/Platforms/Bucket trucks shall conform to requirements identified in Section 22.M.

g. Unless provided by the manufacturer, seat belts are not required at the operator's station on articulating grapple trucks (knuckle boom trucks). If provided by the manufacturer, seat belts are required to be worn. Access ladders shall be a minimum of 12 in (30.5 cm) width with 16 in (40.6 cm) recommended.

10. TRAFFIC CONTROL

a. Traffic control is extremely important on highways, in residential areas, and at construction sites. When traffic may pose a hazard to operations, public roads will be closed. Road closings shall be coordinated in writing with appropriate local agencies. Traffic controls and signage should comply with the DOT Federal Highway Administration's *"Manual on Uniform Traffic Control Devices* (MUTCD)".

b. When a road cannot be closed, the following precautions shall be taken:

(1) "FLAGGER" (MUTCD W-20-7) or "WORKERS AHEAD: (W21-1) or similar appropriate signs shall be placed along the

EM 385-1-1
15 Sep 08

roadway, 1,000 ft (304.8m) and 500 ft (30.5 m) before the work zone, on both sides of the work zone";

(2) Sufficient number of flag persons shall be used to control traffic within the work area;

(3) Flag persons shall be used and shall receive instruction in flagging operations before being placed in traffic (training and certification by the National Safety Council (NSC) is recommended);

(4) All flag persons shall wear high-visibility apparel in accordance with paragraph 05.F, safety-toed footwear and hard hats.

(5) **"STOP/SLOW"** paddles, preferably mounted on a 6 ft staff, will be used for traffic control;

(6) Flag persons shall be able to communicate with each other and with the foreman, and effectively signal/direct the affected public.

(7) Two-way radios shall be used whenever visual contact between flaggers is not maintained.

c. All construction vehicles and all vehicles exceeding 1-1/2 tons (1360.8 kg) shall have a signal person to assist in backing in residential areas.

11. AIR CURTAIN INCINERATOR OPERATIONS AND DEBRIS PILES. Prior to operating an air curtain incinerator, the contractor shall develop a written safe operating procedure. Employees will be briefed on the procedure and the procedure will be readily available for their review.

a. The design of air curtain operations shall provide for efficient burning of materials.

b. Equipment operators feeding and emptying ash from air curtain operations shall <u>be positioned or equipped to provide adequate breathing air. Workers requiring respirators shall be enrolled in the respiratory protection program and all applicable requirements met in accordance with Section 5.</u>

c. Adequate supplies of water or fire extinguishers shall be readily available and fire watches shall be used. <u>A fire watch will be posted at debris reduction sites when the site is not being actively worked and potential exists for spontaneous combustion or other fire hazards. The fire watch shall have the means to expediently communicate with the site supervisor and designated fire response agencies.</u>

d. If a pick-and-drop debris pile is located within the 100 ft (30.5 m) minimum separation zone of the air curtain incinerator, the volume of the pick-and-drop debris pile shall not be more than four times the volume of the incinerator pit.

e. There shall be a 1 ft (0.3 m) high warning barrier the length of the charging side of the pit to warn equipment operators. It shall be constructed of <u>non-</u>combustible material.

f. No hazardous or containerized ignitable material shall be dumped into the pit.

g. Pits must be constructed out of highly compactable material that will hold its shape.

h. <u>Pits will not extend below the water table</u>.

i. Particulate emissions must meet State and EPA standards for burning operations.

j. At least 100 ft (30.5 m) is required between the debris piles and the burn area. At least 1000 ft (304.8 m) is required between the debris piles and the nearest building. At least 1100 ft (335.3 m) is required between the <u>incineration</u> pit and the nearest building. <u>Debris piles shall not be piled directly</u>

EM 385-1-1
15 Sep 08

under transmission lines nor located within 100 ft (30.5 m) of transmission towers.

k. The burn shall be extinguished approximately 2 hours before anticipated removal of the ash mound. The ash mound shall be removed before it reaches 2 ft (0.6 m) below the lip of the incineration pit.

l. The incineration pits shall be made of limestone or equal material, and be reinforced with earth anchors, wire mesh, or other items in order to support the weight of loaders. The edges of the pit shall be checked for integrity on a regular basis to prevent unexpected cave-ins or collapse. There shall be an impervious layer of clay or limestone on the bottom of the pit to attempt to seal the ash from the aquifer. This shall be replaced if scraped by dozers.

m. The length of the pit shall not be more than 6 in (15.2 cm) longer than the blower system at each end. The ends of the pit shall be near vertical and extend to the top of the pit.

n. A 12 in (30.5 cm) soil seal shall be placed on the lip of the incineration pit to seal the blower nozzle. The nozzle should be 3 in (7.6 cm) to 6 in (15.2 cm) from the edge of the pit.

o. The Contractor shall exercise dust control measures while handling ash.

p. Eye wash facilities shall be provided at all burn and grinding operations. **> See Section 06.**

q. For night operations, adequate lighting (5 fc (53.8 lx)) shall be provided in areas surrounding the pits and grinders.

r. Signs shall be posted at entrances to disposal areas indicating "**NOTICE: AUTHORIZED PERSONNEL ONLY**" (USACE SNO-07 or ANSI equivalent).

EM 385-1-1
15 Sep 08

s. The Contractor shall notify the local fire department and arrange for fire suppression support in case of fire beyond the Contractor's firefighting capability.

t. A "<u>Danger/Keep Back</u>" sign shall be posted at the edge of the 100 ft (30.5 m) setback from air curtain incinerators warning unauthorized personnel to keep out (USACE UNS-01 or ANSI-equivalent).

u. All personnel working in debris reduction areas shall wear safety shoes, <u>hard hat, and safety glasses, and have hearing protection available</u>.

v. <u>A minimum 30 ft (9 m) wide fire line, clear of combustible products, shall be maintained at the perimeter, and around critical infrastructures within the perimeter, of debris collection and reduction sites</u>.

12. TEMPORARY ROOFING. <u>During emergency operations that involve residential temporary roofing, RFO Commanders may permit:</u>

a. <u>The use of athletic footwear by workers performing temporary roofing operations only;</u>

b. <u>The removal of hard hats by workers on roof tops;</u>

c. <u>Use of the OSHA's Interim Fall Protection Compliance Guidelines for Residential Construction, STD 03-00-001.</u>

13. DEFENSIVE DRIVING. Personnel involved in emergency operations are at increased risk of motor vehicle accidents due to damaged roadways, debris/hazards in roadways, road closings, malfunctioning or missing traffic control devices, extended duty hours, and driving under challenging environmental conditions. Safe driving programs shall be instituted <u>and those deploying will have current Defensive Driver Training</u>. Personnel operating off-road vehicles shall be trained, prior to operation, in the use of such equipment. **> *See Section 18.C.02; 18.D.***

EM 385-1-1
15 Sep 08

14. PUBLIC SAFETY. Requirements for work area delineation, traffic control devices, and the use of flag persons shall be considered and as per ANSI A10.34. Public service announcements shall be used as needed to promote safety of the public exposed to USACE activities. Barriers and fencing shall be considered in restricting the public from operation sites. It is also necessary for all contact with the public to be handled in a courteous manner. > *See ANSI A-10.34-2001.*

15. HEALTH HAZARD RECOGNITION. Health hazards such as asbestos, lead paint, radiation, and hazardous chemicals shall be identified and controlled through the recommendations of a qualified industrial hygienist(s). Instrumentation, as required, shall be provided for the detection/measurement of health hazards.

16. ACCIDENT REPORTING.

    a. All accidents shall be reported in accordance with AR 385-10 and applicable supplements.

    b. Contractor motor vehicle accidents occurring on public highways shall be reported for trend analysis only and shall not be considered recordable.

    c. The RFO SOH Manager will report accident experience during emergency operations by maintaining an onsite accident log and by creation of a Preliminary Accident Notification (PAN) in ENGLink under the event name for all recordable accidents. This information, as well as information regarding unsatisfactory safety and health performance and/or unresolved safety and health problems, will be periodically reported to the USACE National Program Manager for SOH Emergency Planning and Response.

17. VARIANCES TO SAFETY AND HEALTH REQUIREMENTS. The on-site RFO SOH Manager may recommend variances to the requirements contained within this manual to the Geographic District Safety and Occupational Health Office.

EM 385-1-1
15 Sep 08

a. The Geographic District Safety and Health Office must review the request, concur or non-concur. Geographic District Safety and Occupational Health Offices will exercise prudent judgment in their recommendations for granting variances with due consideration of existing disaster conditions.

b. The recommended variance is then coordinated with the Contracting Officer or his Representative for concurrence and then given to the RFO Commander for approval.

c. The RFO Commander shall have the authority to approve or disapprove requests for variances.

d. All variances granted must be copied to Division and HQ SOHO for information only. The variances approved by the RFO Commander will expire at the end of the emergency operation mission.

APPENDIX C

BLANK

BLANK

EM 385-1-1
15 Sep 08

APPENDIX D

ASSURED EQUIPMENT GROUNDING CONDUCTOR PROGRAM

1. PROGRAM OVERVIEW. If an Assured Equipment Grounding Conductor Program (AEGCP) is used in place of ground-fault circuit interrupters (GFCIs) for ground-fault protection, the AEGCP shall consist of written procedures for equipment inspections, tests, test schedule and results to assure equipment grounding conductors for all cord sets, receptacles that are not a part of the permanent wiring of the building or structure, and equipment connected by cord and plug are installed and maintained to protect employees on construction sites. AEGCP must be in compliance with OSHA, NESC and NEC requirements.

    a. These procedures shall be made available when requested to GDA and affected persons. An AEGCP shall be continuously implemented and enforced at the site by one or more designated persons.

    b. One or more competent persons shall be designated to implement and enforce the AEGCP.

2. VISUAL INSPECTIONS. Visually inspect all cord sets, attachment caps, plugs and receptacles, and any equipment connected by cord and plug **before each day's use** for external damage (i.e., deformed or missing pins, damaged insulation) and for indication of possible internal damage. Ensure flexible cords are being inspected and those arriving onsite between tests are identified and tested.

3. REMOVING EQUIPMENT. Equipment found to be damaged or defective or which fails any of the prescribed inspections or tests shall not be used until repaired or replaced.

EM 385-1-1
15 Sep 08

4. TESTING. Perform two required tests on all electrical equipment: a continuity test and a terminal connection test. Tests are required:

a. Before first use;

b. Before placing back in service following any repairs;

c. Before equipment is used after any incident that can be reasonably suspected to have caused damage (e.g., when a cord set is run over); AND

d. At intervals not to exceed 3 months, except that cord sets and receptacles that are fixed and not exposed to damage shall be tested at intervals not to exceed 6 months.

5. RECORDKEEPING. All inspections and tests shall be documented to identify all equipment that passed the inspection or test, the date of inspection or test, and the individual responsible for the inspection or test.

APPENDIX E

BLANK

BLANK

APPENDIX F

BLANK

BLANK

APPENDIX G

BLANK

BLANK

EM 385-1-1
15 Sep 08

APPENDIX H

BLANK

BLANK

EM 385-1-1
15 Sep 08

APPENDIX I

CRANE TESTING REQUIREMENTS FOR PERFORMANCE TESTS

1. PERFORMANCE TESTING.

a. Performance testing includes both operational performance testing and load performance testing. The following tables and their associated guidelines are of a general nature. For any crane, the manufacturer's guidance has precedence over this general guidance and the manufacturer's guidance shall be followed.

b. The following sequence and limitation shall be complied with when conducting performance tests:

(1) Test rigging first;

(2) Conduct the operational performance test before the load performance test;

(3) Test the main hoist before testing the auxiliary or whip hoists; and

(4) Test loads shall be raised only to a height sufficient to perform the test.

2. OPERATIONAL PERFORMANCE TESTING.
Operational performance testing shall include the tests specified in Table I-1, as defined below.

a. X1 = Load hoist operation and limit switch test.

(1) Raise the load hook through all controller points stopping below the upper limit switch (where applicable);

TABLE I-1

CRANE PERFORMANCE TESTING REQUIREMENTS - NO-LOAD TESTS

Test	Portal	Floating	Tower and derricks	Hammer-head (3)	Mobile (4)	Bridge/ overhead traveling, wall and gantry	Jib, pillar, monorail and fixed hoist
X1	■(1)	■(1)	■(1)	■(1)	■(1)	■(1)	■(1)
X2	■	■	■	■	■(5)		
X3	■	■	■	■			
X4	■	■	■	■			
X5	■	■	■(2)	■			
X6	■	■	■	■			
X7	■	■	■	■			
X8				■		■	■
X9						■	
X10					■		■

Notes:
(1) Conduct for main, auxiliary, and whip hoists, as applicable.
(2) Conduct rotation tests through normal design operating arc.
(3) Conduct hoist tests in combinations such that all structural, mechanical, and electrical components are tested in all possible configurations.
(4) Complete tests shall be performed on each hook. Extend outriggers or stabilizers as specified by the manufacturer. Level the crane as specified by the manufacturer's load chart. Rotate the boom 90° from the longitudinal axis of the crane carrier and position the boom at the minimum working radius.
(5) Conduct fixed boom or telescopic boom, as appropriate.

EM 385-1-1
15 Sep 08

(2) Slowly raise load hook into the upper limit switch to establish that limit switch is operating properly;

(3) Slowly raise hook through the upper limit switch by using limit switch bypass (where applicable);

(4) Lower load hook below the upper limit switch using all the lowering control points;

(5) Slowly lower load hook into the lower limit switch to establish that limit switch is operating properly.

b. X2 = Boom hoist operation and limit switch test, fixed boom.

(1) Raise boom through all controller points, stopping below upper limit switch;

(2) Slowly raise boom into the upper limit switch;

(3) Lower boom below upper limit switch and raise boom through limit switch by using limit switch bypass (where applicable);

(4) Lower boom through all controller points, stopping above lower limit switch (where applicable);

(5) Slowly lower boom into the lower limit switch (where applicable);

(6) Raise boom above lower limit switch and lower boom through limit switch by using limit switch bypass (where applicable).

c. X2t = Boom hoist operation and limit switch test, telescopic boom. In addition to test X2, conduct the following:

(1) Extend and retract telescoping boom sections the full distance of travel;

(2) Check the radius indicator by measuring the radius at the minimum and maximum boom angle.

d. X3 = Luffing drum pawl test.

(1) Check luffing drum pawl for proper engagement in ratchet gear and with limit switch;

(2) Ensure luffing drum pawl is disengaged;

(3) Check the luffing drum pawl limit switch (if installed) for proper operation by operating the boom hoist and manually (at the pawl) activating the limit switch;

(4) Check that boom hoist motor shuts off, brake engages, and indicator lights operate correctly (where applicable). *CAUTION: Do not engage pawl in the ratchet gear.*

e. X4 = Rotation lock test (wind lock, spud lock).

(1) Engage rotation lock and inspect to ensure full engagement;

(2) Check that rotation lock limit switches (clockwise and counterclockwise) prevent engaging rotation drive (where applicable);

(3) Operate rotation lock bypass (clockwise and counterclockwise) to ensure proper operation (where applicable. *CAUTION: Use only enough power to check operation of bypass; ensure rotation lock is disengaged prior to continuing test.*
NOTE: Applicable switches may be operated manually to check for correct operation in lieu of engaging rotation lock.

f. X5 = Rotation test. Rotate clockwise and counterclockwise with boom at minimum radius.

EM 385-1-1
15 Sep 08

g. X6 = Travel test. Conduct operation travel test as prescribed in L14, except without load.

h. X7 = Deadman control test. Test all deadman controls (where installed):

(1) Start each motion;

(2) Release deadman control - motion should stop.

i. X8 = Trolley test.

(1) Trolley the allowable length of the trolley runway using all control points;

(2) Operate trolley into the limit switches at slow speed;

(3) Bring trolley back, and by using the limit switch bypass move trolley into the outboard rail stops;

(4) Repeat above procedure for inboard limit switches and rail stops.

j. X9 = Bridge test.

(1) Operate the bridge travel controller through all points in both directions;

(2) Operate the full distance of the runway and slowly contact the runway rail stops with the crane bridge bumpers.

k. X10 = Other motions test. Test other motions, including swing, by operating through one cycle (one full revolution of major components).

3. LOAD PERFORMANCE TESTING. Load performance testing shall include the tests specified in Table I-2, as defined below.

TABLE I-2

CRANE PERFORMANCE TESTING REQUIREMENTS - AT-LOAD TESTS

Test	Type of Crane						
	Portal (1)	Floating (1)	Tower and derricks (1)	Hammer-head (1)	Mobile (1,5)	Bridge/ overhead traveling, wall and gantry	Jib, pillar, monorail and fixed hoist
L1	■	■	■	■			
L2(2)	■	■	■	■(4)	■(2)	■	■
L3(2)	■	■	■	■(4)	■	■	■
L4(2)	■	■	■	■	■	■	■
L5	■	■	■	■(4)	■(2)		
L6(2)	■	■	■	■(4)	■	■b	■b
L7	■	■	■		■		
L8	■	■	■				
L9(2)	■	■	■	■(4)		■b	■b
L10	■	■	■				
L11	■	■	■(3)	■	■(6)		
L12	■	■	■	■			
L13	■		■	■			
L14	■		■	■			
L15						■b	■b
L16						■	
L17					■		

EM 385-1-1
15 Sep 08

TABLE I-2 (CONTINUED)

CRANE PERFORMANCE TESTING REQUIREMENTS - AT-LOAD TESTS

Test	Type of Crane						
	Portal (1)	Floating (1)	Tower and derricks (1)	Hammer-head (1)	Mobile (1,5)	Bridge/ overhead traveling, wall and gantry	Jib, pillar, monorail and fixed hoist
L18					■		
L19						■	
L20						■	
L21							■

Notes:
(1) All subtests under the test designation are required as applicable.
(2) For variable-rated cranes, perform the applicable variable-rated crane tests in addition to any other required tests.
(3) Conduct for main, auxiliary, jib, and whip hoists.
(4) Conduct rotation tests through normal design operating arc.
(5) Conduct hoist tests in combinations such that all structural, mechanical and electrical components are tested in all possible configurations.
(6) Complete tests shall be performed on each hook. Extend the outriggers or stabilizers as specified by the manufacturer. Level the crane as specified by the manufacturer's load chart. Rotate the boom 90° from the longitudinal axis of the crane carrier and position the boom at the minimum working radius.
(7) Rotate the maximum degrees allowed by the manufacturer. Tests shall be performed with boom fully retracted and fully extended.

EM 385-1-1
15 Sep 08

a. L1 = Stability test. During tests L2m, L3m, L5, and L11, observe roller clearance and roller lift-off from roller path.

b. L1v = Stability test, variable-rated crane. Conduct tests L2m, L3m, and L11 with test load on main hoist at maximum radius of the crane: observe roller clearance and roller lift off from roller path.

c. L2m = Load and boom hoist static test, main hoist.

(1) Raise test load to clear ground and hold for 10 minutes with boom at maximum radius;

(2) Rotate load to check bearing operation;

(3) Do not engage boom or load hoist pawl;

(4) Observe lowering that may occur which indicates malfunction of boom or hoisting components or holding brakes or outriggers;

(5) For all cranes, repeat test (except for step (2)) at minimum radius, maximum load, and boom fully extended, minimum radius, and maximum load for that radius.

d. L2a = Load hoist static test, auxiliary hoist.

(1) Raise test load to clear ground and hold for 10 minutes without hoist pawl engaged;

(2) Rotate load to check bearing operation - observe lowering that may occur which will indicate malfunction of hoisting components or holding brakes.

e. L2w = Load hoist static test, whip hoist.

(1) Raise test load to clear ground and hold for 10 minutes;

EM 385-1-1
15 Sep 08

(2) Rotate load to check operation of bearing - observe lowering that may occur which will indicate malfunction of hoisting components or holding brakes.

f. L3m = Load hoist dynamic test, main hoist.

(1) Raise and lower test load on each hoist controller point and visually observe smooth control between points;

(2) Lower the test load to unload the hoist components, wait 5 minutes, and continue testing.

g. L3a = Load hoist dynamic test, auxiliary hoist. Raise and lower test load on each controller point and visually observe smooth control between points.

h. L3v = Load hoist dynamic test, main hoist, variable-rated crane. Conduct test L3m at the maximum radius of the crane.

i. L3w = Load hoist dynamic test, whip hoist. Raise and lower test load on each controller point and visually observe smooth control between points.

j. L4 = Wire rope test. During either the static or dynamic test, where possible, test the entire working length of the wire rope.

k. L5 = Boom hoist operating test. Visually observe for smooth rotation between boom controller points:

(1) Starting from maximum radius, raise the boom to minimum radius using all boom controller points;

(2) Lower the boom through all controller points.

l. L5z = Boom hoist operating test, mobile crane. Operate the boom from the minimum radius to maximum radius for the load applied; for hydraulic cranes, test shall be performed with boom fully retracted and fully extended; perform test at both maximum test load for crane and for maximum test load at maximum radius of crane.

m. L6 = Hoist foot brake test (hydraulic or mechanical brake). Lower test load, using first control point, then apply the foot brake: this should stop the lowering motion of the test load. ***CAUTION: Not applicable to load-sensitive reactor type hoist controls.***

n. L6b = Hoist load brake.

(1) Raise test load approximately 5 ft (1.5 m);

(2) With hoist controller in the neutral position, release (by hand) the holding brake - the load brake should hold the test load;

(3) Again, with holding brake in the released position, start the test load down (first point) and return the controller to off position as the test load lowers - the load brake should prevent the test load from accelerating.
NOTE: It is not necessary for the load brake to halt the downward motion of the test load.

o. L7 = Boom foot brake test (hydraulic or mechanical brake)

(1) Start with boom near maximum radius and with test load approximately 2 ft (0.6 m) from ground surface;

(2) Lower test load using the first control point of the boom hoist;

(3) Apply the foot brake - this should stop the lowering motion of the boom and load.
CAUTION: Not applicable to load-sensitive reactor type hoist controls.

EM 385-1-1
15 Sep 08

p. L8 = Automatic boom brake (where applicable). This brake is to prevent a "free" boom in case of failure of clutch, boom hoist control, and foot brake:

(1) Raise the boom to minimum radius and with the test load approximately 4 in (10.1 cm) above the ground, set the boom foot brake firmly;

(2) Release the mechanical boom dog;

(3) Release the boom clutch by operating the boom hoist control;

(4) Slowly release the foot brake to the free position;

(5) Hold the test load with automatic brake for 5 minutes, then lower test load by applying the boom hoist clutch and lowering with the controller operation.

q. L8v = Automatic boom brake, variable-rated crane (where applicable). Conduct test L8 at the maximum radius of the crane.

r. L9 = Load hoist loss of power (panic test). This test is designed to test the reaction of a hoisting unit in the event of power failure during a lift:

(1) Hoist the test load approximately 3 m (10 ft) above the ground at maximum allowable radius;

(2) Lower test load at slow speed and with the controller in the slow lowering position, disconnect the main power source by pushing the main power stop button(s);

(3) Return the controller to the neutral position - the test load should stop lowering when the controller is placed in the neutral position.

EM 385-1-1
15 Sep 08

CAUTION: This test is not to be performed on cranes that do not have powered-down boom and load hoists.

s. L9b = Load hoist loss of power (panic test). This test is designed to test the reaction of a hoisting unit in the event of power failure during a lift:

(1) Hoist the test load to convenient distance above the surface;

(2) Lower test load at slow speed and with the controller in the slow lowering position, disconnect the main power source and return the controller to the neutral position - the test load should stop lowering when the controller is placed in the neutral position.
NOTE: Air operated hoists should be vented during this test.

t. L10 = Boom hoist loss of power (panic test). This test is designed to test the reaction of the boom hoist in the event of power failure during a lift:

(1) Hoist the test load approximately 10 ft (3 m) above the ground with the boom near maximum radius;

(2) Lower the boom at slow speed, disconnect the main power source by pushing the main power stop button(s), then return the controller to the neutral position - the boom should stop lowering when the controller is placed in the neutral position.
CAUTION: This test is not to be performed on cranes that do not have powered down boom and load hoists.

u. L11 = Rotation test. Start with the boom at maximum radius, rotate left and right 360°.
NOTE: If test area will not permit, two complete revolutions of the swing pinion <u>are</u> considered adequate.
CAUTION: Care should be exercised when rotating loads over the water and ensure during the initial load-test the floating crane has adequate draft readings per design data.

EM 385-1-1
15 Sep 08

v. L12 = Rotate brake test. Rotate left and right at slow speed and apply brakes, individually, periodically during rotation: each brake should demonstrate its ability to stop the rotating motion in a smooth, positive manner.

w. L13 = Travel motion test. This test shall be conducted with the boom at maximum allowable radius positioned 90° with the crane rails and boom dog engaged.
CAUTION: Operate crane at very slow travel speed; ensure track and supporting foundation are sound and free of any obstructions over the test travel areas (not applicable to floating cranes).

x. L14 = Travel operation test.

(1) With the test load raised to clear the ground and with the boom centered between the crane rails and the boom dog engaged, travel in one direction a minimum of 50 ft (15.2);

(2) Operate the controller through all controller points - the crane should accelerate and decelerate smoothly and all motions should be smooth and positive;

(3) Repeat in the opposite direction.

y. L15 = Trolley motion test.

(1) Raise test load to clear ground and move trolley to the maximum allowable radius - do not move trolley beyond the trolley limit switch;

(2) Hold test load for 10 minutes;

(3) Lower test load to ground until hoist lines are slack;

(4) Wait 5 minutes, raise test load and trolley the allowable length of the trolley runway.

EM 385-1-1
15 Sep 08

z. L15b = Trolley motion test. Operate trolley with test load (if space is available) the full distance of the bridge rails using extreme caution: observe proper brake operation.

aa. L16 = Bridge motion test. Operate bridge with test load (if space is available) the full distance of the runway using extreme caution and observe for any binding of bridge trucks and for proper brake operation.

bb. L17 = Hydraulic crane slippage.

(1) Lift the test load at maximum radius and allow time for fluid and component temperatures to stabilize;

(2) Hold the load for 10 minutes without use of controls by the operator - there shall be no significant lowering of the load, boom, or outrigger beams due to components or systems malfunction or failure during the test.

cc. L18 = Free-rated load test. This is a test to check stability of crane and operation of crane carrier, wheels, tires, tracks, brakes, etc., under load. ***Note: Retract outriggers prior to beginning free-rated load test.***

(1) Hoist maximum free rated test load at its maximum radius over the rear;

(2) Rotate through the "over the rear" working arc and travel a minimum of 50 ft (15.2 m) with test load over the rear of crane with boom parallel to the longitudinal axis of the crane carrier;

(3) Hoist maximum free rated test load at its maximum radius over the side;

(4) Rotate through the full working range and travel a minimum of 50 ft (15.2) with test load over the left and right side of the crane carrier with the boom 90° to the axis of travel.

EM 385-1-1
15 Sep 08

dd. L19 = Primary and secondary holding brakes. For cranes with primary and secondary holding brakes (configuration of crane where a primary brake actuates when controller is returned to the neutral position and secondary brake actuates a few seconds later) and/or eddy current hoist dynamic load brakes):

(1) During either the static or dynamic test, raise the test load and observe the proper timing sequence in the application of the primary and secondary brake when controller is returned to neutral (visually observe both hoist holding brakes to ensure correct position);

(2) Raise test load approximately 1 ft (0.3 m), hold for 10 minutes, and inactivate the secondary holding brake while testing the primary holding brake - observe for noticeable lowering of test load that may occur which will indicate malfunction of hoisting components or brakes;

(3) Re-engage secondary holding brake and release the primary holding brake and hold for 10 minutes - observe for noticeable lowering of test load that may occur which will indicate malfunction of hoisting components or brakes;

(4) Re-engage the primary holding brake - recheck proper operation of time delay and ensure smooth positive stopping.

ee. L20 = Hoist dynamic load brake (eddy current). Check lowering speed against specifications to ensure correct brake operation. ***NOTE: Eddy current brakes will not stop motion.***

ff. L21 = Swing test (where applicable). Swing the test load (where space is available) through the working range at maximum radius, stopping the load at several points: there should be no excessive drift of jib or trolley at any of these points (the significance of drift shall be evaluated).

4. REQUIREMENTS FOR BOOM STOP TESTS. Boom stop tests shall follow these steps.

I-15

Step 1: Check for availability of appropriate operator manual.

Step 2: Make sure crane is level with outriggers (if so equipped) in place.

Step 3: Check boom and boom stops for misalignment, bent parts, and other physical damage.

Step 4: Check boom stop pins (at connections) for lubrication, wear, and damage.

Step 5: Check boom angle indicator with inclinometer for correctness.

Step 6: Check boom hoist disengaging device for proper adjustment and proper angle in accordance with the operator's manual.

Step 7: Check for proper operational setup of the boom stops and boom hoist disengaging device. Physically boom up the boom just to the points listed below as long as the boom does not go beyond the point of operation of the boom hoist disengaging device. It is not the intent of this test to override the boom hoist disengaging device.

a. For cantilever or scissors types, this is the point just before the boom and boom stops touch.

b. For telescoping types, this is the point just prior to compression.

EM 385-1-1
15 Sep 08

APPENDIX J

BLANK

BLANK

APPENDIX K

BLANK

BLANK

APPENDIX L

BLANK

EM 385-1-1
15 Sep 08

APPENDIX M

PROCESS FOR REQUESTING INTERPRETATIONS

The following process will be used for requesting an official interpretation of a requirement contained in this manual. Other DOD Components must submit their requests for interpretations through their chain of command.

1. Official requests for interpretation and all responses shall be in writing.

2. The requester must specifically identify the requirement for which he/she seeks an interpretation. The requester must provide the exact citation and quote the requirement in question. A separate request must be made for each requirement.

3. The requester must state his/her source of confusion regarding the requirement.

4. The requester must provide all the information necessary to understand the context in which the requirement is being applied.

5. The requester must provide his/her interpretation of the requirement and his/her rationale.

6. Every effort shall be made to clarify the requirement at the lowest possible level.

   a. The requester shall work the request for interpretation with the local USACE Command Safety and Occupational Health Office. A Contractor must request interpretation of a requirement from the field office under which they work who will then coordinate with the local Command SOHO to provide a response. The local SOHO must then render a written interpretation of the requirement within 5 working days of receipt.

EM 385-1-1
15 Sep 08

    b. If either the field office or the requester is not satisfied with this response, either may appeal their position in writing to the Division SOHO. The entire package containing the requester's, and the local SOHO's interpretation, rationale, and supporting information shall be sent to the Division SOHO who shall render a written response to the local SOHO within 5 working days of receipt.

    c. If the requester, the field office, or local SOHO is not satisfied with the Division SOHOs response, they may appeal it to the USACE-SO for final resolution. All of the information sent to the Division, the interpretation, rationale, and supporting information shall be provided. Within 5 working days of receipt, USACE-SO will provide a written interpretation to the Division SOHO for dissemination and it shall be final.

7. Interpretations apply ONLY to the specific time and the context in which the requirement is being applied. They may not be used as precedents to determine future applications of the requirement. USACE-SO will make the proper notifications if an interpretation may be applied globally.

8. Unofficial requests for interpretations/clarifications of requirements from local SOHOs may be made via email or telephone. However, the answers provided via this mode will be considered general guidance, not official interpretations.

9. USACE-SO will NOT accept requests for official interpretations from parties outside the USACE structure.

EM 385-1-1
15 Sep 08

APPENDIX N

USACE PROCESS FOR REQUESTING WAIVERS/VARIANCES

The following process shall be used <u>when requesting a waiver or a variance from a requirement</u> contained in this manual. Other DOD Components must submit their requests through their chain of command.

1. Requester shall work the action with the local USACE Command Safety and Occupational Health Office. Waiver/variance request package shall include:

   a. Specification of exact requirement from which relief is being sought, providing the exact citation and quoting the requirement in question. A separate request must be made for each requirement;

   b. Statement as to whether a waiver (total elimination of the requirement) or a variance (retaining the basic requirement, but doing it differently) is being sought;

   c. Details as to why it is not possible or practical to comply with the requirement;

   d. All the information (maps, drawings, references, calculations, change analysis or impact, etc.) necessary to make an informed decision. The burden of proof rests with the requester. Failure to provide the necessary information may be justification for denial of the request. It is not up to the evaluator to defend the requirement being questioned. It is up to the requester to make the case as to why the requirement should be waived or varied;

   e. Identification of specific time period and operation for which the request is being made. A waiver/variance will be granted for specific time periods and operations and may not be used as a

EM 385-1-1
15 Sep 08

defense for failure to comply with a requirement at another time or on another project;

f. Explanation of method they plan to use in lieu of the requirement and how it provides protection equal to or greater than the requirement being challenged. Again, the burden of proof rests with the requester;

g. A detailed AHA addressing the alternate procedure. Risk assessment should be a part of the AHA process;

h. Provision of any other requirements or standards addressing the requirement in question. It is incumbent upon the requester to research the literature to determine if any other requirement or standard exists addressing the requirement from which relief is being sought. If there is another standard(s), the requester must identify it and provide a copy. Requests for waivers/variances will not be processed until this requirement has been met; and

i. A cover letter.

2. Local SOHO shall cover package with their official signed memorandum requesting consideration and including their concurrence or non-concurrence with the request. Package is then sent via mail in hard copy or via e-mail with attached PDF file to HQ USACE-SO with a copy furnished to Division SOH Manager.

3. HQ USACE-SO will then coordinate with Division SOH Manager to evaluate the request. USACE-SO shall have at least 10 working days from date of receipt to consider the request and to render a written decision.

4. A waiver or variance will not be carried over to other operations unless the evaluator extends the scope to include other times and operations. If warranted, HQ USACE-SO may issue a global variance based on an individual request.

EM 385-1-1
15 Sep 08

Appendix O

MANNING LEVELS FOR DIVE TEAMS

NOTE: Manning level tables shown are a minimum. Actual manning levels may increase, as determined by the DDC, after considering the diving support systems, the task at hand, weather conditions, dive platform and location, and other factors. Team members may rotate through the dive team positions as long as the minimum manning levels are maintained and team members are qualified and accepted for the position.

1. SCUBA – Untethered, 0 to 100 ft (0 to 30.5 m)

Untethered SCUBA divers shall always be accompanied by another diver in continuous visual contact.

When depth of dive is 0-100 ft (0-30.5 m), the minimum dive team will be composed as shown in Table O-1:

TABLE O-1 DIVE TEAM COMPOSITION SCUBA - Untethered, 0 to 100 ft (0 to 30.5 m)	
Personnel	Number
Diving Supervisor	1
Divers (in visual contact)	2
Standby Diver*	1
TOTAL TEAM	4

2. SCUBA – Tethered with communications, 0 to 100 ft (0 to 30.5 m)

When depth of the dive is 0-100 ft (0-30.5 m), the minimum dive team will be composed as shown in Table O-2:

EM 385-1-1
15 Sep 08

TABLE O-2 DIVE TEAM COMPOSITION SCUBA – Tethered with communications, 0 to 100 ft (0 to 30.5 m)	
Personnel	**Number**
Diving Supervisor ***	1
Diver in water	1
Standby Diver* (tethered with communications)	1
Tender	1
TOTAL TEAM	4

3. SURFACE SUPPLIED AIR - 0 to 100 ft (0 to 30.5 m)

When surface supplied air is being used as the diving mode, the minimum dive team will be composed as shown in Table O-3:

TABLE O-3 DIVE TEAM COMPOSITION Surface Supplied Air, 0 to 100 ft (0 to 30.5 m) Within No Decompression Limits		
Personnel	**Number**	**Penetration Dive**
Diving Supervisor ***	1	1
Diver	1	2
Standby Diver*	1	1
Tender	1	2
TOTAL TEAM	4	6

Deploying the Standby Diver as a Worker Diver. The Standby diver may be deployed as a working diver provided all of the following conditions are met:

1. Surface-supplied no-decompression dive of 60 fsw or less;

EM 385-1-1
15 Sep 08

2. Same job/location, e.g., working on port and starboard propellers of the same vessel;

3. Prior to deploying the standby diver, the work area shall be determined to be free of hazards (i.e., suctions, discharges) by the first diver on the job site;

4. The dive is NOT a penetration or confined space dive;

5. Each diver has a full-time tender (which brings the minimum number of team members to 5).

4. SURFACE SUPPLIED AIR - 101 to 190 ft (30.8 to 57.9 m)

When surface supplied air is being used as the diving mode, the minimum dive team will be composed as shown in Table O-4:

TABLE O-4
DIVE TEAM COMPOSITION
Surface Supplied Air, 0 to 100 ft Requiring Decompression and All Surface Supplied Air, 101 to 190 ft (30.8 to 57.9 m)

Personnel	Dives within no decompression limits	Dives requiring decompression	Penetration Dive
Diving Supervisor	1	1	1
Chamber Operator**	**/1	****/1	1
Diver	1	1	2
Standby Diver*	1	1	1
Tender	1	1	2
Standby Diver Tender	1	1	1
TOTAL TEAM	5/6	5/6	8

5. SURFACE SUPPLIED MIXED GAS DIVING

For surface supplied mixed gas diving, to include OEA (Nitrox, etc.), the minimum dive team will be composed as shown in Table O-5:

EM 385-1-1
15 Sep 08

TABLE O-5
DIVE TEAM COMPOSITION
Surface Supplied Mixed Gas Diving

Personnel	Dives within no decompression limits	Dives requiring decompression	Penetration Dives
Diving Supervisor	1	1	1
Chamber Operator**	**/1	****/1	1
Diver	1	1	2
Standby Diver*	1	1	1
Tender	1	1	2
Standby Diver Tender	1	1	1
TOTAL TEAM	5/6	5/6	8

Notes:

* The standby diver will be rested and capable of performing emergency rescue assistance. When work is limited to no decompression limits, the standby diver shall be sufficiently free of residual nitrogen to allow for 25 minutes of bottom time at the working depth without exceeding "No Decompression Limits."

** The competent chamber operator may be any non-diving member of the dive team when the chamber is only for emergency use when diving within the no-decompression limits. Saturation diving requires that a life support technician will serve as the chamber operator.

*** The supervisor may be the standby tender for dives under 100 ft (30.5 m).

**** The competent chamber operator may be any non-diving member of the dive team if all diving ceases during chamber decompression.

EM 385-1-1
15 Sep 08

APPENDIX P

SAFE PRACTICES FOR ROPE ACCESS WORK

1. REFERENCES.

a. Society of Professional Rope Access Technicians – Safe Practices for Rope Access Work.

b. Determination of Rope Access and Work Positioning Techniques in Arboriculture.

2. DEFINITIONS.

a. **Competent Person (CP) for Rope Access:** A person with the training, skills, experience and qualifications necessary to assume responsibility for the entire rope access work site, including management and guidance of other Rope Access Technicians on the worksite, who is capable of designing, analyzing, evaluating and specifying rope access systems, and who has the knowledge and experience to direct rescue operations from rope access systems, as well as the skills necessary to perform advanced rescue from rope access systems.

b. **Rope Access Worker:** A person with the appropriate training, skills, and qualifications for performing, under the direct supervision of the CP for Rope Access Lead Technician or Supervisor, standard rope access operations and, at a minimum, has the skills necessary to perform limited rescue from rope access systems.

3. CLIMBING EQUIPMENT.

a. Ropes: Used as working line and safety lines, shall be made of synthetic fiber with a nominal breaking strength of at least 5400 lbs when new. Additionally, elasticity (elongation) shall be limited to 7% with a load of 540 lbs applied.

EM 385-1-1
15 Sep 08

b. Carabineers and snap hooks: Carabineers and snap hooks used for climbing (life support) shall have at least two consecutive, deliberate actions to prepare the gate for opening and shall be rated at 5,000 lbs (22.2kN) and shall meet ANSI Z359.1 standard. Gates shall be rated at 3600 lbs (16kN). Rope snaps and snap hooks shall be self closing and self locking. The use of rope thimbles when attaching rope snaps is recommended to prevent rope fraying.

c. Pulleys/Rope Sleeves: Anti-friction devices are also recommended to prevent rope damage.

d. Rope Blocks/Brakes: Can be used to make the work safer and requires less hands to control heavy loads. When handling limb removal ropes, ground personnel should not wrap the rope around their hands or waist and keep the rope away from their feet to prevent entanglement.

e. Climbers PPE: Appropriate footwear (i.e., climbing boots with safety toes), long pants, work shirt with a minimum 4 in (10.2 cm) sleeve length, eye protection, face shield, hearing protection during chain saw usage, hard hat with chin strap or approved climbers helmet, and fingerless gloves such as mechanics gloves. When the air temperature exceeds 85 °F (29 °C), climbers shall carry a water supply with them.

f. All equipment shall be inspected prior to use and maintained and used in accordance with manufacturer instructions.

g. Employees shall be properly trained in the use of all equipment.

h. Climbing ropes shall not be used to lower limbs or raise equipment.

i. Sharp tools such as hand saws shall be sheathed when not in use.

EM 385-1-1
15 Sep 08

j. Tools used for de-barking, cavity work, cabling, bark tracing, shall be carried in a bag or belt designed for such use, and not carried in pockets or placed in boots.

k. Climbers Saddle: Climbers belts/saddles are only meant to be used as suspension scaffold/equipment. In addition to saddle a fall arrest system is required. Belts shall be equipped with leg straps or seats to take pressure off climbers back.

l. Climbing ropes shall not be spliced to effect repair.

m Ropes shall be coiled and piled, or shall be suspended, so that air can circulate through the coils to aid in drying.

n. Wet ropes shall not be used for electrical work.

o. Ropes shall be inspected before and after each use.

p. If descender devices are used, they shall allow controlled descent, considering weight of worker, length of descent, considerations for safety and need for stopping along working line for purpose of hands-free work.

4. GENERAL PRACTICES.

a. Safety, Secondary, Belay or Backup Line(s).

(1) Safety, Secondary, Belay or Backup line(s) or other appropriate fall arrest devices shall be used in addition to the main line unless the employer can demonstrate that the second line or other fall arrest devices would create a greater hazard or otherwise would not be feasible (See tree climbing exceptions in P.4.a.(2) below).

(2) Safety, Secondary, Belay or Backup line(s) shall not be used alone for tree climbing. The use of a secondary line may pose additional risks and increased difficulties. Careful consideration to the impact of secondary line use should be

EM 385-1-1
15 Sep 08

considered before making a decision on use in tree climbing operations.

(3) Where a safety line is used in conjunction with the main line, each line shall have its own separate anchor and shall be separately fixed to the worker's harness. This does not preclude both lines being attached to a single harness attachment point.

(4) The safety line shall be connected to the dorsal D-ring of the full body harness.

(5) When using safety line, the maximum free-fall distance shall not exceed 6 ft (1.8 m) and the maximum arrest force shall not exceed 1,800 lbs (8 kN).

b. Employer shall insure that anchors have been evaluated in order to ensure that overall system safety factors can be met.

c. Before adopting rope access techniques for a particular job, the contractor shall perform a risk assessment and develop a written AHA, and submit to GDA for acceptance. It would include consideration of the various rope access alternatives available and their respective access advantages and hazards. In particular, attention shall be given to the following aspects:

(1) Ability of the suspended person to safely use materials, equipment or tools necessary for the work and whether the reaction from any tool may place the person at risk;

(2) Whether the work may loosen material which could become a hazard to the worker or others;

(3) Whether the time required for the work at any one location will be such that there may be unacceptable levels of risk;

(4) Whether it would be possible to quickly rescue workers that are using rope access techniques from any position they could be expected to enter.

EM 385-1-1
15 Sep 08

d. The contractor shall make provision for prompt rescue or self rescue and for emergency services.

e. The Rope Access Worker shall:

(1) Have a working understanding of the employer's rope access program and all applicable policy and procedures.

(2) Adjust, inspect, maintain, care for, and properly store rope access equipment.

(3) Inspect and verify the integrity of anchor systems and components.

(4) Recognize worksite hazards and notify the Rope Access Supervisor of any such hazards.

(5) Be capable of identifying work zones and job hazard analyses.

(6) Understand and communicate any written or verbal warnings.

(7) Be familiar with rescue procedures and systems used by the employer, and assist in the performance of rescue from rope access systems.

(8) Utilize appropriate personal protective equipment as designated by the Rope Access Supervisor.

(9) Follow the CP for Rope Access or, where appropriate pursuant to the requirements of the Safe Practices Document, the Rope Access Lead Technician's directions regarding the work to be performed.

(10) Notify the CP for Rope Access if assigned a task or responsibility beyond the Rope Access Worker's training, skills, qualifications, or experience.

BLANK

EM 385-1-1
15 Sep 08

APPENDIX Q

DEFINITIONS

This appendix defines the following terms for the purposes of this manual.

3 Rs: Refers to encountering or suspecting to have encountered, MEC. **RECOGNIZE, RETREAT, REPORT.**

Abrasive blasting: the forcible application of an abrasive to a surface by pneumatic pressure, hydraulic pressure, or centrifugal force.

Abrasive wheel: a cutting tool made of abrasive grains held together by organic (such as resin, rubber, or shellac) or inorganic (such as clay, glass, porcelain, sodium silicate, magnesium oxychloride, or metal) bonds.

Absorbed dose: energy imparted to matter by ionizing radiation per unit mass of irradiated material at the place of interest in that material. The units of absorbed dose are the rad or the Gray (1 Gray equals 1 Joule/Kilogram equals 100 rad).

Accepted/Acceptable: a term denoting when a written procedure, practice, method, program, engineering design, or employee qualification criteria submittal, which, after a cursory review by a GDA, is determined to generally conform to safety and health or contractual requirements. Acceptance or acceptability of such submittals in no way relieves the submitting entity from ensuring employees a safe and healthful work environment or complying with all contractual requirements and good engineering practices.

Accident: an unplanned event that results in injury, illness, death, property damage, mission interruption, or other loss that has a negative effect on the mission.

EM 385-1-1
15 Sep 08

Accident prevention plan (APP): a document that outlines occupational safety and health policy, responsibilities, and program requirements.

Accident, recordable: any accident meeting the definition of an Army accident that involves a Government employee, Contractor, or member of the public that rises to the severity level that they are used to calculate accident experience rates.

Accident, reportable: all USACE and Contractor accidents including occupational illnesses, injuries, and property damage.

Accredited testing laboratory: a laboratory that an accrediting organization has determined has demonstrated the ability to conduct air quality testing according to their standard.

Activity hazard analysis (AHA): a documented process by which the steps (procedures) required to accomplish a work activity are outlined, the actual or potential hazards of each step are identified, and measures for the elimination or control of those hazards are developed.

Adjacent spaces: spaces which border an area on a vessel or vessel section such as, cargo tanks or holds, pump or engine rooms, storage lockers, tanks containing flammable or combustible liquids, gases, or solids, and crawl spaces, in all directions, including all points of contact, corners, diagonals, decks, tank tops, and bulkheads.

Aerial lift/device: any vehicle mounted device, telescoping or articulating, or both, which is used to position/elevate personnel to job sites/activities above the ground. May be made of metal, wood, fiberglass reinforced plastic (FRP) or other; may be powered or manually operated; They include:

- Aerial ladder: an aerial device consisting of a single- or multiple-section extensible ladder;

EM 385-1-1
15 Sep 08

- Articulating boom platform: an aerial device with two or more hinged boom sections;

- Extensible boom platform: an aerial device (except ladders) with a telescopic or extensible boom, including telescopic derricks with personnel platform attachments when used with a personnel platform;

- Insulated aerial device: an aerial device designed for work on energized lines and apparatus.

Related definitions:
- Mobile unit: a combination of an aerial device, its vehicle and related equipment;

- Platform: any personnel-carrying device, basket or bucket, which is a component of an aerial device.

Affected employee: a person whose position requires him/her to operate or use a system that is under lockout or tagout or whose position requires him/her to work in an area where a system that is under lockout or tagout is being serviced or maintained.

Air-purifying respirator: a respirator with an air-purifying filter, cartridge, or canister that removes specific air contaminants by passing ambient air through the air-purifying element.

Air receiver: a tank used for the storage of air discharged from the compressor; used to help eliminate pressure pulsations in the discharge line.

All-Terrain Vehicles (ATVs): ATVs are motorized vehicles intended for off-road use that travel on four low-pressure tires with a seat designed to be straddled by the operator and handlebar for steering control.

Altered: any change to the original manufacturer's design configuration. These are:

EM 385-1-1
15 Sep 08

    a. Replacement of weight-handling equipment parts and components with parts or components not identical with the original (i.e., change in material, dimensions, or design configuration);

    b. The addition of parts or components not previously a part of the equipment;

    c. The removal of components that were previously a part of the load handling equipment; and

    d. Rearrangement of original parts or components.

Ammunition: Generic term related mainly to articles of military application consisting of bombs, grenades, rockets, mines, projectiles and other similar devices or contrivances.

Anchor handling barge: a floating work platform consisting of a pontoon or barge, hoisting equipment, and a fixed A-frame that cannot slew or change radius. An anchor barge is used to extract anchors or buoy weights imbedded in the earth. The load is often unknown and is often not under the tip of the A-frame.

Anchorage (fall protection): a secured point of attachment that can safely withstand the forces exerted by activation of fall protection and rescue equipment. The anchorage is the rigid part of the structure that can be in the form of a beam, girder, column or floor.

Anchorage connector: a component or subsystem by which fall protection or rescue equipment is secured to the anchorage.

Anchorage system: a combination of anchorage and anchorage connector.

Anchored bridging: the steel joist bridging is connected to a bridging terminus point.

EM 385-1-1
15 Sep 08

Anomaly Avoidance. Techniques employed on property known (or suspected) to contain UXO and/or other munitions that may have experienced abnormal environments to avoid contact with potential surface or subsurface explosives or CA hazards to allow entry into the area for the performance of the required operations. Possible examples: Discarded Military Munitions (DMM)), Munitions Constituents (MC) in high enough concentrations to pose an explosive hazard, or chemical agent (CA), regardless of configuration.

Anti-runaway: a safety device to stop a declining conveyor in case of mechanical or electrical failure.

Anti-two blocking (A2B) device: a device that is activated by two-blocking and disengages the particular function whose movement is caused by the two-blocking.

Approach-departure clearance surface: an extension of the primary surface and the clear zone at each end of the runway, first along an inclined plane (glide angle) and then along a horizontal plane, both flaring symmetrically about the runway centerline extended.

Approach-departure clearance zone: the ground area under the approach-departure clearance surface.

Apron conveyor: a conveyor in which a series of apron pans forms a moving bed.

Apron pans: one of a series of overlapping or interlocking plates or shapes that, together with others, form the conveyor bed.

Approved: a method, equipment, procedure, practice, tool, etc., that is sanctioned, confirmed, as acceptable for a particular use or purpose by a person or organization authorized to render such approval or judgment.

EM 385-1-1
15 Sep 08

Arc: a controlled electrical discharge between the electrode and the work piece that is formed and sustained by a gas that has been heated to such a temperature that it can conduct electric current.

Arc cutting: a thermal cutting process that severs or removes metal by melting with the heat of an arc between an electrode and the work piece.

Arc flash: An arc flash is a voltage breakdown of the resistance of air resulting in an arc which can occur where there is sufficient voltage in an electrical system and a path to ground or lower voltage.

Arc welding: a welding process that joins work pieces by heating them with an arc.

Articulating boom crane: a crane with a boom that has sections that are articulated by hydraulic cylinders. The boom may have a telescoping section. The crane can be stationary or mounted on a vehicle, track, locomotive, etc., and is used to lift, swing, and lower loads.

Assigned protection factor (APF): the minimum anticipated protection provided by a properly functioning respirator or class of respirators to a given percentage of properly fitted and trained users.

Associate Safety Professional (ASP): an individual who has achieved an interim designation denoting progress towards the Certified Safety Professional Certification offered by BCSP.

Atmosphere-supplying respirator: a respirator that supplies the respirator user with breathing air from a source independent of the ambient atmosphere, and includes SARs and SCBA units.

Attendant (confined space): an individual stationed outside one or more permit spaces who monitors the authorized entrants and who performs all attendant's duties assigned in the employer's permit space program.

Authorized employee (Hazardous Energy Control): a qualified person who is designated, in writing by the designated authority, to request, receive, implement, and remove energy control procedures.

Authorized entrant (confined space): an employee who is authorized by the employer to enter a permit space.

Automatic circuit re-closer: a self-controlled device for automatically interrupting and re-closing an alternate current circuit with a predetermined sequence of opening and re-closing followed by resetting, hold closed, or lockout operation.

Automatic fire detection device: a device designed to automatically detect the presence of fire by heat, flame, light, smoke, or other products of combustion.

Automatic trap: a device for removing moisture from compressed gas systems.

Available clearance: The distance from the walking working surface to the nearest obstruction that end user might contact during a fall.

Back cut: the final cut in a felling operation, made horizontally on the opposite side from the undercut. > *See definition of notch.*

Backstop: a device to prevent reversal of a loaded conveyor under action of gravity when forward travel is interrupted.

Barricade: a physical obstruction, such as tape, screens, or cones, intended to warn of and limit access to a hazardous area.

Barrier: a physical obstruction that is intended to prevent contact with energized lines or equipment.

Beam platform: a work platform made up of wood beams (oriented vertically).

Bearer: a horizontal member of a scaffold upon which the platform rests and that may be supported by runners.

Bell: an enclosed compartment, pressurized (closed bell) or unpressurized (open bell), which allows the diver to be transported to and from the underwater work area and which may be used as a temporary refuge during diving operations.

Benching: a method of protecting employees from cave-ins by cutting the sides of the excavation in the arrangement of one or more horizontal levels, usually with vertical or near-vertical walls between steps.

Bending moment: the overturning effect at a point which is the product of a force and the distance from the point from which the force is applied.

Blast area: the area in which explosive loading and blasting activities are being conducted and the area immediately adjacent that is within the influence of fly-rock and concussion.

Blast site: the area in which explosive materials are being loaded, or have been loaded, including all holes to be loaded for the same blast for a distance of 50 ft (15.2 m) on all sides.

Blaster: the person(s) authorized to use explosives for blasting purposes.

Blasting agent: any material or mixture, consisting of a fuel and oxidizer, intended for blasting, not otherwise classified as an explosive, and in which none of the ingredients is classified as an explosive, provided that the finished product, as mixed and packaged for use or shipment, cannot be detonated by means of a No. 8 blasting cap when unconfined.

Blasting machine: a device used to supply initiation current to blasting circuits.

EM 385-1-1
15 Sep 08

Boatswain's chair: a suspended seat designed to accommodate one worker.

Boatswain's stand: a suspended stand designed to accommodate one worker in a standing position.

Body belt: a body support comprised of a strap with means for securing about the waist and attaching it to a lanyard, lifeline, or deceleration device.

Body harness, full: straps connected together and secured about a body in a manner that distributes the arresting forces over at least the thighs, waist, chest, shoulders, and pelvis, with provision for attaching a lanyard, lifeline, or deceleration device.

Bolted diagonal bridging: diagonal bridging that is bolted to a steel joist or joists.

Bond: an electrical connection from one conductive element to another to minimize potential differences or providing suitable conductivity for fault current or for mitigation of leakage current and electrolytic action.

Bonding: the permanent joining of metallic parts to form an electrically conductive path that will ensure electrical continuity and capacity to conduct safely any current likely to be imposed.

Bonding jumper: a reliable conductor to ensure the required electrical conductivity between metal parts required to be electrically connected.

Boom: a member hinged to the superstructure or a crane/derrick and used for supporting hoisting tackle.

Boom-angle: the angle above or below the horizontal of the longitudinal axis of the base of the boom section.

Boom-angle indicator: a device that measures the angle of the boom to the horizontal.

Boom hoist mechanism: means for supporting the boom and controlling boom angle.

Boom, live: a boom in which lowering (free-fall) is controlled by a brake without aid from other lowering retarding devices.

Boom stop (crane): a device used to limit the angle of the boom at the highest position.

Bottom time: the total elapsed time, measured in minutes, from the time when the diver leaves the surface in descent to the time that the diver begins ascent.

Braided sling: a sling made from braided rope.

Branch circuit: the circuit conductors between the final over current device protecting the circuit and the outlet(s).

Brazing: a welding process that joins materials by heating them to a temperature that will not melt them but will melt a filler material which adheres to them and forms a joint.

Bricklayers' square scaffold: a scaffold made up of a work platform (planking) supported on bricklayers' squares.

Bridge: that part of a gantry or overhead crane that carries the trolley(s).

Bridging clip: a device that is attached to the steel joist to allow the bolting of the bridging to the steel joist.

Bridging terminus point: a wall, a beam, tandem joists (with all bridging installed and a horizontal truss in the plane of the top chord) or other element at an end or intermediate point(s) of a line of bridging that provides an anchor point for the steel joist bridging.

Bridle sling: multiple-leg-sling; the legs of the sling are spread to distribute the load.

Bucket conveyor: any type of conveyor in which the material is carried in a series of buckets.

Bucking: the act of sawing a felled tree or limbs into smaller sections.

Bus wire: an expendable wire used in parallel or series-in-parallel circuits to which are connected the leg wires of electric blasting caps.

Bushing: an insulating device or lining used to protect a conductor where it passes through an aperture.

Cable: a conductor with insulation, or a stranded conductor with or without insulation and other coverings (single-conductor cable), or a combination of conductors insulated from one another (multiple-conductor cable).

Cable laid endless sling: a wire rope sling made from one continuous length of cable laid rope with the ends joined by one or more metallic fittings.

Cable laid grommet, hand tucked: an endless wire rope sling made from one continuous length of rope formed to make a body composed of six ropes around a rope core. The rope ends are tucked into the body, forming the core. No sleeves are used.

Cable laid rope: a rope composed of several wire ropes laid as strands around a wire rope core.

Cable laid rope sling, mechanical joint: a wire rope sling made from a cable laid wire rope with eyes fabricated by pressing or swaging metal sleeves over the rope junction.

Caisson: a watertight chamber (of wood or steel sheeting or a concrete or steel cylinder) used in construction work underwater or as a foundation. When the bottom of the structure extends below the surface of free water, excavation is performed by workers in a

EM 385-1-1
15 Sep 08

working chamber at an air pressure greater than atmospheric pressure.

Canister or cartridge: a container with a filter, sorbent, or catalyst, or combination of these items, which removes specific contaminants from the air passed through the container.

Capable of being locked: an energy isolating device is considered "capable of being locked out" if it meets the following:

1. Is designed with a hasp or other part to which a lock can be attached (i.e., a lockable electric disconnect switch);

2. Has a locking mechanism built into it; or

3. Can be locked without dismantling, rebuilding, or replacing the energy isolating device or permanently altering its energy control capability (i.e.,using a lock/chain assembly on a pipeline valve, a lockable valve cover, circuit breaker lockout or fuse block-out devices).

Equipment that accepts bolted blank flanges and bolted slip blinds are considered to be capable of being locked out.

Carabiner: a connector component generally consisting of an oval or trapezoidal shaped body with a closed gate or similar arrangement

Carpenter's bracket scaffold: a scaffold made up of a work platform supported on wood or metal brackets.

Catch platform: a temporary structure erected around, attached to and abutting the building being demolished for the purpose of safeguarding and protecting the employees and the public by catching and retaining falling objects or debris.

Cathead: a spool shaped attachment on a winch around which rope is wound for hoisting and pulling.

EM 385-1-1
15 Sep 08

Certified Construction Heath and Safety Technician (CHST): an individual who is currently certified by the Council on Certification of Health, Environmental and Safety Technologists (CCHST).

Certified Health Physicist (CHP): an individual who is currently certified by the American Board of Health Physics.

Certified Industrial Hygienist (CIH): an individual who is currently certified by the American Board of Industrial Hygiene.

Certified Safety Professional (CSP): an individual who is currently certified by the BCSP.

Certified Safety Trained Supervisor (CSTS): an individual who is currently certified by the Council on Certification of Health, Environmental and Safety Technologists (CCHST).

Chain conveyor: any type of conveyor in which one or more chains act as the conveying medium.

Chemical Agent (CA). A chemical compound (to include experimental compounds) that, through its chemical properties, produces lethal or other damaging effects on human beings, and is intended for use in military operations to kill, seriously injure, or incapacitate persons through its physiological effects. Excluded are research, development, test and evaluation solutions; riot control agents; chemical defoliants and herbicides; smoke and other obscuration materials; flame and incendiary materials; and industrial chemicals.

Chemical Warfare Materiel (CWM). Items generally configured as munitions containing a chemical compound that is intended to kill, seriously injure, or incapacitate a person through its physiological effects; includes V- and G-series nerve agents or H-series (mustard) and L-series (lewisite) blister agents in other-than-munitions configurations; and certain industrial chemicals (e.g., hydrogen cyanide (AC), cyanogen chloride (CK), or carbonyl dichloride (called phosgene or CG)) configured as military

EM 385-1-1
15 Sep 08

munitions. CWM does not include: riot control devices; chemical herbicides; industrial chemicals (e.g., AC, CK, or CG) not configured as munitions; smoke and flame producing items; or soil, water, debris or other media contaminated with low concentrations of chemical warfare agents where no CA hazards exist.

Chicken Ladder: See "Crawling Board"

Choker: a sling used to form a slip noose around an object.

Christmas tree lifting – See Multiple Lift Rigging

Class A fire: a fire involving ordinary combustible materials such as wood, paper, clothing, and some rubber and plastic materials.

Class B fire: a fire involving flammable or combustible liquids, flammable gases, greases and similar materials, and some rubber and plastic materials.

Class C fire: a fire involving energized electrical equipment where safety to the employee requires the use of electrically nonconductive extinguishing media.

Class D fire: a fire involving combustible metals such as magnesium, zirconium, sodium, and potassium.

Cleanout: a hole that is put in the concrete masonry unit block to verify that grout goes all the way to the bottom of the cell of blocks in a wall (filling the void cells). The cleanout being in this position keeps employees from under the scaffolding where they are pumping the grout in overhead.

Cleat: a mooring fitting having two horizontal arms to which mooring lines are secured.

Coarse laid rope: 6 x 7 wire rope (6 strands, 7 wires per strand).

Cofferdam: a temporary structure used to keep water (and earth) out of an excavation during construction of the permanent structure.

EM 385-1-1
15 Sep 08

Column: a load-carrying vertical member that is part of the primary skeletal framing system. Columns do not include posts.

Combustible liquid: a liquid having a flash point at or above 100 °F (38 °C). Combustible liquids are subdivided as follows:

a. Class II liquids have flash points at or above 100 °F (38 °C) and below 140 °F (60 °C).

b. Class IIIA liquids have flash points at or above 140 °F (60 °C) and below 200 °F (93 °C).

c. Class IIIB liquids have flash points at or above 200 °F (93 °C).

Command: the USACE Major Subordinate Command, District, Laboratory, or Field Operating Activity with responsibility for a particular activity.

Committed dose equivalent: The dose equivalent to organs or tissues of reference that will be received from an intake of radioactive material by a person during the 50-year period following the intake.

Committed effective dose equivalent: the sum of the products of the weighting factors applicable to each of the body organs or tissues irradiated and the committed dose equivalent to these organs or tissues.

Competent Person: one who can identify existing and predictable hazards in the working environment or working conditions that are dangerous to personnel and who has authorization to take prompt corrective measures to eliminate them.

Competent Person for confined space: A person with thorough knowledge of OSHA's Confined Space Standard, 29 CFR 1910.146, designated in writing by the employer to be responsible for the immediate supervision, implementation and monitoring of the confined space program, who through training, knowledge and experience in confined space entry is capable of identifying, evaluating and addressing existing and potential confined space hazards and, who has the authority to take prompt corrective measures with regard to such hazards.

Competent Person for Confined Space in ships and vessels (CPCSSV): a person who has the knowledge of the designation of spaces where the work is done; ability to understand and follow through on the air sampling, personal protective equipment and instructions of a Marine Chemist, Coast Guard authorized person, or Certified Industrial Hygienist.

Competent Person for Excavation/Trenching: A person meeting the competent person requirements as defined in the definitions of EM 385-1-1 and 29 CFR Part 1926 who has been designated in writing by the employer to be responsible for the immediate supervision, implementation and monitoring of the excavation/trenching program, who through training, knowledge and experience in excavation/trenching is capable of identifying, evaluating and addressing existing and potential hazards and, who has the authority to take prompt corrective measures with regard to such hazards

Competent Person for Fall Protection: a person designated in writing by the employer to be responsible for the immediate supervision, implementation and monitoring of the fall protection program, who through training, knowledge and experience in fall protection and rescue systems and equipment, is capable of identifying, evaluating and addressing existing and potential fall hazards and, who has the authority to take prompt corrective measures with regard to such hazards.

Competent Person for scaffolding: A person meeting the competent person requirements as defined in the definitions of EM 385-1-1 and 29 CFR Part 1926 who has been designated in writing by the employer to be responsible for the immediate supervision, implementation and monitoring of the scaffolding program, who through training, knowledge and experience in scaffolding is capable of identifying, evaluating and addressing existing and

EM 385-1-1
15 Sep 08

potential hazards and, who has the authority to take prompt corrective measures with regard to such hazards

Conductor: a material, usually in the form of a wire, cable, or bus bar, suitable for carrying an electric current.

Conductor shielding: an envelope that encloses the conductor of a cable and provides an equipotential surface in contact with the cable insulation.

Confined space: a space that

    a. Is large enough and so configured that a person can bodily enter and perform assigned work; and

    b. Has limited or restricted means for entry or exit [such that the entrant's ability to escape in an emergency would be hindered (e.g., tanks, vessels, silos, storage bins, hoppers, vaults, and pits are spaces that may have limited means of entry; doorways are not considered a limited means of entry or egress)]; and

    c. Is not designed for continuous worker occupancy.

Confined space on a ship or vessel: a compartment of small size and limited access such as a double bottom tank, cofferdam, or other space which by its small size and confined nature can readily create or aggravate a hazardous exposure.

Connector: an employee who, working with hoisting equipment, is placing and connecting structural members and/or components.

Constructibility: the ability to erect structural steel members in accordance with 29 CFR 1926, Subpart R, without having to alter the over-all structural design.

Construction load: (for joist erection) means any load other than the weight of the employee(s), the joists and the bridging bundle

Container: any vessel of 60 gal (0.23 m^3) or less capacity used for transporting or storing liquids.

Contaminant: any material, that, by nature of its composition or reaction with other materials, is potentially capable of causing injury, death, illness, damage, loss, or pain.

Contractor: any individual or firm under contractual agreement with the government or its subunits for the performance of services and products, such as construction, maintenance, and hazardous waste activities, including subcontractors of a prime contractor.

Controlled Access Zone: a zone to restrict access to unprotected side or edge of a roof or floor.

Controlled decking zone (CDZ): an area in which certain work (e.g., initial installation and placement of metal decking) may take place without the use of guardrail systems, personal fall arrest systems, fall restraint systems, or safety net systems and where access to the zone is controlled.

Controlled load-lowering: lowering a load by means of a mechanical hoist drum device that allows a hoisted load to be lowered with maximum control using the gear train or hydraulic components of the hoist mechanism. Controlled load lowering requires the use of the hoist drive motor, rather than the load hoist brake, to lower the load.

Controlling Contractor: a prime contractor, general contractor, construction manager or any other legal entity which has the overall responsibility for the construction of the project – its planning, quality and completion.

Conveyor: a horizontal, inclined, or vertical device for transporting material in a path predetermined by the design of the device and having points of loading and discharge.

Conveyor, portable: a transportable conveyor that is not self-propelled, usually having supports that provide mobility.

Conveyor, screw: a conveyor screw revolving in a suitably shaped stationary trough or casing fitted with hangers, trough ends, and other auxiliary accessories.

Corrosive: is a substance that can cause destruction of living tissue or damage by chemical action, including acids with a pH of 2.5 or below or caustics with a pH of 11.0 or above.

Crane: a machine for lifting or lowering a load and moving it horizontally, with the hoisting mechanism being an integral part of the machine.

Crane, commercial truck mounted: a crane consisting of a rotating superstructure (center post or turn table), boom, operating machinery, and one or more operator's stations mounted on a frame attached to a commercial truck chassis, usually retaining a payload hauling capability whose power source usually powers the crane.

Crane, crawler: a crane consisting of rotating superstructure with a power plant, operating machinery, and a boom, mounted on a base and equipped with crawler treads for travel.

Crane, floating: a rotating superstructure, power plant, operating machinery, and boom, mounted on a barge or pontoon. The power plant may be installed below decks. The crane's function is to handle loads at various radii.

Crane, floor operated: a crane that is pendant or nonconductive rope controlled by an operator on the floor or an independent platform

Crane, gantry: a crane similar to an overhead crane except that the bridge is rigidly supported on two or more legs running on fixed rails or other runway.

Crane, hammerhead: a lifting machine arranged with a tower (mast), an upper structure that rotates, a horizontally-extended load jib (boom) with trolley, and a counterweight jib extending in the direction opposite of the load jib: neither jib are arranged for luffing. The trolley on the load jib traverses the length of the jib and contains the sheaves and accessory parts which make up the upper load block; the lower load block is suspended from the trolley.

Crane, locomotive: a crane mounted on a base or car equipped for travel on a railroad track.

Crane, luffing jib: a type of jib on a tower crane that is pivoted at the jib foot and supported by luffing cables. The hoist rope usually passes over a sheave at the jib point and the hook radius is changed by luffing, or changing the angle of inclination, of the jib. Rear pivoted luffing jibs are similar but the pivot is towards the rear of the top of the tower rather than at the jib foot.

Crane, mobile: a crane mounted on a truck or crawler.

Crane, overhead: a crane with a single- or multiple-girder movable bridge or fixed hoisting mechanism and traveling on an overhead fixed runway structure.

Crane, pillar: a fixed crane consisting of a vertical member, held in position at its base to resist overturning moment, and normally with a constant-radius revolving boom supported at the outer end by a tension member.

Crane, portal: a crane consisting of a rotating superstructure with operating machinery and boom, all of which is mounted on gantry structure, usually with a portal opening between the gantry columns or legs for traffic to pass through; may be fixed or traveling.

Crane, standby: a crane that is not in regular service but which is used occasionally or intermittently as required.

Crane, tower: similar to a portal crane but with a tower intervening between the upper structure and the gantry or other base structure; typically without a portal. To resist overturning moments, the

EM 385-1-1
15 Sep 08

assembly may be ballasted, fixed to a foundation, or a combination of both. The crane may be either fixed or on a traveling base.

Crane (hoist), under-hung: a crane that is suspended from the bottom flange of a runway track or a single-track monorail system.

Crane, wall: a crane having a jib with or without trolley and supported from a side wall or line of columns of a building. It is a traveling type and operates on a runway attached to the sidewall or columns.

Crane, wheel-mounted (multi-control stations): a crane consisting of a rotating superstructure, operating machinery, and operator's station and boom, mounted on a crane carrier equipped with axles and rubber-tired wheels for travel, a power source(s), and having separate stations for driving and operating.

Crane, wheel-mounted (single control station): a crane consisting of a rotating superstructure, operating machinery, and boom, mounted on a crane carrier equipped with axles and rubber-tired wheels for travel, a power source, and having a single control station.

Crane operator aids: devices that are used to assist a crane operator in the safe operation of the crane, including: two-block warning devices, two-block prevention devices, load and load moment indicator devices, boom angle and radius indicators, boom and jib stops, boom hoist disengaging devices, limit switches, drum rotation indicators, etc.

<u>**Crawling board (chicken ladder**） - a supported scaffold consisting of a plank with cleats spaced and secured to provide footing, for use on sloped surfaces such as roofs.</u>

Cribbing: a system of timbers, arranged in a rectangular pattern, used to support and distribute the weight of equipment.

Critical lift: a non-routine crane lift requiring detailed planning and additional or unusual safety precautions.

Crossbraces: two diagonal scaffold members joined at their center to form an "X", used between frames or uprights or both.

Crotch: to pass a rope through the crotch of a limb, or false crotch, in such a way that the load will be supported by the main leader.

Cumulative trauma disorders: disorders of muscles, tendons, peripheral nerves, or vascular system. These can be caused, precipitated, or aggravated by intense, repeated, or sustained exertions, motions of the body, insufficient recovery, vibration, or cold.

Cylinder manifold: a multiple header for interconnection of gas sources with distribution points.

"DANGEROUS" Placard: A freight container, unit load device, transport vehicle, or railcar that contains non-bulk packages with two or more categories of hazardous materials that require different placards, may be placarded with a DANGEROUS placard instead of the separate placards specified for each of the materials.

Deadman control: a constant-pressure, hand- or foot-operated control designed so that when released, it automatically returns to a neutral or deactivated position.

Debris net: a net designed to catch only debris. It must be used in conjunction with a personnel net if there is any possibility for personnel to fall.

Decelerating device: any mechanism that serves to dissipate energy during a fall.

Decibel (dB): a measure of sound pressure.

dB(A): A-weighted measure of sound pressure used with sound level meters; the weighting causes the sensitivity of the sound level meter to vary with the frequency and intensity of sound and in doing so duplicates the response of the human ear.

EM 385-1-1
15 Sep 08

Decking hole: a gap or void more than 2 in (5.1 cm) in its least dimension and less than 12 in (30.5 cm) in its greatest dimension in a floor, roof, or other walking/working surface. Pre-engineered holes in cellular decking (for wires, cables, etc.) are not included in this definition.

Decompression sickness: a condition with a variety of symptoms which may result from gas or bubbles in the tissues of divers after pressure reduction.

Decompression table: a profile or set of profiles of depth-time relationships for ascent rate and breathing mixtures to be followed after a specific depth-time exposure or exposures.

Derrick: an apparatus consisting of a mast or equivalent member held at the end by guys or braces, with or without a boom, for use with a hoisting mechanism and operating ropes.

Derrick, A-frame: a derrick in which the boom is hinged from a cross member or pedestal between the bottom ends of two upright members spread apart at the lower ends and joined at the top, the boom point secured to the junction of the side members, and the side members are braced or guyed from this junction point.

Derrick, floating: a mast or equivalent member held at the head by guys or braces, with or without a boom, for use with a hoisting mechanism and operating ropes, mounted on a barge or a pontoon. The power plant may be installed below decks.

Derrick, floor: an elevated floor of a building or structure that has been designated to receive hoisted pieces of steel prior to final placement.

Derrick, guy: a fixed derrick consisting of a vertical mast capable of being rotated 360° (but not continuous rotation) supported by guys, and a boom that is pivoted at the bottom and capable of moving in a vertical plane; a reeved rope between the head (top) of the mast and the boom harness (at the boom point) allows lifting

EM 385-1-1
15 Sep 08

and lowering of the boom and a reeved rope from the boom point allows lifting and lowering of the load.

Derrick, stiff leg: a derrick similar to a guy derrick except that the mast is supported or held in place by 2 or more stiff members (stiff legs) which are capable of resisting either tensile or compressive forces. Sills are generally provided to connect the lower ends of the stiff legs to the foot of the mast.

Design load: the maximum intended load: that is, the total of all loads including the worker(s), material, and the equipment placed on the unit.

Designated Dive Coordinator (DDC): a USACE employee assigned the responsibility for organizing, integrating, and monitoring the total dive program within a USACE Command. This individual and an alternate (to perform in the absence of the primary DDC) will be appointed, in writing, by the USACE Commander/Director and will assure adherence to all applicable rules and regulations. At the Major Subordinate Command (MSC) (Division), the Diving Coordinator will provide program guidance and monitor and annually review the MSC dive program at all subordinate levels; at the District, Laboratory, and other field operating activities (FOA) level, the DDC will review and accept all safe practices manuals, dive plans, medical certificates, and dive team qualifications and experience to assure compliance with this manual. For Districts/ labs where diving is performed by USACE divers, the DDC and the alternate shall, as a minimum, successfully complete the HQUSACE approved Diving Safety/ Diving Supervisor Training Course and shall maintain certification by attending the diving refresher course every 4 years. DDCs attending the Diving Safety Course are not required to perform 12 working/training dives unless they are in a dual position as a USACE diver or USACE Diving Supervisor. In all MSCs and in those FOAs where all diving is performed by contractors, the DDC and ADC may alternatively complete the USACE Dive Safety Administrator course and refresher every 4 years. The Dive Safety Administrator course does not certify or re-certify a person as a Dive Supervisor.

EM 385-1-1
15 Sep 08

Designated person: An employee who has been trained or is qualified and assigned the responsibility to perform a specific task.

Detonating cord: a flexible cord containing a center core of high explosives that when detonated will have sufficient strength to detonate other cap-sensitive explosives with which it is in contact.

Detonator: blasting caps, electric blasting caps, delay electric blasting caps, and non-electric delay blasting caps.

<u>**Discarded Military Munitions (DMM).** Military munitions that have been abandoned without proper disposal or removed from storage in a military magazine or other storage area for the purpose of disposal; excludesunexploded ordnance (UXO), military munitions that are being held for future use or planned disposal, or military munitions that have been properly disposed of, consistent with applicable environmental laws and regulations. (10 U.S.C. 2710(e)(2))</u>

Dive location: a surface or vessel from which a diving operation is conducted.

Dive operation: the complete scope of work addressed in a single diving plan.

Dive team: divers and support employees involved in a diving operation, including the diving supervisor.

Dive tender: that individual on the dive team assigned to assist the diver with dressing in and out, entering and exiting the water, and continuously tend the tether or umbilical of the diver while in the water. The dive tender shall have experience and training that encompasses all aspects of tending in order to provide safe and efficient support to the diver.

<u>**Diving, Direct Source Compressor**: Air compressor system used on-site as a direct source to supply air to SSA divers via the receiver tank, manifold, and air line – not compressors used onsite solely to fill SCUBA or other air cylinders.</u>

EM 385-1-1
15 Sep 08

Diving, Heavy Gear: Surface-supplied deep-sea diving gear including helmet (with or without breastplate), dry suit, and weighted shoes, with the helmet directly connected to the dry suit, forming a self-contained pressure envelope for the diver.

Diving Inspector: a USACE employee or other designated qualified person who inspects a Contractor diving operation while work is in progress (not an employee of the dive contractor). USACE Diving inspectors shall be designated in writing by the local Commander upon nomination by the employee's staff level supervisor and with concurrence of the DDC. USACE Diving inspectors must have successfully completed a USACE diving safety/ diving supervisor, Diving Inspector, or Dive Safety Administrator course and shall maintain certification by attending the appropriate HQUSACE-sponsored refresher course every 4 years. Non-USACE Diving monitors/inspectors with other credentials will be considered on a case-by-case basis and may be approved in writing by the DDC with Command notification and concurrence.

Diving Safety Representative (DSR): the Safety and Occupational Health Office representative assigned the responsibility of dive safety. This individual provides dive safety advice to operational elements and actively participates in the review and comment process for diving plans and hazard analyses, as well as on-site monitoring of diving operations. The DSR must successfully complete the USACE diving safety/ diving supervisor, diving inspector, or Dive Safety Administrator course and maintain certification by attending the appropriate HQUSACE-sponsored refresher course every 4 years. Unless required by position, this individual is not required to perform 12 working/ training dives to maintain certification.

Diving supervisor: the employer, or an employee designated by the employer, at the dive location in charge of all aspects of the diving operation that affect the safety and health of dive team members. The diving supervisor shall have experience and training in the conduct of the assigned diving operation.

Dose equivalent: the product of the absorbed dose in tissue, quality factor, and all other necessary modifying factors at the location of interest. The units of dose equivalent are the rem or Sievert (Sv) (1 Sievert equals 100 rem).

Dosimetry: the measure of radiological exposure.

Double-cleated ladder: a ladder, similar to a single cleat ladder but with a center rail, which allows simultaneous two-way traffic for employees ascending or descending.

Double connection: an attachment method where the connection point is intended for two pieces of steel that share common bolts on either side of a central piece.

Double connection seat: a structural attachment that, during the installation of a double connection, supports the first member while the second member is connected.

Dragline: a bucket attachment for a crane that excavates by the crane drawing, with a cable, the bucket towards itself.

Dredge: any vessel fitted with machinery for the purpose of removing or relocating material from or in a body of water.

Drift pin: a pin that is tapered at both ends and used to align holes.

<u>**Drilled Shaft:** a shaft constructed by excavating a cylindrical hole, placing reinforcing steel (if required) and filling the hole with concrete (also called drilled piers or caissons).</u>

Drilling fluid (mud): fluid that is pumped into a drilled hole and used to wash cuttings from the hole: drilling mud is a type of drilling fluid made of a slurry of clay and water and that is used to coat and support the sides of the drill hole and seal off permeable strata.

EM 385-1-1
15 Sep 08

Dry chemical: an extinguishing agent composed of very small particles of chemicals such as sodium bicarbonate, potassium bicarbonate, or potassium chloride supplemented by special treatment to provide resistance to packing and moisture absorption and to provide proper flow capabilities. Does not include dry powders.

Dry location: a location not normally subject to dampness or wetness; a location classified as dry may be temporarily subject to dampness or wetness, as in the case of a building under construction

Dry powder: a compound used to extinguish or control Class D fires.

<u>**Duck Pond**: Openings between stationary vessels or vessels and other structures that create fully enclosed water areas (duck ponds) into which personnel could fall.</u>

Dust: solid particles generated by handling, crushing, grinding, or detonation of organic or inorganic materials.

Duty cycle: operations involving repetitive pick and swing, such as with a dragline, grapple, or clamshell: such operations are conducted primarily for production as opposed to placement.

Duty time: time during which an individual is being compensated for his/her services.

Effective dose equivalent: the sum of the products of the dose equivalent to the organ or tissue and the weighting factors applicable to each of the body organs or tissues irradiated.

Effectively grounded: intentionally connected to earth through a ground connection or connections of sufficiently low impedance and having sufficient current-carrying capacity to prevent the buildup of voltages which may result in undue hazard to connected equipment or to persons.

EM 385-1-1
15 Sep 08

Elevating work platform: a vertically-adjustable, integral chassis, power operated work platforms, which may be horizontally extended or rotated relative to the elevating mechanism; an integral frame boom supported power operated elevating work platforms which either telescope, articulate, rotate, or extend beyond their base dimensions.

Emergency (marine): an unforeseen development that imposes an immediate hazard to the safety of the vessel, the passengers, the crew, the cargo, property, or the marine environment, requiring urgent action to remove or mitigate the hazard.

Emergency situation (respiratory hazard): any occurrence such as, but not limited to, equipment failure, rupture of containers, or failure of control equipment that may or does result in an uncontrolled significant release of an airborne contaminant.

Employee: a Government or Contractor person engaged in work on a USACE project.

Employer: a Government or Contractor organization that has control over employees engaged in work on a USACE project.

Enclosed space: any space, other than a confined space, that is enclosed by bulkheads and overhead. This includes cargo holds, tanks, and quarters, as well as machinery and boiler spaces.

Endless rope: a rope with the ends spliced together.

End-of-service-life indicator (ESLI): a system that warns the respirator user of the approach of the end of adequate respiratory protection (e.g., that the sorbent is approaching saturation or is no longer effective).

End user: <u>a person who has been trained and authorized by the employer on the use of assigned fall protection equipment in a typical fall hazard situation.</u>

EM 385-1-1
15 Sep 08

Energy (shock) absorber: a component whose primary function is to dissipate energy and limit the deceleration forces imposed on the body during fall arrest.

Energy control procedure: a written procedure (including responsibilities, procedural steps for lockout and tagout, and requirements for testing the effectiveness of energy control measures) to be used for the control of hazardous energy.

Energy isolation device: a physical device that prevents the transmission or release of energy. Includes, but is not limited to, manually operated circuit breakers, disconnect switches, slide gates, slip blinds, line valves, blocks, or similar devices, capable of blocking or isolating energy, with a position indicator. The term does not include push buttons, selector switches, and other control circuit type devices.

Energy ratio: a measure of the seismic energy impact of an explosive blast.

Energy source: includes electrical, mechanical, hydraulic, pneumatic, chemical, thermal, nuclear, stored, or other energy.

Engulfment: the surrounding and effective capture by a liquid or finely divided (flow able) solid substance that can be aspirated to cause death by filling or plugging the respiratory system or that can exert enough force on the body to cause death by strangulation, constriction, or crushing.

Enter with restrictions: refers to entry into a confined space when engineering controls, personal protective equipment, and time limitations are imposed by the competent person.

Entry permit (permit): the written or printed document provided to allow and control entry into a permit space and that contains the information specified in ENG Form 5044-R.

Entry supervisor (confined space): the person responsible for determining if acceptable entry conditions are present at a permit

EM 385-1-1
15 Sep 08

space where entry is planned, for authorizing entry and overseeing entry operations, and for terminating entry as required by this manual.

Erection bridging: the bolted diagonal bridging that is required to be installed prior to releasing the hoisting cables from the steel joists.

Escape-only respirator: a respirator intended to be used only for emergency exit.

Exceptional-exposure dive: dives in which the risk of decompression sickness, oxygen toxicity, and or exposure to the elements is substantially greater than normal working dives.

Explosion Proof: this term is usually seen when describing Class I Division 1 equipment. The device must be able to withstand an internal explosion if it should occur and it must work to prevent the spread of the internal explosion to the surrounding saturated atmosphere. Equipment is designed so as not to allow the explosion or other possible sources of ignition to reach the hazardous atmosphere.

Explosive: A substance or a mixture of substances that is capable by chemical reaction of producing gas at such temperature, pressure, and speed as to cause damage to the surroundings; includes all substances known as high explosives and propellants, together with igniters, primers, initiators, and pyrotechnics (e.g., illuminant, smoke, delay, decoy, flare, and incendiary compositions).

Explosive Ordnance Disposal (EOD): Military personnel who have graduated from the Naval School, Explosive Ordnance Disposal; are assigned to a military unit with a Service-defined EOD mission; meet Service and assigned unit requirements to perform EOD duties; have received specialized training to address explosive and certain CA hazards during both peacetime and wartime;are trained and equipped to perform render safe

EM 385-1-1
15 Sep 08

<u>procedures (RSP) on nuclear, biological, chemical, and conventional munitions, and on improvised explosive devices (IED).</u>

Explosive-actuated tool: a tool that uses the expanding gases from a power load to drive a fastener.

Exposure: a measure of the ionizing radiation produced in air by X or gamma radiation, equal to the sum of the electrical charges on all ions of one sign produced per unit mass of air. The special unit of exposure is the Roentgen equal to 2.58×10^{-4} Coulombs per Kilogram of air at standard temperature and pressure.

Exposure hours: the number of paid duty hours. Unpaid hours count as exposure when employees are quartered on-site. Exposures hours are used to calculate accident experience rates.

Exposure (respiratory hazard): exposure to a concentration of an airborne contaminant that would occur if the employee were not using respiratory protection.

Extension trestle ladder: a ladder consisting of a trestle ladder with an additional vertical single ladder, having parallel sides, that is adjustable perpendicularly and is provided with a device to lock it into place.

Extinguisher classification: the letter classification given an extinguisher to designate the classes of fire on which it will be effective.

Extinguisher rating: the numerical rating given to an extinguisher that indicates the extinguishing potential of the unit.

Face: that part of the tunnel or shaft where excavation is in progress or was last done; the vertical surface at the head of a tunnel excavation.

<u>**Fall arrest system**: assembly of equipment, components and subsystems used to arrest a fall.</u>

EM 385-1-1
15 Sep 08

Fall arrestor (rope grab): a device that travels on a lifeline and will automatically engage or lock onto the lifeline in the event of a fall.

False crotch: a pulley, block, sling, lashing, or metal ring, affixed to a tree's leader of limb, through which a load line is passed, to raise or lower limbs or equipment.

Feeder: all circuit conductors between the service equipment, the source of a separately derived system, or other power supply source and the final branch-circuit over-current device.

Figure-four form scaffold: a scaffold consisting of a work platform supported by brackets designed in the shape of a "4."

Filter or air purifying element: a component used in respirators to remove solid or liquid aerosols from the inspired air.

Filtering facepiece (dust mask): a negative-pressure particulate respirator with a filter as an integral part of the facepiece or with the entire facepiece composed of the filtering medium.

Fit factor: a quantitative estimate of the fit of a particular respirator to a specific individual, and typically estimates the ratio of the concentration of a substance in ambient air to its concentration inside the respirator when worn.

Fit test: the use of a protocol to qualitatively or quantitatively evaluate the fit of a respirator on an individual. **> See *Qualitative fit test (QLFT)* and *Quantitative fit test (QNFT).***

Fixed extinguishing system: a permanently installed system that either extinguishes or controls a fire.

Fixed ladder: a ladder that cannot be readily moved or carried because it is an integral part of a building or structure.

Fixed lead: pile driving leads which are rigidly attached to a boom by horizontal struts extending from the leads to extended boom foot

EM 385-1-1
15 Sep 08

pins, thus providing a fixed triangular frame of boom, struts, and leads.

Flammable liquid: a liquid having a flashpoint below 100° F (38° C) and having a vapor pressure not exceeding 40 lbs per square inch absolute (psia) (280 kPa) at 100° F (38° C). Flammable liquids are also categorized as Class I liquids and further defined as follows:

   a. Class 1A liquids have flash points below 73° F (23° C) and have boiling points below 100° F (38° C).

   b. Class 1B liquids have flash points below 73° F (23° C) and have boiling points at or above 100° F (38° C).

   c. Class 1C liquids have flash points at or above 73° F (23° C) and below 100° F (38° C).

Flashback: a recession of the flame into or back of the mixing chamber of the oxy-fuel gas torch.

Fleet angle: the angle between the rope as it leaves the drum (at the extreme end wrap on a drum) for the sheave and an imaginary centerline passing through the center of the sheave groove and a point halfway between the ends of the drum.

Floating plant/vessel: used to transport personnel, work boats, floating cranes and derricks, barges, patrol boats, etc.

Float/ship scaffold: a scaffold hung from overhead supports by means of ropes and consisting of a unit having diagonal bracing underneath: the scaffold rests upon and is securely fastened to two parallel planks bearers at right angles to the span.

Floor arch: the masonry arch shaped filling between steel floor beams or girders, whatever the type of flooring system.

<u>**Floor (roof) hole/opening**: floor or roof holes/openings are any that measure over 2 in (51 mm) in any direction of a</u>

walking/working surface which persons may trip or fall into or where objects may fall to the level below.

Foam: a stable aggregation of small bubbles that flow freely over a burning liquid surface and form a coherent blanket that seals combustible vapors, thereby extinguishing the fire.

Forklift: >*See Powered industrial truck (PIT)*.

Form scaffold: a scaffolding system integrated to formwork.

Freestanding scaffold: a scaffold that is independent of and not rigidly attached to a structure.

Fuel gas: a gas (e.g., acetylene, hydrogen, natural gas, propane) used with oxygen in the oxy-fuel process and for heating.

Full body harness: See "Body Harness, Full".

Full personnel protection: when tagout is used in place of lockout , full personnel protection is provided when:
 a. The tagout device is attached at the same location as the lockout device would have been attached;
 b. All tagout-related requirements of this manual have been complied with; and
 c. Additional means have been taken to provide a level of safety commensurate with that of a lockout device. Such additional means include the removal of an isolating circuit element, blocking of a control switch, opening and tagging an extra (separated by distance) disconnecting device, or the removal of a valve handle to reduce the likelihood of being energized.

Fume: very small suspended solid particles created by condensation from the gaseous state.

Fusible plug: a device designed to relieve pressure and to indicate certain conditions that contribute to low water.

Gangway: any ramp, stairway, or ladder provided for personnel to board/leave a vessel.

Gaseous agent: a fire-extinguishing agent that is in the gaseous state at normal room temperature and pressure and diffuses readily to diffuse itself uniformly throughout an enclosure.

Gas metal arc welding: an arc welding process that uses an arc between a continuous filler metal electrode and the weld pool. Shielding (from the atmosphere) is provided by an externally supplied gas.

Gate: a device or structure by means of which the flow of material may be stopped or regulated.

Generator, mobile: mobile describes equipment, such as vehicle-mounted generators, that is capable of being moved on wheels or rollers.

Generator, portable: portable describes equipment that is easily carried by personnel from one location to another.

Girt (in systems engineered metal buildings): a "Z" or "C" shaped member formed from sheet steel spanning between primary framing and supporting wall material.

Government Designated Authority (GDA): the senior person in charge or his/her appointed representative for the operation being considered.

Grommet: an endless 7-strand wire rope.

Ground: (reference) - that conductive body, usually earth, to which an electric potential is referenced; (as a noun) - a conductive connection whether incidental or accidental, by which an electric circuit or equipment is connected to reference ground; (as a verb) - the connecting or establishing of a connection, whether by intention or accident, of an electric circuit or equipment to reference ground.

Grounded: connected to earth or to some conducting body that serves in place of the earth.

Grounded conductor: a system or circuit conductor that is intentionally grounded.

Grounded system: a system of conductors in which at least one conductor or point (usually the middle wire or neutral point of a transformer or generator windings) is intentionally grounded, either solidly or through a current limiting device (not a current-interrupting device).

Ground fault circuit interrupter: a device used to interrupt the electric circuit to the load when a fault current to ground exceeds some predetermined value that is less than that required to operate the over current protection device of the supply circuit.

Grounding conductor: a conductor used to connect equipment or the grounded circuit of a wiring system to a grounding electrode or electrodes.

Grounding electrode (ground electrode): a conductor embedded in the earth, used for maintaining ground potential on conductors connected to it, and for dissipating into the earth current connected to it.

Grounding electrode conductor (grounding conductor): a conductor used to connect equipment or the grounded circuit of a wiring system to a grounding electrode.

Guarded by location: describes moving parts so protected by their remoteness from the floor, platform, walkway, or other working level, or by their location with reference to frame, foundation, or structure as to reduce the foreseeable risk of accidental contact by persons or objects. Remoteness from foreseeable, regular, or frequent presence of public or employed personnel may in reasonable circumstances constitute guarding by location.

EM 385-1-1
15 Sep 08

Guardrail system: A rail system erected along open-sided floors, openings, and ends of platforms. The rail system consists of a toprail, midrail and their supports.

Halon: a colorless, electrically nonconductive gas that extinguishes fire by inhibiting the chemical chain reaction of fuel and oxygen. Halon 1211 is a liquefied gas, also known as bromochlorodifluromethane. Halon 1301 is also known as bromotrifluoromethane.

Hardware: rigid components or elements such as buckles, D-rings, snap-hooks, and associated devices used to attach the components of a personal fall protection system together.

Hazard: a dangerous condition, potential or inherent, that can bring about an interruption or interfere with the expected orderly progress of an activity. A source of potential injury to person or to property.

Hazardous (physical) agent: noise, non-ionizing and ionizing radiation, and temperature exposure of durations and quantities capable of causing adverse health effects.

Hazardous atmosphere: an atmosphere that may expose persons to the risk of death, incapacitation, impairment of ability to self rescue (i.e., escape unaided from a permit space), injury, or acute illness from one or more of the following causes:

   a. Flammable gas, vapor, or mist in excess of 10% of its lower flammable limit (LFL);

   b. Airborne combustible dust at a concentration that meets or exceeds its LFL;

   c. Atmospheric oxygen concentration below 19.5% or above 23.5%;

EM 385-1-1
15 Sep 08

    d. Atmospheric concentration of any substance for which a dose or PEL is published and which could result in team member exposure in excess of its dose or PEL;

    e. Any other atmospheric condition that is IDLH.

Hazardous energy control plan (HECP): the written plan that clearly and specifically identifies the hazardous energy sources and outlines the scope, purpose, responsibilities, and procedural steps for lockout and tagout and the requirements for testing the effectiveness of energy control measures to be used for the control of hazardous energy from stated sources.

Hazardous environment: an environment with an atmosphere that poses a risk of death, incapacitation, injury, or illness due to flammable or explosive hazards; hazardous substances or agents; oxygen concentrations below 19.5% or above 22%; or any other atmospheric condition recognized as IDLH.

Hazardous substance: any substance defined as a hazardous substance under 29 CFR 1910.120, 29 CFR 1926.65, or 40 CFR 302; any chemical determined to be a hazard as specified in 29 CFR 1910.1200 or 29 CFR 1926.59 to include a chemical (as a gas, liquid, vapor, mist, dust, or fume) which has been identified as causing adverse health effects in exposed employees.

Hazardous, toxic, radioactive waste (HTRW) activity: refers to overall project or worksite involving the investigation, assessment, or clean-up of HTRW or the emergency response to releases of hazardous substances, hazardous waste, or hazardous material at an HTRW site. Includes: activities undertaken for the EPA's Superfund Program, the Defense Environmental Restoration Program (which also includes FUDS and Installation Restoration Program activities), HTRW actions associated with Civil Works projects, and HTRW projects of other Government agencies. Includes, but are not limited to: preliminary assessments/site inspections; remedial investigations; feasibility studies; engineering evaluations/cost analyses; RCRA facility investigations/corrective measures studies/corrective measures implementations/closure

EM 385-1-1
15 Sep 08

plans/Part B permits; or any other pre-design investigations, remedial design, or remedial construction, operation or maintenance at known, suspected, or potential HTRW sites, activities conducted at containerized HTRW sites (leaking PCB transformers and leaking or suspected leaking USTs that contain hazardous substances).

Hazardous, toxic, radioactive waste (HTRW) operation: a specific function on an HTRW site, such as sampling, monitoring, excavation, drum removal, etc.

Hazardous, toxic, radioactive waste (HTRW) site: any facility or location that:

    a. Requires the planned or emergency clean-up of hazardous, toxic, radioactive waste; and

    b. Is designated as an uncontrolled hazardous waste site or covered by the RCRA.

Heating torch: a device for directing the heating flame produced by the controlled combustion of fuel gases.

Heavy gear: diver-worn deep-sea dress, including helmet, in-water stage: a suspended underwater platform that supports a diver in the water. Breastplate, dry suit, and weighted shoes, (e.g., U.S. Navy Mark V gear).

High efficiency particulate air (HEPA) filter: a filter that is at least 99.97% efficient in removing mono-disperse particles of 0.3 µm in diameter. The equivalent NIOSH 42 CFR 84 particulate filters are the N100, R100, and P100 filters.

High radiation area: any area, accessible to personnel, in which there exists radiation at such levels that a major portion of the body could receive in any 1 hour a dose in excess of 100 mrem.

High voltage: is a voltage of 600 volts or greater.

EM 385-1-1
15 Sep 08

Hoist: a machinery unit that is used for lifting or lowering a freely suspended (unguided) load.

Hood (respiratory protection): a respiratory inlet covering that completely covers the head and neck and may also cover portions of the shoulders and torso.

Hopper: a box having a funnel-shaped bottom, or a bottom reduced in size, narrowed, or necked to receive material and direct it to a conveyor, feeder, or chute.

Horizontal lifeline system: A fall arrest system consisting of an assembly of components that uses rope, wire or synthetic cable spanned horizontally between two end anchorages.

Horse scaffold: a scaffold composed of work platforms supported by construction horses.

Hotline tools and ropes: those tools and ropes that are especially designed for work on energized high voltage lines and equipment. Insulated aerial equipment especially designed for work on energized high voltage lines and equipment shall be considered hot line.

Hot tapping: a procedure of attaching connections to equipment in service by welding and drilling.

Hot work: hot riveting, welding, burning, abrasive blasting, or other fire- or spark-producing operations.

Hot work, confined space: hot work in confined space: any activity involving riveting, welding, burning, powder-actuated tools, or similar fire-producing operations. Grinding, drilling, abrasive blasting, or similar spark-producing operations are also considered hot work except when such operations are isolated physically from any atmosphere containing more than 10% of the lower explosive limit of a flammable or combustible substance.

Hot work permit: written authorization to perform operations (for example, riveting, welding, cutting, burning, and heating) capable of providing a source of ignition.

Immediately dangerous to life or health (IDLH–respiratory hazard): an atmosphere that poses an immediate threat to life, would cause irreversible adverse health effects, or would impair an individual's ability to escape from a dangerous atmosphere.

Impulse noise: noise is considered impulse when the variations in sound-pressure level involve peaks at intervals greater than 1 second.

Incidental employee: an employee who, under normal circumstances, would not be in an area where a system is under lockout and tagout but is required to enter or pass through such an area.

Incipient stage fire: a fire that is in the initial or beginning stage and that can be controlled or extinguished by portable fire extinguisher, Class II standpipe, or small hose systems without the need for protective clothing or breathing apparatus.

Independent wire rope core: a small 6 x 7 wire rope with a wire strand core; used to provide greater resistance to crushing and distortion of the wire rope.

Induced current: the generation of a current in a conductor caused by its proximity to a second alternating current source, a moving direct current source (such as a motor), or an extraneous voltage source (such as lightning).

Inside post: the post nearest to the structure against which the scaffold is erected.

Interior structural firefighting: the physical activity of fire suppression, rescue, or both, inside of buildings or enclosed structures that are involved in a fire situation beyond the incipient stage. (See 29 CFR 1910.155)

Intrinsically safe equipment: Equipment and associated wiring incapable of releasing sufficient electrical energy under normal or abnormal conditions to cause ignition of a specific hazardous atmospheric mixture; equipment incapable of igniting the atmosphere surrounding it.

In-water stage: a suspended underwater platform that supports a diver in the water.

Ionizing radiation: electromagnetic and particulate radiation that causes molecular ionization; includes alpha particles, beta particles, gamma rays, x-rays, neutrons, high speed electrons and protons, and other atomic matter.

Isolation: an activity that physically prevents the transmission or release of energy.

Jib: on hammerhead cranes, the horizontal structural member attached to the rotating superstructure of a crane and upon which the load trolley travels; on mobile cranes, an extension attached to the boom to provide added boom length for lifting specified loads.

Job-made ladder: a ladder fabricated by employees, typically at the construction site, and is not commercially manufactured.

Labeled: equipment or materials that has an attached label, symbol, or other identifying mark of an organization that is acceptable to the authority having jurisdiction and concerned with the product evaluation that maintains periodic inspection of production of labeled equipment or materials and by whose labeling the manufacturer indicates compliance with appropriate standards or performance in a specified manner.

Laboratory waste pack: a drum containing individual containers of laboratory materials normally surrounded by cushioning absorbent material.

Ladder: a device incorporating or employing steps, rungs, or cleats on which a person may step to ascend or descend.

Ladder climbing safety device: device that is connected to a harness or belt to prevent falls from ladders.

Ladder, combination: a portable ladder capable of being used either as a stepladder or as a single or extension ladder. It may also be capable of being used as a trestle ladder or a stairwell ladder. Its components may be used as single ladders.

Ladder, extension: a non-self-supporting portable ladder adjustable in length. It consists of two or more sections, traveling guides, or brackets or the equivalent and so arranged as to permit length adjustment.

Ladder, individual-rung/step: a ladder without a side rail or center rail support, made by mounting individual steps or rungs directly to the side or wall of the structure.

<u>**Ladder jack scaffold:** a supported scaffold consisting of a platform resting on brackets attached to ladders. (prohibited)</u>

Ladder, portable: a ladder that can readily be moved or carried, usually consisting of side rails joined at intervals by steps, rungs, cleats, or rear braces.

Ladder, sectional: a non-self-supporting portable ladder, nonadjustable in length, consisting of two or more sections, and so constructed that the sections may be combined to function as a single ladder.

Ladder, side-step, fixed: a fixed ladder that requires a person getting off at the top to step to the side of the ladder side rails to reach the landing.

Ladder, single cleat: a ladder consisting of a pair of side rails connected together by cleats, rungs, or steps.

EM 385-1-1
15 Sep 08

Ladder, single rail: a portable ladder with rungs, cleats, or steps mounted on a single rail instead of the typical two rails.

Ladder, through-step, fixed: a fixed ladder that requires a person getting off at the top to step between the side rails of the ladder to reach the landing.

Ladder, trestle: a self-supporting ladder consisting of two single ladders hinged or joined at the top to form equal angles with the base.

Ladder type: the designation that identifies the working load.

Ladder-type platform: a platform that resembles a ladder covered by planking.

Lagging: timber planks, steel plates, or other structural members used for transferring loads and supporting soil or rock.

Landing area:

   a. The primary surfaces, comprising the surface of the runway, runway shoulders, and lateral safety zones;

   b. The "clear zone" beyond the ends of each runway (i.e., the extension of the primary surface);

   c. All taxiways, and the lateral clearance zones along each side for the length of the taxiways; and

   d. All aircraft parking aprons plus the area extending beyond each edge all around the aprons.

Lanyard: a component consisting of flexible rope, wire rope or strap , which typically has a connector at each end for connecting body support to a fall arrestor, energy absorber, anchorage connector, or anchorage.

Large area scaffold: a scaffold erected over substantially the entire work area. For example: a scaffold erected over the entire floor area of a room.

Laser: a device that produces an intense, coherent, directional beam of light.

Lead: the device on a pile driver that maintains the hammer in position during the driving. A lead typically is made up of two vertical rails or guides, held together by a frame, in which the hammer moves vertically.

Lead (leading) wire: an insulated expendable wire used between the electric power source and the electric blasting cap circuit.

Leader: the upper portion of the primary axis of a tree.

Leading edge: the unprotected side or edge of a floor, roof, or formwork for a floor or other walking/working surface (such as deck) that changes location as additional floor, roof, decking, or formwork sections are placed, formed, or constructed.

Ledger: is a horizontal scaffold member upon which bearers rest. The longitudinal member that joins scaffold uprights, posts, poles, and similar members.

Lifeline: a line (horizontal or vertical) for direct attachment between a worker's personal fall protection equipment and a point of anchorage.

Lift supervisor: the person designated to be in charge of crane lifting; this may be the crane operator or an individual whose function it is to supervise lifting operations.

Limbing: to cut limbs from a tree.

Line-breaking: the intentional opening of a pipe, line, or duct that is or has been carrying flammable, toxic, or corrosive material, an inert gas, or any fluid at a pressure or temperature capable of causing injury.

Liquefied petroleum gas (LP-Gas): any material that is composed predominantly of any of the following hydrocarbons (or mixtures of them): propane, propylene, butanes, and butylenes.

List: the angle of inclination about the longitudinal axis of a vessel.

Listed: equipment, materials, or services included in a list published by an organization acceptable to the authority having jurisdiction (AHJ) and concerned with the evaluation of products or services that maintains periodic inspection of production of listed equipment or materials or periodic evaluation of services and whose listing states either that the equipment, material, or service meets identified standards or has been tested and found suitable for a specified purpose.

Live-boating: The practice of supporting a SSA or mixed gas diver from a vessel that is underway.

Live-line bare-hand technique: a highly specialized technique (usually used on medium- and high-voltage transmission lines) where a qualified employee working from an insulated aerial platform is electrically bonded to an energized line, effectively canceling any electrical potential difference across the worker's body and protecting the employee from electric shock.

Live-line bare-hand work: work that is performed barehanded from an insulated aerial platform, with the linemen in the basket at the same potential as the live conductor on which they are working.

Live-line tools: tools used by qualified employees to handle energized conductors. The tool insulates the employee from the energized line, allowing the employee to perform the task safely. Also known as "hot sticks."

Load block: an assembly of hook or shackle, swivel, pins, and frame.

Load indicator: a device that measures the weight of the load.

Load moment indicator (rated capacity indicator): a device that indicates the bending moment on a crane by measuring both the load on a boom and the horizontal distance from the load (boom point) to the crane's axis of rotation. Load moment indicators are often equipped with warning devices or disengaging devices that are actuated before a crane is overloaded.

Load performance test: a test of a crane's performance, structural competence, and stability while lifting at a percentage of its rated load capacity.

Load-rated: the maximum allowable working load.

Load-working: the external load applied to the crane or derrick, including the weight of load-attaching equipment such as load blocks, shackles, and slings.

Local application system: a fixed fire suppression system that has a supply of extinguishing agent with nozzles arranged to automatically discharge extinguishing agent directly on the burning material to extinguish or control the fire.

Lockout: a form of hazardous energy control using the placement of a lockout device, in accordance with established procedures, on an energy-isolating device to ensure that the energy-isolating device and the system being controlled cannot be operated until the lockout device is removed.

Lockout device: a device that uses a positive means, such as a key or combination lock, to hold an energy-isolating device in the safe position and prevent the energizing of a system.

Long-bed end-dump trailer: a trailer with a length of 30 ft (9.1 m) or more, a length-to-width ratio of or exceeding 4:1, and which is used to transport and dump material.

EM 385-1-1
15 Sep 08

Loose-fitting facepiece: a respiratory inlet covering that is designed to form a partial seal with the face.

Low-slope roof: a roof having a slope less than or equal to 4 in 12 (vertical to horizontal).

Low voltage: voltage less than 600 volts.

Machinery and Mechanized equipment: equipment intended for use on construction sites or industrial sites and not intended for operations on public highways.

Maintenance hole: a surface enclosure that personnel may enter that is used for installing, operating, and maintaining equipment and cable.

Mandrel: a steel shaft and bearings assembly on which a tool, such as an abrasive wheel, is mounted and by which power is transmitted from the machine to the tool.

Manned vessels: vessels that operate with crews, or quartered personnel, or that have work areas that are occupied by assigned personnel during normal work activities.

Marine activities: operations and work involving proximity to or on water.

Mast (derrick): the upright member of the derrick used for support of the boom.

Mast climbing work platform: a hoist having a working platform used for temporary purposes to raise personnel and materials to the working position by means of a drive system mounted on an extendable mast which may be tied to a building.

Material Safety Data Sheet (MSDS): a sheet that provides information on substance identification; ingredients and hazards; physical data; fire and explosion data; reactivity data; health hazard information; spill, leak, and disposal procedures; and special precautions and comments.

Maximum arresting force: the peak force exerted on the boy when a fall protection system arrests or stops a fall.

Metal-clad cable (MC): a factory assembly of one or more conductors, each individually insulated and enclosed in a metallic sheath of interlocking tape or a smooth or corrugated tube.

Metal decking: a commercially manufactured, structural grade, cold-rolled metal panel formed into a series of parallel ribs; this includes metal floor and roof decks, standing seam metal roofs, other metal roof systems, bar gratings, checker plate, expanded metal panels, and similar products.

Military Munitions (MM). All ammunition products and components produced for or used by the armed forces for national defense and security, including ammunition products or components under the control of the DoD, the Coast Guard, the Department of Energy (DoE), and the National Guard. The term includes confined gaseous, liquid, and solid propellants, explosives, pyrotechnics, chemical and riot control agents, smokes, and incendiaries, including bulk explosives and chemical warfare agents, chemical munitions, rockets, guided and ballistic missiles, bombs, warheads, mortar rounds, artillery ammunition, small arms ammunition, grenades, mines, torpedoes, depth charges, cluster munitions and dispensers, demolition charges, and devices and components thereof. The term does not include wholly inert items, improvised explosive devices, and nuclear weapons, nuclear devices, and nuclear components, except that the term does include non-nuclear components of nuclear devices that are managed under the nuclear weapons program of the DOE after all required sanitization operations under the Atomic Energy Act of 1954 (42 U.S.C. 2011 et seq.) have been completed. (10 U.S.C. 101(e)(4)(A) through (C)).

EM 385-1-1
15 Sep 08

Miscellaneous-Type Hooks: Hooks that do not support a load in a direct-pull configuration, such as grab hooks, foundry hooks, sorting hooks and choker hooks.

Misfire: an explosive charge that failed to detonate.

Mixed-gas diving: a diving mode in which the diver breathes mixture other than air, e.g., helium-oxygen, (OEA).

Mobile conveyor: a conveyor supported on a structure that is movable under its own power.

Monorail: a single run of overhead track.

Motor vehicle: <u>a sedan, van, SUV, truck, motorcycle, or other mode of conveyance intended for use on public roadways, and includes construction equipment that is driven on public highways. It is not intended to apply to</u> equipment designed exclusively for use off the highway.

Mud capping (bulldozing, adobe blasting, or dobying): blasting by placing a quantity of explosives against a rock or other object without confining the explosives in a drill hole.

Mudsill: a 2-in x 10-in x 8-in (5.1-cm x 25.4-cm x 20.3-cm) (minimum) wood plate that is used to distribute the scaffolding load over a suitable ground area. The size of the mudsill is determined by the load carried over a particular ground area and by the nature of the soil supporting the sills.

Multi-employer work site: a work site where more than one employer occupies the same work site. The Government considers the Prime Contractor to be the "controlling authority" for all subcontractors.

Multiple-lift rigging (Christmas tree lifting): a rigging assembly manufactured by wire rope rigging suppliers that facilitates the attachment of up to five independent loads to the hoist rigging of a crane.

EM 385-1-1
15 Sep 08

Multipurpose dry chemical: a dry chemical that is approved for use on Class A, Class B, and Class C fires.

<u>**Munitions and Explosives of Concern (MEC).** This term, which distinguishes specific categories of military munitions that may pose unique explosives safety risks means Unexploded ordnance (UXO), Discarded military munitions (DMM), or Munitions constituents (e.g., TNT, RDX), as defined in 10 U.S.C. 2710(e)(3), present in high enough concentrations to pose an explosive hazard.</u>

Negative pressure respirator (tight fitting): a respirator in which the air pressure inside the facepiece is negative during inhalation with respect to the ambient air pressure outside the respirator.

Nitrox Gas (EANx): Any oxygen/nitrogen mixture exceeding the ratio of 21% oxygen/79% nitrogen found naturally occurring in air.

No-decompression limits: the depth-time limits of the "no-decompression limits and repetitive dive group designation table for no-decompression air dives" as specified in the U.S. Navy Diving Manual or equivalent.

Nominal dimension: the dimension of material before it is surfaced and finished.

Non-guided personnel hoist system: a hoist system used to transport personnel in a device that is not attached to fixed tracks or guide ropes (a boatswain's chair is an example of a non-guided personnel hoist).

Non-ionizing radiation: those electromagnetic radiations that do not cause ionization (but may be absorbed) in biological systems; includes low frequency ultraviolet light, infrared light, heat, laser, microwaves, and radio waves.

Nonmetallic-sheathed cable: a factory assembly of two or more insulated conductors having an outer sheath of moisture-resistant, flame-retardant, nonmetallic material.

EM 385-1-1
15 Sep 08

Non-Permit Required Confined Space: a confined space that does not contain, or <u>have the potential to contain an atmospheric hazard capable of causing death or physical harm. The atmosphere should be proven by air monitoring to be free of hazard.</u>

Normally unoccupied remote facility: a facility operated, maintained, or serviced by employees who visit the facility only periodically to check its operation and to perform necessary operating or maintenance tasks. No employees are permanently stationed at the facility. Facilities meeting this definition are not contiguous with, and must be geographically remote from, all other buildings, processes, or persons.

Nosing: that portion of a tread projecting beyond the top of the tread immediately below.

Notch: when cutting a tree to be felled, a notch is cut into the tree on the same side to which the tree is to fall; the notch consists of a horizontal cut (of depth approximately one-third the tree's diameter); the top of the notch is cut at a 45° angle from a height of 2.5 in (6.4 cm) per 1 ft (0.3 m) of diameter above the base of the notch.

OEA: > *See Nitrox Gas*

<u>**OE Safety Specialist.** A USACE employee who is qualified through experience and completion of the U.S. Army Bomb Disposal School, Aberdeen Proving Ground, Maryland, or U.S. Naval EOD School, Indian Head, Maryland ,or Eglin AFB, Florida, and is classified in the GS-0018 job series (CP-12 career series). Performs safety and occupational health support and oversight of projects involving MEC/RCWM.</u>

Open conductors: wires that are run as separate conductors, in contrast to wires run through conduit, cables, or raceways.

Opening: a gap or void 12 in (30.5 cm) or more in its least dimension in a floor, roof, or other walking/working surface.

EM 385-1-1
15 Sep 08

Skylights and smoke domes that do not meet the strength requirements of 29 CFR 1926.754(e)(3) shall be regarded as openings.

Operational performance test: a test, conducted without a test load, to determine the proper operation of a crane.

Outrigger: extendable or fixed structural members with one end attached to the base of a piece of equipment and the other end resting on floats on the ground: used to distribute loads in supporting equipment.

Outrigger float: the pedestal (or bearing pad) on which an outrigger beam is supported.

Outside post: the post away from the structure against which the scaffold is erected.

Overexposure: an exposure to a safety or health hazard above the PEL or, if there is no PEL, above the published exposure levels for the hazard.

Overland conveyor: a single or series of belt conveyors designed to carry material across a distance, usually following the general contour of the load.

Overriding operational necessity: circumstances in which essential work cannot be delayed for safety or environmental reasons, or could not reasonably have been anticipated.

Oxyfuel gas cutting: an oxygen cutting process that uses heat from an oxyfuel gas flame.

Oxyfuel gas welding: a welding process that joins work pieces by heating them with an oxyfuel gas flame

Oxygen deficient atmosphere: an atmosphere with an oxygen content below 19.5% by volume.

EM 385-1-1
15 Sep 08

Oxygen enriched atmosphere: an atmosphere containing more than 23.5% oxygen by volume.

Peak particle velocity: a measure of how fast the ground moves during an explosive blast.

Pendant: a rope or strand of specified length with fixed end connections.

Performance test: a test to determine the proper operation of a crane and the ability of the crane to safely lift loads within its performance rating. A performance test includes operational performance tests and load performance tests.

Perimeter protection: measures taken to prevent personnel, vehicles, and materials from falling into an excavation:

a. **Class I perimeter protection** guarding against personnel falling into an excavation it shall meet the following:

(1) Have the strength, height, and maximum deflection requirements for guardrails;

(2) Provide fall protection equivalent to that provided by a toprail, midrail, and toeboard; and

(3) Have post spacing equivalent to a standard guardrail.

b. **Class I perimeter protection** guarding against traffic (vehicles and/or equipment) falling into an excavation ishall be designed, by a qualified person, to withstand the potential forces and bending moments due to impact by traffic.

c. **Class II perimeter protection**: consists of warning barricades or flagging placed at a distance not closer than 6 ft (1.8 m) from the edge of the excavation: warning barricades or flagging do not have to meet the requirements for Class I perimeter protection but do need to display an adequate warning at an elevation of 3 ft (0.9 m) to 4 ft (1.2 m) above ground level.

d. **Class III perimeter protection**: warning barricades or flagging placed a distance not closer than 6 in (15.2 cm) nor more than 6 ft (1.8 m) from the edge of the excavation: warning barricades or flagging do not have to meet the requirements for Class I perimeter protection but do need to display an adequate warning at an elevation of 3 ft (0.9 m) to 4 ft (1.2 m) above ground level.

Permanent floor: a structurally completed floor at any level or elevation (including slab on grade).

Permit-required confined space (permit space): a confined space that has one or more of the following characteristics:

a. Contains or has the potential to contain a hazardous atmosphere,

b. Contains a material that has the potential for engulfing an entrant,

c. Has an internal configuration such that an entrant could be trapped or asphyxiated by inwardly converging walls or by a floor that slopes downward and tapers to a smaller cross-section, or

d. Contains any other recognized serious safety or health hazard.

Personal Eyewash Units: Personal eyewash units are portable, supplementary units that support plumbed units or self-contained units, or both, by delivering immediate flushing for approximately 15 minutes. May not be used by themselves as eyewash protection.

Personal fall arrest system: an engineered system used to arrest an employee in a fall; consists of an anchorage, connectors, body harness, and may include a lanyard, deceleration device, lifeline, or suitable combination of these.

Personal fall protection system: an engineered system that protects employees from falls.

Physician/ Licensed healthcare professional (PLHCP): an individual whose legally permitted scope of practice (i.e., license, registration, or certification) allows him/her to independently provide, or be delegated the responsibility to provide, some or all of the health care services required by 05.E.08.

Plank platform: a work platform made up of wood boards (oriented horizontally).

Planking: a wood board or fabricated component that is used as a flooring member.

Point of anchorage: a secure point of attachment for lifelines, lanyards, or deceleration devices.

Portable electric tools: electric equipment intended to be moved from one place to another.

Portable ladder: a ladder that can be readily moved or carried.

Portable tank: any closed vessel having a liquid capacity over 60 gal (0.23 m^3) and not intended for fixed installation.

Portal: the entrance to a tunnel.

Position hazard analysis (PHA): a documented process by which the duties (or tasks) of an employee's job position are outlined, the actual or potential hazards of each duty are identified, and measures for the elimination or control of those hazards are developed.

EM 385-1-1
15 Sep 08

Positioning system: a body harness system rigged to allow a worker to be supported on an elevated vertical surface, such as a wall, and work with both hands free while leaning.

Positive-pressure respirator: a respirator in which the pressure inside the respiratory inlet covering exceeds the ambient air pressure outside the respirator.

Potable Water: water which meets the quality standards prescribed in the U.S. Public Health Service Drinking Water Standards, published in 42 CFR Part 72, or water which is approved for drinking purposes by the State or local authority having jurisdiction.

Powered air-purifying respirator (PAPR): an air-purifying respirator that uses a blower to force the ambient air through air-purifying elements to the inlet covering.

Powered industrial truck (PIT): a mobile power propelled truck used to carry, push, pull, lift, stack, or tier materials; Excluded are vehicles used for earth moving and over-the-road hauling; Includes forklifts, pallet trucks, rider trucks, forktrucks, lifttrucks. *> See Forklift*.

Pre-discharge employee alarm: an alarm that will sound at a set time before actual discharge of an extinguishing system so that employees may evacuate the discharge area before system discharge.

Pre-entry briefings: an information briefing given by the site safety and health supervisor to employees before their entry to an HTRW site and instructing employees in the contents of the site-SSHP.

Premises wiring: the interior and exterior wiring, including power, lighting, control, and signal circuit wiring with all of the associated hardware, fittings, and wiring devices, both permanently and temporarily installed, which extend from the load-end of the service lateral conductors to the outlets.

EM 385-1-1
15 Sep 08

Prescribed fire: any fire ignited to meet specific management objectives.

Pressure demand respirator: a positive-pressure, atmosphere-supplying respirator that admits breathing air to the facepiece when the positive pressure is reduced inside the facepiece by inhalation.

Pressure systems: all pipe, tubing, valves, controls, and other devices that operate or are maintained above atmospheric pressure. **> See definition of Vacuum systems.**

Primer: a cartridge or container of explosives into which a detonator or detonating cord is inserted or attached.

Prohibited condition: any condition in a permit space that is not allowed by the permit during the period when entry is authorized.

Protective system: a method of protecting employees from cave-ins, from material falling into an excavation, or from the collapse of adjacent structures; includes benching, sloping, shoring, trench shields, underpinning, rock bolting, etc.

Purlin (in systems-engineered metal buildings): a "Z" or "C" shaped member formed from sheet steel spanning between primary framing and supporting roof material.

Qualified line-clearance tree trimmer: a tree worker who, through related training and on-the-job experience, is familiar with the hazards in line clearance and has demonstrated his/her ability in the performance of the special techniques involved.

Qualified line-clearance tree trimmer trainee: any worker undergoing line-clearance tree trimming training who, in the course of such training, is familiar with the hazards in line clearance and has demonstrated his/her ability in the performance of the special techniques involved.

EM 385-1-1
15 Sep 08

Qualified person: one who, by possession of a recognized degree, certificate, or professional standing, or extensive knowledge, training, and experience, has successfully demonstrated his/her ability to solve or resolve problems related to the subject matter, the work, or the project.

Qualified Person (Electrical): One who has received training in and has demonstrated skills and knowledge in the construction and operation of electrical equipment and installations and the hazards involved. This includes the skills and techniques necessary to distinguish exposed live parts from other parts of electric equipment, to determine the nominal voltage of exposed live parts, the clearance distances and corresponding voltages to which the qualified person will be exposed.
Note 1: Whether an employee is considered to be a "qualified person" will depend upon various circumstances in the workplace, e.g., an individual may be considered "qualified" with regard to certain equipment in the workplace, but "unqualified" as to other equipment.
Note 2: An employee who is undergoing on-the-job training and who, in the course of such training, has demonstrated an ability to perform duties safely at his level of training and who is under the direct supervision of a qualified person is considered to be a qualified person for the performance of those duties.

Qualified person for fall protection: a person with a recognized degree or professional certificate and with extensive knowledge, training, and experience in the fall protection and rescue field who is capable of designing, analyzing, evaluating and specifying fall protection and rescue systems.

Qualified Rigger (Qualified Rigging Supervisor, Qualified Lift Supervisor): an employee that will rig loads or oversee the rigging of loads for hoisting. Employee must be at least 18 years of age; Be able to communicate effectively with the crane operator, the lift supervisor, flagman and affected employees on site; Have basic knowledge and understanding of equipment-operating characteristics, capabilities, and limitations; AND shall be able to demonstrate adequate knowledge and proficiency in the following:

EM 385-1-1
15 Sep 08

<u>Personnel roles and responsibilities; Site preparation (terrain, environment); Rigging equipment and materials; Safe Operating procedures as related to rigging; Principles of safe rigging; Environmental hazards (overhead interferences); Rigging the load, handling the load, common causes of crane-related accidents.</u>

Qualified tree worker: an individual who, through related training and on-the-job experience, is familiar with equipment, techniques, and hazards of tree maintenance and removal and with the equipment used in such operations and has demonstrated his/her ability in the performance of the special techniques involved.

Qualitative fit test (QLFT): a pass/fail fit test to assess the adequacy of respirator fit that relies on the individual's response to the test agent.

Quantitative fit test (QNFT): an assessment of the adequacy of respirator fit by numerically measuring the amount of leakage into the respirator.

Rad: a measure of the dose of ionizing radiation to the body tissue in terms of the energy absorbed per unit of mass of the tissue.

Radiant energy: the energy of electromagnetic waves produced by movement of molecules excited by the heat of an electric arc, gas flame, or the passage of electric current. Includes ultraviolet, visible light, and infrared energy.

Radiation area: any area, accessible to personnel, in which there exists radiation at such levels that a major portion of the body could receive in any 1 hour a dose in excess of 5 mrem, or in any 5 consecutive 8-hour days a dose in excess of 100 mrem.

Radioactive material: any material that emits, by spontaneous nuclear disintegration, electromagnetic or particulate emanations.

Radiological device: machinery or equipment that produces or contains ionizing radiation, such as nuclear density meters and radiographic testing machines.

EM 385-1-1
15 Sep 08

Rails: the side structural members of a ladder to which rungs, cleats, or steps are attached.

Recompression chamber: a pressure vessel for human occupancy such as a surface decompression chamber, closed bell, or deep diving system used to decompress divers to treat decompression sickness.

Reconfiguration: the addition or subtraction of boom, jib, counterweight or, for a fixed crane, a change in foundation.

Red Flag Barge/vessel: a barge/vessel carrying in bulk, hazardous cargoes regulated by SubChapter D (petroleum) and O (chemical) of Chapter I, Title 46 CFR of Certain Dangerous Cargoes (flammable or other hazardous materials) OR Vessels whose primary purpose is the transporting of flammable or other hazardous cargos e.g. oil tankers, chemical parcel tankers, liquid chemical barges, liquefied gas tankers, etc.).

Reeving: a rope system in which the rope travels around drums and sheaves.

Rem (roentgen equivalent in man): a measure of the dose of ionizing radiation to body tissue in terms of its biological effect; the dose required to produce the same biological effect as one roentgen of high-penetration of x-rays.

Rescue system: an assembly of components and subsystems used for self-rescue or assisted-rescue

Residential Type Construction. Regardless of structure size, projects where the materials, methods and procedures are essentially the same as those used in building a typical single-family home or townhouse. Wood framing (not steel or concrete), wooden floor joists and roof structures are characteristic of the materials used, and traditional wood frame construction techniques are used in construction. Structures that use metal studs are considered residential construction if they meet the other criteria for residential construction.

EM 385-1-1
15 Sep 08

Rest: a period of time during which the person concerned is off duty; is not performing work, including administrative tasks; and is afforded the opportunity for uninterrupted sleep. This does not include time for breaks, meals, or travel.

Restraint system: a combination of anchorage, anchorage connector, lanyard (or other mean of connection), and body support that limits travel in such as manner that the user is not exposed to a fall hazard.

Restricted area: when used in conjunction with ionizing radiation, any area to which access is controlled by the employer for purposes of protecting individuals from exposure to ionizing radiation.

Roll out: A process by which a snaphook or carabiner unintentionally disengages from another connector or object to which it is coupled.

Rope Access: a variety of advanced access techniques where roped and specialized equipment are used as the primary method for providing access and support to workers in their jobs at high or hard-to-reach places.

Rope Access Supervisor: A person with the training, skills, experience and qualifications necessary to assume responsibility for the entire rope access work site, including management and guidance of other Rope Access Technicians on the worksite; is capable of designing, analyzing, evaluating and specifying rope access systems and has the knowledge and experience to direct rescue operations from rope access systems, as well as the skills necessary to perform advanced rescue from rope access systems.

Rope Access Worker: A person with the appropriate training, skills, and qualifications for performing, under the direct supervision of a Rope Access Leader, Technician or Supervisor, standard rope access operations and, at a minimum, has the skills necessary to perform limited rescue from rope access systems.

EM 385-1-1
15 Sep 08

Rope grab: see fall arrestor.

Rope-guided personnel hoist system: a hoist system, used to transport personnel in a cage, which is guided by wire ropes as differentiated from a hoist system using anchored rail arrangements.

Rotation resistant rope: a wire rope consisting of an inner layer of strand laid in one direction covered by a layer of strand laid in the opposite direction: this has the effect of counteracting torque by reducing the tendency of the finished rope to rotate.

Runner: a horizontal scaffold member that forms a tie between posts and may also support a bearer.

Runway: a personnel passageway elevated above the surrounding floor or ground level, such as a foot walk along shafting or a walkway between scaffolds.

Saddle-jib: a type of jib on a tower crane that is supported by pendants. The jib is horizontal or nearly horizontal, non-luffing, and the load hook is suspended by a trolley that moves along the jib.

Safe for Workers: denotes a confined space on floating plant that meets the following criteria:

   a. The oxygen content of the atmosphere is at least 19.5 percent and below 22 percent by volume;

   b. The concentration of flammable vapors is below 10 percent of the lower explosive limit (LEL);

   c. Any toxic materials in the atmosphere associated with cargo, fuel, tank coatings, or inerting media are within permissible concentrations at the time of the inspection.

Safety and Occupational Health Office Dive Safety Representative: the Safety and Occupational Health Office

EM 385-1-1
15 Sep 08

representative assigned the responsibility of dive safety. This individual provides dive safety advice to operational elements and actively participates in the review and comment process for all diving plans and hazard analyses, as well as on-site monitoring of diving operations; must successfully complete the USACE diving safety, diving supervisor, or diving inspector course and maintain certification by attending a HQUSACE-sponsored dive inspector course every 4 years. Unless required by position, this individual is not required to perform 12 working/training dives to maintain certification.

Safety belt: See "Body Belt".

Safety can: an approved container, of not more than 5 gal (18.9 L) capacity, having a spring-closing lid and spout cover and designed to safety relieve internal pressures under fire exposure.

Safety deck attachment: an initial attachment that is used to secure an initially placed sheet of decking to keep proper alignment and bearing with structural support members.
Safety factor: the ratio of the ultimate braking strength of a member or piece of material or equipment to the actual working stress or safe working load when in use.

Safety harness: See "Full Body Harness".

Safety Monitoring System: Safety System where Competent Personfor Fall Protection is responsible for recognizing and warning employees of fall hazards.

Safety precaution area: those portions of approach-departure clearance zones and transitional zones where placement of objects incident to contract performance might result in vertical projections at or above the approach-departure clearance or the transitional surface.

Safety Professional: Because of the wide variety of safety, health and environmental responsibilities safety professionals undertake, a simple definition has not been widely accepted within the profession. Instead, industry looks to ANSI Z590.2, Criteria for Establishing the "Scope and Functions of the Professional Safety Position".

Safety relief valves: valves that relieve excess pressure or vacuum (depending on their design) that would otherwise damage equipment or cause injury to personnel.

Safety sign: a visual alerting device in the form of a sign, label, decal, placard, or other marking that advises the observer of the nature and degree of the potential hazard(s) that can cause an accident. It may also provide other directions to eliminate or reduce the hazard and may advise of the probable consequences of not avoiding the hazard.

Safety sign alert symbol: a symbol that indicates a potential personal injury hazard. It is composed of an equilateral triangle surrounding an exclamation mark.

Safety sign message panel: area of the safety sign that contains those words related to: identification of the hazard, how to avoid the hazard, and probable consequences of not avoiding the hazard.

Safety sign panel: area of a safety sign having a distinctive background color different from adjacent areas of the sign or which is clearly delineated by a line or margin.

Safety sign signal word panel: area of the safety panel that contains the signal word.

Safety tag: a device usually made of card stock, paper, paperboard, plastic, or other material on which letters, markings, symbols, or combinations thereof, appear for the purpose of alerting persons to the presence of a temporary hazard or hazardous condition created by situations such as shipment, setup, service, or repair. The tag is removed when the hazard or hazardous condition no longer exists.

EM 385-1-1
15 Sep 08

Scaffold: temporary elevated platform and its supporting structure used for supporting worker(s), materials, or both.

Scaffold, double pole: a scaffold supported from the base by a double row of posts. This scaffold is independent of support from walls and is constructed of posts, runners, horizontal platform bearers, and diagonal bracing (also known as independent pole scaffold).

Scaffold, float: a scaffold hung from overhead supports by means of ropes and consisting of a unit having diagonal bracing underneath. The scaffold rests upon and is securely fastened to two parallel plank bearers at right angles to the span (also known as ship scaffold).

Scaffold, Hanging: A scaffold consisting of a work platform supported by hooks or brackets that are part of the scaffold structure and are directly attached to or hanging on a wall, lock gate, or similar vertical structure, providing an elevated work area for those engaged in repairing or modifying the vertical structure.

Scaffold, horse: a scaffold for light or medium duty that is composed of horses supporting a platform.

Scaffold, interior-hung: a suspended scaffold consisting of a work platform suspended from the ceiling or roof structure by fixed length supports.

Scaffold, ladder jack (PROHIBITED): a light-duty supported scaffold consisting of a platform supported by brackets attached to ladders.

Scaffold, Large area: a scaffold erected over substantially the entire work area. For example: a scaffold erected over the entire floor area of a room.

Scaffold, Lean-to (prohibited): a supported scaffold which is kept erect by tilting it toward and resting it against a building or structure.

Scaffold, load ratings: maximum loadings for the following categories:

   a. **Heavy duty**: a scaffold designed and constructed to carry a working load of 75 lbs per square foot (366.2 kg/m^2), that is intended for stone masonry work, with storage material on the platform.

   b. **Medium duty**: a scaffold designed and constructed to carry a working load of 50 lbs per square foot (244.1 kg/m^2), that is intended for bricklayers or plasterers, with weight of material in addition to workers.

   c. **Light duty**: a scaffold designed and constructed to carry specific working load of 25 lbs per square foot (122.1 kg/m^2), that is intended for workers only, with no material storage other than weight for tools.

   d. **Special duty**: a scaffold designed and constructed to carry specific types of objects, such as palletized materials. The design of planks and other types of scaffold units, the scaffold, and accessories shall be based on categories of load ratings.

Scaffold, manually propelled: a scaffold assembly supported by casters and moved only manually.

Scaffold, mason's multiple-point adjustable suspension: a scaffold having a continuous platform supported by bearers suspended by wire rope hoists from overhead supports.

Scaffold, metal frame: a scaffold consisting of a work platform supported by prefabricated metal frames.

Scaffold, needle-beam: a platform resting on two bearers that is suspended by a line.

Scaffold, outrigger: a scaffold consisting of a work unit supported by outriggers projecting beyond the wall or face of the building or structure, the inboard ends of which are secured inside of such building or structure.

Scaffold, pump jack: a scaffold consisting of a work platform supported by movable support brackets mounted on vertical poles.

Scaffold, single-point suspension: a scaffold supported by a single wire rope from an overhead support so arranged and operated as to permit the raising or lowering of the platform to desired working position.

Scaffold, single pole: a unit resting on bearers or cross beams. The outside ends of this unit are supported on runners secured to a single row of posts or uprights, and the inner ends of this unit are supported on or in the wall.

Scaffold, stonesetters' multiple-point adjustable suspension: a swinging type scaffold having a unit supported by members that is suspended at four points.

Scaffold, system: a scaffold consisting of posts with fixed connection points that accept runners, bearers, and diagonals that can be interconnected at predetermined levels.

Scaffold, tube and coupler: a scaffold consisting of a work platform supported by individual pieces of tubing (uprights, bearers, runners, bracing) connected with couplers.

Scaffold, two-point suspension (swinging scaffold/swinging stage): a suspension scaffold consisting of a platform supported by hangers (stirrups) suspended by two ropes from overhead supports and equipped with means to raise and lower the platform.

Scaffold, window jack: a supported scaffold consisting of a platform supported by a bracket or jack that projects through a window opening.

EM 385-1-1
15 Sep 08

Scaled distance: a scaled factor (ft/lb units) of the potential damage to a structure, based on the distance from the nearest structure to the blast site and the weight of explosives per delay.

Scaling: the removal of loose, overhanging, protruding, or otherwise precariously positioned material from above or along the sides of an excavation.

Scheduled work: Work that is regular and recurring, in that it forms a similar pattern for more than 50% of a working tour.

Scientific Diving: Diving performed solely as a necessary part of a scientific, research, or educational activity by employees whose sole purpose for diving is to perform scientific research tasks. Tasks are light to medium duty, such as environmental or ecological surveys, filming/ recording flora and fauna, biological sample collection, and placement of scientific monitoring equipment. Scientific diving does not include placing or removing heavy objects underwater, regardless of its purpose, or performing any tasks usually associated with commercial diving such as, but not limited to: inspection/ assessment of underwater pipelines, structures and similar objects for structural reasons; construction; demolition; cutting or welding; or the use of explosives.

Scissors lift: a raising/lowering device that is supported or stabilized by one or more pantograph leg sections.

SCUBA: an acronym for self-contained underwater breathing apparatus, in which the supply of breathing mixture carried by the diver is independent of any other source.

Sea-keeping: the aspects of a vessel's design and construction that determine its ability to operate efficiently in the body of water where it will operate (e.g., stability, strength, and speed).

Sea-worthy: a vessel that is fit in all aspects for the anticipated perils of the voyage and will carry the crew and cargo in a safe condition.

Self-contained breathing apparatus (SCBA): an atmosphere-supplying respirator for which the breathing air source is designed to be carried by the user.

Self-retracting lanyard: a deceleration device containing a drum wound line that automatically locks at the onset of a fall to arrest the user, but that automatically pays out from and retracts onto the drum during normal movement of the person to whom the line is attached, , after onset of a fall, automatically locks the drum and arrests the fall.

Separately derived system: a premises wiring system whose power is derived from generator, transformer, or converter winding and has no direct electrical connection, including a solidly connected grounded circuit conductor, to supply conductors originating in another system.

Service: the conductors and equipment for delivering electric energy from the serving utility to the wiring system of the premises served.

Service conductors: the conductors from the service point to the service disconnecting means.

Service drop: the overhead service conductors from the last pole or other aerial support to and including the splices, if any, connecting to the service-entrance conductors at the building or other structure.

Service life: the period of time that a respirator, filter or sorbent, or other respiratory equipment provides adequate protection to the wearer.

Service station (automotive): that portion of property where liquids used as motor fuels are stored and dispensed from fixed equipment into the fuel tanks of motor vehicles or approved containers and shall include any facilities for the sale and service of tires, batteries, and accessories.

EM 385-1-1
15 Sep 08

Service station (marine): that portion of a property where liquids used as fuels are stored and dispensed from equipment on shore, piers, wharves, or floating docks into the fuel tanks of self-propelled craft.

Shackle: a U-shaped metal fitting with a pin through the ends.

Shaft: a passage made from the surface of the ground to a point underground; shafts cut through the ground at an angle greater than 20° to the horizontal. **> See definition of Tunnel.**

Shallow dose equivalent: applies to the external exposure of the skin or an extremity. It is taken as the dose equivalent at a tissue depth of 0.007 cm averaged over an area of 1.6 in^2 (10 cm^2).

Shear connector: headed steel studs, steel bars, steel lugs, and similar devices that are attached to a structural member for the purpose of achieving composite action with concrete.

Sheave: the grooved wheel of a pulley or block over which rope or cable is passed.

Sheeting: **> See Upright**.

Shield: a structure that is designed to withstand the forces imposed on it by the walls of an excavation and prevents cave-ins.

Ship repair: includes any repair of a vessel including, but not restricted to, alterations, conversion, installation, cleaning, painting, and maintenance work. This includes work in confined and enclosed spaces and other dangerous atmospheres in vessels, vessel sections, and on land-side operations regardless of geographic location.

Shoring: a support member that resists compressive forces imposed by a load.

Site control procedures: procedures delineated in the site control program that will be used to minimize any potential contamination

EM 385-1-1
15 Sep 08

of workers, protect members of the public from the site's hazards, and prevent vandalism.

Site Safety and Health Officer (SSHO): the superintendent or other qualified or competent person who is responsible for on-site safety and health.

Site Safety and Health Officer (HTRW): the person on-site with the responsibility for implementation of the APP and SSHP appendix at HTRW activities.

Site Safety and Health Manager (SHM): the CIH, CSP, or CHP responsible for development and enforcement of the APP and SSHP appendix for HTRW activities.

Site safety and health plan (SSHP): an appendix to the APP that describes the site-specific practices.

Site work zones: zones of differing work activities and hazards established to reduce the accidental spread of hazardous substances from a contaminated to an uncontaminated area and to control exposure of personnel to HTRW hazards. There are generally three categories of site work zones:

    a. **Exclusion zones**, where contamination does or could occur,

    b. **Contamination-reduction zones**, which are transition areas between contaminated areas and clean areas and where decontamination takes place, and

    c. **Support zones**, which are uncontaminated areas where administrative and support functions are located.

Sling: an assembly used for lifting when connected to a lifting mechanism at the sling's upper end and when supporting a load at the sling's lower end. *> See Figure 15-4.*

EM 385-1-1
15 Sep 08

Sling - basket: loading with the sling passed under the load with both ends, end attachments, eyes, or handles on the hook or a single master link.

Sling - choker: loading with the sling passed through one end attachment, eye, or handle and suspended by the other.

Sloping: a method of protecting employees from cave-ins by cutting the sides of the excavation in the arrangement of slopes; The angle of the slope needed to prevent cave-in is a function of the soil type, environmental factors such as moisture and freezing weather, and the magnitude and location of any loads and vibration surcharged upon the slopes.

Sling - vertical: a load suspended on a single, vertical, part or leg.

Small hose system: a system of hose, ranging in diameter from 5/8 in (1.6 cm), that is for use by employees and provides a means for the control and extinguishment of incipient stage fire.

Snap hook: a connector comprised of a hook-shaped body with a normally closed gate, or similar arrangement that may be opened to permit the hook to receive an object and, when released, automatically closes to retain the object. The locking type has a self-closing, self-locking keeper that remains locked until unlocked and pressed open for connection or disconnection.

Snap-ties: a concrete wall-form tie, the end of which can be twisted or snapped off after the forms have been removed.

Snow Machine: any vehicle designed to travel over ice and snow using mechanical propulsion in conjunction with skis, belts, cleats or low-pressure tires.

Soldering: a welding process that joins materials by heating them to a temperature that will not melt them but will melt a filler material which adheres to them and forms a joint.

EM 385-1-1
15 Sep 08

Sound pressure: steady state: sound that does not significantly change in intensity or frequency with time.

Specialty Vehicles: all other vehicles not meeting definition of motor vehicle, ATVs, ORVs, Utility Vehicles, machinery or mechanized equipment, dump truck, etc. Examples are golfcarts, Segway HT, snow machines/mobiles, etc.

Specular reflections: reflections from a smooth surface, such as a mirror, glass, metal, etc.

Spindle: a long tapered pin or rod serving as an axis in spinning.

Splice - eye: a splice formed by bending a rope's end back onto itself and splicing it into the rope so that a loop is formed.

Splice - hand tucked: a loop formed in the end of a rope by tucking the end of the strands back into the main body of the rope.

Splice - long: a splice without an appreciable increase of circumference that is used when the rope must run over a sheave or through a hole.

Splice - mechanical: a loop formed in the end of a rope and connected by pressing (swaging) one or more metal sleeves over the junction of the rope.

Splice - short: a splice using less material than a long splice but increasing the circumference.

Springing: the creation of a chamber or pocket in the bottom of a drill hole so that larger quantities of explosives may be inserted; made by the use of a moderate quantity of explosives.

Spring line: an imaginary line connecting the points at which the ceiling (roof) arches begin.

Sprinkler alarm: an approved device installed so that any discharge from a sprinkler system equal to or greater than that from

EM 385-1-1
15 Sep 08

a single automatic sprinkler will result in an audible signal on the premises.

Sprinkler system: a system of piping designed in accordance with fire protection engineering standards and installed to control or extinguish fires. The system includes an adequate and reliable water supply, a network of specialty sized piping and sprinklers that are interconnected, and a control valve and device for actuating an alarm when the system is in operation.

Stable rock: natural solid mineral material that can be excavated with vertical sides and remain intact while exposed.

Standby diver: a diver at the dive location available to assist a diver in the water; standby divers will be dressed for immediate entry into the water.

Standpipe system:

    a. **Class I standpipe system**: a 2-1/2 in (6.4 cm) hose connection for use by fire departments and those trained in handling heavy fire streams.

    b. **Class II standpipe system**: a 1-1/2 in (3.8 cm) hose system that provides a means for the control or extinguishment of incipient stage fires.

    c. **Class III standpipe system**: a combined system of hose that is for use by employees trained in the use of hose operations and that is capable of furnishing effective water discharge during the more advanced stages of fire (beyond the incipient stage) in the interior of workplaces.

Station bill: a placard that designates vessel personnel duties and procedures to be followed in the event of an emergency or emergency drill. Placards are permanently placed in personnel quarters and work areas, and are strategically located throughout the vessel.

Steel erection: the construction, alteration, or repair of steel buildings, bridges, and other structures, including the installation of metal decking and all planking used during the process of erection.

Steel joist: an open web, secondary load-carrying member of 144 ft (43.9 m) or less, designed by the manufacturer, used for the support of floors and roofs. This does not include structural steel trusses or cold-formed joists.

Steel joist girder: an open web, primary load-carrying member, designed by the manufacturer, used for the support of floors and roofs. This does not include structural steel trusses.

Steel truss: an open web member designed of structural steel components by the project structural engineer of record. A steel truss is considered equivalent to a solid web structural member.

Steep-sloped roof: a roof having a slope greater than 4 in 12 (vertical to horizontal).

Stemming: a suitable inert incombustible material or device used to confine or separate explosives in a drill hole or to cover explosives in mud capping.

Step stool: a self-supporting, foldable, portable ladder, non-adjustable in length, 32 in (81.3 cm) or less in height, with flat steps and without a pail shelf, designed to be climbed on the ladder top cap as well as all steps.

Stilts: a pair of poles or similar supports with raised footrests, used for walking above the ground or working surface.

Storage tank: any vessel having a liquid capacity that exceeds 60 gal (227.1 L) is intended for fixed installation and is not used for processing.

EM 385-1-1
15 Sep 08

Stored energy: energy (electrical, mechanical, or chemical) that might be found in a charge capacitor, a loaded spring, chemical solutions, or other similar hazardous form.

Strand laid rope: a wire rope made with strands formed around a fiber core, wire core, or independent wire rope core.

Strong irritant: a chemical that is not corrosive, but causes a strong temporary inflammatory effect on living tissue by chemical action at the site of contact.

Structural steel: a steel member, or a member made of a substitute material (such as, but not limited to, fiberglass, aluminum or composite members). These members include, but are not limited to, steel joists, joist girders, purlins, columns, beams, trusses, splices, seats, metal decking, girts, and all bridging, and cold-formed metal framing which is integrated with the structural steel framing of a building.

Supplied-air respirator (SAR) or airline respirator: an atmosphere-supplying respirator for which the source of breathing air is not designed to be carried by the user.

Support system: a structural means of supporting the walls of an excavation to prevent cave-ins; includes shields, shoring, underpinning, rock bolts, etc.

Surface-supplied air (SSA): a diving mode in which the diver in the water is supplied from the dive location with compressed air for breathing.

Swaged fittings: fittings in which wire rope is inserted and attached by cold flowing method.

Swinger mechanism: the device that rotates a derrick mast.

Swinging (hanging) lead: pile-driving leads that are suspended from an extended boom point sheave pin at the top of the boom. The bottom points of the leads are positioned astride the pile

EM 385-1-1
15 Sep 08

location, the hammer is vertically above the top of the pile. Often the bottoms of the leads are pointed and the weight of the pile leads and hammer force the bottom points into the ground, holding them in position.

Switch: a device for connecting two or more continuous package conveyor lines; an electrical control device; or a mechanism that transfers a trolley, carrier, or truck from one track to another at a converging or diverging section.

System: includes machinery, equipment, and electrical, hydraulic, and pneumatic lines and their subsystems.

Systems-engineered metal building: a metal, field-assembled building system consisting of framing, roof, and wall coverings. Typically, many of these components are cold-formed shapes. These individual parts are fabricated in one or more manufacturing facilities and shipped to the job site for assembly into the final structure. The engineering design of the system is normally the responsibility of the systems-engineered metal building manufacturer.

Tackle: an assembly of ropes and sheaves arranged for lifting, lowering and pulling.

Tagout: a form of hazardous energy control procedure using the placement of a tagout device, in accordance with established procedures, on an energy-isolating device to indicate that the energy-isolating device and the system being controlled may not be operated until the tagout device is removed.

Tagout device: a prominent warning device, such as a tag with a means of attachment, that can be securely attached to an energy-isolating device in accordance with established procedures to indicate that the energy-isolating device and system being controlled may not be operated until the tagout device is removed.

Tailing crane lift: a procedure sometimes used in erecting large pressure vessels or structural elements in which one crane (lead crane) lifts the top of the load and a second crane (tail crane), rigged to the bottom of the load, either secures the bottom of the load from movement or assists in the horizontal positioning of the load.

Take-up: the assembly of the necessary structural and mechanical parts that provides the means to adjust the length of belts, cables, chains, and similar transmission mechanisms to compensate for stretch, shrinkage, or wear, and to maintain proper tension.

Tandem crane lift: the use of two or more cranes to lift a load.
Taut-line hitch: a knot used for securing all workers aloft to their climbing rope, and consisting of either one or two wraps over two wraps.

Threshold limit values (TLV): airborne concentrations of substances and represent conditions under which it is believed that nearly all workers may be repeatedly exposed day after day without adverse health effects. Because of wide variation in individual susceptibility, however, a small percentage of workers may experience discomfort from some substances at concentrations at or below the threshold limit; a smaller percentage may be affected more seriously by aggravation of a pre-existing condition or by development of an occupational illness.

Tied in: the term that describes a tree climber whose climbing line has been properly crotched and attached to the saddle and whose taut-line hitch is tied.

Tight-fitting facepiece: a respiratory inlet covering that forms a complete seal with the face.

Toeboard: <u>a vertical barrier at floor level erected along exposed edges of a floor opening, wall opening, platform, runway, or ramp to prevent materials from falling.</u>

Tool rest (work rest): a device that prevents the tool or work piece from jamming between the abrasive wheel and the wheel guard.

EM 385-1-1
15 Sep 08

Top running bridge: a bridge that travels over top of a runway track.

Toprail: the uppermost horizontal rail of a guardrail system.

Total effective dose equivalent: the sum of the deep-dose equivalent (for external exposures) and the committed effective dose equivalent (for internal exposures).

Total fall distance: The total vertical distance a person falls, when using fall arrest equipment, measured from the onset of a fall to the point where the person comes to rest after the fall is stopped.

Total flooding systems: a fixed suppression system that is arranged to automatically discharge a predetermined concentration of agent into an enclosed space for fire extinguishment or control.

Toxic: pertaining to, or caused by, poison; poisonous; harmful.

Toxic chemical: is a chemical that produces serious injury or illness by absorption through any body surface

Track-guided personnel hoist system: a hoist system used to transport personnel in a car that is attached to fixed tracks or guide members.

Transitional surface: a sideways extension of all primary surfaces, clear zones, and approach-departure clearance surfaces along inclined planes.

Transitional zone: the ground area under the transitional surface (and adjoining the primary surface, clear zone, and approach-departure clearance zone).

Travel restraint system: See "Restraint System".

Travel time (marine): time spent transiting to and from the rest location when not immediately adjacent to or aboard the work site.

EM 385-1-1
15 Sep 08

Trench: an excavation that is narrow in relation to its length; in general, the depth is greater than the width, and the width is not greater than 15 ft (4.6 m).

Trim (floating crane barge): the angle of inclination about the transverse axis of the barge or pontoon.

Trolley: the unit that travels on bridge rails and supports the load block.

Trolley conveyor: a series of trolleys supported from or within an overhead truck and connected by endless propelling means, such as chain, cable, or other linkage, with loads usually suspended from the trolleys.

Trolley line: a horizontal line for direct attachment to a worker's body belt, lanyard, or deceleration device.

Truck (crane): the unit consisting of a frame, wheels, bearings, and axles that supports the bridge girders or trolleys.

Tunnel: an excavation beneath the surface of the ground, the longer axis of which makes an angle not greater than 20° to the horizontal. **> See definition of Shaft.**

Two-block damage prevention device: a system that will stall when two-blocking occurs without causing damage to the hoist rope or crane machinery components.

Two-block warning device: a warning device to alert the operator of an impending two-blocking condition.

Two-blocking: the condition when the lower load block or hook assembly comes in contact with the upper load block, or when the load block comes in contact with the boom tip.

Unexploded Ordnance (UXO). Military munitions that have been

EM 385-1-1
15 Sep 08

primed, fused, armed, or otherwise prepared for action, and have been fired, dropped, launched, projected or placed in such a manner as to constitute a hazard to operations, installation, properties (FUDS sites), personnel, or material and remain unexploded either by malfunction, design, or any other cause (10 U.S.C. 101(e)(5)(A) through (C)).

UXO-Qualified Personnel. Personnel who meet the training requirements for UXO personnel and have performed successfully in military EOD positions or are qualified to perform in the following service contract contractor positions: UXO Technician II, UXO Technician III, UXO Safety Officer, UXO Quality Control Specialist, and Senior UXO Supervisor. Refer to DDESB TP 18 for detailed information for approved contract titles and qualifications

Unfired pressure vessels: vessels that can withstand internal pressure or vacuum but do not have the direct fire of burning fuel or electric heaters (heat may be generated in the vessel due to chemical reactions or the application of heat to vessel contents).

Unmanned vessels: vessels that carry cargo such as materials, supplies, equipment, or liquids, and do not have personnel on board
during normal operations.

Unprotected sides and edges: any side or edge (except at entrances to points of access) of a walking/working surface (e.g., floor, roof, ramp or runway) where there is no wall or guardrail system.

Unsafe Condition: any physical state that is not acceptable or that presents risks to personal safety, or that has the potential to cause personal injury, illness, and/or damage to property. Also, any physical state that contributes to a reduction in the degree of safety normally present.

Upright: a vertical structural support member. In excavation support systems, uprights are placed in contact with the earth and are usually spaced so that individual uprights do not contact one

EM 385-1-1
15 Sep 08

another. Uprights that are spaced such that they are in contact with or interconnected to one another are referred to as sheeting.

USACE Diving Coordinator (UDC): a USACE employee assigned the responsibility for organizing, integrating, and monitoring the total dive program within a USACE Command. This individual and an alternate (to perform in the absence of the primary UDC) shall be appointed, in writing, by the USACE Commander/Director and shall assure adherence to all applicable rules and regulations: at the Major Subordinate Command (MSC) (Division), the Diving Coordinator shall provide program guidance and monitor and annually review the MSC dive program at all subordinate levels; at the District, Laboratory, and FOA level, the Diving Coordinator shall review all safe practices manuals, dive plans, medical certificates, and dive team qualifications and experience to assure compliance with this manual. The UDC and the alternate shall, as a minimum, successfully complete the HQUSACE-approved Diving Safety or Diving Supervisor Training Course and shall maintain certification by attending the diving refresher course every 4 years. UDCs attending the Diving Safety course are not required to perform 12 working/training dives unless they are in a dual position as a USACE diver or USACE Diving Supervisor.

USACE motor vehicle: any vehicle (government-owned; POV or Rental Car if be being used while on-duty in lieu of government-owned vehicle) provided for transportation of government personnel.

Utility Vehicles: Motorized off-highway vehicle capable of maneuvering over uneven terrain, having four or more low pressure tires, designed with side by side seats, seatbelts, steering wheel and optional cab/brush cage (not ROPS). Some offer ROPS as option. (e.g., Rangers, Rhino, M-Gators, Gators, and Mules).

Vehicle-mounted elevating and rotating work platforms: an elevating and rotating work platform mounted on the chassis of a commercial vehicle.

Vertical lifeline system: a vertically suspended flexible line connected from the top to an overhead anchorage and which a fall arrester travels and may also be attached to the bottom anchorage.

Vessel: every type of watercraft or artificial contrivance used, or capable of being used, as a means of transportation on water, including special-purpose floating structures not primarily designed for or used as a means of transportation on water.

Weathervaning: wind induced rotation of a crane superstructure, when out-of-service, to expose minimal surface area to the wind.

Weighting factor: factor that represents the proportion of the total stochastic (cancer plus genetic) risk resulting from irradiation to tissue to the total risk when the whole body is irradiated uniformly.

Wet bulb globe temperature (WBGT) index: a measurement of environmental factors that correlate with human deep body temperature and other physiological responses to heat.

Wet location: installations underground or in concrete slabs or masonry in direct contact with the earth and locations subject to saturation with water or other liquids, such as vehicle washing basins, and locations exposed to weather and unprotected.

Whaler: a horizontal structural member; in excavation support systems, whalers are placed parallel to the face of the excavation and bear against uprights or the excavation wall.

Whipline (runner or auxiliary line): a separate hoist rope system usually of a lighter load capacity than the main hoist.

Wild land fire: a planned or an unplanned fire in wild land fuels.

Work positioning system: See "Positioning System".

BLANK

EM 385-1-1
15 Sep 08

APPENDIX R

METRIC CONVERSION TABLE

Unit A Measure	To convert Unit A to B Measure multiply by:	To convert Unit B to A multiply by:	Unit B Measure
ACCELERATION			
Foot/second^2	0.3048	3.2808	Meter/second^2
ANGLES			
Mils (circular) true	0.0572	17.45	Degree, angular
Mils (circular) Russian	0.06	16.67	Degree, angular
Mils (circular) U.S. military	0.0562	17.78	Degree, angular
AREA			
Acre	4,047	2.471x10^{-4}	Meter^2
Acre	1.563x10^{-3}	640	Square miles
Acre	43,560		Square feet
Foot^2	0.0929	10.764	Meter^2
Inch^2	6.452	0.155	Centimeters^2
Mile^2 (US Statute)	2,589,988	3.861x10^{-7}	Meter^2
Yard^2	0.8361	1.1960	Meter^2
BENDING MOMENT (Torque)			
Kilogram-force-meter	9.8067	0.102	Newton-meter
Pound-force-foot	1.356	0.7376	Newton-meter

Unit A Measure	To convert Unit A to B Measure multiply by:	To convert Unit B to A multiply by:	Unit B Measure
CAPACITY (See Volume)			
DENSITY (See Mass/Volume)			
ENERGY (Includes Work)			
Foot-pound	0.001285	778.17	BTU
Foot-Pound	3.766×10^{-7}	2655224	Kilowatt-hours
Foot-pound-force	1.356	0.7376	Joule
Kilowatt-hour	3,600,000	2.778×10^{-7}	Joule
Kilowatt-hour	3412		BTU
Watt-second	1.000	1.000	Joule
FLOW (See Mass/Time or Volume/Time)			
FORCE			
Kilogram-force	9.8067	0.1020	Newton
Kip	4448	0.0002248	Newton
Pound-force (avoirdupois)	4.488	0.2248	Newton
FORCE/AREA (See Pressure)			
FORCE/LENGTH			
Pound-force/foot	14.59	0.06852	Newton/meter
LENGTH			
Angstrom	1.0×10^{-10}	1.0×10^{10}	Meter
Fathom	1.829	0.5468	Meter
Feet	0.3048	3.281	Meter
Feet	0.167	6	Fathoms
Inch	2.54	0.3937	Centimeter

EM 385-1-1
15 Sep 08

Unit A Measure	To convert Unit A to B Measure multiply by:	To convert Unit B to A multiply by:	Unit B Measure
Mil	2.540×10^{-5}	39370.1	Meter
Mile – Nautical	1852.000	0.0005	Meter
Mile – Statute	1609	0.0006	Meter
Mile – Statute	0.869	1.152	U.S. Nautical Mile
Mile –Statute	5,280	1.894×10^{-4}	Feet
Mile-Statute	1.6093	.6214	kilometers
LIGHT			
Foot candle	10.76	0.09290	Lumen/meter^2 (Lux)
MASS			
Grain	0.0648	15.43	Grams
Ounce (avdp)	0.02835	35.27	Kilogram
Ounce	.0625	16	Pound
Ounce (avdp)	437.5	0.002286	Grains
Ounce (troy)	480.0	0.00208	Grains
Pound (avdp)	0.0005	2240	Long or Gross Ton
Pound (avdp)	.4536	2.2046	Kilogram
Slug	14.59	0.06852	Kilogram
Ton (Long, 2240 lbs)	1016	0.0009842	Kilogram
Ton (Meter)	1000.00	0.001	Kilogram
Ton (Short, 2000 lbs)	907.2	0.001102	Kilogram
Ton (Net or short-tons)	0.8929	1.12	Ton (long or gross)

Unit A Measure	To convert Unit A to B Measure multiply by:	To convert Unit B to A multiply by:	Unit B Measure
MASS/AREA			
Pound-mass/foot^2	4.882	0.2048	Kilogram/meter^2
MASS/CAPACITY (See Mass/Volume)			
MASS/TIME (Includes Flow)			
Cubic feet per second	448.8	0.002228	US Gallons/min
Pound-mass per second	0.4536	2.205	Kilogram/second
Ton (short, mass) per hour	0.2520	3.968	Kilogram/second
MASS/VOLUME			
Pound-mass/foot^3	16.02	0.06243	Kilogram/meter^3
Pound-mass/inch^3	27680	3.613×10^{-5}	Kilogram/meter^3
Ton (long,mass)/yard^3	1329	0.0007525	Kilogram/meter^3
POWER			
Foot-pound-force/hour	3.766×10^{-4}	2655	Watt
Horsepower	550	0.001818	Foot-pounds per sec
Horsepower (550 ft-lb/s)	745.7	0.001341	Watt
Horsepower (water)	746.0	.001340	Watt

EM 385-1-1
15 Sep 08

Unit A Measure	To convert Unit A to B Measure multiply by:	To convert Unit B to A multiply by:	Unit B Measure
Horsepower (US)	1.014	0.9863	Horsepower (metric)
PRESSURE OR STRESS (Force/Area)			
Atmospheres (mean) 4^0 C.	33.90	0.02950	Feet of water
Atmospheres (mean)	14.70	0.0680	Pounds per sq inch
Atmospheres (mean)	29.92	0.03342	Inches of mercury
Feet of Water	62.43	0.01602	Pounds per sq foot
PSI	2.036	0.4912	Inches of mercury
SHIPPING			
Cubic feet	0.010	100.0	Register tons
Cubic feet	0.0250	40.0	US shipping tons
Cubic feet	0.0238	42.0	British shipping tons
SPEED (See Velocity)			
STRESS (See pressure)			
TEMPERATURE			
Degree Fahrenheit	t°C= (t°F-32)/1.8	t°F =1.8 t°C +32	Degree Celsius
Degree Fahrenheit	-17.22	33	Degree Celsius
TORQUE (See Bending Moment)			
VELOCITY (Includes Speed)			
Feet/second	0.3048	3.281	Meter/second
Feet/section	.6818	1.467	Miles/hour

Unit A Measure	To convert Unit A to B Measure multiply by:	To convert Unit B to A multiply by:	Unit B Measure
Kilometer/hour	0.2778	3.600	Meter/second
Knot (Int'l)	0.5144	1.944	Meter/second
Miles/hour	1.467	0.6818	Feet/second
Miles/hour			Kilometers/hour
Miles/hour (statute)		1.151	knots
VOLUME			
Board foot	0.0024	423.8	Meter^3
Foot^3	0.0283	35.31	Meter^3
Foot^3	1728	0.000579	Inches^3
Foot^3	7.481	0.1337	Gallons (US)
Gallon (Canadian)	0.0046	219.97	Meter^3
Gallon (US)	0.0038	264.2	Meter^3
Gallon (US)	0.8327	1.201	Gallons (Imperial)
Gallon (US)	3.7853	0.2642	Liter
Inch^3	1.6387x10^{-5}	61,024	Meter^3
Liter	0.0010	1000	Meter^3
Ton (register)	2.832	0.3532	Meter^3
Yard^3	.7646	1.308	Meter^3
VOLUME/TIME (Includes Flow)			
Foot^3/minute	4.719x10^{-4}	2,118.9	Meter^3/second
Yard^3/minute	0.0127	78.48	Meter^3/second
Gallon (U.S. liquid)/minute	6.309x10^{-5}	15,850	Meter^3/second

Unit A Measure	To convert Unit A to B Measure multiply by:	To convert Unit B to A multiply by:	Unit B Measure
WEIGHT, LINEAR			
Pounds/foot	1.488	0.672	Kilogram per meter
Pounds/yard	0.496	2.016	Kilogram per meter
WORK (See Energy)			

BLANK

EM 385-1-1
15 Sep 08

APPENDIX S

REFERENCES AND RESOURCES

SECTION A. REFERENCES

1. NUMBERED PUBLICATIONS

ACI 347	Guide to Formwork for Concrete
ANSI 01.1	Woodworking Machinery
ANSI A10.3	Safety Requirements for Powder-Activated Fastening Systems
ANSI A10.4	Safety Requirements for Personnel Hoists and Employee Elevators for Construction and Demolition Operations
ANSI A10.5	Safety Requirement for Material Hoists
ANSI A10.6	Safety Requirements for Demolition
ANSI A10.7	Safety Requirements for Commercial Explosives and Blasting Agents
ANSI A10.8	Safety Requirements for Scaffolding
ANSI A10.22	Safety Requirements for Rope-Guided and Non Guided Worker's Hoists
ANSI A10.34	Protection of the Public on or Adjacent to Construction Sites
ANSI A14.1	Ladders – Wood – Safety Requirements

ANSI A14.2	Ladders – Portable Metal – Safety Requirements
ANSI A14.3 -2008	Ladders – Fixed – Safety Requirements
ANSI A14.4	Safety Requirements for Job Made Wooden Ladders
ANSI B74.2	Specifications for Shapes and Sizes of Grinding Wheels, and for Shapes and Sizes and Identifications of Mounted Wheels
ANSI C95.4	Radio Frequency Antennas When Using Electric Blasting Caps During Explosive Operations
ANSI D6.1	Manual on Uniform Traffic Control Devices for Streets and Highways
ANSI Z41	Personnel Protection – Protective Footwear
ANSI Z80.3	Requirements for Nonprescription Sunglasses and Fashion Eyewear
ANSI Z88.2	Practices for Respiratory Protection
ANSI Z89.1	Personal Protection - Protective Headwear for Industrial Workers
<u>ANSI Z117.1</u>	<u>Confined Spaces</u>
ANSI Z136.1	Safe Use of Lasers
<u>ANSI Z244.1</u>	<u>Personnel Protection – Lockout/Tagout of Energy Sources</u>

ANSI Z308.1	Minimum Requirements for Workplace First Aid Kits
ANSI Z358.1	Emergency Eyewash and Shower Equipment
<u>ANSI Z490.1</u>	<u>Accepted Practices for Safety, Health and Environmental Training</u>
ANSI Z535.1	Safety Color Code
ANSI Z535.2	Environmental and Facility Safety Signs
ANSI Z535.5	Accident Prevention Tags (for temporary hazards)
ANSI/ACDE-01	Divers – Commercial Diver Training – Minimum Standard
ANSI/AGA GPTC Z380.1	GPTC Guide for the Gas Transmission and Distribution Piping System
ANSI/API 2C	Specification for Offshore Cranes
ANSI/ASME A13.1	Scheme for the Identification of Piping Systems
ANSI/ASME A17.1	Safety Code for Elevators and Escalators
ANSI/ASME B30.2	Overhead and Gantry Cranes, Top Running Bridge, Single or Multiple Girder, Top Running Trolley Hoist
ANSI/ASME B30.3	Construction Tower Cranes
ANSI/ASME B30.4	Portal, Tower, and Pedestal Cranes

ANSI/ASME B30.5	Mobile and Locomotive Cranes
ANSI/ASME B30.6	Derricks
ANSI/ASME B30.8	Floating Cranes and Floating Derricks
ANSI/ASME B30.9	Slings
<u>ANSI/ASME B30.10</u>	<u>Hooks</u>
ANSI/ASME B30.11	Monorails and Underhung Cranes
ANSI/ASME B30.12	Handling Loads Suspended from Rotorcraft
ANSI/ASME B30.17	Overhead and Gantry Cranes (Top Running Bridge, Single Girder, Underhung Hoist)
ANSI/ASME B30.22	Articulating Boom Cranes
<u>ANSI/ASME B30.26</u>	<u>Rigging Hardware</u>
ANSI/ASME B31.1	Power Piping
ANSI/ASME B56.1	Safety Standard for Low Lift and High Lift Trucks
<u>ANSI/ASSE A10.38</u>	<u>Basic Elements of an Employer's Program to Provide a Safe and Healthful Work Environment</u>
<u>ANSI/ASSE A10.44</u>	<u>Control of Energy Sources (Lockout/Tagout) for Construction and Demolition</u>

ANSI/ASSE Z87.1	Practice for Occupational and Educational Eye and Face Protection
<u>ANSI/ASSE Z359</u>	<u>Fall Protection Code</u>
<u>ANSI/ASSE Z359.0</u>	<u>Definitions and Nomenclature Used for Fall Protection and Fall Arrest</u>
<u>ANSI/ASSE Z359.1</u>	<u>Safety Requirements for Personal Fall Arrest Systems, Subsystems and Components</u>
<u>ANSI/ASSE Z359.2</u>	<u>Minimum Requirements for a Comprehensive Managed Fall Protection Program</u>
<u>ANSI/ASSE Z359.3</u>	<u>Safety Requirements for Positioning and Travel Restraint Systems</u>
<u>ANSI/ASSE Z359.4</u>	<u>Safety Requirements for Assisted-Rescue and Self-Rescue systems, Subsystems and Components</u>
ANSI/AWS D1.0	Code for Welding in Building Construction
ANSI/AWS D1.1	Structural Welding Code - Steel
ANSI/AWS F4.1	Recommended Safe Practices for Preparation for Welding and Cutting of Containers and Piping
ANSI/AWS Z49.1	Safety in Welding, Cutting and Allied Processes
ANSI/IEEE C95.2	Standard for Radio Frequency Energy and Current Flow Symbols

ANSI/IESNA RP-1	Practice for Office Lighting
ANSI/IESNA RP-8	Roadway Lighting ANSI Approved
ANSI/IESNA RP-12	Marine Lighting
ANSI/ISEA 105	Hand Protection Selection Criteria
ANSI/ISEA 107	High Visibility Safety Apparel
ANSI/SIA A92.2	Vehicle-Mounted Elevating and Rotating Aerial Devices
ANSI/SIA A92.3	Manually Propelled Elevating Aerial Platforms
ANSI/SIA A92.5	Boom-supported Elevated Working Platforms
ANSI/SIA A92.6	Self-Propelled Elevating Work Platforms
ANSI/UL 1313	Nonmetallic Safety Cans for Petroleum Products
AR 11-9	The Army Radiation Safety Program
AR 11-34	The Army Respiratory Protection Program
AR 40-5	Preventive Medicine
AR 95 Series	Aviation
AR 200-1	Environmental Protection and Enhancement
AR 385-10	The Army Safety Program

AR 385-11	Ionizing Radiation Protection
AR 385-40	Accident Reporting and Records
AR 385-55	Prevention of Motor Vehicle Accidents
AR 700-136	Tactical Land Based Water Resources Management in Contingency Operations
ASCE 7-98	Guide to the Use of Wind Load Provisions
ASTM D120	Standard Specification for Rubber Insulating Gloves
ASTM D1051	Standard Specification for Rubber Insulating Sleeves
ASTM F496	Standard Specification for In-Service Care of Insulating Gloves and Sleeves
ASTM F696	Standard Specification for Leather Protectors for Rubber Insulating Gloves and Mittens
ASTM F852	Standard Specification for Portable Gasoline Containers for Consumer Use
ASTM F976	Standard Specification for Portable Kerosine Containers for Consumer Use
ASTM F1117	Standard Specification for Dielectric Overshoe Footwear

ASTM F1166	Standard Practice for Human Engineering Design for Marine Systems, Equipment and Facilities
ASTM F1236	Standard Guide for Visual Inspection of Electrical Protective Rubber Products
ASTM F1506	Standard Performance Specification for Flame Resistant Textile Materials for Wearing Apparel for Use by Electrical Workers Exposed to Momentary Electric Arc and Related Thermal Hazards
ASTM F1897	Standard Specification for Leg Protection for Chain Saw Users
<u>ASTM F2412</u>	<u>Standard Test Methods for Foot Protection</u>
<u>ASTM F2413</u>	<u>Standard Specification for Performance Requirements for Foot Protection</u>
CGA C6	Standard for Visual Inspection of Steel Compressed Gas Cylinders
CGA C8	Standard for Requalification of DOT-3HT, CTC-3HT, and TC-3HTM Seamless Steel Cylinders
CGA G7.1	Commodity Specification for Air
CMAA 70	Multiple Girder Electric Overhead Traveling Cranes

DDESB TP No. 18	Minimum Qualifications for UXO Technicians and Personnel, Dec 2004
DFARS Subpart	Drug-Free Work Force 252.223-7004
DOD 6055.09-STD	DOD Ammunition and Explosives Safety Standards, Feb 08
DODI 4715.5-G	Overseas Environmental Baseline Guidance Document
DODI 6055.1	DOD Safety and Occupational Health Program
DODI 6055.3	Hearing Conservation
DODI 6055.12	DOD Hearing Conservation Program
EM 385-1-97	Munitions and Explosives Response Actions
EO 12196	Occupational Safety and Health Programs for Federal Employees
EP 75-1-2	Unexploded Ordnance (UXO) Support During Hazardous, Toxic and Radioactive Waste (HTRW) and Construction Activities
EP 75-1-3	Recovered Chemical Warfare Materiel (RCWM) Responses
EP 310-1-6A	Sign Standards Manual, Volume 1
EP 310-1-6B	Sign Standards Manual, Volume 2

EP 385-1-95a	Basic Safety Concepts and Considerations for OE Operations
EP 385-1-95b	Explosives Safety Submissions
EP 1130-2-500	Inspection and Certification Agreement Appendix L Between USACE and USCG
EP 1130-2-540	Project Operations and Environmental Stewardship Operations and Maintenance Guidance and Procedures
ER 95-1-1	Control and Use of Aircraft
ER 385-1-6	Standard Color and Markings for Hardhats
ER 385-1-91	Training, Testing, and Licensing of Boat Operators
ER 385-1-95	Safety and Health Requirements for Munitions and Explosives of Concern (MEC) Operations
FAR Clause 52.236-13	Accident Prevention
Federal Aviation Regulation 91	General Operating and Flight Rules
Federal Aviation Regulation 133	Rotorcraft External-Load Operations
Federal Aviation Regulation 135	Operating Requirements: Commuter and On Demand Operations and Rules Governing Persons On Board Such Aircraft

EM 385-1-1
15 Sep 08

FM 10-52	Water Supply in Theaters of Operations
FM 21-10/	Field Hygiene and Sanitation MCRP 4-11.1D
MIL-STD 101B	Color Code for Pipelines and for Compressed Gas Cylinders
NAVMED P-5010-	Manual of Naval Preventive Medicine 010-LP-207-1300
NAVSEA S9074-AQ	Requirements for Welding GIB-010/248 Brazing Procedure and Performance Qualifications
NEC 250	Grounding
NEC 250.30	Grounding of Transformers and Generators
NEC 250.34	Grounding of Services Equipment
NEC 410	Lighting Fixtures, Lampholders, Lamps, and Receptacles
NEC 502	Class II Locations
NFPA 10	Portable Fire Extinguishers
NFPA 30	Flammable and Combustible Liquids Code
NFPA 30A	Automotive and Marine Service Station Code

NFPA 51	Standard Design and Installation of Oxygen-Fuel Gas Systems for Welding, Cutting, and Allied Processes
NFPA 58	Liquefied Petroleum Gas Code
NFPA 70E	Standard for Electrical Safety Requirements for Employee Workplaces
NFPA 101	Life Safety Code
NFPA 241	Safeguarding Construction, Alteration, and Demolition Operations
NFPA 295	Wildfire Control
NFPA 302	Pleasure and Commercial Motor Craft
NFPA 327	Cleaning or Safeguarding Small Tanks and Containers without Entry
NFPA 386	Portable Shipping Tanks for Flammable and Combustible Liquids
NFPA 1977	Protective Clothing and Equipment for Wildland Fire Fighting
NIST Voluntary Product	American Softwood Lumber Standard Standard DOC PS 20
Power Crane and	Draglines Shovel Association Standard No. 4
SAE J167	Overhead Protection for Agricultural Tractors - Test Procedures and Performance Requirements

EM 385-1-1
15 Sep 08

SAE J220	Crane Boom Stops
SAE J231	Minimum Performance Criteria for Falling Object
SAE J386	Operator Restraint System for Off-Road Work Machines
SAE J1040	Performance Criteria for Rollover Protective Structures (ROPS) for Construction, Earthmoving, Forestry, and Mining Machines
SAE J1042	Operator Protection for General-Purpose Industrial Machines
SAE J1043	Minimum Performance Criteria for Falling Object Protective Structure (FOPS) for Industrial Machines
SAE J1084	Operator Protective Structure Performance Criteria for Certain Forestry Equipment
SAE J1194	Roll Over Protective Structures (ROPS) for Wheeled Agricultural Tractors
SAE J1366	Rating Lift Cranes Operating on Platforms in the Ocean Environment
TB MED 577	Sanitary Control and Surveillance of Field Water Supplies
UFGS 01525	Safety Requirements
UL 943	Ground-Fault Circuit-Interrupters

EM 3851-1
15 Sep 08

5 CFR 293	Personnel Records
10 CFR 20	Standards for Protection Against Radiation
10 CFR 20	Assigned Protection Factors for Appendix A Respirators
10 CFR 20	Annual Limits on Intake (ALIs) and Appendix B Derived Air Concentrations (DACs) of Radionuclides for Occupational Exposure; Effluent Concentrations; Concentrations for Release of Sewerage
10 CFR	Energy
10 CFR 20	Quantities of Licensed Material Appendix C Requiring Labels
10 CFR 20.1906	Procedures for Receiving and Opening Packages
14 CFR	Aeronautics and Space
14 CFR 91	General Operating and Flight Rules
14 CFR 133	Rotorcraft External-Load Operations
14 CFR 135	Operating Requirements: Commuter and On Demand Operations and Rules Governing Persons On Board Such Aircraft
27 CFR	Alcohol, Tobacco Products and Firearms
27 CFR 555	Commerce in Explosives

EM 385-1-1
15 Sep 08

29 CFR	Labor
29 CFR 1904	Recording and Reporting Occupational Injuries and Illnesses
29 CFR 1910	Occupational Safety and Health Standards
29 CFR 1910	Commercial Diving Operations Subpart T
29 CFR 1910.94	Ventilation
29 CFR 1910.25	Portable Wood Ladders
29 CFR 1910.95	Noise Exposure Computation Appendix A
29 CFR 1910.109	Explosives and Blasting Agents
29 CFR 1910.119	Process Safety Management of Highly Hazardous Chemicals
29 CFR 1910.120	Hazardous Waste Operations and Emergency Response
29 CFR 1910.134	Respiratory Protection
29 CFR 1910.134	User Seal Check Procedures Appendix B-1
29 CFR 1910.134	OSHA Respirator Medical Evaluation Appendix C Questionnaire
29 CFR 1910.134	Information for Employees Using Appendix D Respirators When Not Required Under the Standard

29 CFR 1910.141	Sanitation
29 CFR 1910.145	Specifications for Accident Prevention Signs and Tags
29 CFR 1910.146	Permit-Required Confined Spaces
29 CFR 1910.155	Scope, Application and Definitions Applicable to Subpart L
29 CFR 1910.178	Powered Industrial Trucks
29 CFR 1910.213	Woodworking Machinery Requirements
29 CFR 1910.219	Mechanical Power-Transmission Apparatus
29 CFR 1910.1000	Air contaminants
29 CFR 1910.1000	Mineral Dusts Table Z-3
29 CFR 1910.1001	Asbestos
29 CFR 1910.1020	Access to Employee Exposure and Medical Records
29 CFR 1910.1025	Lead
29 CFR 1910.1030	Bloodborne Pathogens
29 CFR 1910.1096	Ionizing Radiation
29 CFR 1910.1200	Hazard Communication
29 CFR 1915	Occupational Safety and Health Standards for Shipyard Employment

29 CFR 1915	Confined and Enclosed Spaces for Subpart B Other Dangerous Atmospheres in Shipyard Employment
29 CFR 1918.66	Cranes and Derricks Other Than Vessel's Gear
29 CFR 1926	Safety and Health Regulations for Construction
29 CFR 1926	Excavations Subpart P
29 CFR 1926	Steel Erection Subpart R
29 CFR 1926	Blasting and the Use of Explosives Subpart U
29 CRF 1926.35	Employee Emergency Action Plans
29 CFR 1926.59	Hazard Communication
29 CFR 1926.62	Lead
29 CFR 1926.64	Process Safety Management of Highly Hazardous Chemicals
29 CFR 1926.65	Hazardous Waste Operations and Emergency Response
29 CFR 1926.754	Structural Steel Assembly
29 CFR 1926.803	Compressed Air
29 CFR 1926.1101	Asbestos
29 CFR 1960	Basic Program Elements for Federal Employees OSHA

EM 3851-1
15 Sep 08

30 CFR	Mineral Resources
30 CFR 36	Approval Requirements for Permissible Mobile Diesel-Powered Transportation Equipment
30 CFR 56	Safety and Health Standards--Surface Metal and Nonmetal Mines
30 CFR 57	Safety and Health Standards--Underground Metal and Nonmetal Mines
30 CFR 70	Mandatory Health Standards--Underground Coal Mines
30 CFR 71	Mandatory Health Standards--Surface Coal Mines and Surface Work Areas of Underground Coal Mines
33 CFR	Navigation and Navigable Waters
33 CFR 88.13	Lights on Moored Barges
33 CFR 88.15	Lights on Dredge Pipelines
33 CFR 155	Oil or Hazardous Material Pollution Prevention Regulations for Vessels
33 CFR 155.320	Fuel Oil and Bulk Lubricating Oil Discharge Containment
33 CFR 156	Oil and Hazardous Material Transfer Operations
33 CFR 156.120	Requirements for Transfer
33 CFR 183	Boats and Associated Equipment

EM 385-1-1
15 Sep 08

40 CFR	Protection of Environment
40 CFR 61	National Emission Standard for Subpart M Asbestos
40 CFR 141	National Primary Drinking Water Regulations
40 CFR 143	National Secondary Drinking Water Regulations
40 CFR 302	Designation, Reportable Quantities, and Notification
42 CFR	Public Health
42 CFR 84	Approval of Respiratory Protective Devices
46 CFR	Shipping
46 CFR 25.30-15	Fixed Fire Extinguishing Systems
46 CFR 45.115	Bulwarks and Guardrails
46 CFR 58.50-10	Diesel Fuel Tanks
46 CFR 64	Marine Portable Tanks and Cargo Handling Systems
46 CFR 98.30	Handling and Storage of Portable Tanks
46 CFR 160	Lifesaving Equipment
46 CFR 173	Special Rules Pertaining to Vessel Use

EM 3851-1
15 Sep 08

49 CFR	Transportation
49 CFR	U.S. DOT Hazardous Materials Chapter 1 Regulations
49 CFR 171	General Information, Regulations, and Definitions
49 CFR 172	Hazardous Materials Table, Special Provisions, Hazardous Materials Communications, Emergency Response Information and Training Requirements
49 CFR 173	Shipping Container Specification Regulations of the Department of Transportation
49 CFR 174	Carriage by Rail
49 CFR 175	Carriage by Aircraft
49 CFR 176	Carriage by Vessel
49 CFR 177	Carriage by Public Highway
49 CFR 177.835	Class 1 (Explosive) Materials
49 CFR 178	Specifications for Packaging
49 CFR 179	Specifications for Tank Cars
49 CFR 192	Welding of Steel in Pipelines
49 CFR 571	Federal Motor Vehicle Safety Standards

2. UNNUMBERED PUBLICATIONS

ABS, *Guide for Certification of Cranes.*

ACGIH, *Threshold Limit Values and Biological Exposure Indices.*

AIHA, *Welding Health and Safety: A Field Guide for OEHS Professionals.*

ASME, *Boiler and Pressure Vessel Code.*

ASME, *Code for Unfired Pressure Vessels.*

DOT Federal Highway Administration's, *Manual on Uniform Traffic Control Devices for Streets and Highways.*

ILO International Classification of Radiographs of Pneumoconioses, most recent edition.

National Classification Committee, *National Motor Freight Classification,* National Motor Freight Traffic Association, Alexandria, VA.

NBBI, *National Board Inspection Code.*

NIOSH, *Respirator Decision Logic.*

NIOSH, *Work Practice Guide for Manual Lifting.*

Occupational Safety and Health Act of 1970.

Oil Pollution Act of 1990.

Uniform Classification Committee, *Uniform Freight Classification*, National Railroad Freight Committee, Atlanta, GA.

United Nations, *Recommendations on the Transport of Dangerous Goods*, United Nations, New York, 1995.

EM 3851-1
15 Sep 08

U.S. Navy Diving Manual.

3. FORMS

ENG Form 5044-R	USACE Entry Permit (LRA)
NRC Form 3	Notice to Employees
NRC Form 241	Report of Proposed Activities in Non-Agreement States, Areas of Exclusive Federal Jurisdiction, or Offshore Waters
OSHA 300 Form	Log of Work-Related Injuries and Illnesses
OSHA 300A Form	Summary of Work-Related Injuries and Illnesses
SF 46	U.S. Government Motor Vehicle Operator's Identification Card
USCG Form 835	Notice of Merchant Marine Inspection Requirements

SECTION B. RESOURCES

Acoustical Society of America (ASA), 2 Huntington Quadrangle, Suite 1N01, Melville, NY 11747-4502; (516) 576-2360, (516) 576-2377 (fax)

American Association of State Highway and Transportation Officials (AASHTO), 444 N. Capitol St., N.W., Washington, DC 20001; (202) 624-5800, (202) 624-5806 (fax)

American Bureau of Shipping (ABS), 16855 Northchase Dr., Houston, TX 77060; (281) 877-5800

EM 385-1-1
15 Sep 08

American Concrete Institute (ACI), 38800 Country Club Dr., Farmington Hills, MI 48331; (248) 848-3700, (248) 848-3701 (fax)

American Conference of Governmental Industrial Hygienists (ACGIH), 1330 Kemper Meadow Dr., Cincinnati, OH 45240; (513) 742-2020

American Gas Association (AGA), 400 N. Capitol St., N.W., Washington, DC 20001; (202) 824-7000, (202) 824-7115 (fax)

American Industrial Hygiene Association (AIHA), 2700 Prosperity Ave, Suite 250, Fairfax, VA 22031; (703) 849-8888, (703) 207-3561 (fax)

American Institute of Steel Construction (AISC), One East Wacker Dr., Suite 3100, Chicago, IL 60601-2001; (312) 670-2400, (312) 670-5403 (fax)

American Institute of Timber Construction (AITC), 7012 S. Revere Pkwy, Suite 140, Englewood, CO 80112; (303) 792-9559, (303) 792-0669 (fax)

American National Standards Institute (ANSI), 25 West 43rd St., New York, NY 10036; (212) 642-4900, (212) 398-0023 (fax)

American Petroleum Institute (API), 1220 L St., NW, Washington, DC 20005-4070; (202) 682-8000, (202) 682-8232 (fax)

American Society of Civil Engineers (ASCE), 1801 Alexander Bell Dr., Reston, VA 20191-4400; (703) 295-6300, (703) 295-6222 (fax)

American Society of Heating, Refrigerating and Air-Conditioning Engineers (ASHRAE), 1791 Tullie Circle, N.E., Atlanta, GA 30329-2305; (404) 636-8400, (404) 321-5478 (fax)

American Society of Mechanical Engineers (ASME), Three Park Ave., New York, NY, 10016-5990; (212) 591-7722, (212) 591-7674 (fax)

EM 3851-1
15 Sep 08

American Society of Safety Engineers (ASSE), 1800 E. Oakton St., Des Plaines, IL 60018-2187 ; (847) 699-2929, (847) 768-3434 (fax)

American Society for Testing and Materials (ASTM), 100 Barr Harbor Dr., West Conshohocken, PA 19428-2959; (610) 832-9585, (610) 832-9555 (fax)

American Welding Society (AWS), 550 LeJeune Rd., N.W., Miami FL 33126; (305) 443-9353, (305) 443-7559 (fax)

Association of Diving Contractors (ADC), 5206 FM 1960 West, Suite 202, Houston, TX 77069; (281) 893-8388, (281) 893-5118 (fax)

Compressed Air and Gas Institute (CAGI), 1300 Sumner Ave., Cleveland, OH 44115-2851; (216) 241-7333, (216) 241-0105 (fax)

Compressed Gas Association (CGA), 4221 Walney Rd., 5th Floor, Chantilly, VA 20151-2923; (703) 788-2700, (703) 961-1831 (fax)

Concrete Reinforcing Steel Institute (CRSI), 933 Plum Grove Rd., Schaumberg, IL 60173; (847) 517-1200, (708) 517-1206 (fax)

Conveyor Equipment Manufacturers Association (CEMA), 6724 Lone Oak Blvd, Naples, FL 34109; (239) 514-3441, (239) 514-3470 (fax)

Gas Piping Technology Committee (GPTC, ANSI Z380.1), American Gas Association, 400 N. Capitol Street, N.W., Washington, DC 20001; (202) 824-7000

Grinding Wheel Institute (GWI), 30200 Detroit Rd., Cleveland, OH 44115-1967; (216) 899-0010, (216) 892-1404 (fax)

Hardwood Plywood and Veneer Association. 1825 Michael Faraday Dr., Reston, VA 20195-0789; (703) 435-2900, (703) 435-2537 (fax)

EM 385-1-1
15 Sep 08

Human Factors and Ergonomics Society, P.O. Box 1369, Santa Monica, CA 90406-1369; (310) 394-1811, (310) 394-2410 (fax)

Illuminating Engineering Society of North America (IESNA), 120 Wall St., Floor 17, New York, NY 10005; (212) 248-500, (212) 248-5017 (fax)

Institute of Electrical and Electronics Engineers (IEEE), 3 Park Ave, 17th Floor, New York, NY 10016-5997; (212) 419-7900, (212) 752-4929 (fax)

Institute of Makers of Explosives (IME), 1120 19th St., N.W., Suite 310, Washington, DC 20036; (202) 429-9280, (202) 293-2420 (fax)

International Organization for Standardization, 1, rue de Varembé, Case postale 56, CH-1211 Geneva 20, Switzerland; +41 22 749 01 11, +41 22 7333 34 30 (fax)

International Safety Equipment Association, 1901 N. Monroe St., Arlington, VA 22209-1762; (703) 525-1695, (703) 528-2148 (fax)

Material Handling Institute (MHI), 8720 Red Oak Blvd., Suite 201, Charlotte, NC 28217; (704) 676-1190, (704) 676-1199 (fax)

Mine Safety and Health Administration (MSHA), 1100 Wilson Blvd., 21st Floor, Arlington, VA 22209-3939; (202) 693-9400, (202) 693-9401 (fax)

National Association of Marine Surveyors, P.O. Box 9306, Chesapeake, VA 23321-9306; (757) 488-9538, (757) 488-0584 (fax)

National Association of Safe Boating Law Administrator (NASBLA), 1500 Leestown Rd., Suite 330, Lexington, KY 40511; (859) 225-9487, (859) 231-6403 (fax)

EM 3851-1
15 Sep 08

National Board of Boiler and Pressure Vessel Inspectors (NBBI), 1055 Crupper Ave., Columbus, OH 43229; (614) 888-8320, (614) 888-0750 (fax)

National Bureau of Standards (NBS). See National Institute for Standards and Technology (NIST)

National Electrical Manufacturers Association (NEMA), 1300 N. 17th St., Suite 1847, Rosslyn, VA, 22209; (703) 841-3200, (703) 841-5900 (fax)

National Fire Protection Association (NFPA), 1 Batterymarch Park, P.O. Box 9101, Quincy, MA 02169-7471; (617) 770-3000, (617) 770-0700 (fax)

National Institute for Occupational Safety and Health, 200 Independence Ave, S.W., Rm 715H, Washington, DC 20201; (202) 401-6997

National Institute for Standards and Technology (NIST), 100 Bureau Dr., Stop 3460, Gaithersburg, MD 20899-6478; (301) 975-6478, (301) 975-2128 (fax)

National Safety Council (NSC), 1121 Spring Lake Dr., Itasca, IL 60143-3201; (630) 285-1121, (630) 285-1315 (fax)

Naval Sea Systems Command (NAVSEA), 1333 Isaac Hull Ave, S.E., Washington Navy Yard, DC 20376; (202) 781-000

Occupational Safety and Health Administration (OSHA), 200 Constitution Avenue, NW, Washington, DC 20210; 1-800-321-6742

Power Tool Institute (PTI), 1300 Sumner Ave, Cleveland, OH 44115-2851; (216) 241-7333, (216) 241-0105 (fax)

Scaffold Industry Association (SIA), 20335 Ventura Blvd., Suite 420, Woodland Hills, CA 91364; (818) 610-0320, (818) 610-0323 (fax)

EM 385-1-1
15 Sep 08

Scaffold, Shoring, and Forming Institute (SSFI), 1300 Sumner Ave, Cleveland, OH 44115-2851; (216) 241-7333, (216) 241-0105 (fax)

Society of Automotive Engineers (SAE), 400 Commonwealth Dr., Warrendale, PA 15096-0001; (724) 776-4841, (724) 776-0790 (fax)

Underwriters Laboratory (UL). 333 Pfingsten Rd., Northbrook, IL 60062; (847) 282-8800, (847) 407-1395 (fax)

United States Government Printing Office (GPO), Superintendent of Documents, U.S. Government Printing Office, Washington, DC 20402; (202) 512-1530, (202) 512-1262 (fax)

BLANK

EM 385-1-1
15 Sep 08

APPENDIX T

BLANK

BLANK

EM-385-1-1
15 Sep 08

APPENDIX U

FLOATING PLANT AND MARINE ACTIVITIES DIAGRAMS

FIGURE U-1

TYPE A RAILING

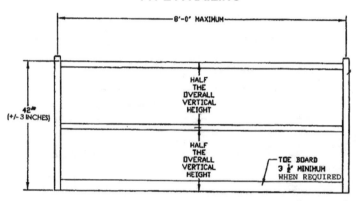

MARINE RAILING TYPE A, TWO TIER RIGID FALL PROTECTION RAILING

FIGURE U-2

TYPE B RAILINGS

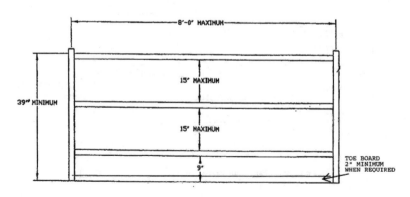

MARINE TYPE B THREE TIER RIGID RAILING

FIGURE U-2 (CONTINUED)

TYPE B RAILINGS

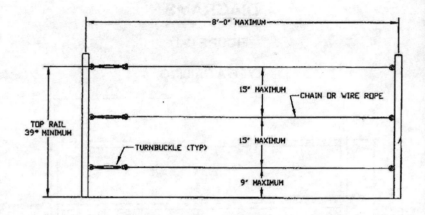

MARINE TYPE B THREE TIER TENSIONED RAILING

FIGURE U-3

TYPE C RAILINGS

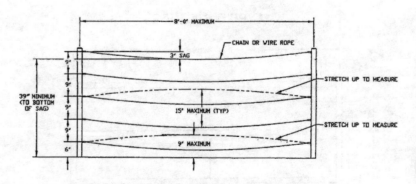

MARINE TYPE C NON-TENSIONED RAILING (3" SAG SHOWN)

EM-385-1-1
15 Sep 08

FIGURE U-3 (CONTINUED)

TYPE C RAILINGS

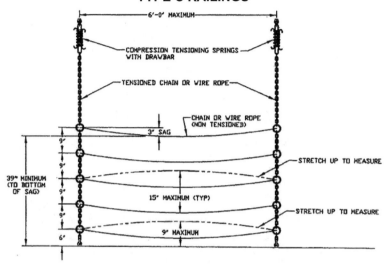

MARINE TYPE C FLEXIBLE/ SWING-AWAY RAILING
WITH FLEXIBLE TIERS (3" SAG SHOWN)

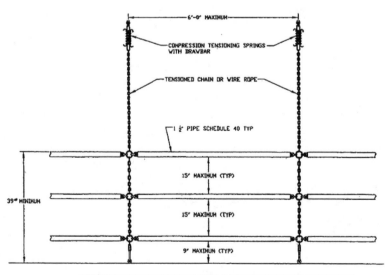

MARINE TYPE C FLEXIBLE/ SWING-AWAY RAILING WITH RIGID TIERS

BLANK

EM 385-1-1
15 Sep 08

ACRONYMS

3 Rs	Recognize, Retreat, Report
A2B	Anti-two Blocking
AAUS	American Academy of Underwater Scientists
ABS	American Bureau of Shipping
ACDE	Association of Commercial Diving Educators
ACGIH	American Conference of Governmental Industrial Hygienists
ACI	American Concrete Institute
ACM	asbestos-containing material
ADC	Association of Diving Contractors
ADCI	Association of Diving Contractors International
AED	automatic external defibrillator
AEGCP	Assured Equipment Grounding Conductor Program
AFFF	aqueous film foaming foam
AGA	American Gas Association
AHA	activity hazard analysis/analyses
AHA	American Heart Association
AIHA	American Industrial Hygiene Association
ALARA	as low as is reasonably achievable
ALI	annual limits on intake
ANSI	American National Standards Institute
APF	assigned protection factor
API	American Petroleum Institute
APP	accident prevention plan
AR	Army Regulation
ARA	Army Radiation Authorization
ARC	American Red Cross
ASCE	American Society of Civil Engineers
ASHRAE	American Society of Heating, Refrigeration and Air-Conditioning Engineers
ASME	American Society of Mechanical Engineers
ASP	Associate Safety Professional
ASSE	American Society of Safety Engineers
ASTM	American Society for Testing and Materials
ATV	all terrain vehicles
AWG	American Wire Gauge
AWS	American Welding Society

EM 385-1-1
15 Sep 08

BCD	buoyancy compensation device
BCSP	Board of Certified Safety Professionals
BRAC	base realignment and closure
Btu	British thermal units
<u>CA</u>	<u>chemical agent</u>
<u>CAIS</u>	<u>chemical agent identification set</u>
<u>Cd</u>	<u>conductive footwear</u>
CDC	Centers for Disease Control
CDZ	controlled decking zone
CERCLA	Comprehensive Environmental Response, Compensation, and Liability Act
cfm	Cubic Feet per Minute
CFR	Code of Federal Regulations
<u>CG</u>	<u>chemical agent-Phosgene or Carbonyl Dichloride</u>
CGA	Compressed Gas Association
CHP	Certified Health Physicist
CHST	Certified Construction Health and Safety Technician
CIH	Certified Industrial Hygienist
cm	centimeter
cm^2	square centimeter
CMAA	Crane Manufacturer's Association of America
CO_2	carbon dioxide
CO	carbon monoxide
CONUS	continental United States
COR	Contracting Officer's Representative
CPCSSV	Competent Person for Confined Spaces on Ships and Vessels
CPR	cardiopulmonary resuscitation
CRZ	contamination reduction zone
<u>CS</u>	<u>riot control agent</u>
CSCP	Confined Space Competent Person
CSP	Certified Safety Professional
CSTS	Certified Safety Trained Supervisor
<u>CWM</u>	<u>chemical warfare materiel</u>
DA	Department of the Army
DA Pam	Department of the Army Pamphlet
DAC	derived air concentration
dB	decibel

dB(A)	decibels A-weighed
°C	degrees Celsius
°F	degrees Fahrenheit
DAN	Divers Alert Network
DDC	District Diving Coordinator
DFARS	Defense Federal Acquisition Regulation Supplement
DMM	discarded military munitions
DOD	Department of Defense
DODI	Department of Defense Instruction
DOE	Department of Energy
DOT	Department of Transportation
DSR	Dive Safety Representative
EANx	nitrox gas
ECP	entry control point
ELSA	emergency life support apparatus
EM	Engineering Manual
EMR	Electromagnetic Radiation
EMR	experience modification rate
EMS	emergency medical services
EMT	emergency medical technician
EO	Executive Order
EOD	explosive ordnance disposal
EP	Engineering Pamphlet
EPA	Environmental Protection Agency
ER	Engineering Regulation
ERP	emergency response plan
ERT	emergency response team
ESLI	end-of-service life indicator
ETS	environmental tobacco smoke
EZ	exclusion zone
FAA	Federal Aviation Administration
FAR	Federal Acquisition Regulation
fc	footcandle
FCAW	flux cored arc welding
FDA	Food and Drug Administration
FEV(1)	forced expiratory volume at 1 second
FGS	Final Governing Standards
FM	Field Manual

FOA	field operating activities
FOPS	falling object protective structures
FRP	fiberglass-reinforced plastic
ft	foot
ft^3	cubic foot
ft^2	square foot
ft/min	Feet per Minute
FUDS	formerly used defense sites
FUSRAP	formerly used sites remedial action program
FVC	forced vital capacity
gal	gallon
GDA	Government Designated Authority
GFCI	ground fault circuit interrupter
GMAW	gas metal arc welding
GPTC	Gas Piping Technology Committee
H	chemical agent-Mustard
H-3	Tritium
HAV	Hepatitis A virus
HAZCOM	hazardous communication
HAZWOPER	hazardous waste operations and emergency response
HBV	Hepatitis B virus
HCV	Hepatitis C virus
HD	chemical agent-Distilled Mustard
HE	high explosives
HECP	Hazardous Energy Control Program
HEPA	high efficiency particulate air
HIV	human immuno-deficiency virus
HLL	horizontal life line
hp	horsepower
HQUSACE	Headquarters, U.S. Army Corps of Engineers
HTRW	hazardous, toxic, and radioactive waste
HVAC	heating, ventilation, and air conditioning
HS	chemical agent-Mustard
Hz	hertz
IAQ	indoor air quality
IDLH	immediately dangerous to life and health
IEEE	Institute of Electrical and Electronics Engineers
IESNA	Illuminating Engineering Society of North America

EM 385-1-1
15 Sep 08

ILO	International Labor Office
IME	Institute of Makers of Explosives
in	inch
in^2	square inch
IRP	Installation Restoration Program
IRSC	Ionizing Radiation Safety Committee
ISEA	International Safety Equipment Association
ISO	International Organization of Standardization
kA	kiloamp
kg	kilogram
kHz	kilohertz
km	kilometers
<u>kN</u>	<u>kiloNewton</u>
kPa	kilopascal
kV	kilovolt
lb	pound
L	liter
LBD	lead-based paint
LCDS	ladder climbing devices
LEL	lower explosive limit
LFL	lower flammable limit
LID	load indicating device
LLD	load limiting device
lm	lumens
LMI	load moment indicating
LP-Gas	liquefied petroleum gas
LP	licensed physician
LPA	licensed physician's assistant
LPN	licensed practical nurse
L/s	liters per second
lx	lux
m	meter
<u>M S</u>	<u>Military Munitions Support Services</u>
m^3	cubic meter
m^2	square meter
MC	metal-clad cable
<u>MC</u>	<u>munitions constituents</u>
MCRP	Marine Corps Reference Publication
<u>MEC</u>	<u>munitions and explosives of concern</u>

Acronyms-5

mg	milligram
mi	miles
MILCON	Military Construction
MIL-STD	Military Standard
<u>MM</u>	<u>military munitions</u>
mm	millimeters
MMAD	mass median aerodynamic diameters
MOA	Memorandum of Agreement
<u>MOOTW</u>	<u>Military Operations Other Than War</u>
MOU	Memorandum of Understanding
mph	miles per hour
mrem	millirems
<u>MRS</u>	<u>munitions response site</u>
m/s	meters per second
MSC	major subordinate command
MSDS	material safety data sheet
MSHA	Mine Safety and Health Administration
MSS	motion stopping safety system
<u>MT</u>	<u>metric ton</u>
MUTCD	Manual on Uniform Traffic Control Devices for Streets and Highways
µSv	microsieverts
mSv	millisieverts
MVA	megavolt-amperes
NAMS	National Association of Marine Surveyors
NASBLA	National Association of Safe Boating Law Administrators
NAUI	National Association of Underwater Instructors
NAVFAC	Naval Facilities
NAVMED	Navy Medical
NAVSEA	Naval Sea Systems Command
NBBI	National Board of Boiler and Pressure Vessel Inspectors
NEC	National Electrical Code
NEMA	National Electrical Manufacturers Association
NESC	National Electrical Safety Code
NESHAP	National Emissions Standards for Hazardous Air Pollutants
NFPA	National Fire Protection Association

NIOSH	National Institute for Occupational Safety and Health
NIST	National Institute of Standards and Technology
NMFC	National Motor Freight Classification
NOAA	National Oceanic and Atmospheric Administration
NPDWR	National Primary Drinking Water Regulation
NPRCS	non-permit required confined space
NRC	Nuclear Regulatory Commission
<u>NREMT</u>	<u>Nationally Registered Emergency Medical Technician</u>
NRR	noise reduction rating
NSC	National Safety Council
NVLAP	National Voluntary Laboratory Accreditation Program
OCONUS	outside continental United States/overseas
<u>OE</u>	<u>ordnance and explosives</u>
OEA	oxygen enriched air
OEBGD	overseas environmental baseline guidance document
OEL	occupational exposure limit
OEM	original equipment manufacturer
OJT	on-the-job training
OSHA	Occupational Safety and Health Administration
Pa	pascal
<u>PA</u>	<u>Physician's Assistant (licensed and/or registered)</u>
PADI	Professional Association of Diving Instructors
PAN	preliminary accident notification
PAPR	powered-air purifying respirator
PCB	polychlorinated biphenyls
pCi/L	picocuries per liter
PDT	project delivery team
PEL	permissible exposure limit
PFD	personal floatation device
PHA	position hazard analysis
PIT	powered industrial truck
PLHCP	Physician-Licensed Healthcare Professional
<u>POC</u>	<u>Point of Contact</u>
PM	Project Manager
PMP	Project Management Plan
POL	petroleum, oil, and lubricants

PPE	personal protective equipment
ppm	parts per million
PRCS	permit-required confined spaces
PrgMP	Program Management Plan
PRT	Planning and Response Teams
<u>PS</u>	<u>chemical agent-Chloropicrin</u>
psf	pounds per square foot
psi	per square inch
psia	per square inch absolute
<u>QA</u>	<u>quality assurance</u>
<u>QASP</u>	<u>Quality Assurance Surveillance Plan</u>
QC	quality control
QLFT	qualitative fit test
QNFT	quantitative fit test
<u>QCP</u>	<u>Quality Control Plan</u>
<u>QCS</u>	<u>Quality Control Supervisor</u>
<u>RAC</u>	<u>Risk Assessment Code</u>
RCRA	Resource Conservation and Recovery Act
RDS	respirable dust standard
REL	recommended exposure limit
REM	roentgen equivalent in man
RF	radio frequency
RFO	Recovery Field Office
RN	registered nurse
ROPS	rollover protective structure
RPE	registered professional engineer
RSC	radiation safety committee
RSO	radiation safety officer
RSSO	USACE Radiation Safety Staff Officer
SAE	Society of Automotive Engineers
SAMS	Society of Accredited Marine Surveyors
SAR	supplied-air respirator
SCBA	self-contained breathing apparatus
SCUBA	self-contained underwater breathing apparatus
SHM	safety and health manager
SIA	Scaffold Industry Association
SMS	safety monitoring system
<u>SOHO</u>	<u>Safety and Occupational Health Office</u>
SOP	standard operating procedure

SPF	sun protection factor
SSA	surface-supplied air
SSHO	site safety and health officer
SSHP	site safety and health plan
Sv	sieverts
SZ	support zone
TB MED	Technical Bulletin, Medical
T&M	time and materials
TEDE	total equivalent dose exposure
TIP	tie-in point
TLV	threshold limit value
TSD	treatment storage and disposal
TWA	time-weighted average
UDC	USACE Command Diving Coordinator
UFC	Uniform Freight Classification
UFGS	Unified Facilities Guide Specification
UL	Underwriters Laboratory
USACE	U.S. Army Corps of Engineers
USCG	U.S. Coast Guard
USEPA	U.S. Environmental Protection Agency
UST	underground storage tank
UV	ultraviolet
UVA	ultraviolet A-region
UVB	ultraviolet B-region
UXO	unexploded ordnance
VLL	vertical life line
WBGT	wet bulb globe temperature
WLS	warning line system
WP	White Phosphorous

BLANK

EM 385-1-1
15 Sep 08

INDEX

-A-

Abrasive blasting 112-117, 276-277
    equipment 276
Access 575
    Haul roads 46-47
    Ladder 522
    Route 43
Accident prevention
    plan 2, 4, 13, 638, A-1
    signs, tags, labels 143-144, 150, 152, 158-160, 166
Accidents 1, 14, 17, 20, 47, 107, 289
Activity hazard analysis (See also hazard analysis) 2, 10, 114, 654, 724
Aerial lift 251, 252, 387, 492, 509-512,
.... 557-559, 748, 751, 760, B-8
Aircraft 18, 113, 126, 700, 763, 766, 779, 781
Airfield operations 763
Alarm systems
    Emergency 685
    Fire 197-198
    General 451
    Monitor 739
All terrain vehicles (ATVs) 409, 422, 437-439
Anchor Handling Barge 370
Antimony 295
Arc welding and cutting 203, 212, 213
    cables and connectors ....
Arc Flash 72, 75, 216, 219, 220, 504
    Incident/Accident 18
Arsenic 129, 205
Asbestos 5, 90, 92, 565
Assured equipment grounding conductor program 226-227, D-1
Attachment plugs and receptacles 218
Automatically darkening lenses ....
Automatic External Defibrillator (AED) 39, 40, 718
Automatic feeding devices 271

-B-

Backup alarms (Reverse signal alarms) 309, 411, 412
Barium 205
Batteries and battery charging 232, 234, 450, 451, 701, 709
Beryllium 205, 206
Blasting 435, 626, 629, 635, 636, 639-642, 695-697, 699, 700, 704-715, 728, 739

Blind (in one eye)	58
Body belt/harness systems	506/72, 396, 493, 503, 504, 508, 510, 544, 749
Boiler and Pressure Vessel Code	477, 485, 486
Boilers	485, 486
Boom - see cranes and derricks	
Brush chippers	756, 757
Brush removal and chipping	755
Bulletin Board, Safety and Health	1
Burning operations	169, 208, 633

-C-

Cadmium	6, 205
Cage boom guards	232
Caissons - see underground construction	
Carabiners/Snaphooks	505
Carbon monoxide	118, 739, 740
Carbon tetrachloride	192
Cardiopulmonary resuscitation (CPR)	6, 33, 38, 39, 42, 474, 684, 718, 745
Caution signs	62, 146, 147, 195
Cement	129, 281, 283
Certified Welder	204, 390
For ROPs	388, 417
Chain	295-297, 300, 384, 424, 465, 466, 545, 578
Conveyors	401
Lockers	326, 329, 368
Chain saws	51, 276, 751, 752, 759-761
Change rooms	
Chemical agent	770, 782, 786
Chopping tools	761
Christmas tree lifting (See Multiple Lifting/Rigging)	
Chromium	129, 130, 205, 206, 214
Circuit breaker	225, 226, 241
Classified locations (See also Hazardous (classified) Locations	234, 236
Cobalt	205
Code for Unfired Pressure Vessels	481
Cofferdams	491, 590, 602, 705
Collateral Duty Safety Officer (CDSO)	13
Combustible liquid	174, 177
Communication facilities	256
Compressed air	116, 481, 484, 485, 713, 718
blasting	520, 529, 535
cleaning	136, 482
work/work plan	16, 17, 637, 638, 639, 641
Compressed gas	211
cylinders	168, 486, 488, 489

EM 385-1-1
15 Sep 08

Compressors 225, 481, 482, 625, 738, 739
Confined space (See also Permit-required confined space 117, 186, 205, 435
.... 589, 595, 613, 683, 688, 689, 789-796
    Marine Facilities.. 795-796
Construction areas 63, 141, 152, 311, 431, 620
Contact lenses 57
Contract diving operations.. 719
    air compressor systems... 718
    altitude dive tables 723, 738
    bell 735-737
    breathing air supply hoses.. 740
    briefing 729
    decompression sickness/pulmonary barotraumas 728
    dive log 727
    dive operations plan 720-722, 725
    dive teams. 729, 720, 724, 729, 738, 741, O-1
    divers 454, 512, 717-745
    emergency and first aid equipment. 743
    equipment. 726
    mixed-gas diving 737
    power tools 743
    pre-dive conference... 719, 724, 725
    safe practices manual... 720, 721
    SCUBA diving operations 733-734
    surface supplied air 717-743
Control of hazardous energy (See also Hazardous Energy).... 257, 260, 399, 724
Controlled Access Zone (CAZ) 495
Conveyors.. 399-407, 621, 631
Copper 113, 205, 243
Covers (hole)... 499
Cranes and derricks 307
    anti-two block (upper limit) device 337-339, 381, 392
    boom, angle/radius indicator 336, 339, 392
    boom, assembly and disassembly 253, 357
    boom, hoist disengaging device 328
    boom, stops 328, 335
    communication 310, 315, 347, 355, 360, 376
    crawler-, truck-, wheel-, and ringer-mounted cranes.................... 357
    critical lifts 289, 311, 319-320, 343, 347, 353, 355, 367, 387, 653, 731
    derricks 245, 256, 307, 319, 322, 326, 329,
    .... 334-337, 356, 363-368, 373-375, 656, 657
    drum rotation indicators 340
    duty cycle 337, 338, 340, 380, 461
    and electricity 222, 230, 232, 245, 255, 256
    environmental considerations 356
    floating 307, 326, 334, 338, 341, 363, 451

    gantry 230, 307, 319, 334, 343, 345, 352, 354, 371, 587
    helicopter 153, 375-377, 379
    inspection criteria 321-344, I-1
    inspections, frequent 325, 326
    load indicating device 340
    load moment indicator 340
    load performance test 341, 342, 397
    luffing jib 337, 339
    mobile 307, 359
    monorails 307, 319, 320, 373
    multiple lifting (multiple lift rigging)..
    on-rubber rating 359
    operators 312, 313, 316-320
    operational performance test 316, 328, 386, 387, 417
    operators, examination and qualification 311-321
    outriggers 251, 324, 340, 354, 358, 359, 383, 393
    overhead 319, 334, 343, 345, 352, 354, 360, 372
    periodic inspections 262, 267, 326, 380
    pillar 334, 359
    portal 307, 319, 359
    tandem/tailing crane lifts 347, 356
    testing requirements 396, I-1
    tower(hammerhead) 307, 319, 324, 334, 359-362
    underhung 319, 320, 373
Cumulative trauma prevention 125
Cutting, arc and gas 55, 207

-D-

D-rings 504, 505, 506, 509
Dead Man (Kill) Switch 469
Debris nets 284, 285, 500, 501
Deficiency Tracking Log 2
Demolition 565
    engineering survey 565
    mechanical 572
    plan 565
Derricks - see cranes and derricks
Detonating cord 697, 709, 710
Dielectric test 232
Diesel fuel 632-633
Disconnects 221, 240, 241
Dive tables 723, 738
Diving Operations 717, O-1
    See also Contract Diving Operations
Dose Limits 100-101

Dosimetry... 99, 101, 102
Double insulated 224
Dredging 471
    Disposal Sites.. 473
    Hopper dredges... 473
Drilling equipment 433-435, 707
Drilling machines 634
Drinking water 21-23, 120, 473
Dump trucks... 410, 424, 430, 431
Dust 136, 170, 197, 235, 236, 237, 283, 377, 437, 630, 641, 696, 763

-E-

Electrical 215; 6, 16, 40, 51, 57, 63, 73-76, 170, 203
    conductors 213, 516, 575, 644
    conductors, overhead 230
    conductors, stringing 247, 248
    electrical protective equipment... 73, 74
    isolation... 215, 260-264, 792
    overload protection 221, 361
    qualified person.. 215
    substations 243, 255, 256
    storms 251, 436, 447, 677
    temporary wiring and lighting.. 227-229
    underground electrical installations 254
Electrician, Qualified Person... 215
Electrician, verifiable credentials... 215
Electromagnetic 110, 111, 256, 704, 773
Elevating work platform 389, 556
Emergency
    descent devices 516
    eye wash...87, 88
    lighting and power systems 450
    medical technician 40
    operations 20, 51, 325, B-1
    planning 19, 449, 684, 691
    response 4, 14, 20, 33, 63, 86, 93, 100, 440, 615, 616, 654, 681
    ....688-691, 693
    Shower..87
Enclosed spaces 204, 268, 456, 795
Engineering/administrative controls 7, 49, 85, 91, 92, 98, 103, 104, 110, 115,
....................................129, 130, 135-137, 214, 683, 687, 689, 792, 795
Environmental monitoring... 92, 123
Epoxy resins 35
Examiner...313, 314, 316, 427
Excavations 9, 427, 492, 589, 764

```
    Class I perimeter protection..................................................................595
    Class II perimeter protection .................................................................595
    Class III perimeter protection.................................................................596
    inspection and testing..........................................................................590
    mobile equipment and motor vehicle precautions.................................594
    protection from falling material ............................................................594
    protection from water...........................................................................593
    protective systems......................................................................590-592, 599
    qualified person.....................................................................................
    shield systems.......................................................................................600
    sloping and benching............................................................. 597, 605-610
    trenching................................................................................. 6, 589, 601
Explosive-actuated tools..................................................................... 274, 275
Explosives................... 51, 192, 353, 419, 421, 566, 590, 617, 635, 639, 695, 767
Eye and face protection.............................................................51, 52, 57, 58, 74
```

-F-

```
Face masks and hoods ........................................................58, 96, 117, 119, 270
Fall protection ..................9, 72, 76, 77, 387, 394, 396, 461, 464, 474, 491, 515,
                         543, 559, 562, 576, 581, 583, 590, 643, 650, 674, 749
    warning line systems ...........................................310, 493, 510, 577, 584
    .personal fall arrest systems and positioning devices.......... 394, 491, 502
    ................................................................. 504, 508, 650, 674, 675, 749
    safety nets ................................................................................ 77, 284, 491,
    Fall Plan.................................................................................494-495
    Controlled Access Zones...................................................................495
    Self-Retracting Lifeline (SRL)............................................................505
    Horizontal LifeLine (HLL)..................................................................507
    Vertical LifeLine (VLL).......................................................................507
    Restraint Systems.............................................................................508
    Safety Monitoring System (SMS)......................................................511
    Full Body Harnesses (See Body Belts/Harnesses)
Falling object protective structures.............................................................415
Fencing ................................................................................... 43, 400, 618
Fiberglass-Reinforced Plastic (FRP)............................................................76
Fire
    alarm systems; watches ...................................................197, 198, 623
    blankets ............................................................................................192
    detection systems.............................................................................197
    extinguishers ..........................93, 149, 190, 411, 423, 469, 621, 631, 702
    extinguishers, approved ...................................................................190
    extinguishing, chlorobromomethane .................................................192
    extinguishing systems, fixed.............................................................195
    fighting equipment .......................149, 160, 170, 192, 196, 199, 201, 616
```

```
    fighting organizations, training and drilling ........................................... 198
    lanes ................................................................................................... 170
    patrols ................................................................................................ 199
    prevention and protection ............................................................ 167, 630
    prevention and protection plan .................................................... 167, 630
    protection, first response .................................................................... 190
    protection, in the construction process .............................................. 170
    protection, standpipe and hose system .............................................. 193
    suppression systems, fixed ..................................................... 160, 195
First aid ..................... 6, 18, 20, 33-41, 96, 121, 141, 149, 159, 160, 199, 201,
    ................................................. 411, 474, 616, 684, 692, 725, 731, 743, 745
    attendant .............................................................................................. 40
    facilities ............................................................................................. 616
    kits ............................................................................................. 36, 411
    station ................................................................................ 34, 39, 616
Fit testing - see respirators
Flag Person ............................................................................................ 154, 712
Flammable
    atmosphere ........................................................................................ 207
    gases ................................................................................. 207, 622, 628
    liquid ................... 27, 89, 90, 95, 160, 170, 172, 175, 176, 189, 213, 796
    materials .................................................... 208, 421, 476, 483, 566
Flammable and combustible liquids ................................. 172, 175-177, 284
    Diking/curbing ............................................................................. 176, 593
    portable tanks .............................................................................. 173, 177
    storage cabinets and areas ... 174, 176, 182, 199, 280, 577, 617, 630, 632
    storage tanks ............................................................................... 174, 479

Flashlight ............................................................................................... 709
Flexible cords ........................................................................................ 217
Float Plans ............................................................................................. 470
Floating cranes and derricks - see cranes and derricks
Floating plant ....................... 78, 153, 221, 228, 232, 329, 429, 445, 491, 495, 796
    Access ...............................................................................................
    escape hatches and emergency exits ............................................. 452
    inspection and certification ............................................................. 445
    personnel qualifications .................................................................. 446
        See Dredging and Launches, Motorboats, and Skiffs
Floor and wall holes and openings .................. 491, 570, 571, 575, 584, 659, 660,
Floor removal ........................................................................................ 571
Fluorine ................................................................................................. 206
Flying objects, protection against .............................................. 75, 376, 414, 415
Foodservice ..................................................................................... 29, 30
Forklift (PITs) ........................................................................................ 431
Formwork ......................................................... 170, 492, 549, 646, 647, 650
Fueling ................................................................ 187, 308, 422, 428, 633
```

Fuses	218, 222, 703, 773
Fusible Plugs	486

-G-

Gas metal arc welding	59, 214
Gassy operations	622-630
Generators	
Portable	223, 226
vehicle-mounted	222, 223
Glare-resistant glasses	58
Grinding and abrasive machinery	55, 112, 269, 270, 655
Ground/grounding	222
Electrode	223, 225
frame grounding	213, 223
protective	224, 263

Guardrails, standard ... 77, 309, 310, 413, 390, 421-22, 455. 459, 491-493, 495 499, 507, 510, 525, 545, 550, 561, 563, 568, 582, 596, 602, 634, 644, 650, 678

-H-

Hand protection	51
Hand signals	153, 289, 319, 347, 349, 355, 379, 443
Hand tools	225, 516, 267
Hand-arm vibration	125
Hand lamps, portable	219
Handrails	329, 460, 515, 582, 655
Harmful plants, animals, and insects	96
Haul roads	46-48, 429
Hazard analysis	
Activity Hazard Analysis	2, 114
Arc Flash Analysis	654, 724
Diving	729
Position hazard analysis	4, 6, 7, 10
Hazard communication	85
Hazardous classifications	622
Hazardous locations	170, 234, 402, 457, 617
Hazardous energy, control	257
Program (HECP) /Procedures	259, 265, 724, 731
Hazardous materials	173, 174, 203, 209, 353, 475, 476
Hazardous substances, agents, environments	87, 595, 683, 691, 692
Hazardous, toxic, and radioactive waste	6, 681
Head protection	63, 74, 441, 442, 761
Hearing	
conservation	60, 62
protection	60-62, 116-118, 761
Heat/cold stress monitoring plan	119, 730

Heating devices 93, 94, 184, 185
    Fuel-combustion space 186
    Melting Kettles... 93
    open-flame heating devices.. 185
Herbicides 28
High Visibility Apparel/Vests 66, 67, 154, 423, 594
Hoisting 95, 246, 273, 287, 295, 303
    Equipment 16, 280, 290, 307
        Class IIIA 320
        Class IIIB 321
        Operators.. 321
            Inspection 321
        Employees 389
        Wire ropes 345
Hooks 288, 297, 301-304, 323, 348, 374, 383, 389, 391
.... 456, 501, 521, 535, 543, 545, 582, 621, 637, 657, 749, 759, 761
Hot or molten substances 58
Hot stick distances 240
Hot tapping 209
Hot work permits 93, 207
Housekeeping 21, 91, 92, 135, 149, 159, 167, 168, 283, 377, 500
Hydraulic
    fluid 632
    tools 243
Hydrocarbons 236, 740
Hydrogen sulfide 625-627
Hydrostatic testing 477

-I-

Impalement hazards 492, 595, 643
Inclement weather 119, 421, 468
Indoctrination 13
Industrial hygienist 84-87, 126, 685, 795
Infirmaries 39, 40, 141
Inflatable PFDs 77, 78, 448, 733
Insecticides 28
Insects 6, 31, 96
Insulating/insulation
    links 232
    mats 218
Interpretations M-1
Intrinsically safe 234, 451
Ionizing radiation 97, 101, 107, 160, 682, 685
    warning signs, labels, signals 150, 160

-J-

Jumbos 634, 635

-K-

Kill Switch (Dead Man)...469

-L-

Labels 104, 143, 150, 151, 329, 502, 557, 579
Ladder Climbing Device..509
Ladders....................... 95, 141, 203, 204, 243, 245, 324, 383, 385, 421, 455, 458, 459, 482, 491, 508, 509, 515, 516, 522, 547, 558, 559, 561, 567, 575, 576, 578-582, 596, 597, 636, 638, 655, 748..
Lanyards 72, 502, 505, 506, 508, 510, 544, 749
Lasers 108, 110
Launches, motorboats, and skiffs.. 77, 457, 468-470
Lead 5, 90, 91, 98, 121, 205, 233, 243, 565
Licensed physician 16, 17, 34, 39, 133, 719, 745
Licensed physician's assistant 40
licensed practical nurse 40
Lifeline 493, 494, 498, 507, 510, 544, 577, 752
Life ring 78, 80
Life saving and safety skiffs.. 79, 464
Lift trucks (Aerial).. 244
Lift trucks (PITs)..432
Lift-slab operations 651, 652
Lifting - see safe lifting
Lighting 4, 40, 48, 78, 139-141, 170, 227-229, 235, 237, 357, 450, 615-617, 632, 640, 793
Lime 281, 283
Limited access zone 676
Limited Service Contract..12, A-1
Lineman's equipment.. 72, 504
Liquefied petroleum gas (LP-Gas) 179, 180, 182-189, 470, 632
Live-line bare-hand... 240, 250-252
Lockout and tagout (Control of Hazardous Energy)...........152, 216, 258-261, 323, 426, 479, 724, 728
Locks/Tags...262
Long-bed end-dump trailers 417

-M-

Machinery and mechanized equipment..................................... 409, 422, 424, 426
Maintenance Vehicles..421

Manganese 205
Manned/Unmanned Vessels... 461, 462
Manual on Uniform Traffic Control Devices (MUTCD)......................... 48, 144
Marine activities 445, 456
Masonry construction 644, 676, 677
Material
    handling, storage, disposal.. 279
    hoists 334, 348, 377, 380, 382, 417
Material Safety Data Sheets.. 7, 86, 89, 433

Medical 33
    facilities 14, 33, 685
    examinations 69, 107, 133, 317
    surveillance........91, 93, 107, 115, 125, 130, 133, 135, 201, 683, 688-691
Medically qualified... 15
Melting kettles.. 93, 94
Mercury 205
Methane 622, 623, 625-628, 740
MILCON Transformation.. 3
Motor vehicles 16, 181, 409, 410, 414, 422, 423
    Activities while driving.. 418
    Contractor.. 417
    USACE... 417
    Operating Limits – 10/12 hour rule..16
Multiple Lift Rigging... 289-291, 354
Munitions and Explosives of Concern (MEC)..767-768

-N-

National Board of Boiler and Pressure Vessel Inspectors 447
Navigation locks 80, 475
Nickel 114, 205
Noise hazard areas 62
Nonlonizing radiation...108
Nonmetallic 168, 617, 757
Non-sparking tools...268

-O-

Open hooks, pelican...303, 456
Operators................... 16, 274, 276, 311-321, 343, 364, 370, 373, 386, 409, 413,
.... 415, 417, 418, 420, 421, 427, 696
    ATVs..438
    Boat, Motorboat...446, 471
    PITs (forklifts, lift trucks)... 432
    Utility Vehicles (UVs)... 439, 441

Outrigger beams 535-537, 542
Overcurrent device/protection 221
Overhead guards 414
Oxyfuel gas cutting and welding 209, 211
Oxygen cylinders 209, 489
Oxygen deficient atmosphere 111
Oxygen enriched atmosphere 207, 738
Ozone.. 205

-P-

Paint barges 174
Paints 6, 28, 129, 176, 204, 206, 273
Perimeter Protection ....
    Floating Plant, Main Deck PP 461-466, U-1
    Excavations 595-596
Permit-required confined space 789-796
    entry procedures 790
    program 791
Personal fall protection - see fall protection
Personal flotation devices 77-79
    lights 78
Personal protective equipment
    .... 4, 7, 49, 110, 116, 117, 289, 687, 689, 792
    clothing 29, 58, 70, 75, 91, 97, 110, 135, 137, 220
    footwear 65, 66
    see specific type
Photogrey Lenses (Auto-darkening) 58
Physical qualifications 15, 317
Physicians - see licensed physician
Pile driving 339, 382, 385, 463, 603
PITs (See Forklift)
Planking 381, 518, 519-521, 530, 531, 542, 554, 572, 576, 587
Plants, poisonous 96, 97
Platforms ... 21, 80, 141, 218, 309, 310, 377, 381, 389-392, 394, 413, 458,
.... 491, 509-522, 534-555, 557, 560, 576, 587, 634, 638, 678, 749
Position Hazard Analysis 4, 6, 7
Positioning device - see fall protection
Post-tensioning 644
Potentially gassy operations 622, 623
Power Driven Nailers, Staplers 277
Pre-cast concrete operations 643, 650, 651, 655
Preparatory inspection 258, 434
Preservative coatings 204
Pressurized equipment and systems 477, 479
Process safety management 89

Project safety and health plan 3, 4, 8, 63, 65, 119
Public 44, 46, 48, 99, 103, 104, 106, 112, 126, 143, 148, 150, 153,
....................182, 198, 200, 228, 258, 259, 263, 402, 406, 412, 416, 422,
....................438, 441, 443, 445, 446, 512, 594, 677, 695, 700, 702, 705

-Q-

Qualified Rigger...288, 290, 657
Qualified Operator..274
Qualified Person..............9, 10, 13, 14, 88, 167, 172, 215, 218, 219, 302, 307,
....................322, 326, 327, 330, 332, 333, 341, 343, 346, 355, 358, 360,
....................361, 364, 367-369, 373, 380, 392, 409, 436, 445, 501-507,
.... 512, 534, 556, 558, 593, 618, 620, 653, 663-665, 672-677, 747

-R-

Radiant energy 58, 214
Radiation...(See also Ionizing and NonIonizing)..
    Electromagnetic...704, 773
    monitoring 101
    optical.. 55-57
    Safety Committee (RSC)...99
    safety officer 98
    safety program... 98, 99,100, 106
Radio frequency (FF).. 110, 163
Radio, two-way & communications 33, 119, 153, 198, 319, 347, 355,
.... 393, 426, 446, 464, 728, 765, 766
Radioactive Waste Disposal... 105
Rail clamps 335, 362, 383
Railing (See also guardrails and handrails)...575
    Marine..464
Ramps. 459, 587, 596
Registered nurse 40
Reinforcing steel.. 282, 643, 645
Rescue 15, 18, 19, 449, 450, 455, 464, 493, 494, 511, 595, 614,
.... 615, 654, 692, 725, 750, 791, 794
Residential-Type Construction...491, 643, 678
Respirators 67, 85, 204, 615
    atmosphere-supplying 69
    dust masks...67
    emergency use self-rescuer devices... 615
    fit testing 69-72
    medical evaluation...69
    program..68
    program administrator..68
    self-contained breathing apparatus...71

Reverse-flow check valve 211
Reverse signal alarm (see also back-up alarm) 411
Rigger (see also Qualified Rigger) 389, 312, 315, 346, 355, 356, 357
Rigging 287, 248
    Drums 301, 303, 345
    fiber rope 297, 298
    slings 299, 307, 387, 488, 534, 545
    wire rope 291, 330, 334, 391, 498
Ring buoys 78-79
Rodents 31
Rollover protective structures (ROPS) 309, 415-417, 441
Roofing 677, 584, 655, 678
    brackets 562
    clothing for roofers 95
    nailers 277
    Warning Line System 511
Rope - see rigging or wire rope
Runways 95, 280, 372, 373, 381, 382, 575, 587, 763

-S-

Safe lifting techniques 279
Safety
    Blocks, floating, ... 80
    Control, primary 187
    Conveyor 399
    devices 179, 203, 267, 273, 275, 309, 315, 323, 324, 328,
    .... 335, 361, 368, 370, 395, 448, 485, 645
    equipment 49, 441, 728
    harness 734, 743
    lashing 273, 480
    nets – debris 284
    nets – fall protection 77, 491, 500, 501, 512
    skiff 79, 464
    tire rack/cage 414
    (relief)valves 480
Safety and health program 1, 12, 13
Sampling 84, 131, 207, 795
    Air Compressors 739
    Chromium 129
    Hydrogen Sulfide 626
    Mold 128
    Program 683
Sanitation 21, 29, 136, 137, 149, 159, 639
Saws - see woodworking machinery
Scaffolds 280, 482, 492, 516, 517, 677, 679

EM 385-1-1
15 Sep 08

    access 80, 245
    base/mudsills 520
    bracket 523, 549
    capacities 245, 517
    carpenter's bracket 523
    design 517, 527
    erection/dismantling 509, 515
    fall protection 492, 509, 510, 576
    form 549
    hanging 544
    horse 552
    independent pole scaffolds 532
    inspection of 516
    lean-to and prop-scaffolds 516
    manually-operated hoists 538
    manually propelled mobile scaffolds 527
    metal 524
    metal frame 526
    operations 547
    pump jack 552
    stilts 562
    suspended 213, 510, 533
    suspended, mason's multiple-point adjustable 536, 542
    suspended, stonesetters, multiple-point adjustable 543
    suspended, support devices 535
    suspended, support ropes 534
    tube and coupler scaffolds 524
    wood pole 528
Scaffolds, platforms, or temporary floors 491, 516
Scows/Barges 474, 459, 463, 461
Seatbelts 414, 440, 441
Selenium 205
Service/refueling/lubrication areas 189, 178
Severe weather 447-449, 119, 677
Shackles 288-289, 302, 501, 537
Shafts - see underground construction
Sheaves 305, 328
Sheet Pile Stirrups 491
Shoring 204, 515, 568, 589, 592, 593, 601, 618, 641, 645, 650
Showers 28, 29
SignalPerson 46, 153, 154, 318, 319, 338, 346-348, 355,
.... 377, 392, 394, 412, 420
Signal systems, procedures 153, 154
        see spotter
Signs. 1, 44, 62, 103, 104, 108, 120, 143-166, 217, 254, 285,
.... 400-406, 420, 434, 455, 456, 472, 493, 557, 568, 613,

	618, 623, 631, 644, 696, 708, 713
Silica	112-137, 437
Site Safety & Health Officer (SSHO)	6, 11, 12, 67, 120, 686, 691
Slings - see rigging	
Slip forms	649, 650
Sloping/benching - see excavation	
Slow-moving vehicle emblem	150, 165, 441
Smoke alarms	451
Smoking	126, 135, 168, 172, 254, 475, 487, 623, 631, 683, 703
Snaphooks/carabiners	505
Snorkeling	744
Soap	24, 28, 29, 97, 136, 187
Solar radiation	121
Solvents	6, 126, 176, 214, 236, 286
Sound-pressure	60-63
Specialty Vehicles	409, 442
Spotter	337-339, 420, 434, 512
see signalperson	
Spray guns	273
Sprinkler head	209
Stairways	585, 171, 176, 182, 191, 203, 283, 567
railings	585-586
Standard guardrails and handrails – see Guardrails, Handrails	
Static electricity	276
Steel	
erection	643, 492, 491
removal	572
Sump Pumps	228
Stilts	562
Sun screen	121
Switches	221, 240, 256, 361, 402
Blasting	640

-T-

Tag lines	245, 351, 375, 386, 755
Tank cars/trucks	178, 179
Temporary	
building spacing	43, 170
facilities	43
floors	491, 516
heating devices - see heating devices	
lighting	140, 228, 229
power distribution systems	227
project fencing	44

sleeping quarters	45, 46, 451, 452
structures	43
Throw bags	79
Tire service vehicles	429
Toe boards	309, 383, 413, 459, 461, 496, 498, 499, 550, 551, 583
Toilets	24-27, 141
Tools	
hand	225, 516
pneumatic	241, 268, 273
power	225, 267, 269, 678, 743
Torch valves	211
Torches	170, 210, 211
Towels	25, 29
Towing	420, 424, 431, 443, 444
Vessels	446, 448, 450, 468, 474
Toxic or corrosive materials (flushing facilities)	34
Traffic flagging procedures	153
Trailer anchoring systems	43
Trainer	13, 261, 437, 438, 494
Training	4, 7, 10, 12, 13-15, 20, 35
Transportation	3, 26
Of Personnel	421
Of Explosives	700
Tree maintenance and removal	747, P-1
brush chippers	756
brush removal	755
cant hooks, cant dogs, tongs, and carrying bars	761
chopping tools	761
felling	753
limbing and bucking	758
power saws	271, 760
pruning and trimming	757
rope access	750, P-1
tree climbing	750, P-1
trucks	748, 757, 759, 760
wedges and chisels	762
Trenching - see excavations	
Tubing, polyvinyl chloride and aluminum	179
Tunnels	34, 141, 228, 402, 458, 613, 639
see underground construction	

-U-

UFGS	3
Ultraviolet degradation	64
Underground construction	387, 613

```
        air monitoring requirements..................................................................624
        air quality standards ................................................................ 624, 626
        caissons................................................................................ 613, 637, 638
        fire prevention and protection............................................................. 630
        ground support systems ........................................................................ 619
        rescue teams ....................................................................................... 614, 615
        shafts ................................................................................ 613, 614, 635-637
        ventilation............................................................................... 624, 628, 639
Unexploded ordnance ........................................................................... 66, 433, 767
Unmanned Vessel............................................................................................461, 462
Utilities ............................................................................ 360, 433, 456, 566, 590, 595, 750
Utility Vehicles...................................................................................................409, 439
```

-V-

```
Vanadium.................................................................................................................. 205
Variances (& Waivers)...............................................................................................N-1
Vehicle-mounted elevating and rotating work platforms ...................................... 557
Vent pipes ................................................................................................................. 186
Ventilation and exhaust systems ............................................................... 111, 629
Vermin control ........................................................................................................... 31
Vessel  ........................................................................................365-371, 445-476
Visitors  ................................................................................................ 14, 65, 102, 213
```

-W-

```
Waivers (& Variances)..............................................................................................N-1
Wall
        openings - see floor and wall holes and openings
        removal ........................................................................................................ 570
Warning Line System (WLS).................................................................................510
Warning signs ..................................................... 44, 108, 145, 254, 400, 696, 713
Washing facilities .................................................................... 24, 28, 88, 129, 136
Waste disposal .......................................................................................................... 30
Welder, Certified.................................................................................................204, 388
Welding and cutting ................................................................................................. 203
Wet locations, electrical ................................................................................. 222, 228
Wild land fire control ............................................................................................. 199
        plan ................................................................................................................ 199
        teams and operations ................................................................................... 201
Windshields ............................................................................... 309, 415, 423, 428
Wire rope - see rigging
Woodworking
        machinery and saws..................................................................................... 271
        machinery guarding....................................................................................... 271
Work Clothing, minimum.............................................................................................50
```

Work platforms..	491, 512, 515
Crane-Supported...	389
Movable..	509
Elevating..	510, 555, 557
Scissors Lift..	510
Work practice controls	85, 87, 206, 214
Work/warm-up regimen	121
Working alone at night...	77
Working alone in remote locations...	20
Working in Crane-Supported Work Platform, over water......	387, 394
Working in temporary field conditions.....................................	28
Working over/above water...	394
Working over/near water...	512
Working underground..	626
Working under loads..	643

BLANK